AF660833

Rank File in Nursing

Rank File in Nursing

Complete Preparatory Guide for Various Competitive Exams/Interviews in Nursing

Sona PS MSc (Nsg)
Assistant Professor
Government College of Nursing
Thiruvananthapuram
Kerala, India

Foreword
B Ekbal

JAYPEE

JAYPEE BROTHERS MEDICAL PUBLISHERS (P) LTD

New Delhi • London • Philadelphia • Panama

Jaypee Brothers Medical Publishers (P) Ltd

Headquarters

Jaypee Brothers Medical Publishers (P) Ltd
4838/24, Ansari Road, Daryaganj
New Delhi 110 002, India
Phone: +91-11-43574357
Fax: +91-11-43574314
Email: jaypee@jaypeebrothers.com

Overseas Offices

J.P. Medical Ltd
83, Victoria Street, London
SW1H 0HW (UK)
Phone: +44-2031708910
Fax: +02-03-0086180
Email: info@jpmedpub.com

Jaypee-Highlights Medical Publishers Inc
City of Knowledge, Bld. 237, Clayton
Panama City, Panama
Phone: +1 507-301-0496
Fax: +1 507-301-0499
Email: cservice@jphmedical.com

Jaypee Medical Inc
The Bourse
111 South Independence Mall East
Suite 835, Philadelphia, PA 19106, USA
Phone: +1 267-519-9789
Email: jpmed.us@gmail.com

Jaypee Brothers Medical Publishers (P) Ltd
17/1-B Babar Road, Block-B, Shaymali
Mohammadpur, Dhaka-1207
Bangladesh
Mobile: +08801912003485
Email: jaypeedhaka@gmail.com

Jaypee Brothers Medical Publishers (P) Ltd
Bhotahity, Kathmandu, Nepal
Phone: +977-9741283608
Email: kathmandu@jaypeebrothers.com

Website: www.jaypeebrothers.com
Website: www.jaypeedigital.com

© 2014, Jaypee Brothers Medical Publishers

The views and opinions expressed in this book are solely those of the original contributor(s)/author(s) and do not necessarily represent those of editor(s) of the book.

All rights reserved. No part of this publication may be reproduced, stored or transmitted in any form or by any means, electronic, mechanical, photocopying, recording or otherwise, without the prior permission in writing of the publishers.

All brand names and product names used in this book are trade names, service marks, trademarks or registered trademarks of their respective owners. The publisher is not associated with any product or vendor mentioned in this book.

Medical knowledge and practice change constantly. This book is designed to provide accurate, authoritative information about the subject matter in question. However, readers are advised to check the most current information available on procedures included and check information from the manufacturer of each product to be administered, to verify the recommended dose, formula, method and duration of administration, adverse effects and contraindications. It is the responsibility of the practitioner to take all appropriate safety precautions. Neither the publisher nor the author(s)/editor(s) assume any liability for any injury and/or damage to persons or property arising from or related to use of material in this book.

This book is sold on the understanding that the publisher is not engaged in providing professional medical services. If such advice or services are required, the services of a competent medical professional should be sought.

Every effort has been made where necessary to contact holders of copyright to obtain permission to reproduce copyright material. If any have been inadvertently overlooked, the publisher will be pleased to make the necessary arrangements at the first opportunity.

Inquiries for bulk sales may be solicited at: jaypee@jaypeebrothers.com

Rank File in Nursing

First Edition: **2014**

ISBN 978-93-5090-773-3

Printed at Repro India Limited

Dedicated to

My Beloved Father

Foreword

I am happy to introduce an innovative and comprehensive preparatory guide for practicing nurses appearing for various competitive examinations and interviews. The guide is prepared in such a way as to meet the challenges and intricacies of the present selection criteria based upon objective tests.

It is necessary in the present evaluation system that the candidates have an insight into the complexities and fundamentals of the subject matter. Ms Sona PS has taken this as a challenge and organized the book in such a way as to help the nurses to get a clear understanding of the fundamentals of medical science from a practical point of view. The book is presented in a highly user-friendly manner focusing on diseases affecting different systems, stressing always on the basic concepts of scientific nursing practices.

She has taken exceptional care to see that all the subjects under nursing syllabus have been included in the book in an easily understandable and in-depth manner. The subject matter is presented in a highly readable manner with the key points being emphasized and highlighted in boxes for easy retention and recollection. This will help the readers to revise the topic effectively just before the competitive examinations and viva. Multiple choice questions have been included at the end of each chapter for easy review of the topics discussed earlier. Simulated examinations done at the end of the book, will be very helpful to the users for self-assessment and building up self-confidence.

I am sure that this book will be very informative and useful for undergraduate, graduate and postgraduate nurses for preparing various competitive examinations and for improving their nursing skills.

B Ekbal MS (Gen Surg) MCh (Neurosurg)
Retired Professor of Neurosurgery
Former Vice-Chancellor
University of Kerala
Thiruvananthapuram, Kerala, India

Preface

I am extremely happy to present a novel rank file for all the nurses who are dedicated to patient care. Nowadays, objective tests are preferred in competitive examinations to distinguish the qualifiers and non-qualifiers and even could pick-up the outstanding in the group. Attempting and qualifying objective tests require insight into the subject matter. I have tried to organize the chapters in a user-friendly manner under different specialties so that it will be easy for the users to assimilate and utilize the information. Almost all the subjects under nursing syllabus have been included in a simplified but in-depth manner. The key points are emphasized and highlighted in boxes for easy retention and recollection. It will help for a quick revision on the eve of viva examinations, competitive examinations, etc. Multiple choice questions (MCQs) have been added as much as possible after each chapter for better understanding and review. Mock examinations at the end of the book will strengthen the users indeed. This book will be useful for undergraduate, graduate and postgraduate nurses for preparing themselves and for ensuring high rank in various competitive examinations and face-to-face interviews.

I hope that this text will be provoking and stimulating the nursing community and enjoyable at the same time. An honest attempt had been taken to include all the possible MCQs commonly asked in the competitive examinations in nursing; but in the midst of all, errors may be possible. I am not asserting or claiming any perfection in this venture.

Constructive criticisms and suggestions are most welcome to the email address *feedback.nursing2010@gmail.com* which will be assimilated in the coming editions.

Sona PS

Acknowledgments

I express my deep obligation to my parents and teachers who shaped my character and career and guided me in publishing this book.

Dr B Ekbal, renowned Neurosurgeon and former Vice-Chancellor of University of Kerala, has been my guide and inspiration throughout my life. My sincere thanks to you Sir, for writing the foreword for this book.

My gratitude to God Almighty for enabling me to complete this work in time.

No words are sufficient to express my acknowledgment to my best friend and husband Mr Shine S Babu, my loving children Ms Aiswarya Shine and Master Adithya Shine, for their wonderful support and care given to me during the preparation of this book, without which this book would have never been a reality.

Thanks to Mr Rontgen and Mr Venu for assisting me with the DTP work.

Sincere thanks to M/s Jaypee Brothers Medical Publishers (P) Ltd, New Delhi, India, who readily accepted for publishing this book.

Special thanks to M/s Jaypee Brothers Medical Publishers, Kochi Branch for coordinating and accomplishing this task in right time.

Contents

1. Medical Surgical Nursing 1

Basic Concepts 1

Infection 1; Infection Chain 1; Infection Control 1; Physical and Chemical Control of Microorganisms 2; Barrier Nursing 2; Antimicrobial Drugs 3; Antitubercular Drugs 4; Antifungal Drugs 4; Anthelmintics 4; Pain 4; Analgesics 4; Fluid and Electrolyte Balance 5; Electrolytes 6; Acid-Base Balance 6; Acid-Base Imbalances 8; Nutrition 8; Shock 8

Diseases and Disorders of the Central Nervous System 13

Overview of Anatomy and Physiology of CNS 13; Vision 15; Hearing 15

Diseases and Disorders of the Nervous System 16

Increased Intracranial Pressure (ICP) 16; Cerebrovascular Accident (CVA) 17; Parkinson's Disease 17; Myasthenia Gravis 17; Spinal Cord Injury 18; Meningitis 18; Encephalitis 18; Brain Abscess 19; Trigeminal Neuralgia (Tic-Douloureux) 19; Bell's Palsy 19; Guillain-Barre Syndrome 20

Disorders of the Eye 20

Cataract 20; Glaucoma 20; Retinal Detachment 21

Disorders of the Ear 21

Otosclerosis 21; Meniere's Disease 21

Diseases and Disorders of the Cardiovascular System 24

Overview of Anatomy and Physiology of CVS 24; Blood 25; Blood Clotting Process 27; Blood Circulation 27; Lymphatic System 29

Diseases and Disorders of the Cardiovascular System 29

Coronary Artery Disease (CAD) 29; Angina Pectoris 30; Myocardial Infarction 30; Coronary Artery Bypass Graft (CABG) 30; Dysrhythmias 30; Sinus Tachycardia 30; Sinus Bradycardia 30; Atrial Fibrillation (AF) 31; Premature Ventricular Contraction (PVC) 31; Ventricular Tachycardia (VT) 31; Congestive Cardiac Failure (CCF) 31; Left Sided Heart Failure 31; Right Sided Heart Failure 31; Pulmonary Edema 31; Cardiac Tamponade 32; Hypertension 32; Antihypertensive Therapy (AHT) 32; Thromboangiitis Obliterans (TAO) or Buerger's Disease 33; Thrombophlebitis 33; Cardiovascular Drugs 33; Antianginal Drugs 33; Peripheral Vasodilators 33; Beta Blockers 34; Cardiac Stimulants 34; Anticoagulants 34; Thrombolytic Drugs 36; Antilipemic Agents 36

Diseases and Disorders of the Respiratory System 43

Review of Anatomy and Physiology 43; Mechanism of Respiration 43; Gas Exchange 43; Lung Volumes 43

Diseases and Disorders of the Respiratory System 44

Chronic Obstructive Pulmonary Disease (COPD) 44; Pulmonary Tuberculosis 44; Chest Trauma 44; Flail Chest 45; Pneumothorax/Hemothorax 45; Atelectasis 45; Pleural Effusion 45; Chest Drainage Systems 45; Pneumonia 46; Cancer of the Larynx 46; Oral Cancer 47

Diseases and Disorders of the Gastrointestinal System 53

Review of Anatomy and Physiology 53; Physiology of Digestion and Absorption 54

Diseases and Disorders of the Gastrointestinal System 54

Stomatitis 54; Oral Cancer 54; Cancer of the Esophagus 54; Esophageal Varices 54; Hiatus Hernia 55; Gastritis 55; Gastric Ulcers 55; Duodenal Ulcer 55; Gastric Surgery 55; Dumping Syndrome 56; Cancer of the Stomach 56; Ulcerative Colitis 56; Cancer of the Colon/Rectum 56; Bowel Surgery 57; Peritonitis 57; Hemorrhoids 57

Disorders of the Liver 58

Hepatitis 58; Cirrhosis of Liver 58; Ascites 58; Hepatic Encephalopathy 59

Disorders of the Gallbladder 59

Cholecystitis 59; Cholelithiasis 59

Disorders of the Pancreas 59

Pancreatitis 59; Cancer of the Pancreas 60

Diseases and Disorders of the Genitourinary System 63

Review of Anatomy and Physiology 63; Urinary System 63

Disorders of the Urinary Tract 63

Cystitis 63; Nephrolithiasis/Urolithiasis 63; Glomerulonephritis 63; Acute Renal Failure 64; Chronic Renal Failure 64; Surgery of Urinary System 64

Disorders of the Reproductive System 65

Epididymitis 65; Prostatitis 65; Benign Prostatic Hypertrophy (BPH) 65; Prostatic Surgery 65; Dialysis 65

Diseases and Disorders of the Musculoskeletal System 68

Review of Anatomy and Physiology 68

Diseases and Disorders of the Endocrine System 73

Review of Anatomy and Physiology 73; Hormone Regulation 73

2. Nursing Foundations 77

Nursing 77; Communication 77; Essentials of Communication Process 77; Ethical Aspects of Nursing 77; Nursing Process 77 Medical and Surgical Asepsis 78; Assessment of Client 79; Specimen Collection and Testing 80; Personal Hygiene 82; Pressure Sore (Bed Sore and Decubitus Ulcer) 82; Vital Signs 83; Temperature 83; Fever 83; Pulse 84; Respiration 84; Blood Pressure 85; Body Mechanics 85; Immobility 85; Exercise 86; Comfort Measures 86; Enema 86; Hot and Cold Applications 87; Administration of Medications 87

3. Mental Health Nursing 94

Personality 94; Anxiety and Behavior 94 Defense Mechanisms 95; Deviant Patterns of Behavior 95; Basic Principles in Psychiatric Nursing 95; Therapeutic Nurse-Patient Relationship 96; Drugs in Emotional Disorders 96; Mental Retardation 98; Pervasive Developmental Disorders 98; Disruptive Behavior Disorders 98; Eating Disorders 99; Gender Identity Disorders 99; Tic Disorders 100; Elimination Disorders 100; Speech Disorders 100; Organic Mental Syndromes and Disorders 101; Alzheimer's Disease and Dementa of the Alzheimers Type 102; Psychoactive Substance-Induced Organic Mental Disorders 102; Psychoactive Substance Use Disorders 102

4. Child Health Nursing 130

The Newborn 130; Preterm (Premature) or Low Birth Weight Infant 130;

Special Conditions in the Neonate 131

Hyperbilirubinemia 131; Hemolytic Disease of the Newborn (Erythro Blastosis Foetalis) 131; Neonatal Sepsis 132; Hypoglycemia 132; Growth and Development 132; Child with Chromosomal Abnormalities 133

Disorders of Gastrointestinal System 133
Cleft Lip 133; Cleft Palate 133; Tracheoesophageal Anomalies 133; Intestinal Obstruction 134; Pyloric Stenosis 134; Intussusception 134; Omphalocele (Exomphalus) 134; Hirschsprung's Disease (Congenital Aganglionic Megacolon) 134; Appendicitis 135; Imperforate Anus 135

Disorders of the Neurosensory System 135
Increased ICP 135; Spina Bifida (Myelodysplasia) 136; Reyes Syndrome 136; Seizure Disorders 136; Cerebral Palsy 137

Disorders of the Eye 137
Blindness 137; Conjunctivitis 137

Disorders of the Ear 138
Deafness 138; Otitis Media 138

Diseases and Disorders of the Cardiovascular System 138
Normal Changes in Fetal Circulation After Birth 138; Congestive Cardiac Failure 139; Congenital Heart Defects 139; Acyanotic Heart Defects 139; Cyanotic Heart Defects 140; Rheumatic Fever 141

Diseases and Disorders of the Hematologic System 141
Anemias 141; Idiopathic Thrompocytopenic Purpura (ITP) 142; Hemophilia 142

Diseases and Disorders of the Respiratory System 142
Tonsillitis 143; Acute Spasmodic Laryngitis (Croup) 143; Bronchial Asthma 143

Diseases and Disorders of the Genitourinary System 143
Urinary Tract Infection (UTI) 143; Vesicoureteral Reflux 143; Undescended Tests (Cryptorchidism) 144; Hypospadias 144; Acute Glomerulonephritis 144; Nephrotic Syndrome (Nephrosis) 144; Hydronephrosis 145

Diseases and Disorders of the Musculoskeletal System 145
Congenital Dislocation of the Hip (CDH) 145; Clubfoot (Talipes) 146; Osteogenesis Imperfecta 146; Scoliosis 146

Diseases and Disorders of the Endocrine System 147
Diabetes Mellitus 147; Congenital Hypothyroidism (Cretinism) 147; Hypopituitarism (Pituitary Dwarfism) 147; Hyperpituitarism (Gigantism) 148

5. Community Health Nursing 160

Primary Health Care 160; Maternal and Child Health 160; Health Problems of India 161; Health Programs of India 161; Environmental Health 162; Air 164; Ventilation 164; Lighting 164; Noise 164; Refuse 164; Mosquito Borne Diseases 164; Epidemiology of Disease 164; Disease Cycle 165; Levels of Prevention 165; Terminology Related to Epidemiology 165; Disease Transmission 166; Immunity 166; Immunizing Agents 167; National Immunization Schedule 167; Cold Chain 168; Portals of Exit 168; General Measures for the Control of Infectious Diseases 168; Disinfection 168

Communicable Diseases 169
Smallpox (Variola) 169; Chickenpox (Varicella) 169; Measles (Rubeola) 169; German Measles (Rubella) 170; Mumps 170; Diphtheria 170; Whooping Cough 171; Severe Acute Respiratory Syndrome (SARS) 171; Tuberculosis (TB) 171; Meningococcal Meningitis 172; Poliomyelitis 172; Hepatitis A 173; Hepatitis B 173; Hepatitis C 173; Hepatitis E 173; Cholera 173; Food Poisoning 174; Sexually Transmitted Diseases (STDs) 175; Acquired Immunodeficiency Syndrome (AIDS) 175; Hospital Acquired Infections 175

Demography and Family Welfare 176
Demography 176; Family Planning 176; Occupational Health 176; Occupational Diseases 177; Health Statistics 177; Health Education 178

Health and Social Services in India **179**
The Bhore Committee 179; The Mudaliar Committee 179; The Chadha Committee 179;
The Mukherji Committee 179; Kartar Singh Committee 179; Shrivastav Committee 180;
National Health Policy 180
Five Year Plans **180**
International Health Agencies **180**
World Health Organization (WHO) 180;
UNICEF (United Nations International Children's Emergency Fund) 180;
The World Bank 181

6. Maternity Nursing **193**

Puberty 193; Menstruation 193; Development of the Embryo 194;
Placenta 194; Umbilical Cord 194; Fetal Circulation 194;
Physical and Physiological Changes in the Mother during Pregnancy 194; Labor 197;
Clinical Findings Prior to Labor 197; Clinical Findings of True Labor 197;
Mechanism of Labor 197; Stages of Labor and Maternal Changes 197; Oxytocics 198;
Maternal Analgesia and Anesthesia during Labor 198; Postpartum Period 198;
The Newborn 199; Pregnancy-induced Hypertension (PIH), Pre-Eclampsia and Eclampsia 200;
Bleeding during the First Trimester 200; Antepartum Hemorrhage (APH) 201;
Postpartum Hemorrhage (PPH) 202; Multiple Pregnancy 202; Polyhydramnios 202;
Oligohydramnios 202; Vomiting In Pregnancy 202; Abnormalities of Placenta and Cord 203;
Heart Disease in Pregnancy 203; Gestational Diabetes 203; Anemia during Pregnancy 204;
Induction of Labor 204; Premature Rupture of Membranes (PROM) 204;
Preterm or Premature Labor 204; Postterm or Post Date Labor 204;
Difficult Labor or Dystocia 205; Precipitate Labor 205; Episiotomy 205
Family Planning **205**
Contraceptive Methods 205; Medical Termination of Pregnancy (MTP) 206; Menopause 206

7. Gynecologic Nursing **210**

Related Anatomy and Physiology 210; External Genitalia 210
Internal Genital Organs **210**
Vagina 210; The Uterus 210; Fallopian Tubes (Uterine Tubes) 211; Ovary 211;
Pelvic Floor 212; Perineum 212; Pelvic Peritoneum 212; Broad Ligament 212
Neuroendocrinology of Reproduction **213**
Hypothalamus 213; Anterior Pituitary 213; Posterior Pituitary 213; Ovary 213;
Hypothalamic Pituitary Ovarian Axis 214
Gynecological Diseases and Disorders **214**
Precocious Puberty 214; Delayed Puberty 214; Puberty Menorrhagia 215;
Pelvic Infections 215; Pelvic Inflammatory Disease (PID) 215
Pelvic Infection Following Delivery and Abortion **216**
Abortion 216; Genital Tuberculosis 217; Sexually Transmitted Diseases 217; Acute Gonorrhea 217;
Syphilis 218; Herpes Genitalis 218; Acquired Immunodeficiency Syndrome (AIDS) 219
Disorders of Mentstrual Cycles **219**
Dysmenorrhea 219; Mittelschmerz's Syndrome (Ovulatory Pain) 220; Premenstrual Syndrome (PMS) 220
Abnormal Menstrual Bleeding **220**
Menorrhagia 220; Epimenorrhea (Polymenorrhea) 221; Metrorrhagia 221;
Oligomenorrhea 221; Hypomenorrhea 221; Dysfunctional Uterine Bleeding (DUB) 221;
Displacement of the Uterus 222; Retroversion 222; Genital Prolapse 222; Infertility 223;
Assisted Reproductive Technology (ART) 224
Benign Lesions of the Cervix **224**
Cervical Erosion 224; Cervical Eversion (Ectropion) 225; Cervical Tear 225;
Cervical Cysts 225; Elongation of the Cervix 225

Benign Lesions of the Uterus 225
Fibroid 225; Benign Lesions of the Ovary 226; Follicular Cyst 226; Corpus Luteum Cyst 226; Lutein Cyst 227; Polycystic Ovarian Syndrome (PCOS) 227; Endometrial Cyst 227; Ovarian Tumors 227; Classification of Ovarian Tumor 227; Mucinous Cyst Adenoma 228; Serous Cyst Adenoma 228; Dermoid Cyst 228; Endometriosis 228; Cervical Intraepithelial Neoplasia (CIN) 229; Carcinoma Cervix (Ca Cervix) 229; Malignant Ovarian Tumors 230; Genital Fistula 231

Intersexuality 232
Female Intersex 232; Disorders of Gonadal Development 233; Male Intersex 233; Klinefelter's Syndrome 234; True Hermaphroditism 234; Diagnosis of Intersex 234; Management of Intersex 234; Menopause 234

8. Nutrition 245
Functions of Food 245; Constituents of Food 245; Classification of Foods 245; Nutrients 245; Proteins 246; Functions of Proteins 246; Sources of Proteins 246; Protein Requirements 246; Effects of Protein Deficiency 246

Fats 246
Classification of Fats 246; Carbohydrates 247; Vitamins 247; Vitamin A 248; Vitamin D 249; Vitamin E 249; Vitamin B_1 or Thiamine 249; Vitamin B_2 or Riboflavin 250; Niacin 250; Vitamin B_6 or Pyridoxine 250; Folic Acid 250; Vitamin B_{12} 250; Vitamin C or Ascorbic Acid 250; Minerals 251

9. Objective Questions on Nursing Research 254

Appendices 261
Normal Values 261
Abbreviations 263

Previous Solved Question Papers Staff Nurse (Kerala Public Service Commission) 264
Staff Nurse (Insurance Medical Service) 264
Junior Public Health Nurse - Grade II (Municipal Common Service) 270
Staff Nurse (Health Department) 275
Staff Nurse (State Farming Corporation) 280
Staff Nurse Grade II (Health Department) 285
Staff Nurse (Plantation Corporation) 290
Staff Nurse (48/2008) 295
Qualifying Examination for KNMC Registration 301
Qualifying Examination for KNMC Registration 307
Qualifying Examination for KNMC Registration 312
Senior Lecturer in Nursing-Kerala PSC 318
Rank Making Points 324
Model Question Papers 327
Model Question Paper I 327
Model Question Paper II 332
Model Question Paper III 337
Model Question Paper IV 342

Index 347

Abbreviations

Abbreviation	Expansion
ACT	Activated Clotting Time
ADH	Antidiuretic Hormone
AHG	Antihuman Globulin
AHTR	Acute Hemolytic Transfusion Reaction (also HTR)
AIDS	Acquired Immunodeficiency Syndrome
ALT	Alanine Aminotransferase
ANA	Antinuclear Antibody
ANH	Acute Normovolemic Hemodilution
anti-HBc	Antibody to Hepatitis B Core Antigen
anti-HCV	Antibody to Hepatitis C Virus
anti-HTLV-I/II	Antibody to Human T-cell Lymphotropic Virus type I/II
aPPT	Activated Partial Thromboplastin Time
ARDS	Acute Respiratory Distress Syndrome
AST	Aspartate Aminotransferase
ATIII	Antithrombin III
CHD	Coronary Heart Disease
CJD	Creutzfeldt-Jakob Disease (see nvCJD)
CMV	Cytomegalovirus
CPD	Citrate, Phosphate, Dextrose (solution)
CPDA-1	Citrate, Phosphate, Dextrose-Adenine (solution)
C/T	Crossmatch-to-Transfusion ratio (C:T)
DDAVP	1-Desamino-8-D-Arginine Vasopressin (desmopressin)
DIC	Disseminated Intravascular Coagulation
EACA	Epsilon-Aminocaproic Acid
FDA	Food and Drug Administration
FFP	Fresh Frozen Plasma
FNHTR	Febrile Nonhemolytic Transfusion Reaction
GGTP	Gamma Glutamyl Transpeptidase (GGT)
GHVD	Graft-Versus-Host Disease
HAM	HTLV-I-Associated Myelopathy
HB	Hemoglobin
HBOC	Hemoglobin-Based Oxygen Carrier
HBsAg	Hepatitis B Surface Antigen
HCT	Hematocrit
HBV	Hepatitis B Virus
HCV	Hepatitis C Virus
HDN	Hemolytic Disease of the Newborn
HES	Hydroxyethyl Starch
HH	Hemochromatosis
HIV	Human Immunodeficiency Virus
HLA	Human Lymphocyte Antigen

HTLV-I/II	Human T-cell Lymphotropic Virus type I/II
HTR	Hemolytic Transfusion Reaction (also AHTR)
IAD	Intraoperative Autologous Donation
IFG	Impaired Fasting Glucose
IgA	Immunoglobulin A
ITP	Idiopathic Thrombocytopenic Purpura
LD	Lactate Dehydrogenase
MAC	*Mycobacterium avium* Complex
MCH	Mean Corpuscular Hemoglobin
MCHC	Mean Corpuscular Hemoglobin Concentration
MCV	Mean Corpuscular Volume
MPV	Mean Platelet Volume
NAT	Nucleic Acid Amplification Testing
nvCJD	New Variation Creutzfeldt-Jakob Disease (CJD)
PABD	Preoperative Autologous Blood Donation
PABT	Preoperative Autologous Blood Transfusion
PFC	Perfluorochemical(s)
PLTs	Platelets
PMNs	Polymorphonuclear Leukocytes
PPF	Purified Protein Fraction
PRP	Platelet-Rich Plasma
PT	Prothrombin Time
PTP	Post-transfusion Purpura
PTT	Partial Thromboplastin Time
Q-T	from QRS complex to end of T wave (interval)
RBCs	Red Blood Cells
Rh	Rhesus Factor
STS	Serologic Test for Syphilis
T&S	Type and Screen
TA-GVHD	Transfusion-Associated Graft-Versus-Host Disease
TEG	Thromboelastograph
TRALI	Transfusion-Related Acute Lung Injury
TSE	Transmissible Spongiform Encephalopathies
TSH	Thyroid Stimulating Hormone
TSP	Tropical Spastic Paraparesis
TTP	Thrombotic Thrombocytopenic Purpura
TTTS	Twin to Twin Transfusion Syndrome
TXA	Transexamic Acid
vWd	von Willebrand's Disease
WBCs	White Blood Cells

Chapter 1

Medical Surgical Nursing

Basic Concepts

INFECTION

Infection is the invasion of the body by pathogenic organisms that multiply and produce harmful effects. Communicable disease is an infectious disease that may be transmitted from one person to another. Incubation period is the time period from the entry of an infectious organism into the body to the development of various signs and symptoms of the disease. Carrier is an agent that transmits the infectious agent from one person to another.

Incubation period is the time period from the entry of an infectious organism into the body to the development of various signs and symptoms of the disease.

Carrier is an agent that transmits the infectious agent from one person to another.

In a patient already suffering from a disease, a new infection is set up from another source or host is known as **Cross infection.**

INFECTION CHAIN

A. **Causative agent**: Invading organism (e.g. bacteria, virus, fungi, etc.).

B. **Reservoir**: Environment in which the invading organisms live and multiply.

C. **Portal of exit**: Mode of escape from reservoir (e.g. respiratory tract, gastrointestinal tract, etc.).

D. **Mode of transmission**: Method by which invading organism is transported to a new host.(e.g. direct contact, air, food).

E. **Portal of entry**: Means by which organisms enters new host (e.g. respiratory tract, gastrointestinal tract, broken skin).

F. **Susceptible host**: Susceptibility is determined by factors such as number of invading organisms, duration of exposure, age, state of health, nutritional status, etc. (Fig. 1.1).

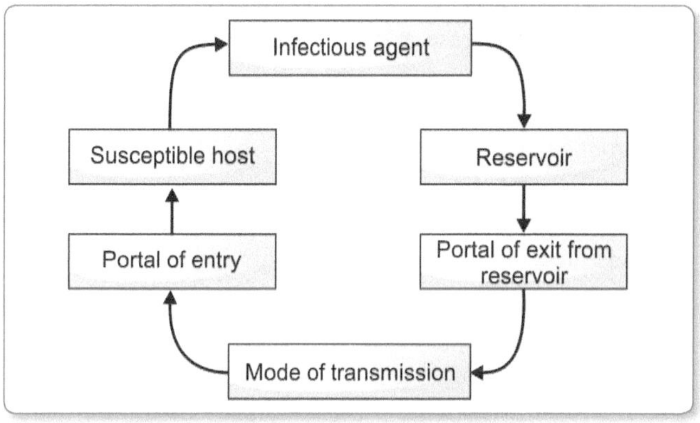

Fig. 1.1: Infection chain

INFECTION CONTROL

Related Terminology

1. **Asepsis:** Freedom from infection or prevention of contact with microorganisms.
2. **Antiseptic**: An agent that will inhibit the growth and development of microorganisms without necessarily killing them.
3. **Bacteriostat**: An agent that inhibit the growth of bacteria.
4. **Bacteriostasis**: It is a state in which bacterial growth is checked without necessarily killing him.
5. **Bacteriocide**: An agent that has the power to kill micro-organisms.
6. **Culture**: Process of growth of microorganisms or other living cells using a culture medium.
7. **Contamination**: Act of soiling or making impure by contact.
8. **Cross infection**: Infection transmitted between individuals infected with different pathogenic organisms.
9. **Carrier**: A person who harbors the pathogenic organisms without showing the signs and symptoms of particular disease.
10. **Colonization**: Microorganisms invade a host, grow and multiply but do not cause infection or disease.

11. **Disinfection**: Destroying of all the pathogenic organisms.
12. **Concurrent disinfection**: Immediate disinfection of all contaminated articles and bodily discharges during the course of the disease.
13. **Terminal disinfection**: The disinfection of the client's unit at the end with all the articles used by the client upon his discharge, death or release from isolation.
14. **Disinfectant:** An agent which kills the pathogenic organisms.
15. **Droplet infection**: Infection of the individuals by means of fine particles of saliva and mucus that are expelled from mouth and nose of another person during coughing, sneezing or speaking.
16. **Fomites:** Objects that have been in contact with a contagious disease and are capable of transmitting that disease.
17. **Infection**: The entry and multiplication of a disease producing agent in the body.
18. **Nosocomial infection or hospital acquired infection**: The client develops an infection that was not present or was incubating at the time of admission to the hospital.
19. **Quarantine**: Isolation of well persons who have come in contact with an infectious disease for a period of time equal to the longest incubation period of that disease.
20. **Isolation**: Separation of infected persons from the non-infected persons for the period of communicability under conditions which will prevent the transmission of infection to others.
21. **Sepsis**: Infection of the body by pus forming bacteria.
22. **Transmission**: Transfer of disease from one person to another.
23. **Sterilization**: Destruction of all microorganisms pathogenic and non-pathogenic including their spores.
24. **Autoclaving**: Process of sterilization of articles by steam under pressure using autoclave.
25. **Immunization**: Act of creating immunity artificially against a particular disease.

PHYSICAL AND CHEMICAL CONTROL OF MICROORGANISMS

Physical Methods

A. Heat sterilization:

a. Moist heat

i. Steam under pressure or autoclave: Usually operated at 250°F (121°C), 15 lb pressure; time needed for the procedure depend on the articles to be sterilized.

ii. Boiling water: Object to be sterilized immersed in water and boiled for 15 minutes.

b. Dry heat (hot air oven): Operating temperature 310–338°F (160 to 170°C) usually for two hours.

c. Pasteurization: Disinfection of milk and other substances by moderate heat, two methods holding method and flash method.

B. Radiation: All types of radiation are injurious to microbes; gamma rays and ultraviolet lights are used.

C. Filtration: Removal of microbes from liquids by means of porous materials; used to sterilize drugs, culture media, etc.

D. Refrigeration: Low temperature inhibits microbial multiplication; used for food preservation.

E. Hypertonicity: By their osmotic effects, hypertonic solutions inhibit microbial multiplication.

F. Desiccation: Removal of water, bacterial spores and certain vegetable cells resistant to such treatment, commonly used for food preservation.

Chemical Methods

A. Many terms are used to describe the action of chemical agents like antiseptic, disinfectant, germicide, bactericide, fungicide, viricide, etc.

B. Type and number of microbes, concentration, time needed, temperature, presence of organic matter all these will affect the action of chemical agents.

C. Commonly used chemical agents are:

a. Ethyl alcohol 70%
b. Isopropyl alcohol 80%
c. Benzalkalonium chloride
d. Hydrogen peroxide
e. Silver nitrate
f. Iodine and iodine releasing compounds
g. Chlorine and chlorine releasing compounds
h. Cresols
i. Ethylene oxide.

BARRIER NURSING

Barrier nursing or isolation technique is intended to confine the microorganisms within a given and recognized area. There are a number of isolation techniques and precautions used to prevent the spread of infection.

1. **Respiratory isolation**: Indicated where the pathogens are spread by droplet from the respiratory tract. Aspects include:
    a. Keep a distance from the infected person.
    b. Wear masks.

c. Wear gowns when caring for clients who has drooling of saliva.
d. Ask clients to cover mouth with hand kerchief or provide mask to the client.
e. Restrict visitors.
f. A person suffering from respiratory disease/low immunity should not attend the infected person.

2. **Enteric isolation**: Indicated when the pathogens are transmitted in feces. Aspects are:
   a. Handwashing; both infected person and carer should perform.
   b. Wear gloves and gowns while handling soiled items.
   c. Soiled article/linen should be disinfected before washing/cleaning.
3. **Wound and skin isolation**: Indicated for pathogens which are found in wounds and can be transmitted by the contact with the wounds or by contact with the articles contaminated by the wound discharges. Techniques are:
   a. Wear gloves and gown.
   b. Safe disposal of dressings and discharges from the wounds.
   c. Proper disinfection of articles used for wound dressing.
   d. Keep separate articles for the client.
   e. Handwashing.
   f. Avoid cuts and abrasions on the hand of the carer.
4. **Blood isolation**: Intended to prevent transmission of pathogens that are found in blood. Aspects are:
   a. Wear gloves and gown, and goggles if chance for eye splashes.
   b. Disinfect articles used for infected client.
   c. Handwashing.
   d. Use separate articles for the infected client.
   e. Avoid cuts and abrasions on the hand of the carer.
5. **General precautions:**
   a. Maintain high degree of cleanliness.
   b. Health teaching about disease transmission.
   c. Restrict visitors.
   d. Emphasize on handwashing.
   e. Keep toilet articles separate for each person.
   f. Immunization against common communicable diseases if facilities available.
   g. Protect persons with lower resistance.
   h. Follow isolation techniques when needed.

Disinfection: Destruction or removal of all pathogenic organisms.

Sterilization: Destruction or removal of all pathogenic organisms including their spores.

ANTIMICROBIAL DRUGS

Drugs that prevent multiplication and growth of organisms (bacteriostatic) or kills the organisms (bactericidal).

Antimicrobial drugs are drugs that prevent multiplication and growth of organisms (bacteriostatic) or kill the organisms (bactericidal).

1. **Penicillins**: Bactericidal, inhibit cell wall synthesis of microorganisms. Used in systemic infections caused by gram-positive organisms, prophylaxis for rheumatic fever and bacterial endocarditis.

Side effects: Hypersensitivity reaction, gastrointestinal (GI) upsets, anemia, thrombocytopenia, leucopenia, nephritis, irritation at injection site.

2. **Cephalosporins**: Bactericidal, inhibit bacterial cell wall synthesis. Used in systemic infections caused by gram positive organisms, prophylactic use in surgery, intra-abdominal infections.

   First generation cephalosporins: For example, cephazolin sodium.

   Second generation cephalosporins: For example, cefoxitine sodium.

   Third generation cephalosporins: For example, cefotaxime.

Side effects: Phlebitis at IV site, diarrhea, pseudomembranous colitis, hypersensitivity reactions, fungal overgrowth, discomfort at IM injection site, nephrotoxicity, hepatotoxicity, bone marrow depression.

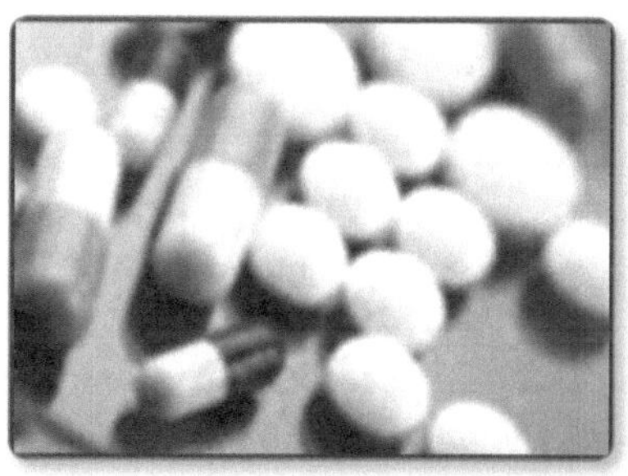

3. **Aminoglycosides**: Bactericidal, acts by suppressing protein synthesis in the bacterial cell wall. Used in serious gram-negative bacterial infections, eye and ear infection.

> ***Side effects:*** Ototoxicity, nephrotoxicity, neuromuscular blocks, hypersensitivity, photosensitivity with topical preparation.

4. **Tetracyclines**: Broad spectrum antibiotic with bacteriostatic action, at higher doses bactericidal in action, used in *Chlamydia, Mycoplasma, Rickettsia*, acne vulgaris, gonorrhea, spirochetes.

> ***Side effects:*** Headache, dizziness, neutropenia, nausea, vomiting, diarrhea, colitis, abdominal cramps, hepatotoxicity, photosensitivity, hypersensitivity and superinfections, chelating to teeth and new bone.

5. **Chloramphenicol**: A synthetic broad spectrum agent, primarily bacteriostatic, but is bactericidal in higher doses. Inhibits protein synthesis. Used in *H. influenzae* meningitis, *Rickettsiae, S. typhi*, Mycoplasma, bacteroids, typhoid fever.

> ***Side effects:*** Aplastic anemia, neurotoxicity, gray-baby syndrome, abdominal distension, vomiting, palor, hypersensitivity, enterocolitis and super-infections.

6. **Vancomycin:** Bacteriostatic and bactericidal effects, interferes with cell membrane synthesis, used in staphylococcal infections, pseudomembranous colitis, gram-positive organisms.

> ***Side effects:*** Ototoxicity, nephrotoxicity, hypersensitivity, thrombophlebitis, red-neck syndrome (flushing and hypotension from rapid IV infusions) and superinfections.

ANTITUBERCULAR DRUGS

Drugs to treat tuberculosis. Drugs commonly used are isoniazid, ethambutol, rifampicin, streptomycin, and pyrazinamide.

Isoniazid (INH): Side effects are peripheral neuritis (numbness and tingling in hands and feet) and hepatitis.

Ethambutol: Side effect is optic neuritis, a loss of red-green color discrimination.

Rifampicin: Side effects include orange discoloration of body fluids like urine, tears, saliva, etc. hepatitis and flu like syndrome.

Streptomycin: Side effects include eighth nerve damage causing vertigo, tinnitus, dizziness and roaring in ears, loss of hearing and renal toxicity.

Pyrazinamide: Side effect is excess uric acid levels which can cause gout and hepatitis.

ANTIFUNGAL DRUGS

For example, amphotericin B, nystatin, griseofulvin, clotrimazole, fluconazole.

Fungicidal or fungiostatic in action, alters fungal cell membrane permeability.

Adverse effects include febrile reactions, nausea, vomiting, nephrotoxicity, hypokalemia, thrombophlebitis, tachycardia, hypotension and hypersensitivity reactions.

ANTHELMINTICS

These are group of drugs that affect various systems within the worms causing them to die. Most of these drugs are poorly absorbed in the gastrointestinal tract (GIT) and remains effective as it passes through the GIT and is excreted in the feces, e.g. mebendazole and albendazole.

PAIN

Pain is an unpleasant sensation, entirely subjective that produces discomfort, distress or suffering.

> Pain is an unpleasant sensation, entirely subjective that produces discomfort, distress or suffering.

Gate control theory: Substantia gelatinosa in the dorsal horn of the spinal cord acts as a gate, mechanisms that can close to keep pain impulses from reaching the brain or can open to allow pain impulses to ascend to the brain.

Acute pain is of short duration, may last from split seconds to about six months, usually associated with autonomic nervous system symptoms like increased BP, pulse, sweating and pallor.

Chronic pain: Prolonged duration lasts for 6 months or longer and rarely accompanied by autonomic nervous system activity.

> **Acute pain** is of short duration, may last from split seconds to about six months, usually associated with autonomic nervous system symptoms like increased BP, pulse, sweating and pallor.

> **Chronic pain** is of prolonged duration lasts for 6 months or longer and rarely accompanied by autonomic nervous system activity.

ANALGESICS

Analgesics are drugs used for pain control.

Narcotic Analgesics

Acts on opiod receptors in central nervous system (CNS) and induces sedation, analgesia and euphoria, e.g. morphine sulfate, codeine and meperidine.

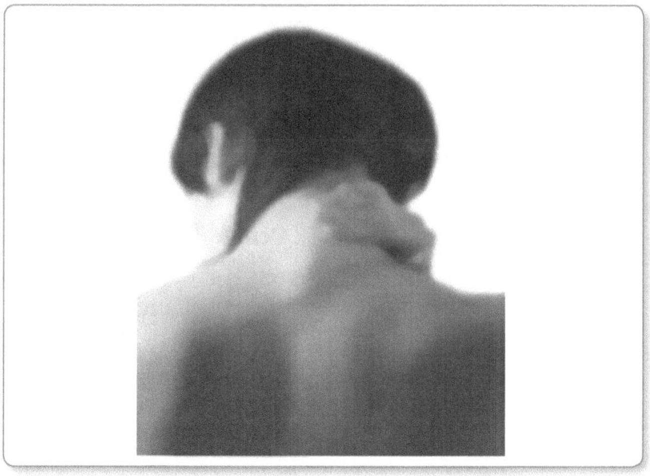

Uses

Used in the relief of moderate to severe pain, pre-operative medication, pain relief in MI, relief of dyspnea occurring in pulmonary edema or acute LVF (left venticular failure).

Adverse Effects

Sedation, confusion, euphoria, impaired coordination, dizziness, urinary retention, hyperglycemia, respiratory depression, tachycardia, hypotension, nausea, vomiting, constipation, allergic reactions, tolerance, physical and psychological dependence and pupil constriction.

> Antidote of morphine is naloxone hydrochloride.

Non-narcotic Analgesics

Inhibits formation of prostaglandins involved with pain. Analgesia also occurs by action of hypothalamus and blocking generation of pain impulses. Also has antipyretic, anti-inflammatory and antiplatelet action. For example, aspirin (acetyl salicylic acid), indomethacin, ibuprofen, paracetamol.

Adverse Effects

Tinnitus, confusion, dizziness (symptom of salicylism), drowsiness, epistaxis, bleeding, bruising, edema, hypertension, nausea and vomiting, diarrhea, gastritis, hypersensitivity, hypoglycemia, impaired renal function, respiratory alkalosis and metabolic acidosis.

> Tinnitus, confusion and dizziness are symptoms of salycylism.

Adjuvants

Includes several classes of drugs that may either potentiate the effect of narcotic or non-narcotic analgesics or have independent analgesic properties in certain situations. For example, hydroxyzine, amitriptyline.

FLUID AND ELECTROLYTE BALANCE

Fluids

Water constitutes about 50% of individual's body weight; water is the single largest component of human body.

> Water is the single largest component of human body and constitutes about 50% of individual's body weight.

Body water is divided into two compartments:

1. **Intracellular**: Within the cells.
2. **Extracellular**: Outside the cells; further divided into interstitial and intravascular fluid.

> Fluids in two compartments move among cells, tissue spaces and plasma.

Major avenues by which water enters and leaves the body

a. Water enters the body through digestive tract both in liquids (drinking) and in foods (preformed water).
b. Water is formed in the body by metabolism of foods (oxidative water).
c. Water leaves the body via the kidneys (as urine), intestines (with feces) and lungs and skin (insensible water losses).

Distribution of total body water in a normal 70 kg person

Compartment	% Body weight
Total body water	60
• Intracellular fluid (ICF)	40
• Extracellular fluid (ECF) (Plasma 5%, interstitial, transcellular fluid, etc. 15%)	20

Mechanism that maintain total fluid volume

A. Osmoreceptor system

a. Regulates water output volume to balance fluid intake volume.
b. Most important mechanism for the regulation of water output because other fluid losses through the skin, lungs and gastrointestinal system have no feedback mechanism relative to water loss.
c. Cells in the hypothalamus synthesize anti-diuretic hormone (ADH), which is then stored in the posterior pituitary before release into the circulation.
d. Osmoreceptors respond to dehydration by increasing the frequency of nerve impulses to the posterior pituitary, resulting in an increase in the ADH released, this increases water reabsorption in the kidney tubules and decreases urinary output.

e. Osmoreceptors respond to overhydration by decreasing nerve impulses to the posterior pituitary, which decreases the release of ADH, resulting in an increase in the urinary output.

B. Interaction of the circulatory system

a. Regulation of blood volume (extracellular fluid volume).
b. Increase fluid intake increases the blood volume.
c. Increased blood volume results in an increase in the cardiac output, blood pressure, and therefore glomerular filtration.
d. Increased glomerular filtration results in an increase in urinary output and a decrease in blood volume.

C. Regulation of fluid intake: Thirst mechanism

a. Dehydration of cells in the thirst center of the hypothalamus gives rise to thirst sensation.
b. Thirst sensations are also induced by dryness of the oral mucosa.
c. Fluid intake stretches the stomach and moistens the mouth and throat; these sensations cancel thirst sensation before the actual hydration of body fluids.

D. Various factors such as hyperventilation, hypoventilation, vomiting, diarrhea and circulatory failure may alter the volume of fluid lost from the body.

ELECTROLYTES

Electrolytes are salts or minerals in extracellular or intracellular body fluids. If positively charged, called cations and if negatively charged called anions.

Positively charged electrolytes are called cations and negatively charged ones are called anions.

Common Electrolytes

a. Sodium: 135 to 148 mEq/L
b. Potassium: 3.5 to 5 mEq/L
c. Calcium: 9 to 11 mg%
d. Magnesium: 1.3 to 2.1 mEq/L
e. Chloride: 98 to 106 mEq/L

Mechanisms that Maintain Electrolyte Concentrations

A. Aldosterone feedback mechanism

a. Adrenal cortex secretes the steroid hormone aldosterone when extracellular fluid sodium concentration decrease or potassium concentrations increase.
b. Aldosterone stimulates kidney tubules to reabsorb sodium; potassium reabsorption decreases as sodium reabsorption increases; sodium is salvaged while potassium is excreted.
c. This mechanism help preserve normal sodium and potassium concentrations in extracellular fluid.
d. Secondary effects of aldosterone:
   i. Chloride conservation with sodium.
   ii. Water conserved because it is reabsorbed by osmosis as tubules reabsorb salt.

B. Parathyroid regulation of calcium

a. Parathyroid glands secretes parathormone when extracellular fluid calcium concentrations decrease.
b. Parathormone stimulates the release of calcium from the bone, calcium reabsorption in the small intestine (vitamin D required), and calcium reabsorption in the kidney tubules.
c. Increased extracellular fluid calcium concentrations results in decreased secretion of parathormone and gradual loss of excess calcium.

ACID-BASE BALANCE

- Acids are substances that can donate H^+ ion in a solution and bases are substances that can accept H^+ ions.
- pH is the H^+ ion concentration of a solution. Normal pH of the human blood is 7.4 (7.35–7.45).

pH is the H^+ ion concentration of a solution. Normal pH of the human blood is 7.4 (7.35–7.45).

- Buffer or control systems maintain normal pH. Kidneys secrete acids and reabsorbs bicarbonate while the respiratory system gives off carbon dioxide in acidic states. In alkalosis, the kidneys excrete bicarbonate and the respiratory system retains carbonic acid.

Buffer mechanisms for maintaining acid-base balance

A. The buffer mechanism consists of chemicals called buffers, which are present in the blood and other body fluids and which combine with relatively strong acids or bases to convert them to weaker acids or bases; hence, buffers function to prevent marked changes in blood pH levels when either acids or bases enter the blood.

B. A buffer is often referred to as buffer pair because it consists not one but two substances; the chief buffer pair in the blood consists of the weak acid, carbonic acid (H_2CO_3) and its basic salts, collectively called base bicarbonate (HCO_3); sodium bicarbonate ($NaHCO_3$) is the most abundant base bicarbonate present in blood plasma.

C. When the body is in a state of acid base balance, blood contains 27 mEq base bicarbonate per liter and 1.35 mEq carbonic acid per liter and this is expressed as a ratio as base bicarbonate/carbonic acid ratio, i.e. 27/1.35 or 20:1.

Etiology and manifestations of major fluid and electrolyte disturbances		
Fluid/Electrolyte Imbalance	**Etiology**	**Signs and Symptoms**
Extracellular fluid (ECF) deficit	Decreased fluid intake Prolonged fever Vomiting Excessive use of diuretics	Increased thirst Dry skin and mucous membrane Increased temperature Flushed skin Rapid, thready pulse Increased Hct, Na^+ and specific gravity
Extracellular fluid (ECF) excess	Congestive heart failure Liver disease Malnutrition Renal disease Excessive parenteral fluids	Weight gain Crackles Edema Ascites Confusion Weakness Decreased Hct
Hypokalemia	Diarrhea Vomiting Diabetic acidosis Diuretics Inadequate intake	Loss of muscle tone Cardiac arrhythmias Abdominal distention Vomiting Decreased serum K^+
Hyperkalemia	Advanced kidney disease Severe burns Tissue trauma Excessive dose of potassium	Cardiac irregularities Weakness Diarrhea Nausea Irritability Increased serum K^+
Hyponatremia	Diuretics Electrolyte free IVF Diarrhea GI suction Excessive perspiration with increased water intake	Abdominal cramps Convulsions Oliguria Decreased serum sodium and specific gravity
Hypernatremia	Diabetes insipidus Excessive sodium chloride IVF intake	Dry, sticky mucous membrane Oliguria Firm tissue turgor Dry tongue Increased serum Na^+ and specific gravity
Hypocalcemia	Removal of parathyroid glands Administration of electrolyte free solution	Tingling of extrimities Tetany Cramps Convulsions
Hypercalcemia	Hyperparathyroidism Prolonged immobility Excessive intake of Ca^+ or vitamin D	Flank pain (renal calculi) Deep bone pain Relaxed muscles

D. Whenever the base bicarbonate/carbonic acid ratio of blood equals 20/1, the blood pH equals 7.4.

> When the body is in a state of acid base balance, the base bicarbonate/carbonic acid ratio is 20:1 and the blood pH will be 7.4

The pH of body fluids shifts below the ideal of 7.35–7.45 for several reasons:

1. Glucose, used by almost all body cells, is oxidized; as a result energy, water and carbon dioxide are produced; the CO_2 combines with water to produce carbonic acid (H_2CO_3).
2. Metabolism of sulfur amino acids results in the formation of sulfuric acid.
3. Metabolism of phospholipids and phosphor-proteins results in formation of phosphoric acid.
4. Muscle metabolism under anerobic conditions produces lactic acid.
5. Rapid weight loss results in extra fat metabolism, producing ketone bodies.
6. The acid produced by the normal mechanisms just mentioned requires neutralization to avoid acidosis, coma and death.

ACID-BASE IMBALANCES

a. **Metabolic acidosis**: A primary deficit in the concentration of base bicarbonate in the ECF; decreased pH and bicarbonate. Seen in diabetic ketoacidosis (DKA), uremia, starvation, diarrhea, severe infections and renal tubular necrosis.
b. **Metabolic alkalosis**: A primary excess of base bicarbonate in the ECF; elevated pH and bicarbonate. Seen in severe vomiting, nasogastric suctioning, diuretic therapy, excessive ingestion of sodabicarb and biliary drainage.
c. **Respiratory acidosis**: A primary excess of carbonic acid in the ECF with decreased pH and elevated PCO_2, seen in COPD, sedative overdose, acute airway obstruction and weakness of respiratory muscles.
d. **Respiratory alkalosis**: A primary deficit of carbonic acid in ECF with elevated pH and decreased PCO_2, seen in hyperventilation, mechanical over ventilation and encephalitis.

Imbalances	Acidosis	Alkalosis
Respiratory	pH decrease, PCO_2 increase	pH increase, PCO_2 decrease
Metabolic	pH decrease, HCO_3^- decrease	pH increase, HCO_3^- increase

NUTRITION

Essential Nutrients

Carbohydrates, fats, proteins, minerals, vitamins and water that must be supplied to the body in specific amounts. Foods are the sources of nutrients and provide energy to build, repair and maintain tissue and regulate body processes. Imbalances of required nutrients results in malnutrition.

Carbohydrates

Major source of food energy; gives 4 kcals/gm. Exists as monosaccharides, disaccharides and polysaccharides.

Dietary Sources

Grains, fruits, vegetables, nuts, milk and sugars.

Lipids

Most concentrated source of energy and gives 9 kcals/gm. Include fats, oils, resins, waxes and fat like substances such as glycerides, phospholipids, sterols and lipoproteins. Lipids also help for insulation and padding of body organs and carrier of the fat soluble vitamins viz. A, D, E and K.

Dietary Sources

Oil from seeds of grains, nuts, vegetable oils, milk fat, butter, cream, cheese, fat in meat, fish oil and egg yolk.

Proteins

Compounds that are composed of amino acids, gives 4 kcals/gm. Proteins are necessary for growth and continuous replacement of cells throughout life, has a role in immune process, participate in regulating body processes like fluid balance, muscle contraction, mineral balance, iron transport and buffer actions.

Dietary Sources

Meat, fish, egg, milk, cheese, poultry, grains, nuts and legumes.

> Deficiency causes kwashiorkor (protein malnutrition) and marasmus (protein energy malnutrition).

SHOCK

An abnormal physiological state where an imbalance exists between the amount of circulatory blood volume and the size of the vascular system resulting in circulatory failure and lack of oxygen and nutrients to the tissues.

Classification of Shock

a. **Hypovolemic**: Due to decreased circulating blood volume (hemorrhage, burns, vomiting, diarrhea).

b. **Cardiogenic**: Failure of the heart to pump the blood properly (MI, CCF, cardiac arrhythmias, tension pneumothorax).
c. **Septic**: Release of bacterial toxins due to infection as in septicemia.
d. **Neurogenic**: Failure of arteriolar resistance, leading to massive vasodilatation (extreme pain, spinal cord injury, spinal anesthesia, head injury).
e. **Anaphylactic**: Release of histamine and related substances resulting from allergic reaction (insect venom, snake venom, medications, dyes used in radiological studies).

> Shock is an abnormal physiological state where an imbalance exists between the amount of circulatory blood volume and the size of the vascular system resulting in circulatory failure and lack of oxygen and nutrients to the tissues.

Clinical Features

a. **Skin:** Cool, pale, moist in hypovolemic and cardiogenic shock; warm, dry and pink in septic and neurogenic shock.
b. **Pulse:** Tachycardia, weak and thread pulse.
c. **Blood pressure:** BP may be normal in early stages due to compensatory mechanisms, BP drops in later stages.
d. **Respiration:** Rapid and shallow due tio tissue anoxia and excessive amounts of carbon dioxide.
e. **Level of consciousness:** Restlessness and apprehension, progress to coma.
f. **Urinary output:** Decreased due to impaired renal perfusion.
g. **Temperature:** Decreases in severe shock (except septic shock).

> Skin may be cool, pale, moist in hypovolemic and cardiogenic shock but may be warm, dry and pink in septic and neurogenic shock.

Drugs in Shock

a. **Dopamine:** Dilates renal, mesenteric and splanchnic vessels which in turn increases renal perfusion and urinary output.
b. **Dobutamine:** Increases myocardial contractility, vasodilator.
c. **Isoproterenol:** Increases myocardial contractility, causes peripheral vascular dilatation.
d. **Norepinephrine:** Improves cardiac contractility and cardiac output, potent vasoconstrictor.
e. **Sodium nitro prusside (SNP):** Vasodilator, decreases peripheral vascular resistance and work load of heart, used in cardiogenic shock.
f. **Digitalis preparations:** Improves cardiac performance.
g. **Corticosteroids:** Used in septic shock, decrease inflammatory response.
h. **Antibiotics:** Used in septic shock to treat infection.

REVIEW QUESTIONS

1. **Invasion of the body by pathogenic organisms:**
   a. Inflammation b. Infection
   c. Sepsis d. Carrier
2. **Agent that transmit infection from one person to another without showing signs and symptoms of the disease:**
   a. Agent b. Case
   c. Carrier d. Host
3. **Environment in which the invading organisms live and multiply:**
   a. Portal of entry b. Reservoir
   c. Portal of exit d. Environment
4. **Means by which a disease producing organism enters a new host:**
   a. Portal of entry b. Reservoir
   c. Portal of exit d. Environment
5. **An agent that inhibit the growth and development of microorganisms without necessarily killing them:**
   a. Asepsis b. Antibiotic
   c. Antiseptic d. Disinfectant
6. **In a patient already suffering from a disease, a new infection set up from another source or host known as:**
   a. Sepsis b. Cross infection
   c. Iatrogenic infection d. Contamination
7. **An agent that inhibit the growth of bacteria:**
   a. Antiseptic b. Bactericide
   c. Fungicide d. Bacteriostat
8. **An agent that has the power to kill the bacteria:**
   a. Antiseptic b. Bactericide
   c. Fungicide d. Bacteriostat

9. Act of soiling or making impure by contact:

a. Sepsis b. Contamination
c. Colonization d. Culture

10. Invasion and growth of microorganisms in a host without causing infection or disease:

a. Sepsis b. Contamination
c. Colonization d. Culture

11. Immediate disinfection of all contaminated articles and bodily discharges during the course of the disease:

a. Bactericide b. Terminal disinfection
c. Concurrent disinfection d. Sterilization

12. The disinfection of the client's unit at the end with all the articles used by the client upon his discharge:

a. Bactericide b. Terminal disinfection
c. Concurrent disinfection d. Sterilization

13. Infection of the individuals by fine particles of saliva and mucus from mouth and throat of another person:

a. Fomite infection b. Droplet infection
c. Nosocomial infection d. Iatrogenic infection

14. The entry and multiplication of a disease producing agent in the body:

a. Asepsis b. Infection
c. Inflammation d. Injury

15. Separation of infected persons from the non-infected persons for the period of communicability:

a. Quarantine b. Isolation
c. Reverse isolation d. Contamination

16. Infection in a client that was not present or was incubating at the time of admission to the hospital:

a. Fomite infection b. Droplet infection
c. Nosocomial infection d. Iatrogenic infection

17. Isolation of well persons for a period of time equal to the longest incubation period of a disease:

a. Quarantine b. Isolation
c. Reverse isolation d. Contamination

18. Destruction of all microorganisms including their spores:

a. Immunization b. Terminal disinfection
c. Concurrent disinfection d. Sterilization

19. Act of creating immunity artificially against a particular disease:

a. Sterilization b. Disinfection
c. Immunization d. Isolation

20. Steam under pressure sterilization is also known as:

a. Disinfection b. Pasteurization
c. Autoclaving d. Incineration

21. The best method of destroying hospital waste is:

a. Disinfection b. Pasteurization
c. Autoclaving d. Incineration

22. Best method used for disinfection of milk:

a. Boiling b. Pasteurization
c. Autoclaving d. Desiccation

23. Removal of microbes from liquids by means of porous materials:

a. Desiccation b. Boiling
c. Pasteurization d. Filtration

24. Drying method used in food preservation:

a. Boiling b. Pasteurization
c. Autoclaving d. Desiccation

25. Enteric isolation is indicated if the transmission is by:

a. Respiratory route b. Feco-oral route
c. Parenteral route d. Sexual contact

26. Destruction or removal of all pathogenic organisms:

a. Disinfection b. Sterilization
c. Autoclaving d. Boiling

27. Drugs given for the prophylaxis of rheumatic fever:

a. Cephalosporins b. Aminoglycosides
c. Penicillins d. Tetracyclines

28. A third generation cephalosporin:

a. Cefazolin sodium b. Cefepine
c. Cefoxitine d. Cefotaxime

29. Ototoxicity is seen with:

a. Tetracyclines b. Penicillins
c. Aminoglycosides d. Chloramphenicol

30. Gray-baby syndrome is seen with the administration of:

a. Tetracyclines b. Penicillins
c. Aminoglycosides d. Chloramphenicol

31. Red neck syndrome is a side effect of:

a. Streptomycin b. Vancomycin
c. Chloramphenicol d. Tetracycline

32. Peripheral neuritis is an adverse effect of which of the anti-TB drugs:

a. Isoniazid b. Ethambutol
c. Streptomycin d. Pyrazinamide

33. Orange discoloration of body fluids is seen with:
a. Isoniazid b. Ethambutol
c. Streptomycin d. Rifampicin

34. Eighth nerve damage is a serious complication of:
a. Rifampicin b. Ethambutol
c. Pyrazinamide d. Streptomycin

35. Mebendazole is an:
a. Antibiotic b. Antiviral drug
c. Fungicide d. Anthelmintic

36. Pain associated with autonomic nervous system changes:
a. Chronic pain b. Acute pain
c. Visceral pain d. Referred pain

37. A narcotic analgesic:
a. Paracetamol b. Acetaminophen
c. Acetyl salicylic acid d. Morphine sulphate

38. Antidote of morphine is:
a. Protamine sulfate b. Naloxone
c. BAL d. N-acetyl cystine

39. Important cation of ECF:
a. Sodium b. Potassium
c. Calcium d. Chloride

40. Important cation of ICF:
a. Calcium b. Potassium
c. Chloride d. Sodium

41. The normal serum sodium level is:
a. 120–130 mEq/L b. 130–140 mEq/L
c. 135–148 mEq/L d. 150–158 mEq/L

42. The normal serum potassium level is:
a. 2–3 mEq/L b. 2.3–3 mEq/L
c. 3.5–5 mEq/L d. 5–7.4 mEq/L

43. Normal blood calcium level is:
a. 5–7 mg% b. 8–9 mg%
c. 9–11 mg% d. 12–12.5 mg%

44. Normal pH of human blood is:
a. 7–7.2 b. 7.35–7.45
c. 7.2–8.4 d. 7.6–8.1

45. A primary deficit in the base bicarbonate in the ECF:
a. Metabolic alkalosis b. Metabolic acidosis
c. Respiratory alkalosis d. Respiratory acidosis

46. Thirst center is situated in the:
a. Anterior pituitary b. Posterior pituitary
c. Hypothalamus d. Medulla oblongata

47. The hormone that maintain fluid balance is:
a. Antidiuretic hormone b. Prolactin
c. Oxytocin d. GnRH

48. Hormone secreted by adrenal cortex that maintains electrolyte balance:
a. ADH b. GHRH
c. Aldosterone d. Renin

49. The normal bicarbonate/carbonic acid ratio in the human body:
a. 1:20 b. 20:1
c. 1:27 d. 27:1

50. The buffer mechanisms maintaining acid-base balance of the body consists of the following except:
a. Base bicarbonate b. Soda bicarb
c. Carbonic acid d. Carbon dioxide

51. pH and bicarbonates decrease in:
a. Metabolic alkalosis b. Metabolic acidosis
c. Respiratory alkalosis d. Respiratory acidosis

52. pH and bicarbonates increase in:
a. Metabolic alkalosis b. Metabolic acidosis
c. Respiratory alkalosis d. Respiratory acidosis

53. Cardiac arrhythmias occurs in:
a. Hyponatremia b. Hypernatremia
c. Hypokalemia d. Hypocalcemia

54. Tetany is a classical finding in:
a. Hyponatremia b. Hypernatremia
c. Hypokalemia d. Hypocalcemia

55. A primary excess of base bicarbonate is in the ECF:
a. Metabolic alkalosis
b. Metabolic acidosis
c. Respiratory alkalosis
d. Respiratory acidosis

56. A primary excess of carbonic acid in the ECF:
a. Metabolic alkalosis
b. Metabolic acidosis
c. Respiratory alkalosis
d. Respiratory acidosis

57. Compounds composed of amino acids:

a. Carbohydrates
b. Fats
c. Proteins
d. Minerals

58. Energy yield form carbohydrates:

a. 4 Kcals/gm
b. 6 Kcals/gm
c. 9 Kcals/gm
d. 7 Kcals/gm

59. Marasmus is:

a. Protein malnutrition
b. Protein-energy malnutrition
c. Vitamin deficiency
d. Deficiency of fatty acids

60. Histamine and related compounds are responsible for:

a. Hypovolemic shock
b. Cardiogenic shock
c. Anaphylactic shock
d. Neurogenic shock

61. Warm, dry, pink skin is seen in:

a. Hypovolemic shock
b. Cardiogenic shock
c. Anaphylactic shock
d. Neurogenic shock

62. A drug used in shock:

a. Mebendazole
b. Dopamine
c. Acyclovir
d. Isoniazid

ANSWER KEY

1. b	2. c	3. b	4. a	5. c	6. b	7. d	8. b	9. b	10. c	11. c	12. b
13. b	14. b	15. b	16. c	17. a	18. d	19. c	20. c	21. d	22. b	23. d	24. d
25. b	26. a	27. c	28. d	29. c	30. d	31. b	32. a	33. d	34. d	35. d	36. b
37. d	38. b	39. b	40. b	41. c	42. c	43. c	44. b	45. b	46. c	47. a	48. c
49. b	50. d	51. b	52. a	53. c	54. d	55. a	56. d	57. c	58. a	59. b	60. c
61. d	62. b										

Diseases and Disorders of the Central Nervous System

OVERVIEW OF ANATOMY AND PHYSIOLOGY OF CNS

The Nervous System

The nervous system consists of the central nervous system (CNS) which involves brain and the spinal cord and the peripheral nervous system (PNS) which includes the cranial and spinal nerves. The autonomic nervous system (ANS) is a subdivision of the PNS that automatically controls body functions such as breathing and heart beat. It is further divided into sympathetic and parasympathetic nervous systems (Fig. 1.2).

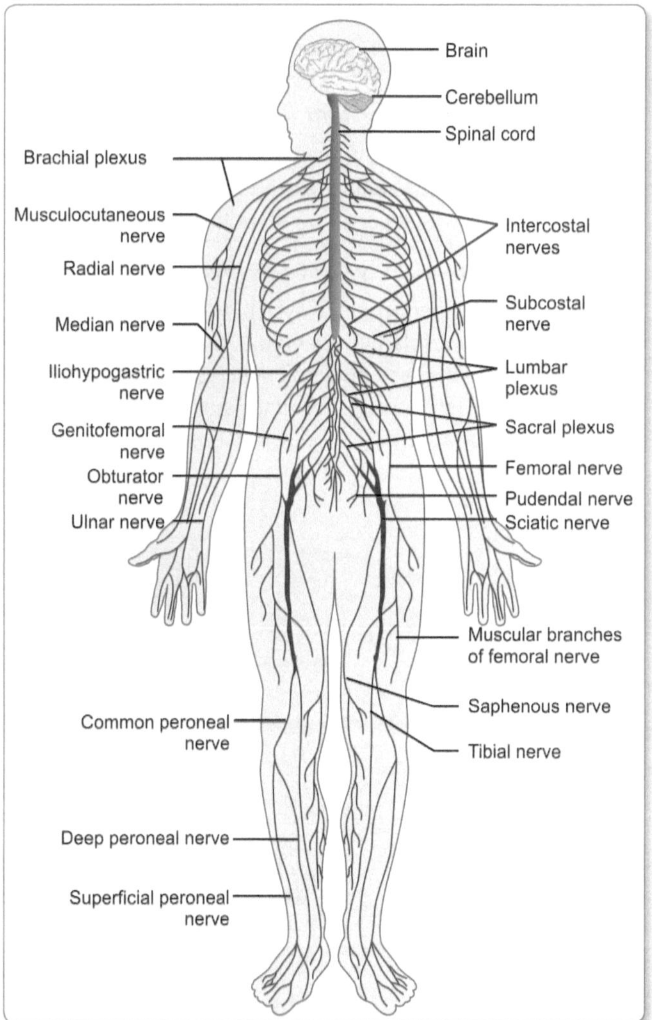

Fig. 1.2: The nervous system

The Neurons

Neurons are the primary component of the nervous system composed of cell body, axon and dendrites. Axons transmit impulses away from the cell body and dendrites conduct impulses towards the nerve cell body.

- **Synapse**: Synapse is the junction between neurons where an impulse is transmitted.
- **Neurotransmitters**: Chemical agents (e.g. acetylcholine, norepinephrine) involved in the transmission of impulse across the synapse.
- **Afferent neurons or sensory neurons**: Transmit impulses from peripheral receptors to the CNS.
- **Efferent neurons (motor neurons)**: Conduct impulses from CNS to muscles and glands.
- **Interneuron**: Connecting link between afferent and efferent neuron.

Brain

- Brain consists of the cerebrum, diencephalon, brainstem and cerebellum (Fig. 1.3).
- **Cerebrum**: It has right and left cerebral hemispheres which are divided into four lobes. Frontal lobe is considered with higher intellectual functions, personality, behavior and motor function. Specialized motor speech area (Brocas area) is situated in the frontal lobe. Parietal lobe registers general sensation. Temporal lobe is concerned with hearing, taste, smell, understanding and formulation of language. The occipital lobe is concerned with vision.

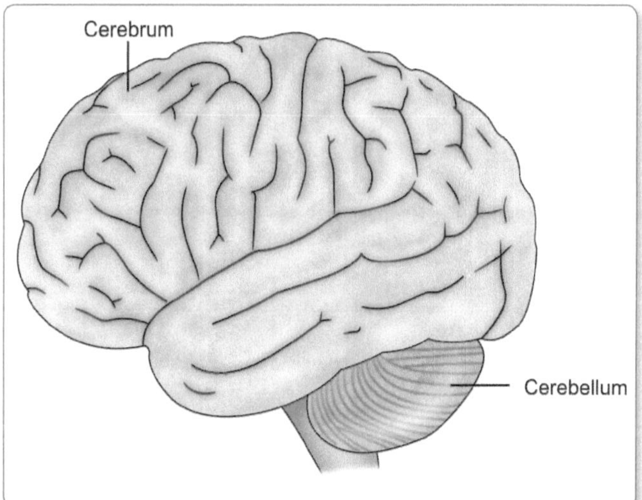

Fig. 1.3: The brain

- **Corpus callosum**: Large fiber tract that connects the two cerebral hemispheres.
- **Basal ganglia**: Islands of gray matter within white mater of the cerebrum.
- **Diencephalon**: Connects cerebrum to brain stem. Contains thalamus and hypothalamus.
- **Thalamus**: It is the relay station for discrimination of sensory signals. Controls primitive emotional responses.
- **Hypothalamus**: Plays a major role in the regulation of vital functions such as BP, sleep, food and water intake and body temperature. Act as control center for pituitary gland and affect both divisions of the autonomic nervous system.
- **Brainstem**: Consists of midbrain, pons and medulla oblongata. Contains vital centers of the cardiac, respiratory and vasomotor functions.
- **Cerebellum**: Coordinates muscle tone and movements and maintains equilibrium.

Spinal Cord

Spinal cord serves as a connecting link between the brain and the periphery. Extends from foramen magnum to the second lumbar vertebrae. Consists of 'H' shaped gray matter in the center surrounded by white matter. The white matter contains sensory pathways and motor pathways. Spinal cord is concerned with reflex reaction, consisting of involuntary response to a stimulus occurring over a neural pathway which is not relayed to and from the brain (Fig. 1.4).

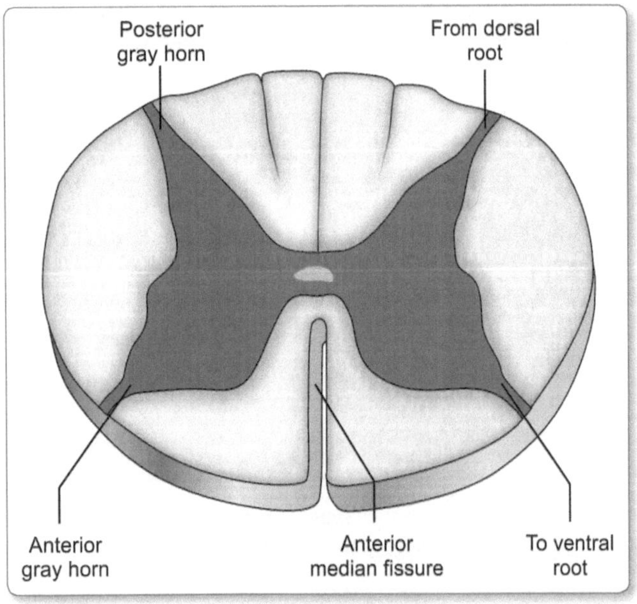

Fig. 1.4: Spinal cord

Meninges

Meninges is the membrane covering brain consisting of three layers viz. dura matter, arachnoid matter and pia mater, pia mater being the inner most layer. The area between dura and arachnoid mater is called subdural space the area between arachnoid and pia mater is called subarachnoid space.

Ventricles

Four fluid filled cavities connecting with one another and the spinal cord. Concerned with the production and circulation of the spinal fluid (Fig. 1.5).

Cerebrospinal Fluid (CSF)

Surrounds brain and spinal cord which offers protection by functioning as a shock absorber. CSF is produced from the choroid plexus.

> Cerebrospinal fluid (CSF) is produced from the choroid plexus.

Peripheral Nervous System (PNS)

Peripheral nervous system consists of 31 pairs of spinal nerves which carry impulses to and from the spinal cord and 12 pairs of cranial nerves which carry impulses to and from the brain.

Autonomic Nervous System (ANS)

ANS is part of peripheral nervous system which regulates cardiac muscle, smooth muscle and glandular functions. Consists of sympathetic nervous system which generally accelerates some body functions in response to stress and parasympathetic nervous system which controls normal body functions.

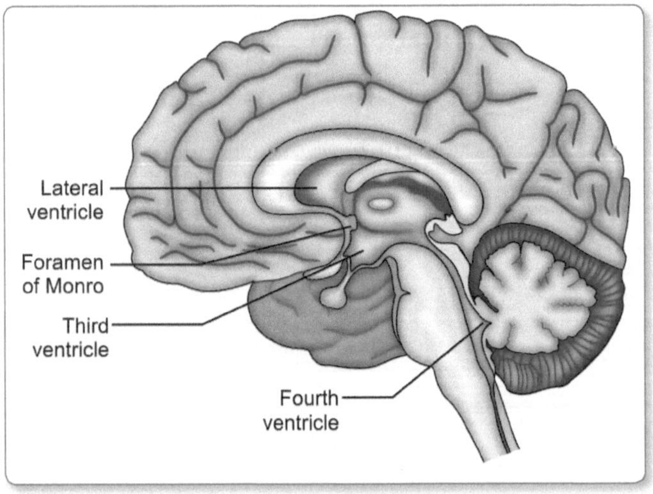

Fig. 1.5: Ventricles of brain

Cranial nerves and their functions		
Number	**Cranial Nerve**	**Nature**
I	Olfactory	Sensory
II	Optic	Sensory
III	Oculomotor	Motor
IV	Trochlear	Motor
V	Trigeminal	Mixed
VI	Abducens	Motor
VII	Facial	Mixed
VIII	Vestibulo-cochlear	Sensory
IX	Glossopharyngeal	Mixed
X	Vagus	Mixed
XI	Accessory	Motor
XII	Hypoglossal	Motor

Autonomic nervous system (ANS) is a part of peripheral nervous system which regulates cardiac muscle, smooth muscle and glandular functions.

VISION

Eyes are the organs of vision which consist of external structures and internal structures.

- External structures are eyelids, conjunctiva and lacrimal apparatus.
- Internal structure of the eye: There are three layers of the eyeball. Outer sclera and cornea, middle choroid, ciliary body and iris and inner layer retina (Fig. 1.6).
- Sclera is a tough white connective tissue (white of the eye).
- Cornea is a transparent tissue through which light enters the eye.
- Choroid is a highly vascular layer nourishing retina.
- Ciliary body secretes aqueous humor; ciliary muscles change the shape of the lens.
- **Iris:** Pigmented membrane behind cornea which gives color to the eye. Pupil is a circular opening in the middle of the iris.
- **Retina:** It is light sensitive layer composing of rods and cons. Optic disk or blind spot is the area in the retina for the entrance of the optic nerve where there are no photoreceptors.
- In the central region of the retina is a yellowish spot called the "macula lutea". It has a depression in its center called the "fovea centralis." This depression is the region of the retina that produces the sharpest vision. Toward the center of the fovea centralis is an area called the "optic disk." The nerve fibers leave the eye at this point to become parts of the optic nerve. A central artery and vein also pass through at the optic disk to supply blood to the cells of the inner layer of the eye.
- **Visual pathway:** Retina translates light waves into nerve impulses that travel over the optic nerves. Optic nerves for each eye meet at the optic chiasma; fibers from the median half of the retina cross her and travel to the opposite side of the brain as optic tracts. Optic tracts reach the occipital lobe of the cerebrum where visual impulses are perceived and interpreted (Fig. 1.7).

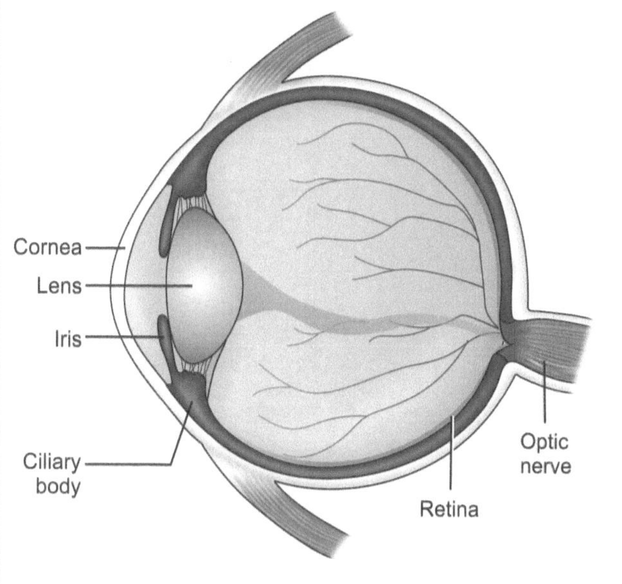

Fig. 1.6: Structure of the eye

Optic disk or blind spot is the area in the retina for the entrance of the optic nerve where there are no photoreceptors.

HEARING

Ears are the organ of hearing and consist of external ear, middle ear and inner ear.

- External ear consists of the auricle or pinna, the external auditory canal and tympanic membrane (Fig. 1.8).
  - Middle ear has ear ossicles or three small bones (viz. malleus, incus and stapes) and Eustachian tube. Sound waves are conducted between the middle ear and inner ear through the ear ossicles.
  - Eustachian tube connects nasopharynx and middle ear, thus equalizing pressure on both sides of the ear drum.

- Inner ear consists of the cochlea and the vestibular apparatus (Fig. 1.9).
- Cochlea contains organ of Corti, the receptor end organ of hearing which transmits sound waves and initiates nerve impulses carried by the eighth cranial nerve to the temporal lobe of the cerebrum.
- Vestibular apparatus is the organ of balance and composed of three semicircular canals and the utricle.

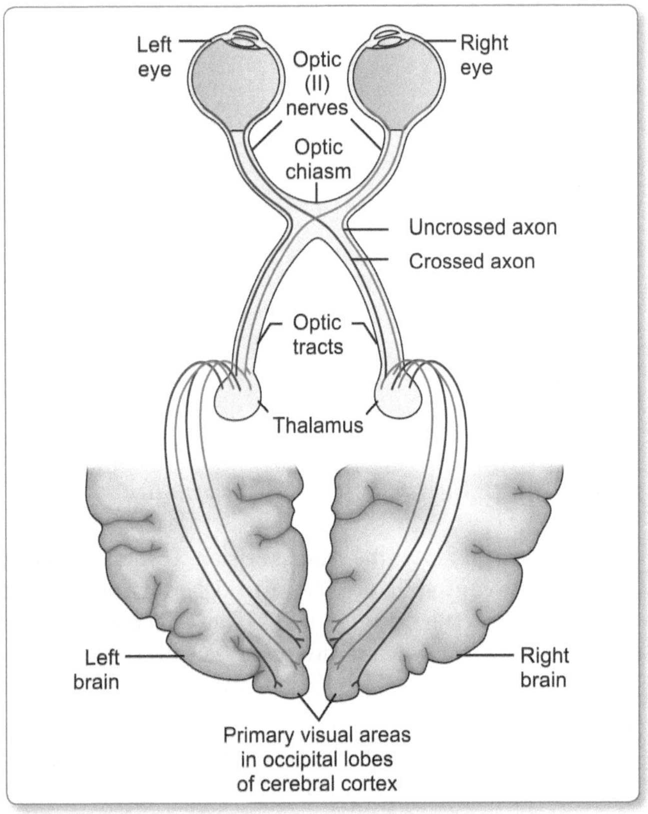

Fig. 1.7: Visual pathway

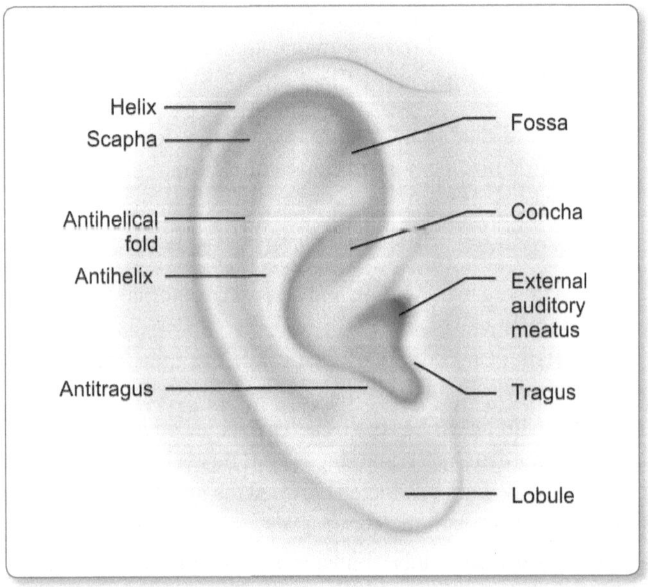

Fig. 1.8: External ear

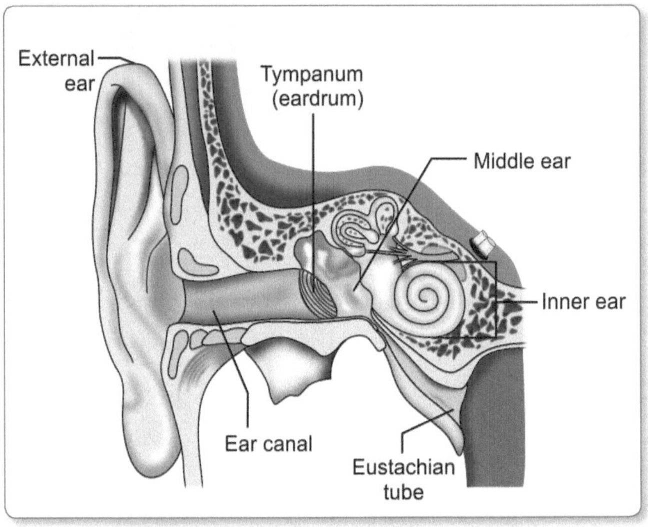

Fig. 1.9: Parts of the ear

Eustachian tube connects nasopharynx and middle ear, thus equalizing pressure on both sides of the ear drum.

DISEASES AND DISORDERS OF THE NERVOUS SYSTEM

INCREASED INTRACRANIAL PRESSURE (ICP)

Increase in the ICP can occur due to an increase in any of the major intracranial components viz. brain tissue, CSF or blood. Increased ICP may be caused by tumors, abscesses, hemorrhage, edema, hydrocephalus, inflammation, etc. Untreated increased ICP can lead to displacement of the brain tissue (herniation) and it is a life-threatening situation because of pressure on vital structures in the brainstem, nerve tracts and cranial nerves.

Clinical Signs

- **Earliest sign:** Decrease in the level of consciousness (LOC); progress from restlessness to confusion and disorientation to lethargy and coma and changes in vital signs.
- Systolic BP rises without rise in diastolic BP (widening of pulse pressure). Pulse rate slows abnormal respiratory patterns (Cheyne-Stokes respiration) and elevated body temperature. Other signs include ipsilateral (same side) dilation of pupil, contralateral (opposite side) hemiparesis, headache, projectile vomiting and papilledema.

Treatment

a. Maintain patent airway and adequate ventilation. Hypoxia increases ICP. Hyperventilate client with 100% oxygen before suctioning.
b. Monitor vital signs and neuron checks.
c. Fluid restriction.
d. Position with head elevated to 30–45°.
e. Avoid excessive coughing, sneezing, vomiting and constipation to prevent increase in ICP.
f. **Drugs:** Hyperosmotic agents (mannitol), corticosteroids, diuretics, anticonvulsants and analgesics.
g. Surgical management, if indicated.

CEREBROVASCULAR ACCIDENT (CVA)

- Destruction of brain cells due to reduction in cerebral blood flow and oxygen (infarction).
- Caused by thrombosis, embolism and hemorrhage.
- **Risk factors**: Include hypertension, diabetes, athero-sclerosis, arteriosclerosis and cardiac diseases.
- **Stages of development of CVA**
    i. **Transient ischemic attack (TIA)**: Warning sign of impending CVA, brief period of neurological deficit lasting less than 30 seconds.
    ii. **Stroke in evolution**: Progressive development of stroke symptoms for a period of hours to days.
    iii. **Complete stroke**: Neurological deficit remains unchanged for a longer period.
- **Clinical features**: Headache, dizziness, confusion, disorientation, nuchal rigidity, fever, bounding pulse, Cheyne-Stokes respiration, hemiparesis, hemiplegia.
- **Diagnosis:** By CT, MRI, EEG, cerebral angiography.

> **Transient ischemic attack (TIA)** is a warning sign of impending CVA; it is a brief period of neurological deficit lasting less than 30 seconds.

- **Treatment**
    - Maintain patent airway and adequate ventilation
    - Monitor vital signs, neuro-checks and signs of increased ICP
    - Maintain nutrition by IVF or NG feeding.
    - Measures to prevent increased ICP
    - Drugs: Hyperosmotic agents, corticosteroids, anticonvulsants, thrombolytics, anticoagulants and antihypertensives
    - Rehabilitation for hemiplegics.

PARKINSON'S DISEASE

- A progressive disease with the degeneration of the nerve cells in the basal ganglia resulting in generalized decline in muscular function; disorder of the extrapyramidal system and usually occurs in older population.
- **Cause**: Unknown, sometimes disorder is post-encephalitic, toxic, atherosclerotic, and traumatic or drug induced.
- Results in degeneration of the dopamine producing neurons in the substantia nigra in the midbrain.
- Depletion of dopamine results in the degeneration of the basal ganglia.

> Parkinson's disease is a progressive disease with the degeneration of the nerve cells in the basal ganglia resulting in generalized decline in muscular function.

- **Findings**
    - Tremor, mainly of the upper limbs, 'pill rolling', resting tremor
    - Cogwheel rigidity
    - Slowness of movement (brady kinesis)
    - Stooped posture, shuffling, propulsive gait
    - Mask face with decreased blinking of the eye
    - Increased salivation, drooling
    - Emotional lability, monotonous speech
    - Autonomic symptoms like excessive sweating, seborrhea, lacrimation and constipation.
- **Treatment**
    - Drugs
        - L dopa—increases the level of dopamine in the brain, avoid multiple vitamin preparations containing vitamin B_6 and foods high in vitamin B_6.
        - Carbi dopa—levodopa
        - Amantadine
        - Anticholinergic drugs (benztropine, trihexy-phenidyl)—used in combination with L dopa for controlling tremor and rigidity.
    - Antihistamines—diphenhydramine
    - Bromocryptine
        - Safe environment
        - Physiotherapy and speech therapy
        - Adequate nutrition, avoid constipation
        - Psychological support.

MYASTHENIA GRAVIS

- A neuromuscular disorder in which there is a disturbance in the transmission of impulses from nerve to muscle cells at the neuromuscular junction causing extreme muscle weakness.
- An autoimmune disorder whereby antibodies destroy acetylcholine receptor sites on the post-synaptic membrane of the neuromuscular junction.
- Voluntary muscles are affected, especially those innervated by cranial nerves.

- **Findings**
  - Diplopia, dysphagia
  - Extreme muscle weakness, increases with activity and reduces with rest
  - Ptosis, mask face
  - Weak voice, hoarseness
  - Tensilon test: IV injection of tensilon provides spontaneous relief of symptoms
  - EMG and serum antibodies are also used for diagnosis.

> Myasthenia gravis is a neuromuscular disorder in which there is a disturbance in the transmission of impulses from nerve to muscle cells at the neuromuscular junction causing extreme muscle weakness.

- **Treatment**
  - Drugs

    Anticholinesterase drugs: Neostigmine, pyridostigmine, blocks the action of cholinesterase and increases the level of acetylcholine, causes excessive salivation and sweating, abdominal cramps, nausea, vomiting, diarrhea and fascciculations.
  - **Thymectomy:** Thymus is thought to be involved in the production of acetylcholine receptor antibodies.
  - **Plasmapheresis:** Removes circulating acetylcholine receptor antibodies.

SPINAL CORD INJURY

- Injury to the spinal cord can occur due to motor vehicle accidents, diving in shallow water, falls, industrial accidents, sports injuries, gunshot or stab wounds. Nontraumatic causes include tumors, hematomas, aneurysms, congenital defects like spina bifida. Lavel of injury can be cervical, thoracic or lumbar.
- **Findings**
  - Spinal shock characterized by absence of reflexes below the level of the lesion, flaccid paralysis, lack of temperature control in affected parts, hypotension with bradycardia, retention of urine and feces.
  - Symptoms depend on the level and the extent of the injury. Can be quadriplegia, respiratory paralysis, paraplegia, loss of voluntary movement and sensation below the level of the injury, reflex activity below the level of the lesion may return after spinal shock resolves, permanent flaccid paralysis.
- **Diagnosis**: CT and MRI
- **Treatment**
  - Immobilization and normal spinal alignment to promote healing
  - **Surgery:** Decompression laminectomy, spinal fusion.

> Spinal shock characterized by absence of reflexes below the level of the lesion, flaccid paralysis, lack of temperature control in affected parts, hypotension with bradycardia, retention of urine and feces.

MENINGITIS

- Inflammation of the meninges of the brain and spinal cord.
- Caused by bacteria, virus or other microorganisms
- Infection may reach CNS by direct extension from adjacent cranial structures, by oral or naso-pharyngeal route or via the blood, CSF or lymph.
- Most common organisms are *Meningococcus*, *Pneumococcus*, *H. influenzae* and *Streptococcus.*
- **Findings**
  - Headache, malaise, photophobia, irritability, vomiting.
  - Chills and fever.
  - Signs of meningeal irritation like nuchal rigidity, Kernig's sign, opisthotonus and Brudzinski's sign.
  - **Kernig's sign:** Contraction or pain in the hamstring muscle while attempting to extend the leg when hip is flexed.
  - **Opisthotonus:** Head and heels bend backward and body arched forward.
  - **Brudzinski's sign:** Flexion at the hip and knees in response to forward flexion of the neck.
- Seizures and decreased level of consciousness
- **Diagnosis** by LP and CSF studies
- **Treatment**
  - Antibiotics
  - Symptomatic treatment
  - Maintain fluid and electrolyte balance
  - Monitor vital signs and neuro-checks.

> Signs of meningeal irritation in meningitis include signs like nuchal rigidity, Kernig's sign, opisthotonus and Brudzinski's sign.

> **Kernig's sign:** Contraction or pain in the hamstring muscle while attempting to extend the leg when hip is flexed.

ENCEPHALITIS

- Inflammation of the brain caused by virus (herpes simplex virus/arbovirus are common)
- May occur as a sequelae of other diseases such as measles, mumps and chickenpox.
- **Findings**
  - Headache, vomiting

- Fever, chills
- Seizures, altered level of consciousness.

- **Treatment**
  - Monitor vital signs and neuro-checks
  - Symptomatic treatment
  - Maintain fluid and electrolyte balance.

BRAIN ABSCESS

- Collection of free or encapsulated pus within the brain tissue.
- Usually follows an infectious process elsewhere in the body (ear, sinuses, mastoid bone).
- **Findings**
  - Headache, vomiting
  - Malaise, anorexia
  - Signs of increased ICP
  - Focal neurological deficits (hemiparesis, seizures).
- **Treatment**
  - Antibiotics
  - Monitor vital signs and neuro-checks
  - Symptomatic treatment
  - Craniotomy and drainage of the abscess.

TRIGEMINAL NEURALGIA (TIC-DOULOUREUX)

- Disorder of the fifth cranial nerve
- Causes disabling and recurring attacks of severe pain along the sensory distribution of one or more branches of the trigeminal nerve.

> Trigeminal neuralgia is a disorder of the fifth cranial nerve causing disabling and recurring attacks of severe pain along the sensory distribution of one or more branches of the trigeminal nerve.

- **Findings**
  - Sudden attack of severe shooting pain in one side of the face.
  - Attacks are usually triggered by a cold breeze, foods and fluids of extreme temperature, toothbrushing, chewing, talking or touching the face
  - Twitching, grimacing and frequent blinking, tearing of the eye during the attack.
- **Treatment**
  - Pain management techniques.
  - Teach to avoid triggering factors.
  - Anticonvulsants.
  - **Nerve block:** Injecting alcohol to one or more branches of the trigeminal nerve.
  - Avulsion of branches of the trigeminal nerve
  - **Rhizotomy:** Total severance of sensory root of trigeminal nerve.
  - Microsurgery, percutaneous radiofrequency trigeminal gangliolysis and microvascular decompression of trigeminal nerve.

BELL'S PALSY

- Disorder of seventh cranial nerve.
- Results in the loss of ability to move the muscles on one side of the face.
- Cause may be viral or autoimmune.
- **Findings**
  - Loss of taste over anterior two-third of the tongue on affected side.
  - Complete paralysis of one side of the face.
  - Loss of expression, displacement of mouth towards unaffected side and inability to close eyelid on affected side.
  - Pain behind the ear.
- **Treatment**
  - **Drugs:** Corticosteroids, mild analgesics
  - Soft diet, instruct to chew on unaffected side, avoid hot fluids/foods.
  - Dark glasses for protection, artificial tears to prevent drying of the cornea and eye patch at night.

> Bell's palsy is a disorder of seventh cranial nerve resulting in the loss of ability to move the muscles on one side of the face.

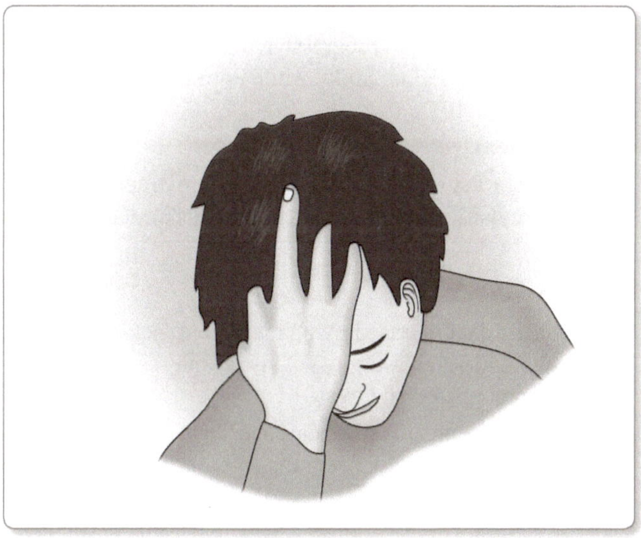

GUILLAIN-BARRE SYNDROME

- Disorder characterized by symmetrical, bilateral, peripheral polyneuritis characterized by ascending paralysis.
- Cause may be autoimmune.
- Precipitated by antecedent viral infections and immunizations.
- **Findings**
  - Clumsiness, mild sensory changes
  - Progressive, ascending, muscle weakness in more than one limb
  - Cranial nerve involvement (dysphagia)
  - Respiratory paralysis
  - Absence of deep tendon reflexes (DTR)
  - Autonomic dysfunction.
- **Treatment**
  - Mechanical ventilation if respiratory paralysis.
  - Plasmapheresis to reduce circulating antibodies.
  - Atropine in bradycardia and propranolol in tachycardia.
  - Symptomatic treatment.

> Guillain-Barre syndrome is a disorder characterized by symmetrical, bilateral, peripheral polyneuritis characterized by ascending paralysis.

DISORDERS OF THE EYE

CATARACT

- Disorder caused by the opacity of the ocular lens.
- Usually occurs in old age (senile cataract) or may develop secondary to trauma, radiation, infection and certain drugs (corticosteroids).
- **Findings**
  - Blurred vision, progressive decrease in vision, glare in bright lights, milky white appearance of the pupil (Fig. 1.10).
- **Treatment**
  - Cataract surgery (extracapsular extraction/phaco-emulsification with intraocular lens implantation).

GLAUCOMA

- Disorder characterized by increased intraocular pressure, resulting in progressive loss of vision, may cause blindness if not recognized and treated.
- **Risk factors** include advancing age, diabetes, hypertension, heredity, history of previous eye surgery, trauma or inflammation.

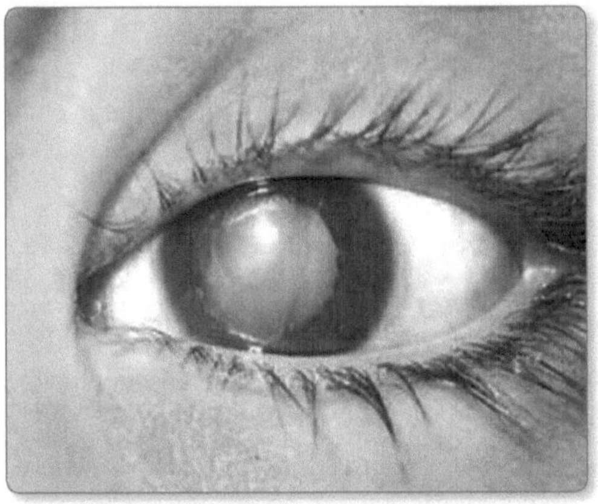

Fig. 1.10: Milky white appearance of the pupil

- **Types**
  - **Chronic open angle glaucoma:** Common type, due to obstruction of the out flow of aqueous humor, characterized by impaired peripheral vision (tunnel vision) progressing to loss of central vision, halos around lights.
  - **Acute closed angle glaucoma:** Due to forward displacement of the iris against the cornea obstructing the outflow of aqueous humor, occurs suddenly, characterized by severe eye pain, blurred cloudy vision, halos round lights, nausea and vomiting, steamy cornea, moderate papillary dilatation.
  - **Chronic closed angle glaucoma**: Similar to acute closed angle glaucoma with the potential for an acute attack; characterized by transient blurred vision, slight eye pain, halos around light.

> Chronic open angle glaucoma is the common type of glaucoma and is due to obstruction of the out flow of aqueous humor, characterized by impaired peripheral vision (tunnel vision) progressing to loss of central vision.

- **Treatment of chronic open angle glaucoma**
  - **Drugs:** One or more combination of pilocarpine, epinephrine, acetazolamide and timolol maleate. Pilocarpine increase the out flow of aqueous humor; epinephrine decreases aqueous humor production and increases outflow; acetazolamide decreases aqueous humor production; timolol decreases intraocular pressure.
  - **Surgery:** If no improvement with the drugs. Procedures done are trabeculectomy, trephining, laser trabeculoplasty.

> Trabeculectomy, trephining, laser trabeculoplasty are the surgical procedures done for chronic open angle glaucoma.

- **Treatment of acute closed angle glaucoma**
  - **Drugs:** Pilocarpine (miotic), oral glycerin and mannitol to reduce IOP, and narcotic analgesics for pain.
  - **Surgery:** Peripheral iridectomy and laser therapy.
- **Treatment of chronic closed angle glaucoma**
  - **Drugs:** Pilocarpine.
  - **Surgery:** Bilateral peripheral iridectomy to prevent acute attacks.

> **Pilocarpine** increase the out flow of aqueous humor; **Epinephrine** decreases aqueous humor production and increases outflow; **Acetazolamide** decreases aqueous humor production; **Timolol** decreases intraocular pressure.

RETINAL DETACHMENT

- Detachment of the sensory retina from the pigment epithelium of the retina.
- **Caused** by trauma, ageing process, severe myopia, post-cataract extraction, severe diabetic retinopathy.
- Tear in the retina allow vitreous humor to sweep behind the sensory retina and separate it from the pigment epithelium.
- **Findings**
  - Flashes of light
  - Visual field loss; veil like curtain coming across field of vision.
- **Treatment** is by surgical correction viz. photocoagulation by argon laser, cryosurgery/diathermy and sclera buckling.

> Veil like curtain coming across field of vision is a classical sign in retinal detachment.

DISORDERS OF THE EAR

OTOSCLEROSIS

- Disorder characterized by formation of new spongy bone in the labyrinth of the ear causing fixation of the stapes in the oval window preventing transmission of the auditory vibration to the inner ear.
- **Findings:** Progressive loss of hearing, tinnitus.
- **Diagnosis** by audiometry, Weber's and Rinne's test.
- **Treatment**: Stapedectomy, i.e. removal of the diseased portion of the stapes and replacement with a prosthesis to conduct vibration from middle ear to inner ear.

> Otosclerosis is a disorder characterized by formation of new spongy bone in the labyrinth of the ear causing fixation of the stapes in the oval window preventing transmission of the auditory vibration to the inner ear.

MENIERE'S DISEASE

- Disease of the inner ear resulting from the dilatation of the endolymphatic system and increased volume of endolymph and characterized by recurrent and progressive triad of symptoms viz. vertigo, tinnitus and hearing loss.
- **Findings**
  - Sudden attack of vertigo lasting for hours or days
  - Nausea, tinnitus, progressive hearing loss
  - Vomiting, nystagmus.
- **Treatment**
  - **Acute cases:** Atropine (decrease autonomic system activity), diazepam and fentanyl.
  - **Chronic cases:** Vasodilators (nicotinic acid), diuretics, mild sedatives or tranquilizers (diazepam), antihidstamines (diphenhydramine).
  - **Surgery:** Surgical destruction of the labyrinth causing loss of vestibular and cochlear function; endolymphatic sac decompression or shunt to equalize pressure in endolymphatic space.

> **Meniere's disease** is a disease of the inner ear resulting from the dilatation of the endolymphatic system and characterized by recurrent and progressive **triad of symptoms viz. vertigo, tinnitus and hearing loss.**

REVIEW QUESTIONS

1. **Method to reduce cerebral edema by constricting cerebral vessels:**
   a. Dexamethazone
   b. Mechanical hyperventilation
   c. Mannitol
   d. Ventriculotomy

2. **Glasgow coma scale is a systematic neurological assessment tool that evaluates all of the following except:**
   a. Eye opening
   b. Motor response
   c. Papillary reaction
   d. Verbal performance

3. **A patient's Glasgow coma scale is indicative of coma. His score is:**
   a. Zero b. Two
   c. Ten d. Six
4. **Posture with the flexion of the upper extremities, extension of the lower extremities and plantar flexion denotes:**
   a. Decorticate rigidity b. Decerebrate rigidity
   c. Scissor gait d. Shuffling gait
5. **A symptom of retinal detachment:**
   a. Diplopia b. Severe eye pain
   c. Sudden blindness d. Bright flashes of light
6. **Normal CSF pressure is:**
   a. 80–180 mm of Hg b. 160–220 mm of Hg
   c. $<$ 80 mm of Hg d. $>$ 200 mm of Hg
7. **CSF is secreted by:**
   a. Foramen magnum b. Cerebral aqueduct
   c. Choroid plexus d. Foramen of Luschka
8. **Normal CSF protein level:**
   a. 60–80 mg% b. 100–120 mg%
   c. 30–60 mg% d. 15–45 mg%
9. **A state in which the client has continuous seizures in rapid succession without regaining consciousness in between and lasting for at least 30 minutes is:**
   a. Tonic clonic seizures b. Status epilepticus
   c. Focal seizures d. Jacksonian seizures
10. **An invasive procedure to study CSF:**
    a. Myelogram b. CT scan
    c. MRI scan d. Cerebral angiogram
11. **An X-ray study in which contrast material is injected into subarachnoid space is:**
    a. CT scan b. MRI scan
    c. Cerebral angiogram d. Myelogram
12. **Signs of increased ICP include the following except:**
    a. Tachycardia
    b. Bradycardia
    c. Hypertension
    d. Widening of pulse pressure
13. **Amount of blood received by brain per minute:**
    a. 500–600 mL b. 750–900 mL
    c. 1000–1200 mL d. 1500 mL
14. **Stimulation of vagus nerve causes:**
    a. Bradycardia b. Tachycardia
    c. Hypertension d. Hypotension
15. **Equilibrium of the body is maintained by:**
    a. Cerebrum b. Cerebellum
    c. Medulla oblongata d. Pons
16. **An arterial anastomosis present at the base of the brain:**
    a. Volar arch b. Brachiocephalic trunk
    c. Circle of Willis d. Brachial plexus
17. **The most commonly occurring type of brain tumor:**
    a. Pituitary adenoma b. Neurofibroma
    c. Glioma d. Meningioma
18. **The part of the ear that contains the receptors for hearing:**
    a. Middle ear b. Cochlea
    c. Utricle d. Sacule
19. **Crossing of optic nerves in the cranial cavity:**
    a. Macula lutea b. Blind spot
    c. Optic tract d. Optic chiasma
20. **A necessary component of rhodopsin:**
    a. Vitamin A b. Vitamin B_6
    c. Vitamin C d. Vitamin D
21. **A procedure done to relieve intractable pain in the upper torso:**
    a. Chondrectomy b. Cordotomy
    c. Rhizotomy d. Wolfgang's procedure
22. **The ear ossicles are located in:**
    a. External ear b. Middle ear
    c. Inner ear d. Eustachian tube
23. **Labyrinthectomy is the treatment for:**
    a. Otosclerosis b. Otitis media
    c. Meniere's disease d. Trigeminal neuralgia
24. **Labyrinthectomy results in:**
    a. Absence of pain b. Permanent deafness
    c. Anosmia d. Reduction in tinnitus
25. **Reflex control of respiration occurs in the:**
    a. Pons and medulla b. Cerebral cortex
    c. Hypothalamus d. Cerebellum
26. **Nerve deafness results from damage to:**
    a. Cochlear nerve b. Vestibular nerve
    c. Trigeminal nerve d. Vagus nerve

27. **The medulla is the center for:**
   a. Control of sexuality
   b. Temperature regulation
   c. Water balance
   d. Control of breathing and heart beat

28. **A disorder of fifth cranial nerve:**
   a. Bell's palsy b. Nerve deafness
   c. Trigeminal neuralgia d. Myasthenia gravis

29. **A disorder of seventh cranial nerve:**
   a. Bell's palsy b. Nerve deafness
   c. Trigeminal neuralgia d. Myasthenia gravis

30. **Pill rolling movement is characteristic of:**
   a. Myasthenia gravis b. Parkinsonism
   c. Bell's palsy d. Trigeminal neuralgia

31. **A focal neurological deficit lasting less than 24 hours:**
   a. Stroke b. Stroke in evolution
   c. TIA d. Hypertensive crisis

32. **Drug of choice in parkinsonism:**
   a. L-dopa b. Dilantin
   c. Acetaminophen d. Pyridoxine

33. **Slow, shuffling gait is a characteristic feature of:**
   a. Myasthenia gravis
   b. Multiple sclerosis
   c. Guillain-Barre syndrome
   d. Parkinsonism

34. **The treatment that removes circulating acetyl-choline antibodies:**
   a. Thymectomy
   b. Plasmapheresis
   c. Anticholinesterase drug therapy
   d. Radiotherapy

35. **Anticholinesterase drugs produce the following side effects except:**
   a. Excessive salivation b. Abdominal cramps
   c. Diarrhea d. Constipation

36. **Cervical spinal cord injuries at C1-C8 level causes:**
   a. Quadriplegia b. Paraplegia
   c. Hemiplegia d. Hemiparesis

37. **Disorder of fifth cranial nerve causing excruciating pain:**
   a. Bell's palsy b. Facial palsy
   c. Trigeminal neuralgia d. Lou Gehrig's disease

38. **Opacity of the ocular lens due to ageing:**
   a. Cataract b. Glaucoma
   c. Myopia d. Hypermetropia

39. **Disorder characterized by increased intraocular pressure:**
   a. Cataract b. Glaucoma
   c. Myopia d. Hypermetropia

40. **Trabeculectomy is the surgical treatment for:**
   a. Chronic open angle glaucoma
   b. Acute closed angle glaucoma
   c. Chronic closed angle glaucoma
   d. Detached retina

41. **Scleral buckling is the surgical management for:**
   a. Chronic open angle glaucoma
   b. Acute closed angle glaucoma
   c. Chronic closed angle glaucoma
   d. Detached retina

42. **Surgical treatment for otosclerosis:**
   a. Myringotomy b. Tympanoplasty
   c. Labyrinthectomy d. Stapedectomy

43. **Disease of the inner ear causing dilation of the endolymphatic system:**
   a. Menier's disease b. Otosclerosis
   c. Otitis media d. Nystagmus

44. **Disorder characterized by formation of new spongy bone in the labyrinth causing fixation of the stapes:**
   a. Menier's disease b. Otosclerosis
   c. Otitis media d. Nystagmus

45. **An important postoperative care for a patient undergone stapedectomy:**
   a. Check gag reflex
   b. Encourage independence
   c. Instruct the client not to blow the nose
   d. Position the client on the operative side

ANSWER KEY

1. b	2. c	3. d	4. a	5. d	6. a	7. c	8. d	9. b	10. a	11. d	12. a
13. b	14. a	15. b	16. c	17. c	18. b	19. d	20. a	21. c	22. b	23. c	24. b
25. a	26. a	27. d	28. c	29. a	30. b	31. c	32. a	33. d	34. b	35. d	36. a
37. c	38. a	39. b	40. a	41. d	42. d	43. a	44. b	45. c			

Diseases and Disorders of the Cardiovascular System

OVERVIEW OF ANATOMY AND PHYSIOLOGY OF CVS

Heart

The heart is a muscular pump which pumps blood into the arterial system and receives blood from the venous system maintaining circulation throughout the body.

Heart wall is composed of pericardium, myocardium and endocardium. The heart has two atria and two ventricles; the right atrium receives systemic venous blood from the superior vena cava and left atrium receives oxygenated blood from the lungs through the pulmonary veins. Lie below the atria are the ventricles; right ventricle contracts and propels deoxygenated blood into the pulmonary circulation via the aorta during ventricular systole.

The mitral valve or bicuspid valve is located between the left atrium and the left ventricle. The tricuspid valve is located between the right atrium and the right ventricle. Attached to mitral and tricuspid valve, there are chorde tendinae which prevent eversion of the valve during systole. Semilunar valves are present at the origin of the aorta and pulmonary artery. Closure of the semilunar valves produce the second heart sound (S2) and the closure of the bicuspid and tricuspid valve produces the first heart sound (S1).

Conduction System of the Heart

Cardiac conductions start at the sinoatrial (SA) node which is the pacemaker of the heart. The cardiac impulses initiated in the SA node spread across the atria into the atrioventricular (AV) node. From the AV node impulses are conducted to bundle of His and Purkinje fibers. Electrical activity of the heart can be visualized by attaching electrodes to the skin and recording activity by electrocardiograph (ECG). The total duration of the cardiac cycle is 0.8 seconds.

> SA node is the pacemaker of the heart.

> Electrical activity of the heart can be visualized by attaching electrodes to the skin and recording activity by electrocardiograph (ECG).

> The total duration of the cardiac cycle is 0.8 seconds.

Coronary Arteries

The coronary arteries branch off at the base of the aorta and supply blood to the myocardium and the conduction system. The major function of the blood vessel is to supply the tissues with blood, remove wastes and carry unoxygenated blood back to the heart. This is achieved by means of the arteries, arterioles, capillaries, venules and veins.

Cardiac Enzymes

The cardiac enzymes will be elevated with myocardial infarction (MI).

a. Creatinine phosphokinase (CPK)—50–325 mu/mL
b. CPK-MB—0%
c. Lactic acid dehydrogenase (LDH)—100–225 mu/mL
d. Aspartate aminotransferase (AST); also called SGOT—7–40 u/mL

> **The cardiac enzymes** and their normal values
> - Creatinine phosphokinase (CPK)—50–325 mu/mL
> - CPK-MB—0%
> - Lactic acid dehydrogenase (LDH)—100–225 mu/mL
> - Aspartate aminotransferase (AST); also called SGOT—7–40 u/mL

Serum Electrolytes

a. **Sodium (Na^+)**—135–148 mEq/L; reflects the relative fluid balance; hyponatremia indicates fluid excess and hypernatremia indicates fluid excess.
b. **Potassium (K^+)**—3.5–5.4 mEq/L; increased potassium (hyperkalemia) and decreased potassium (hypokalemia) levels can cause dysrhythmias.
c. **Magnesium (Mg^{++})**– 1.3 to 2.1 m Eq/L; decreased levels can cause dysrhythmia.
d. **Caicium (Ca^{++})**– 4.5 to 5.3 mEq/L or 9 to 11 mg%; calcium is necessary for blood clotting and neuromuscular activity; decreased levels cause teteny; increased levels may cause muscle atony; increased and decreased levels can cause dysrhythmias.

> **Serum Electrolytes**
> Sodium (Na^+)—135–148 m Eq/L
> Potassium (K^+)—3.5–5.4 mEq/L
> Magnesium (Mg^{++})—1.3–2.1 mEq/L
> Calcium (Ca^{++})—4.5–5.3 mEq/L or 9–11 mg%.

Serum Lipids

a. **Total cholesterol**—150 to 200 mg/dL; elevated levels predispose to atherosclerotic plaque formation.

b. **High density lipids (HDL)**—30 to 85 mg/dL; low levels predispose to cardiovascular disease.
c. **Low density lipids (LDL)**—50 to 140 mg/dL; high levels predispose to cardio vascular disease.
d. **Triglycerides**—10 to 150 mg/dL; high levels increase the risk of atherosclerotic heart disease.

> **Serum Lipids**
> Total cholesterol—150–200 mg/dL
> High density lipids (HDL)—30–85 mg/dL
> Low density lipids (LDL)—50–140 mg/dL
> Triglycerides—10–150 mg/dL.

Electrocardiogram (ECG): Noninvasive test that produces a graphic record of electrical activity of the heart. Holtor monitoring provides continuous monitoring of ECG for up to 24 hours.

> **Electrocardiogram (ECG)** is a noninvasive test that produces a graphic record of electrical activity of the heart.

Exercise ECG (Treadmill test or Stress test): The ECG is recorded during prescribed escalated exercise; stress test may show heart disease when resting ECG does not.

Echocardiogram: Noninvasive recording of the cardiac structures using ultrasound.

Cardiac catheterization: Invasive, but often diagnostic test for cardiac disease. A catheter is inserted into the right or left side of the heart to measure intracardiac pressures and oxygen levels in various parts of the heart, with injection of the dye, it allows visualization of heart chambers, blood vessels and course of blood flow (angiography).

Coronary angiography: Visualization of the coronary arteries by injection of radiopaque contrast dye to evaluate cardiac disease. Coronary angiography and stenting may be performed along with angiography to treat atherosclerotic plaques in the coronary arteries.

> **Coronary angiography** is the visualization of the coronary arteries by injection of radiopaque contrast dye to evaluate cardiac disease.

Central venous pressure (CVP): Obtained by inserting a catheter into the external jugular, antecubital or femoral vein. The catheter is attached to an IV infusion and water manometer by a three way stop cock. Provide information about the blood volume adequacy of central venous return, provides an IV route for drawing blood samples, administering fluids and medications and possibly inserting a pacing catheter. Normal CVP is 4 to 10 cm of water; elevation indicates hypervolemia and decreased level indicates hypovolemia.

> Normal CVP is 4—10 cm of water.

BLOOD

Blood Components

1. **Serum:** Plasma with fewer or no coagulating factors
2. **Plasma:**
   - Plasma consists of water (90%), electrolytes, proteins, nitrogenous substances, lipids, hormones, vitamins and enzymes.
   - Proteins act as buffers, albumin is the largest component of plasma proteins.
   - Albumin is principally responsible plasma colloid osmotic pressure. It reversibly combines with and transports certain lipids, bilirubin, thyroxin and certain drugs such as barbiturates.
   - Globulin also helps to establish colloid osmotic pressure. Transport certain vitamins, iron, copper and cortisol; helps in hemostasis.
   - Gamma globulins are antibodies found in plasma.
   - Plasma also contains glucose which is a prime oxidative metabolite of body cells.

> The proteins which the plasma contains give the blood the sticky consistency called viscosity.

3. **Blood cells or corpuscles**

a. **Erythrocytes or red blood cells (RBCs)**
   - Pliable biconcave disk that maximizes the surface area for ease of diffusion of respiratory gases
   - Number—males 4.5–6.2 lakh/mm^3; females 4.0–5.5 lakh per mm^3.
   - RBC is formed in the red bone marrow of the vertebrae, sternum, ribs, iliac crests, clavicle, scapulae and skull (Fig. 1.11).

> Formation of RBC in the red bone marrow is termed as erythropoiesis.

   - Under conditions of low oxygen tension, liver and kidneys secrete proteins into the blood that combine to form erythropoietin which stimulates erythrocyte production.

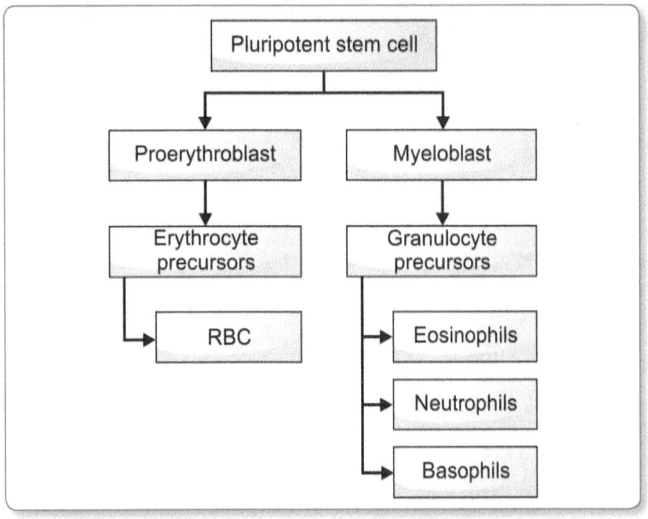

Fig. 1.11: Formation of RBCs and granulocytes

- Hemoglobin (Hb) is hem molecules combined with globulin, formed within the erythrocytes utilizing copper, cobalt, iron, nickel and vitamin B_6.
- Erythrocytes live for about 120 days; old or deteriorated ones are removed by reticulo-endothelial cells of the liver, spleen and bone marrow; hem is converted to bilirubin which is excreted from the liver as part of the bile.

b. **Leukocytes or white blood cells (WBCs)**
   - Types
     1. Granulocytes: Originate in red bone marrow and consist of neutrophils (50–70%), eosinophils (1–4%) and basophils (0–1%).
     2. Agranulocytes: Originate in red bone marrow and lymphatic tissue and consist of monocytes (3–8%) and lymphocytes (25–40%).
   - Functions of WBC include phagocytosis, antibody synthesis and destruction of transplanted tissues and cancer cells by T lymphocytes.
   - Leukocytes live for a few hours or days.

Differential leukocyte count and absolute count in normal adults

WBCs	DC (%)	Absolute count per mm^3
Neutrophils	40–75	2000–7500
Eosinophils	1–6	40–440
Basophils	0–1	0–100
Lymphocytes	20–40	1500–4000
Monocytes	2–10	500–800

c. **Thrombocytes or platelets**
   - Anucleate cellular fragments associated with hemostasis.
   - Originated by fragmentation of megacaryocytes in bone marrow
   - Number: 1,50,000 to 5,00,000 cells/mm^3.
   - Function in blood coagulation by adhering to damaged areas to decease blood loss and releasing chemicals that constrict damaged blood vessels.

Physical Properties of Blood

1. Volume: Males 5 to 6 liters
   Females 4.5 to 5.5 liters.
2. Hematocrit: Percent blood volume occupied by RBC (normal 36–45%).
3. Specific gravity: 1.05–1.06.

Blood Groups

- Name of blood groups indicate the type of antigen in RBC. For example, group A has A antigen in RBC, group B has B antigen in RBC, group O has no antigen and group AB has both antigens A and B in the RBC.

> Blood group O is the universal donor and blood group AB is the universal recipient.

- Every person's blood belong to one of the four blood groups—Group A, B, AB and O and is either Rh positive or Rh negative.
- Plasma normally contains no antibodies against antigen present on its own RBC, but does contain antibodies against other antigens not present in RBC, e.g. Group A plasma contains antibodies against B antigen and does not contain antibodies against A antigen.
- Blood does not normally contain anti-Rh antibodies; Rh positive blood never contains them; Rh negative blood will contain anti-Rh antibodies if the individual has been transfused with Rh positive blood or has carried an Rh positive fetus.

Blood groups

Blood group	Antigen in RBC	Antibody in plasma	Transfusion possible
A	A	B	A, O
B	B	A	B, O
AB	A and B	None	Any group
O	None	anti-A, anti-B	Group O only

Blood Vessels

- **Arteries:** Vessels that carry blood away from the heart, arteries branch into arterioles and then into capillaries.
- **Veins:** Vessels that carry blood towards the heart, veins branch into venules which collect blood from capillaries.
- **Capillaries:** Microscopic vessels that carry blood from arterioles to venules and venules unite to form veins; exchange of substances between blood and interstitial fluid occurs in capillaries.
- **Covering of blood vessels**
  - Arteries are lined by three layers of membrane; outer being a fibrous coat called tunica adventitia, middle being smooth muscle called tunica media and inner lining of endothelium called tunica intima.
  - Veins have the same three coats; but thinner and fewer elastic fibers.
  - Capillaries have only tunica intima.

> Pulmonary artery is the only artery in the human body that carries deoxygenated blood.

> Pulmonary veins are the only veins in the body that carries oxygenated blood.

BLOOD CLOTTING PROCESS

Hemostasis

Hemostasis or arrest of bleeding may be achieved by the following processes.

a. Vasoconstriction: Reflex spasm in the cut or ruptured vessel's smooth muscles.
b. Aggregation of platelets: Platelets adhere to the damaged blood vessel walls forming plugs.
c. Blood coagulation or clotting: Blood becomes gel as soluble fibrinogen is converted into insoluble fibrin; process brought about by at least a dozen different clotting factors operating in sequence.
d. Both prothrombin and fibrinogen are soluble proteins normally present in blood in adequate amounts for clotting to occur at the normal rapid rate.
e. Fibrin is an insoluble protein formed from the soluble protein fibrinogen, in the presence of the enzyme thrombin, fibrin appears as a tangled mass of threads, blood cells becomes entrapped within these threads and RBCs give the clot its red color (Fig. 1.12).

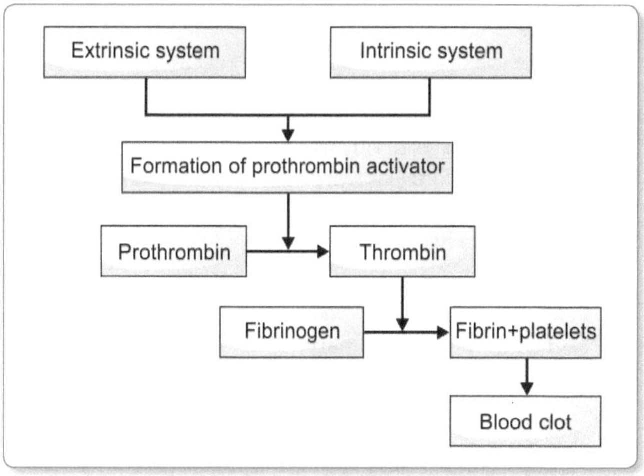

Fig. 1.12: Blood clotting process

BLOOD CIRCULATION

The circulation of blood is divided into three:

A. The systemic circulation
B. The pulmonary circulation
C. The portal circulation

Systemic Circulation

Arteries

The vessels that carry blood from the left ventricle through the body generally and back to the right atrium are those which constitute the systemic circulation.

Aorta is the main artery of systemic circulation, arises from the upper part of the left ventricle, goes as ascending aorta, arch of aorta and descending aorta and enters the abdominal cavity to become the abdominal aorta. Then it divides into two main branches viz. left and right common iliac arteries (Fig. 1.13).

> Firmness of outer tunica adventitia makes arteries stand open instead of collapsing when cut; but veins collapse when cut.

The branches of abdominal aorta are:

1. Phrenic arteries
2. Coeliac trunk consisting of left gastric artery, the hepatic artery and the splenic artery
3. Superior mesenteric arteries
4. Adrenal arteries
5. Renal arteries

6. Ovarian arteries in the female and testicular arteries in the male
7. Inferior mesenteric arteries.

The main two branches of abdominal aorta viz. the two common iliac arteries divide as follows:

The ascending aorta has two branches; right and left coronary arteries, which supply the heart wall.

The arch of aorta has three branches:

1. The brachiocephalic trunk which divides into right common carotid artery and right subclavian artery
2. Left common carotid artery
3. Left subclavian artery.

The common carotid arteries supply the head and neck. The branches are external carotid artery and internal carotid artery which leads to their own branches.

Branches of external and internal carotid arteries are as follows (Fig. 1.14):

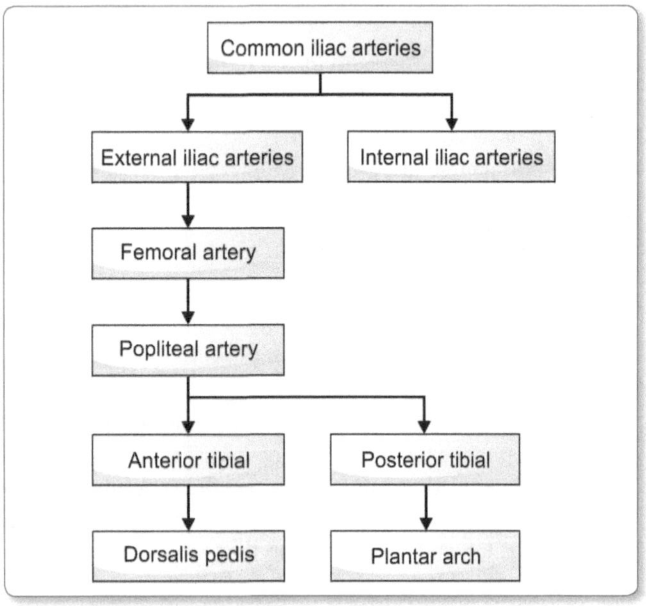

Fig. 1.13: Branches of common iliac arteries

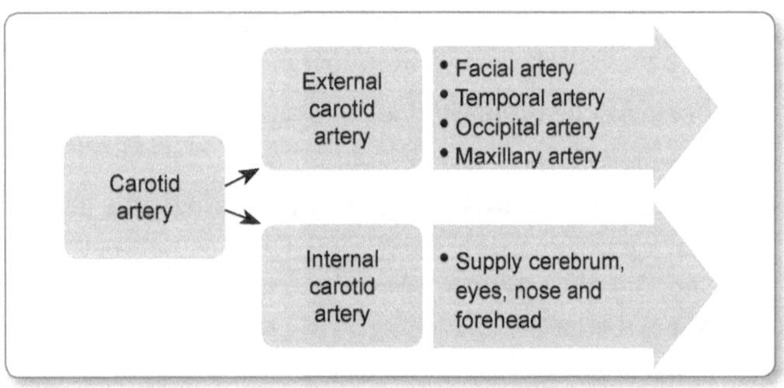

Fig. 1.14: Branches of carotid artery

The vertebral arteries arising from the subclavian arteries goes up and enter the skull, the two vertebral arteries join together to form the basilar arteries.

Circle of Willis: The brain is supplied by a circle of arteries viz. Circle of Willis or circulus arteriosus. This circle is situated at the base of the brain. In front, the two anterior cerebral arteries are joined by the anterior communicating artery. Behind, the basilar artery divides into two posterior cerebral arteries each of which is joined to the internal carotid arteries by the posterior communicating artery. Middle cerebral arteries also join with the network.

Blood is supplied to the upper limb through one main artery viz. subclavian artery which then becomes the axillary artery as far as the middle third of the humerus and the brachial artery as far as the back of the radius where it divides into radial and ulnar arteries. The ulnar artery forms the superficial palmar arch to supply the digits.

Veins

The veins, which return venous blood to the heart, are either superficial veins or deep veins. Deep veins usually accompany arteries. The veins can be described in two groups:

1. The veins of the head, neck, upper limbs and thorax which all end in superior vena cava.
2. The veins of the lower limbs, abdomen and pelvis, which all end in inferior vena cava.

The venous return form head and neck is accomplished by the internal jugular veins and the external jugular veins. At the root of the neck, the internal jugular veins join with the subclavian veins to form the brachiocephalic veins which in turn unite to form the superior vena cava through which blood is returned to the right atrium.

The superficial and deep veins of the upper limb are:

- Superficial veins: The cephalic, basilic and median veins and their tributaries.
- Deep veins: These pour their blood into the axillary veins, which is a continuation of the basilic veins and which becomes continuous with the subclavian veins.

The veins of the lower limb are:

- Superficial veins: The short and long saphenous veins, which empty into the deep popliteal vein at the back of the knee.
- Deep veins: The anterior and posterior tibial veins, the popliteal vein and the femoral vein.

The femoral veins end at the inguinal ligament by becoming the external iliac vein. The internal iliac vein, returning blood from the pelvis, unite with the external iliac vein to become the common iliac vein, one on either side of the body. These unite to form the inferior vena cava. Inferior vena cava also receives venous blood from the renal veins, ovarian/testicular veins and hepatic veins.

The vena cavae pour all venous blood into the right atrium except that from the coronary circulation which is conveyed by the coronary sinus directly into the right atrium.

Pulmonary Circulation

These vessels are concerned with carrying deoxygenated blood from the heart to the lungs and oxygenated blood from the lungs back to the heart. The pulmonary trunk carries venous blood from the right ventricle, and it divides into right and left pulmonary arteries to carry blood to the lungs. The four pulmonary veins return the oxygenated blood from the lungs to the left atrium, two vessels from each lung.

Portal Circulation

The portal system includes all the veins which drain blood from the abdominal part of the digestive system and from the spleen, pancreas and gallbladder. The blood from these organs is carried to the liver by the portal vein, which ends in vessels like capillaries called sinusoids. The blood is then conveyed by the hepatic vein into the inferior vena cava. The liver also receives oxygenated blood and this is conveyed to it by the hepatic artery.

LYMPHATIC SYSTEM

Lymphatic system consists of lymph vessels, lymph, lymph nodes and spleen.

a. **Lymph vessels**
   - Lymph capillaries similar to blood capillaries in structure, larger lymphatic similar to veins but are thinner walled, have more valves and have lymph nodes in certain places along their course.
     - Right lymphatic duct drains lymph form the upper right quadrant into the right subclavian vein.
     - Lymphatics return fluid and proteins to blood from interstitial fluid; adequate lymph return is essential for maintaining homeostasis.
     - Interference of the return of proteins to the blood results in edema caused by the loss of protein and changes in colloid osmotic pressure.

b. **Lymph nodes**
   - Lymphatic tissue separated into compartments by fibrous partitions; afferent lymphatic vessels enter each node and one efferent vessel drains lymph out of node.
   - Usually seen in clusters, important ones are:
     a. Submental or submaxillary group in the floor of the mouth.
     b. Superficial cervical nodes in neck along sternocleidomastoid muscle.
     c. Superficial cubital nodes at bend of elbow.

> Largest lymphatic is known as thoracic duct, drains lymph from entire body, except upper right quadrant, into the left subclavian vein.

     d. Axillary nodes in armpit.
     e. Inguinal nodes in groin.
   - Functions include defence of the body against injurious substances by filtering them out of lymph thereby preventing their entry into the bloodstream.
   - Lymphatic tissue of lymph nodes forms T and B lymphocytes.

c. **Lymph**
   - Fluid in lymphatics
   - Interstitial fluid; formed by plasma filtering out of blood enters the lymphatic capillaries to become lymph.

d. **Spleen**
   - A lymphatic tissue similar to lymph node.
   - It is a deep, purplish red color organ, lies high up at the back of the abdomen on the left side behind the stomach.
   - The fibrous tissue of spleen contains cells which help to produce fresh white cells, engulf the red blood cells that are beginning to wear out and break them down.
   - Also thought to assist in fighting infection, as it becomes enlarged in certain diseases where the blood is infected, e.g. malaria and typhoid fever.

DISEASES AND DISORDERS OF THE CARDIOVASCULAR SYSTEM

CORONARY ARTERY DISEASE (CAD)

- Coronary artery disease refers to a variety of pathologic conditions that cause narrowing or obstruction of the coronary arteries, resulting in decreased blood supply to the myocardium.
- Atherosclerosis is the major causative factor.
- May manifest as angina pectoris or myocardial infarction (MI).

- Risk factors for CAD include family history of CAD, elevated serum lipoproteins, cigarette smoking, diabetes mellitus, and hypertension, and obesity, sedentary and stressful lifestyle.

ANGINA PECTORIS

- Transient, paroxysmal chest pain produced by insufficient blood flow to the myocardium resulting in ischemia.
- Precipitating factors include physical exertion, consumption of heavy meal, extremely cold weather, strong emotions, cigarette smoking and sexual activity.
- **Findings**
  1. Pain: Substernal with possible radiation to the neck, jaw, back and arms and relieved by rest
  2. Palpitations, tachycardia
  3. Dyspnea
  4. Diaphoresis
  5. Increased serum lipid levels
  6. ECG-ST segment depression and T inversion during pain.
- **Treatment**
  1. Drugs: Nitrates, beta adrenergic blocking agents, calcium channel blockers, lipid lowering drugs if dyslipidemia present.
  2. Sugery: Angioplasty or coronary artery bypass graft (CABG).

> Commonly used nitrate is sublingual nitrogly-cerine. Relax for 15 minutes after taking tablet to prevent dizziness. If no relief with one tablet, take an additional one at 5 minutes, but not more than three tablets within a period of 15 minutes. Transient headache is the frequent side effect of nitroglycerine.

MYOCARDIAL INFARCTION

- The death and necrosis of the myocardial cells from inadequate oxygenation, often caused by a sudden complete blockage of a coronary artery.
- Risk factors include atherosclerosis, CAD, thrombus formation, hypertension and diabetes mellitus.
- **Findings**
  1. Substernal pain with radiation to the neck, arm, jaw or back, severe and crushing with sudden onset unrelieved by rest or nitrates.
  2. Nausea, vomiting, dyspnea
  3. Skin cool and clammy
  4. BP decrease; restlessness
  5. Elevated WBC, CPK and CPK-MB, SGOT, LDH (LDH 1 and LDH 2) and ESR.
  6. ECG-T wave inversion, ST wave changes with myocardial ischemia.

CORONARY ARTERY BYPASS GRAFT (CABG)

Done in clients with CAD, new supply of blood brought to diseased or occluded coronary artery bypassing the obstruction with a graft that is attached to the aorta proximally and to the coronary artery distally. Internal mammary artery and great saphenous artery are used for the graft.

> Internal mammary artery and great saphenous artery are used for the coronary artery bypass graft.

DYSRHYTHMIAS

An arrhythmia is a disruption in the normal events of cardiac cycle. It may take a variety of forms.

SINUS TACHYCARDIA

- A heart rate of over 100 beats/minute; originating in SA node.
- May be caused by fever, apprehension, physical activity, anemia, hyperthyroidism, drugs (epinephrine, theophylline), myocardial ischemia and caffeine use.
- The heart rate will be 100–160 beats per minute (bpm), rhythm regular, P wave, PR interval, QRS complex normal in ECG.
- Treatment is correction of underlying cause, elimination of stimulus, sedatives and propranolol.

> In sinus tachycardia, the heart rate will be 100 to 160 beats per minute, rhythm regular, P wave, PR interval, QRS complex normal in ECG.

SINUS BRADYCARDIA

- A slowed heart rate by SA node
- Caused by excessive vagal tone/decreased sympathetic tone, MI, intracranial tumors, meningitis, myxedema, cardiac fibrosis and in well trained athletes.
- Heart rate is less than 60 bpm, rhythm regular, P wave, PR interval, QRS complex normal in ECG.
- Treatment not needed in majority of cases.
- Atropine or isoproterenol may be given.
- A pacemaker may be inserted if the cardiac output is inadequate.

In sinus bradycardia, heart rate is less than 60 bpm, rhythm regular, P wave, PR interval, QRS complex normal in ECG.

ATRIAL FIBRILLATION (AF)

- An arrhythmia in which ectopic foci cause rapid, irregular contractions of the heart.
- Commonly seen in patients with rheumatic mitral stenosis, thyrotoxicosis, cardiomyopathy, hypertensive heart disease, pericarditis and coronary heart disease.
- Atrial rate varies between 350 to 600 bpm and ventricular varies between 100 to 160 bpm.
- Rhythm is regularly irregular, no definite P wave, PR interval not measurable, QRS complex normal.
- **Treatment**
  a. It is by digitalis preparations, propranolol or verapamil with digitalis.
  b. Cardioversion.

In atrial fibrillation (AF), atrial rate varies between 350–600 bpm and ventricular varies between 100–160 bpm; rhythm is regularly irregular, no definite P wave, PR interval not measurable, QRS complex normal.

PREMATURE VENTRICULAR CONTRACTION (PVC)

- Irritable impulses originate in the ventricle, caused by electrolyte imbalance, digitalis therapy, myocardial disease, caffeine drugs (epinephrine, isoproterenol), hypoxia and CCF.
- Rate varies, rhythm irregular, P wave normal but often lost in QRS complex, PR interval not measurable and QRS complex wide and distorted.
- Treatment is by lidocaine 50–100 mg IV followed by IV drip at 1 to 4 mg/minute.

In premature ventricular contraction (PVC), the heart rate varies, rhythm irregular, P wave normal but often lost in QRS complex, PR interval not measurable and QRS complex wide and distorted.

VENTRICULAR TACHYCARDIA (VT)

- Ectopic focus is in ventricles
- Caused by CAD, MI, digitalis toxicity and hypokalemia.
- Atrial rate 60 to 100 bpm and ventricular rate 110 to 250 bpm, P wave often lost in QRS complex, PR interval not measurable, QRS complex is wide.
- Treated with lidocaine (50–100 mg IV, then IV drip of lidocaine at the rate of 1–4 mg/minute), propranolol and cardioversion.

In ventricular tachycardia (VT), atrial rate 60–100 bpm and ventricular rate 110–250 bpm, P wave often lost in QRS complex, PR interval not measurable, QRS complex is wide.

CONGESTIVE CARDIAC FAILURE (CCF)

Inability of the heart to pump an adequate blood to meet the metabolic needs of the body.

LEFT SIDED HEART FAILURE

- Left ventricular damage causes blood to back up through the left atrium into the pulmonary veins causing pulmonary congestion.
- Findings include dyspnea, orthopnea, paroxysmal nocturnal dyspnea (PND), tiredness, muscle weakness, cough, tachycardia and increased PCO_2.

In left sided heart failure, the findings include dyspnea, orthopnea, paroxysmal nocturnal dyspnea (PND), tiredness, muscle weakness, cough, tachycardia and increased PCO_2.

RIGHT SIDED HEART FAILURE

- Weakened right ventricle unable to pump blood into the pulmonary system, systemic venous congestion causes pressure build up.
- Findings include anorexia, nausea, weight gain, dependant edema, jugular venous distention bounding pulses, oliguria, elevated CVP, decreased PCO_2 and increased SGPT.

In right sided heart failure, the findings include anorexia, nausea, weight gain, dependant edema, jugular venous distention bounding pulses, oliguria, elevated CVP, decreased PCO_2 and increased SGPT.

Medical management of all cases includes digitalis preparations, diuretics and vasodilators. If drug therapy is not successful, intra-aortic balloon pump (IABP), mechanical heart or heart transplantation may be needed for survival.

PULMONARY EDEMA

- A medical emergency resulting from left sided heart failure
- The capillary pressures within the lungs become so great that there is oozing of blood into the alveoli, bronchi and bronchioles.
- **Caused** by left sided heart failure or rapid administration of IV fluids.

- **Management** by oxygen therapy, endotracheal intubation and drugs.
- **Drugs:** Morphine sulfate to induce vasodilatation, digitalis to improve cardiac output and frusemide (lasix) to relieve fluid retention, aminophylline to relieve bronchospasm, vasodilators like nitroglycerine and isosorbide dinitrate to dilate the blood vessels.

CARDIAC TAMPONADE

- An emergency situation characterized by an accumulation of fluid/blood in the pericardium that prevents adequate ventricular filling.
- Caused by blunt or penetrating chest trauma, malignant pericardial effusion or can occur as a complication of cardiac surgery.
- **Findings** include chest pain, hypotension, distended neck veins, tachycardia, muffled heart sounds, paradoxical pulse and pericardial friction rub, elevated CVP and decreased Hb.
- **Treatment.**

HYPERTENSION

- Persistent elevation of the systolic BP above 140 mm of Hg and diastolic BP above 90 mm of Hg.
- **Types:** Essential HT, secondary HT
- **Essential HT:** Elevation in BP is due to loss of elastic tissue and arteriosclerotic changes in the aorta and large vessels.
- **Secondary HT:** BP is elevated as a result of other diseases such as renal parenchymal disease, Cushing's disease, pheochromocytoma, primary aldosteronism and coarctation of aorta.
- **Findings:** Pain similar to angina pain, intermittent claudication, occipital headache, nocturia, fatigue, dizziness, epistaxis and dyspnea on exertion.
- **Medical management:** By diet, weight reduction, life style changes along with antihypertensive drugs.

Stepped up care with antihypertensives

- Step I: Thiazide diuretics, beta blockers, calcium channel blockers or ACE inhibitors.
- Step II: Thiazide diuretics, beta blockers, calcium channel blockers or ACE inhibitors, alpha blockers or centrally acting antihypertensives.
- Step III: Add or replace with direct acting vasodilators.
- Step IV: ACE inhibitors, adrenergic blockers.

ANTIHYPERTENSIVE THERAPY (AHT)

1. **Centrally acting AHT**

For example: **Clonidine, m-dopa**

- Blocks sympathetic nerve impulses in the brain.
- Adverse effects include orthostatic hypotension, drowsiness, behavioral changes, peripheral edema, urinary retention, dry mouth and constipation.

2. **Alpha adrenergic receptor blocker**

For example: **Prazosin**

- Blocks alpha receptors in the arterial smooth muscles.
- Adverse effects include postural hypotension, syncope and reflex tachycardia.

3. **Peripheral acting adrenergic neuron blockers**

For example: **Reserpine**

- Blocks norepinephrine centrally and peripherally.
- Adverse effects include depression, drowsiness, nasal obstruction, decreased cardiac output, postural hypotension, diarrhea and increased gastric secretions.

4. **Angiotensin converting enzyme (ACE) inhibitors**

For example: **Enalapril, captopril**

- Act by inhibiting angiotensin converting enzyme which inhibit the vasoconstrictor angiotensin II.
- Adverse effects include blood dyscrasias, hypotension, proteinuria, hyperkalemia, and loss of taste perception.

5. **Direct acting vasodilators**

For example: **Hydralazine, sodium nitroprusside (SNP)**

- Act by direct relaxation of arteriolar smooth muscle causing vasodilation.
- Adverse effects include headache, dizziness, depression, tachycardia, angina, palpitations, weight gain, sodium retention, anorexia, nausea and vomiting.

6. **Beta adrenergic blockers**

For example: **Propranolol, metoprolol**

- Blocks beta adrenergic receptors resulting in decreased BP and heart rate and force of contraction.
- Side effects include drowsiness, light headedness, lethargy, cramping, nausea and bradycardia.

7. **Diuretics**

a. Thiazide diuretics, e.g. chlorothiazide, hydrochlorothiazide
b. Loop diuretics, e.g. frusemide
c. Potassium sparing diuretics, e.g. spironolactone

- Diuretics are used along with AHT. All these drugs inhibit sodium re-absorption producing decreased BP.

THROMBOANGIITIS OBLITERANS (TAO) OR BUERGER'S DISEASE

- Acute inflammatory disorder affecting medium and smaller arteries and veins of the lower extremities, resulting in occlusion of a vessel.
- High incidence is seen among smokers.
- Findings include intermittent claudication, sensitivity to cold, decreased or absent peripheral pulse, ulceration and gangrene.
- Treatment is by vasodilators (e.g. isoxsuprine), analgesics to relieve ischemic pain and anticoagulants to prevent thrombus formation.
- Bypass grafting, endarterectomy, balloon catheter dilatation, lumbar sympathectomy may also be done if medical management fails.

> TAO is an acute inflammatory disorder affecting medium and smaller arteries and veins of the lower extremities, resulting in occlusion of a vessel.

THROMBOPHLEBITIS

- Inflammation of the vessel wall of the vein with formation of a clot.
- Most frequent veins affected are the saphenous, femoral and popliteal veins.
- Results in damage to the surrounding tissues, ischemia and necrosis.
- **Findings**
  a. Pain, tenderness, redness, induration along the course of the vein if superficial vein is affected.
  b. If deep vein is affected, swelling, venous distension of the limb, tenderness over involved vein, positive Homan's sign and cyanosis.
  c. Elevated WBC and ESR.
- Medical management is by anticoagulant therapy.
- (Heparin, warfarin) or by surgical management like vein ligation and stripping, thrombectomy, insertion of umbrella filter into the inferior vena cava.

CARDIOVASCULAR DRUGS

Cardiac Glycosides

For example: **Digoxin**

- **Action:** It ncreases force of myocardial contraction (positive inotropic effect), decreases the rate of conduction (negative chronotropic effect), while increasing the refractory period of AV node. Positive inotropic effect improves blood supply to vital organs and kidneys, providing a diuretic effect
- **Uses:** CCF, atrial fibrillation, atrial flutter, paroxysmal atrial tachycardia
- **Side effects**
  a. Anorexia, nausea, vomiting, diarrheas
  b. Headache, fatigue, confusion, insomnia, convulsions
  c. Visual disturbances, blurred vision
  d. Toxicity may lead to arrhythmias and bradycardia.

> - Therapeutic serum digoxin level is 0.5–2.0 ng/mL
> - Digoxin toxicity is increased in the presence of hypokalemia
> - Digoxin should not be administered to an adult patient if the apical pulse rate is less than 60 beats per minute.

ANTIANGINAL DRUGS

For example: **Nitrites and nitroglycerine**

- **Actions:** Dilates the peripheral vascular smooth muscles of smaller vessels, which decreases cardiac preload and afterload leading to decreased myocardial oxygen needs. Selectively dilates large coronary arteries, which helps to decrease angina pain and hypoxia of the myocardium.
- **Uses:** Treatment and prophylaxis of angina pectoris; IV nitroglycerine manages CCF associated with acute MI and controls intraoperative hypotension or manages hypertension.
- **Side effects**
  a. Headache, usually disappears with long-term therapy
  b. Flushing, hypotension, dizziness
  c. Reflex tachycardia.

> The most common complaint of a patient on nitrates is headache, which usually disappears with long-term therapy.

PERIPHERAL VASODILATORS

- Group of direct acting vasodilators, causes relaxation of smooth muscle of the blood vessels.
- Used to treat peripheral vascular disorders such as Reynaud's disease and Burger's disease, diabetic vascular disease and varicose ulcers.
- Related drug is dipyridamole (persantine).
- Potent vasodilator that also decreases platelet aggregation and clotting time. Selectively dilates small resistance vessels of coronary vascular bed.

Direct acting vasodilators	
Drug	**Adverse effects**
Cyclandelate	Flushing, headache, weakness, heartburn, tachycardia
Isoxsuprine hydrochloride	Hypotension, tachycardia, chest pain, nausea, vomiting, abdominal distress, weakness, rash
Papaverine hydrochloride	Malaise, dizziness, hypertension, flushing of face, tachycardia, nausea, abdominal distress, anorexia, rash

- Used to treat chronic angina attacks, prevention of thromboembolism after cardiac valve replacement surgery.
- Adverse effects include headache, dizziness, weakness, hypotension, GI distress, flushing and skin rashes.

Dipyridamole or persantine is used to treat peripheral occlusive vascular disorders (POVD) such as Reynaud's disease and Burgers' disease, diabetic vascular disease and varicose ulcers.

BETA BLOCKERS

For example: **Propranolol metoprolol**

- **Actions:** Beta adrenergic blocker that decreases heart rate, force of contraction, myocardial irritability, conduction velocity and depresses automaticity.
- **Uses:** Cardiac arrhythmias caused by excessive cardiac stimulation of sympathetic nerve impulses, digitalis induced arrhythmias, essential hypertension, angina pectoris, preoperative management of pheochromocytoma, prevention of migraine headaches.
- **Adverse effects:** Dizziness, drowsiness, insomnia, depression, hypoglycemia, bronchospasm, bradycardia, heart block, hypotension and rash.
- **Related drugs:** Esmolol, nadolol, pinolol and timolol.

CARDIAC STIMULANTS

Cardiac stimulants are autonomic nervous system drugs, e.g. atropine sulfate and isoproteronol.

Atropine Sulfate

- Blocks vagal stimulation of SA node in the heart, thus increasing the heart rate.
- Acts systemically to block cholinergic activity throughout the body.
- **Cardiac uses:** Treatment of sinus bradycardia or asystole, management of symptomatic sinus bradycardia.
- Adverse effects are related to blocking of cholinergic activity in the body.

Isoproterenol

- Stimulates beta 1 adrenergic receptors in heart to increase cardiac output, also act as a bronchodilator.
- **Cardiac uses:** Cardiac standstill, carotid sinus hypersensitivity, Stokes-Adams syndrome, ventricular arrhythmias.
- **Side effects:** Headache, palpitations, dry mouth, flushing, sweating and bronchial edema.

ANTICOAGULANTS

Anticoagulants hinder one or more steps of the coagulation process. They do not dissolve existing blood clots but prevent further coagulation from occurring.

Common drugs in use are heparin and warfarin sodium.

Heparin Sodium

- **Actions:** Blocks conversion of prothrombin to thrombin and fibrinogen to fibrin, action is immediate.
- **Uses**
  1. Prophylaxis and treatment of thrombosis and embolism
  2. Anticoagulation for vascular and cardiac surgery
  3. Prevention of clotting in blood samples and during dialysis
  4. Treatment of disseminated intravascular coagulation (DIC)
  5. Adjunctive treatment of coronary occlusion in acute MI.
- **Adverse effects**
  1. Hemorrhage, bruising and thrombocytopenia
  2. Alopecia
  3. Osteoporosis
  4. Suppression of renal function with long-term high dose use
  5. Allergic reactions: Fever, chills, urticaria, bronchospasm.
  6. Elevated AST and ALT.

Antidote of heparin is protamine sulfate.

Lidocaine is used in ventricular arrhythmias viz. VT, VF and PVCs. Therapeutic serum lidocaine levels range between 1.5–5 mcg/mL.

Antiarrhythmic drugs		
Drug	**Action**	**Adverse effects**
Quinidine	Depress myocardial excitability, slows conduction time in atria and ventricles, prolongs PR interval and QRS complex, prolongs refractory period, depress myocardial contractility, reduces vagal tone used in AF, atrial flutter and VT	Hematologic: Agranulocytosis, thrombocytopenia, purpura, urticaria CNS: Vertigo, blurred vision, diplopia, confusion, syncope GIT: Vomiting, cramping CVS: AV heart block, atrial or ventricular arrhythmias, hypotension, severe bradycardia, arterial embolism
Procainamide	Depress ectopic pacemakers; action on the heart similar to quinidine. Used to treat PVCs, VT and some atrial arrhythmias	Same as quinidine plus severe hypotension with parenteral route
Lidocaine	Suppresses automaticity of ectopic pacemaker, shortens refractory period, decreases duration of action potential in Purkinje fibers, local anesthetic action. Used for acute ventricular arrhythmias	CNS: Dizziness, slurred speech, apprehension, muscle twitching, tremors, convulsions CVS: Hypotension, bradycardia Dermatological: Urticarial rash, peripheral edema
Disopiramide	Increases action potential duration and refractory period of the atria and the ventricles which decrease automaticity and conduction velocity Useful for PVCs and episodes of VT	CVS: Hypotension, precipitation or aggrevation of CHF GU: Urinary hesistancy CNS: Dry mouth, blurred vision, fatigue, headache, malaise, dizziness GIT: Nausea, constipation
Verapamil Nifedipine Diltiazem	Calcium channel blockers, inhibit the reflux of extracellular calcium ions into cardiac and smooth muscle cells. Antianginal effects include dilation of coronary arteries. Verapamil also decreases the influx of calcium into the cardiac contractile and conduction cells SA and AV node. Useful in the management of chronic, stable angina and treatment of SVT	CVS: Hypotension, bradycardia, palpitations, peripheral edema CNS: Flushing, weakness, dizziness, light headedness GIT: Nausea, cramping, heartburn, constipation with verapamil RS: Dyspnea, cough, wheezing
Digitalis	Stimulates the force of cardiac contraction with improvement of cardiac output. Decreases cardiac oxygen demands, diastolic heart rate Useful in the treatment of CHF, and certain arrhythmias such as AF and atrial flutter	Digitalis toxicity CNS: Headache, fatigue, malaise, drowsiness, muscle weakness, insomnia, agitation, seizures, paresthesias of hands and feet, personality changes, impaired memory and hallucinations CVS: Arrhythmias Eyes: Yellow, green halos GIT: Nausea, vomiting, abdominal distention and pain

Warfarin Sodium (Coumadin)

- **Actions:** Blocks prothrombin synthesis, action takes 2 to 5 days to occur.
- **Uses**
  1. Prophylaxis and treatment of thrombosis and embolism
  2. Atrial fibrillation with embolization
  3. Adjunct in treatment of coronary occlusion
- **Adverse effects**
  1. Hemorrhage from any tissue or organ
  2. Anorexia, nausea, vomiting, diarrhea
  3. Hypersensitivity, dermatitis, urticaria, fever
  4. Jaundice, hepatitis
  5. Paralytic ileus, skin necrosis of toes, tip of nose, buttocks, thighs and abdomen in overdose.

Antidote of warfarin sodium is vitamin K.

- Laboratory tests used to monitor heparin therapy: Partial thromboplastin time (PTT)
- Laboratory tests used to monitor warfarin therapy: Prothrombin Time (PT) and INR.

THROMBOLYTIC DRUGS

For example: **Streptokinase, urokinase, alteplase**

- **Actions:** Transforms plasminogen to plasmin which degrades fibrinogen, fibrin clots and other plasma proteins.
- **Use:** Pulmonary emboli, coronary artery thrombosis, deep vein thrombosis, arteriovenous cannula occlusion.
- **Adverse effects:** Bleeding, arrhythmias and allergic reactions.

Antidote for streptokinase is aminocaproic acid.

ANTILIPEMIC AGENTS

- Statin groups, e.g. simvastatin, atorvastatin and rosuvastatin, etc.
- **Actions:** Statins block the pathway for synthesizing cholesterol in the liver. This is significant because most circulating cholesterol comes from internal manufacture rather than the diet. When the liver can no longer produce cholesterol, levels of cholesterol in the blood will fall.

Cholesterol synthesis appears to occur mostly at night, so statins with short half-lives are usually taken at night to maximize their effect.

- **Other effects**
  - Improve endothelial function
  - Modulate inflammatory responses
  - Maintain plaque stability
  - Prevent thrombus formation.
- **Uses**
  - Dyslipidemia
  - Primary and secondary prevention of coronary heart disease
  - Have a favorable effect: Colon cancer, inflammation, dementia, lung cancer, nuclear cataracts and hypertension.
- **Side effects**
  - Myalgias, muscle cramps
  - Liver enzyme derangements
  - Polyneuropathy
  - Acute renal failure.

REVIEW QUESTIONS

1. **The chest pain resulting from inadequate blood supply to the myocardium:**
   a. Myocardial infarction b. Angina pectoris
   c. Atherosclerosis d. Arteriosclerosis
2. **The most common site of acute myocardial infarction:**
   a. Posterior wall of right ventricle
   b. Posterior wall of left ventricle
   c. Anterior wall of right ventricle
   d. Anterior wall of left ventricle
3. **The amount of blood ejected from the ventricle with each contraction:**
   a. Cardiac output b. Cardiac volume
   c. Stroke volume d. Cardiac capacity
4. **Antidote of heparin:**
   a. Protamine b. Promethazine
   c. Probenecid d. Warfarin
5. **Drug of choice for patients with heart failure:**
   a. Propranolol b. Lasix
   c. Heparin d. Digoxin
6. **Average weight of the heart in human beings:**
   a. 100 gm b. 300 gm
   c. 500 gm d. 750 gm
7. **Abnormal heart rhythms are:**
   a. Dysrhythmias
   b. Tachycardia
   c. Bradycardia
   d. Paroxysmal nocturnal dyspnea
8. **Sinus tachycardia is heart rate more than:**
   a. 100 beats per minute
   b. 120 beats per minute
   c. 140 beats per minute
   d. 150 beats per minute

9. Sinus bradycardia is heart rate less than:
a. 50 beats per minute b. 60 beats per minute
c. 70 beats per minute d. 72 beats per minute

10. Heart is covered by:
a. Peritoneum b. Pleura
c. Pericardium d. Perimetrium

11. The pacemaker of the heart:
a. SA node b. AV node
c. Bundle of His d. Purkinje fibers

12. Blood vessels supplying myocardium:
a. Mammary arteries b. Pulmonary arteries
c. Coronary arteries d. Iliac arteries

13. Drug used to relieve pain in MI:
a. Digoxin b. Morphine sulfate
c. Heparin d. Sodium nitroprusside

14. The cardiac enzyme that is very specific and sensitive indicator of MI:
a. Troponin I b. SGOT
c. SGPT d. ALT

15. Functional disorder of the heart in which the heart cannot pump blood to meet the metabolic needs of the body:
a. Myocardial infarction b. Angina pectoris
c. RVH d. Heart failure

16. Contractile musculature of the heart:
a. Pericardium b. Myocardium
c. Endocardium d. Epicardium

17. The amount of energy used for defibrillation:
a. 100 J b. 200 J
c. 350 J d. 500 J

18. Delivering electric voltage of preset voltage to the heart during cardiac arrest:
a. Cardioversion b. Defibrillation
c. Cardiomyopathy d. Angiopathy

19. The depth of chest compression given in CPCR:
a. 1 inch b. 1½ inches
c. 2 inches d. 2½ inches

20. Compression ventilation ratio in CPCR:
a. 15:2 b. 20:2
c. 20:1 d. 15:1

21. Most severe form of AV block:
a. I degree block b. II degree block
c. III degree block d. Mobitz type I

22. A potent vasodilator that decrease both preload and afterload without directly affecting the heart rate:
a. Digoxin b. Dobutamine
c. Morphine sulfate d. Sodium nitroprusside

23. A fibrinolytic agent:
a. Dopamine b. Amiodarone
c. Streptokinase d. Sodium nitroprusside

24. A vasodilator drug:
a. Sorbitrate b. Streptokinase
c. Urokinase d. Metoprolol

25. The most serious complication occurring after cardiac surgery:
a. Dysrhythmias b. Cardiac tamponade
c. Hypertension d. Bleeding

26. A cardiac glycoside:
a. Nifedipine b. Lidocaine
c. Procainamide d. Digoxin

27. Paroxysmal nocturnal dyspnea is seen in:
a. Right sided heart failure
b. Left sided heart failure
c. Cardiac arrest
d. Cardiac arrhythmia

28. Dependant edema and hepatomegaly is seen in:
a. Right sided heart failure
b. Left sided heart failure
c. Cardiac arrest
d. Cardiac arrhythmia

29. Pink frothy sputum is a clinical sign of:
a. Myocardial infarction b. Angina pectoris
c. Pulmonary edema d. Cardiac arrhythmia

30. Accumulation of fluid/the pericardium preventing ventricular filling:
a. Cardiac tamponade b. Pulmonary edema
c. Myocardial infaraction d. Angina pectoris

31. Electronic devise that provides repetitive electrical stimulation to the heart muscle:
a. ECG b. Pacemaker
c. Defibrillator d. Intra-aortic balloon pump

32. An oral anticoagulant:
a. Heparin
b. Streptokinase
c. Cyanocobalamin
d. Warfarin

33. A major side effect of lipid lowering drugs:
a. Nephrotoxicity
b. Hepatotoxicity
c. Ototoxicity
d. Impaired vision

34. Normal CVP is:
a. 4–10 cm of water
b. 10–15 cm of water
c. 25–30 mm of Hg
d. 10–20 mm of Hg

35. A definite sign of thrombophlebitis:
a. Brudszinski's sign
b. Murphy's sign
c. Positive Homan's sign
d. Cullen's sign

36. An elevated potassium level in the blood:
a. Hypokalemia
b. Hyponatremia
c. Hypernatremia
d. Hyperkalemia

37. A positive Trendelenburg test is diagnostic of:
a. Carditis
b. Varicose vein
c. Phlebitis
d. DVT

38. An inflammatory occlusion of the peripheral arteries impairing the peripheral circulation:
a. Buerger's disease
b. Raynaud's disease
c. Aneurysm
d. Varicose vein

39. Malignant increase in the number of erythrocytes:
a. Anemia
b. Thalassemia
c. Polycythemia vera
d. Thrombocytopenia

40. The normal pH of arterial blood:
a. 7.0
b. 7.30
c. 7.42
d. 7.50

41. Pacemaker serves the function normally performed by the:
a. Accelerator nerves to the heart
b. AV node
c. Bundle of His
d. SA node

42. A side effect of digoxin:
a. Hyperkalemia
b. Hypokalemia
c. Hypocalcemia
d. Hypercalcemia

43. Angina pectoris is a sign of:
a. Myocardial ischemia
b. Myocardial infarction
c. Coronary thrombosis
d. Mitral insufficiency

44. 0.45% of sodium chloride is:
a. Isotonic
b. Hypertonic
c. Hypotonic
d. Isometric

45. Blood clotting is the function of:
a. RBC
b. Platelets
c. WBC
d. Erythrocytes

46. Blood clotting requires the presence of:
a. Iron
b. Calcium
c. Fluoride
d. Chloride

47. Pulse pressure is:
a. Diastolic pressure
b. Systolic pressure
c. Difference between diastolic and systolic pressure
d. Pressure in the pulmonary veins

48. Edema is due to:
a. Increased permeability of capillary walls
b. Reduced return of lymph
c. Increased capillary pressure
d. All the above

49. Signs and symptoms of salycilate toxicity include:
a. Chest pain
b. Pink colored urine
c. Slow pulse rate
d. Ringing in ears

50. Antibiotics are the drugs used to treat:
a. Infection
b. Inflammation
c. Pain
d. Itching

51. Reason for chest pain associated with myocardial infarction:
a. Decreased oxygen in heart muscle
b. Left ventricular overload
c. Circulatory collapse
d. Electrolyte imbalance

52. A patient receiving warfarin should report to the doctor:
a. Hematuria
b. Constipation
c. Dyspnea
d. Pruritus

53. Side effect of morphine include:
a. Increased blood pressure
b. Decreased respiratory rate
c. Reduced mucus secretion
d. Visual disturbance

54. What is the compression-ventilation ratio for two rescuers CPR?:

a. 4:2 b. 5:1
c. 5:2 d. 15:2

55. The best indication that fluid replacement for the client in hypovolemic shock is adequate:

a. Skin feels warm
b. Systolic BP above 100 mm Hg
c. Diastolic BP above 90 mm Hg
d. Urine output more than 30 mL/hr

56. Automatic rhythmic contractility is characteristic of:

a. Cardiac tissue b. Nervous tissue
c. Connective tissue d. Muscular tissue

57. World Heart Day is observed on:

a. 21 September b. 28 September
c. 10 October d. 14 August

58. A medication given to a patient with angina:

a. Digoxin b. Sorbitrate
c. Metoprolol d. Lidocaine

59. The chest pain resulting from inadequate blood supply to myocardium:

a. Right heart failure b. Myocardial infarction
c. Angina pectoris d. Left heart failure

60. Normal hemoglobin level:

a. 4 – 8 gm% b. 1 – 5 gm%
c. 15 – 25 gm% d. 10 – 14 gm%

61. Digoxin toxicity occurs when serum level of digoxin exceeds:

a. 1.5 mg/dL b. 1.8 mg/dL
c. 2.0 mg/dL d. 2.5 mg/dL

62. The drug given to relieve pain in myocardial infarction:

a. Acetyl salicylic acid b. Tramadol
c. Diclofenac sodium d. Morphine sulphate

63. Inflammation of the parietal and visceral pericardium:

a. Cardiac tamponade b. Myositis
c. Pericarditis d. Angina

64. The amount of blood ejected from the ventricles during each heart beat:

a. Cardiac output b. Tidal volume
c. Vital capacity d. Stroke volume

65. The amount of blood ejected per minute by rhythmic ventricular contraction:

a. Cardiac output b. Tidal volume
c. Vital capacity d. Stroke volume

66. Duration of cardiac cycle is:

a. 0.4 seconds b. 0.6 seconds
c. 0.8 seconds d. 0.08 seconds

67. The conscious awareness of rapid heartbeat experienced by a person:

a. Tachycardia b. Palpitation
c. Bradycardia d. Syncope

68. Diagnostic procedure done in heart disease:

a. EEG b. USG
c. EMG d. ECG

69. Feeling with hand to note the size of internal organs:

a. Auscultation b. Percussion
c. Palpation d. Vibration

70. Tachycardia is:

a. Elevated BP b. Rapid pulse
c. Elevated temperature d. Rapid respiration

71. The following is an iron chelating agent:

a. Chlorpheniramine b. Deferoxamine
c. Sulfonamide d. EDTA

72. The drug used for morphine induced respiratory depression is:

a. Pethidine hydrochloride
b. Calcium gluconate
c. Magnesium sulphate
d. Naloxone

73. In acidosis, pH of blood will be:

a. Less than 7.35 b. 7.35–7.45
c. More than 7.45 d. Between 7.0–7.45

74. Streptokinase is:

a. Anti-ischemic agent b. Antithrombotic agent
c. Fibrinolytic agent d. Vasodilator

75. Blood clots floating in the circulating blood:

a. Emboli b. Thrombus
c. Plaque d. Aneurysm

76. The apical pulse is located at:

a. 2nd intercostal space b. 3rd intercostal space
c. 5th intercostal space d. 7th intercostal space

77. **Drug used to treat bradycardia:**
a. Morphine b. Sodium nitroprusside
c. Verapamil d. Atropine

78. **An ototoxic drug:**
a. Aspirin b. Digoxin
c. Chlorpromazine d. Dapson

79. **The second heart sound is due to closure of:**
a. Aortic valve b. Mitral valve
c. Tricuspid valve d. Foramen ovale

80. **Full volume but rapidly collapsing pulse:**
a. Bounding pulse b. Bigeminal pulse
c. Water hammer pulse d. Dicrotic pulse

81. **Sign of hypocalcemia:**
a. Cullen's sign b. Homan's sign
c. Goodell's sign d. Trousseau's sign

82. **Relex elicited by stroking the sole of the foot with a sharp instrument:**
a. Patellar reflex b. Achilles reflex
c. Triceps reflex d. Plantar reflex

83. **The position used to treat shock and decreased blood pressure:**
a. Lithotomy position
b. Genupectoral position
c. Dorsal recumbent position
d. Trendelenberg position

84. **Absence of recognizable 'QRS' complex in ECG indicates:**
a. Atrial fibrillation
b. Ventricular fibrillation
c. Sinus arrhythmias
d. Paroxysmalventricular tachycardia

85. **Pressure exerted by plasma protein is called:**
a. Hydrostatic pressure
b. Filtration pressure
c. Systolic blood pressure
d. Oncotic pressure

86. **Human albumin is an example of:**
a. Crystalloid b. Amino acid solution
c. Colloid solution d. Fat emulsion

87. **Stimulation of alpha adrenergic receptors produces:**
a. Vasodilatation
b. Increased heart rate
c. Increased myocardial contractility
d. Vasoconstriction

88. **Deficiency of clotting factor IX leads to:**
a. Hemophilia b. Thrombocytopenia
c. Christmas disease d. Thalassemia

89. **The following parameter should be monitored in patients after heart valve replacement:**
a. Prothrombin time b. Clotting time
c. Bleeding time d. Platelet count

90. **Examination with the help of stethoscope is called:**
a. Percussion b. Palpation
c. Auscultation d. Inspection

91. **When pulse rate is less than 60 beats per minute it is called:**
a. Bradycardia b. Bradypnea
c. Tachycardia d. Tachypnea

92. **Nitroglycerine is given sublingually to relieve pain by vasodilatation of:**
a. Pulmonary artery b. Coronary artery
c. Aortic artery d. Carotid artery

93. **Normal bleeding time is:**
a 1–3 mt b. 6–10 mt
c. 3–6 mt d. 10–12 mt

94. **The most common cause of heart disease in adolescence or young adult is:**
a. Rheumatic fever b. Congenital heart disease
c. Anemia d. CCF

95. **Right ventricular enlargement due to pulmonary problem is called:**
a. Cardiac tamponade b. Corpulmonale
c. Cardiomyopathy d. Emphysema

96. **An antifungal agent:**
a. Amphotericin B b. Adenocine arabinocide
c. Adriamycin d. Amantidine

97. **Which part of the heart is responsible for circulating blood through the lungs?:**
a. Left ventricle b. Right ventricle
c. Left atrium d. Right atrium

98. **Function of vitamin K is:**
a. Helps in wound healing
b. Helps in formation of healthy bones and teeth
c. Helps for clotting of blood
d. Helps in calcium absorption from the intestine

99. **The longest vein in the body is:**
a. Femoral vein b. Cephalic vein
c. Long saphenous vein d. Umbilical vein

100. Scheduled dose of digoxin is with held and notify physician when the adult patient's pulse rate drop below:

a. 50/mt b. 60/mt
c. 70/mt d. 80/mt

101. Which of the following drug is to be infused fast?:

a. Aminophylline b. Mannitol
c. Dopamine d. Potassium chloride

102. The most important electrolyte of intracellular fluid is:

a. Sodium b. Potassium
c. Chloride d. Calcium

103. Infection with Group A beta hemolytic streptococci is associated with:

a. Hepatitis b. Rheumatoid arthritis
c. Rheumatic fever d. Meningitis

104. Hypotension in postoperative period leads to:

a. Hypoxia b. Hypovolemia
c. Cardiac arrhythmias d. TAO

105. Normal CVP is:

a. 4–10 cm of water b. 60–120 cm of water
c. 20–40 cm of water d. 40–60 cm of water

106. Anasarca is:

a. General malaise b. Periorbital edema
c. Pitting edema d. Generalized edema

107. The valve that lies between right atrium and right ventricle:

a. Tricuspid valve b. Bicuspid valve
c. Mitral valve d. Aortic valve

108. The most reliable investigation in CAD is:

a. Cardiac catheterization
b. Echocardiography
c. Coronary angiography
d. Computerized tomography

109. SLE is a disease of:

a. Bone b. Erythrocytes
c. Connective tissue d. Joints

110. Platelets should not be administered under which of the following conditions:

a. The platelet bag is cold
b. The platelets are 2 days old
c. The platelet bag is at room temperature
d. The platelets are 12 hours old

111. Aspirin is administered to the client experiencing an MI because of its:

a. Antipyretic action b. Antithrombotic action
c. Antiplatelet action d. Analgesic action

112. During the first 24 hours after thrombolytic treatment for an ischemic CVA, the primary goal is to control the clients:

a. Pulse b. Respiration
c. Blood pressure d. Temperature

113. An ECG mainly gives information about the:

a. Excitation of the myocardium
b. Perfusion of the myocardium
c. Contractile force of the myocardium
d. Integrity of the myocardium

114. There is one heart beat and two arterial pulsations giving the sensation of a double beat is called:

a. Paradoxical pulse b. Bigeminal pulse
c. Dicrotic pulse d. Intermittent pulse

115. The blood group contains no antibodies:

a. A b. B
c. O d. AB

116. The cells that are responsible for the production of antibodies are:

a. Red blood cells b. Platelets
c. Plasma d. White blood cells

117. A method of making the victim to breath passively:

a. Artificial respiration b. Spontaneous respiration
c. Deep breathing d. Kussmaul's breathing

118. A red pigment in the blood cells which combines with oxygen and carbon dioxide for carrying them:

a. Red blood cells b. Hemoglobin
c. Platelet d. Plasma

119. Characteristic of the blood flow due to arterial bleeding is the following except:

a. Bright red in color
b. Spurts at each contraction of the heart
c. Flow is pulsatile
d. Dark red in color

120. The primary goal for the client with Buerger's disease is to prevent:

a. Embolus formation
b. Fat embolus formation
c. Thrombus formation
d. Thrombophlebitis

121. Which symptom is an early indicator of hypoxia in the unconscious client:

a. Cyanosis b. Decreased respirations
c. Restlessness d. Hypotension

122. How many main openings are there in the diaphragm?:

a. 1 b. 2
c. 3 d. 4

123. The action of epinephrine is:

a. Relax bronchial spasm
b. Liquefy respiratory secretions
c. Increase antibody formation
d. Reduce airway diameter

124. A large nodule of lymphoid tissue:

a. Liver b. Gallbladder
c. Spleen d. SVC

125. Small pouch at the beginning of thoracic duct:

a. Right lymphatic duct b. Palatine tonsil
c. Appendix d. Cisterna chyli

ANSWER KEY

1. b	2. d	3. c	4. a	5. d	6. b	7. a	8. a	9. b	10. c	11. a	12. c
13. b	14. a	15. d	16. b	17. b	18. b	19. b	20. a	21. c	22. d	23. c	24. a
25. a	26. d	27. b	28. a	29. c	30. a	31. b	32. d	33. b	34. a	35. c	36. d
37. b	38. a	39. c	40. c	41. d	42. b	43. a	44. c	45. b	46. b	47. c	48. d
49. d	50. a	51. a	52. a	53. b	54. b	55. d	56. a	57. b	58. b	59. b	60. d
61. c	62. d	63. c	64. d	65. a	66. c	67. b	68. d	69. c	70. b	71. b	72. d
73. a	74. c	75. a	76. c	77. d	78. a	79. a	80. c	81. d	82. d	83. d	84. b
85. d	86. c	87. d	88. c	89. a	90. c	91. a	92. b	93. b	94. a	95. b	96. a
97. b	98. c	99. c	100. b	101. b	102. b	103. c	104. c	105. a	106. d	107. a	108. c
109. c	110. a	111. c	112. c	113. a	114. c	115. d	116. c	117. a	118. b	119. d	120. c
121. c	122. c	123. a	124. c	125. d							

Diseases and Disorders of the Respiratory System

REVIEW OF ANATOMY AND PHYSIOLOGY

Upper Respiratory Tract

Upper respiratory tract include the nose, pharynx and the larynx.

Nose consists of the nasal cavities separated by the septum. The major functions of the nose are warming, moistening and filtering of the air.

Nose is continuous with the pharynx which is divided into nasopharynx, oropharynx and laryngopharynx. Larynx is otherwise called 'voice box' which connects the upper and lower airways. The opening of the larynx is called the glottis. Vocal cords of the larynx permits speech and are involved in the cough reflex.

> The thyroid cartilage of the larynx is formed of two flat pieces of cartilage fused together in the front to form laryngeal prominence or "Adam's apple".

Lower Respiratory Tract

Lower respiratory tract consists of the trachea, bronchi, bronchioles, the lungs and other associated structures.

Trachea or 'windpipe' extends from the larynx and divided into bronchi before entering into the lungs. The tracheobronchial tree ends at the terminal bronchioles and alveolar epithelium.

Lungs are the major organ of respiration which is divided into lobes; three in right lung and two in left lung. Pleura is the serous membrane covering the lungs. The lungs and the associated structures are protected by the rib cage and intercostals muscles. There are 12 pairs of ribs. The main function of lung is gas exchange and alveoli of the lungs are responsible for gas exchange.

> Pleura is the serous membrane covering the lungs.

MECHANISM OF RESPIRATION

Respiration consists of inspiration and expiration. The chest expands during inspiration owing to movement of the diaphragm and intercostals muscles. When the diaphragm contracts during inspiration, it is flattened and lowered and the thoracic cavity is increased in length. The lung expands to fill the space and the air is sucked into the bronchial tree.

During expiration, the diaphragm relaxes and assumes its original dome shape. The intercostals muscles relax and the ribs revert to their previous position. The lungs recoil and air is driven out through the bronchial tree.

GAS EXCHANGE

The exchange of gases within the body takes place both in the lungs, where it is called external respiration and in the tissues where it is called internal respiration.

> The exchange of gas between the alveoli of the lungs and the blood capillaries is termed as external respiration and those between the blood and the body tissues is termed as internal respiration.

> Respiration is controlled by the respiratory center in the medulla oblongata.

LUNG VOLUMES

1. **Tidal volume:** Amount of air breathed in and out during normal quiet breathing. Normal tidal volume is about 500 mL.
2. **Inspiratory capacity:** After a normal expiration, the amount of air taken in during forced inspiration is called the inspiratory capacity. The normal inspiratory capacity is about 3 liters.
3. **Expiratory reserve volume:** The amount of air forcefully expelled out from the lungs after a quiet expiration. The expiratory reserve volume comes around 1000 mL.
4. **Residual volume:** The amount of air left in the respiratory passages after the deepest possible expiration is called residual volume. It comes around 1100 mL.
5. **Vital capacity:** Vital capacity is the largest volume of air expired after the deepest possible inspiration. The normal vital capacity is about 4 liters.
6. **Forced expiratory volume (FEV):** The amount of air forcefully expired from the lungs in one second. FEV normally measures 75 to 80% of the vital capacity.

LUNG VOLUMES

Lung Volume	Normal
Tidal volume	500 mL
Inspiratory capacity	3 liters
Expiratory reserve volume	1000 mL
Residual volume	1100 mL
Vital capacity (VC)	4 liters
Forced expiratory volume	70–80% of VC

DISEASES AND DISORDERS OF THE RESPIRATORY SYSTEM

CHRONIC OBSTRUCTIVE PULMONARY DISEASE (COPD)

Group of respiratory conditions that produce obstruction of the airflow; includes emphysema, bronchitis, bronchiectasis and bronchial asthma.

Emphysema

- Enlargement and destruction of the alveolar, bronchial and bronchiolar tissue with resultant loss of recoil, air trapping, thoracic overdistension, sputum accumulation and loss of diaphragmatic muscle tone.
- **Findings** include anorexia, fatigue, weight loss, feeling of breathlessness, cough, sputum production, flaring of the nostrils, use of accessory muscles of respiration, increased rate and depth of breathing and dyspnea.
- **Treatment:**

  Drugs: Bronchodilators (aminophylline, terbutaline, isoproterenol, theophylline); antibiotics and corticosteroids.

Bronchitis

- Excessive production of mucus in the bronchi with accompanying persistent cough.
- Characteristic changes include hyperplasia and hypertrophy of the mucus secreting glands in the bronchi; chronic inflammation and narrowing of the smaller airways.
- **Findings:** Productive cough, dyspnea on exertion, use of accessory muscles of respiration, scattered rales and rhonchi, cyanosis, distended neck veins and ankle edema.
- **Management:** Drugs like bronchodilators, antibiotics and expectorants.

Bronchiectasis

- Permanent, abnormal, dilatation of the bronchi with destruction of muscular and elastic structure of the bronchial wall.
- Usually caused by bacterial infection, recurrent, lower respiratory tract infection, etc.
- **Findings** include chronic cough with production of mucopurulent sputum, hemoptysis, exertional dyspnea, wheezing, anorexia, fatigue, weight loss.
- **Management** is same as for emphysema.

Bronchial Asthma

- Obstructive disease of the lower respiratory tract often caused by an allergic reaction.
- Allergy results in histamine release which produce edema of the mucous membrane, spasm of the smooth muscles of the bronchi and bronchioles, accumulation of tenacious secretions.
- **Findings** include shortness of breath (SOB), expiratory wheeze, air trapping, use of accessory muscles of respiration and diaphoresis.
- **Management:** Bronchodilators (theophylline, aminophylline, terbutaline), corticosteroids and antibiotics.

PULMONARY TUBERCULOSIS

- Bacterial infectious disease caused by *Myco-bacterium tuberculosis*
- Spread via air-borne droplets when infected persons cough, sneeze or laugh.
- Infection spread via the lymph and circulatory system.
- **Findings:** Cough (yellow, mucoid sputum), dyspnea, hemoptysis, rales or crackles, anorexia, malaise, weight loss, evening low grade fever, palor, pain, fatigue, night sweats.

> Pulmonary TB is the bacterial infectious disease caused by *Mycobacterium tuberculosis*

- Diagnostic tests
  - Chest X-ray
  - Skin test (Mantoux test) with purified protein derivative (PPD) is positive.

> An area of induration 10 mm or more in Mantoux test is interpreted as positive.

  - Sputum positive for acid fast bacilli (AFB) in three consecutive sputum samples.

> Sputum samples should be collected in the early morning before brushing and taking oral fluids.

  - **Treatment:** Antitubercular drugs used are isoniazid (INH), ethambutol, rifampicin, streptomycin and pyrazinamide.

CHEST TRAUMA

- Most common chest injury from blunt trauma is fractured ribs.

> Ribs 4–8 are most commonly fractured in chest trauma because they are least protected by chest muscles.

- Displaced fractured ribs may penetrate the pleura and the lungs.

- **Findings:** Pain on inspiration, tenderness and bruising at injury site, splinting with shallow respirations, apprehensiveness
- **Treatment:** Drug therapy consists of narcotics and intercostals nerve block for pain relief.

FLAIL CHEST

- Fracture of several ribs and resultant inability of the affected chest wall.
- The flail portion and the underlying tissues move paradoxically to the rest of the chest cage and lungs.
- The flail portion is sucked in on inspiration and bulges out on expiration.
- **Findings** include severe dyspnea, grunting, paradoxical chest motion, cyanosis, neck vein distention, tachycardia, and hypotension.
- Narcotics and sedatives are given for pain relief.
- If respiratory function is worse, ventilation may be necessary.

PNEUMOTHORAX/HEMOTHORAX

- Partial or complete collapse of the lungs due to an accumulation of air/fluid in the pleural space.
- **Types**
  - **Spontaneous pneumothorax:** Rupture of a small bleb on the visceral pleura produces this type of pneumothorax.
  - **Open pneumothorax:** Air enters the pleural space through an opening in the chest wall, usually caused by stabbing or gunshot wound.
  - **Tension pneumothorax:** Air enters the pleural space with each inspiration but cannot escape; causes increased intrathoracic pressure and shifting of mediastinal contents to the unaffected side (mediastinal shift).
  - **Hemothorax:** Accumulation of blood in the pleural space, frequently found in an open pneumothorax, resulting in a hemo-pneumothorax.
- **Assessment findings:** Sudden, sharp pain in the chest, dyspnea, diminished or absent breath sounds on affected side, decresed respiratory excursion on affected side, decreased vocal fremitus, tracheal shift to the opposite side, weak, rapid pulse; anxiety and diaphoresis.
- **Treatment**
  - Administer narcotics/analgesics/sedatives for pain relief
  - Position in high Fowler's position
  - Thoracentesis: Putting needle/tube into the thoracic cavity to remove the air/fluid/blood.

ATELECTASIS

- Collapse of part or all of a lung due to bronchial obstruction.
- May be caused by intrabronchial obstruction/ extrabronchial compression or endobronchial disease.
- **Findings** include dyspnea, decreased breath sounds on affected side, decreased respiratory excursion, dullness to flat upon percussion over affected area, cyanosis, tachycardia, tachypnea, elevated temperature, pain over affected area.
- **Treatment:** Antibiotics, bronchodilators and symptomatic management.

PLEURAL EFFUSION

- Collection of fluid in the pleural space may be produced by a variety of causes like liver/kidney disease, pneumonia, tuberculosis, lung abscess, bronchial carcinoma, trauma, pulmonary edema, etc.
- **Findings:** Dyspnea, dullness over affected area upon percussion, absent or decreased breath sounds over affected area, pleural pain, dry cough, pleral friction rub, palor, fatigue; fever and night sweats with empyema.
- **Treatment**
  - Thoracentesis
  - Treat underlying cause
  - Antibiotics
  - Fibrinolytic agents to dissolve fibrin clots
  - Closed chest drainage.

CHEST DRAINAGE SYSTEMS

- Involves the use of tubes and suction to return the negative pressure to the intrapleural space
- The chest tube is placed in the second or third intercostals space to drain air from the intra-pleural space
- The chest tube is placed in the eighth or ninth intercostals space to drain blood or fluid from the intrapleural space.

> The chest tubes are usually placed in the second or third intercostal space to drain air and placed in the eighth or ninth intercostal space to drain blood or fluid.

Types of Drainage Systems

- **One bottle system:** Allows air or fluid to drain from the pleural cavity by gravity via a glass rod which extends approximately 2 cm below the surface of the water within the collection bottle.

- **Two bottle system:** Involves one bottle that act as a collection chamber and provides a water seal while a second bottle can be connected to a suction apparatus; the bubbling of water within the second bottle indicates that the desired suction is maintained.
- **Three bottle system:** Involves one bottle that serves as a collection chamber, one act as a water seal chamber and one that controls suction.
- Commercially prepared plastic unit designed for closed chest suction are also available.

> In 1967, Deknatel introduced the first integrated disposable chest drainage unit based on the three bottle system.

- The water level in the small arm of the water seal raises as intrapleural pressure becomes more negative. If there is no air leak, the water level should rise and fall with the patient's respirations, reflecting normal pressure changes in the pleural cavity.
- During spontaneous respirations, the water level should rise during inhalation and fall during exhalation. If the patient is receiving positive pressure ventilation, the oscillation will be just the opposite—the water level should fall with inhalation and rise with exhalation. This oscillation is called tidaling and is one indicator of a patent pleural chest tube.

> Bubbling in the water seal chamber indicates an air leak.

> Vigorous milking or stripping can create dangerously high negative pressures.

Clamping the Chest Tube

- If there has been no bubbling in the water seal, there is no air leak from the lung. Therefore, the tube may be clamped for the short time it takes to re-establish drainage.
- If there has been bubbling and there is an air leak from the lung, one must not clamp the chest tube. Doing so will cause air to accumulate in the pleural cavity since the air has no means of escape. This can rapidly lead to tension pneumothorax.
- The few times to clamp a chest tube:
  1. You are performing a physician ordered procedure such as sclerosing
  2. Assessing for a leak
  3. Prior to removing the chest tube to determine if the patient can do without the chest tube (with a physician's order).
- In pleural chest drainage, the major hazard is tension pneumothorax. The most likely cause is obstructed tubing. Quickly assess the tubing's patency and notify the doctor immediately.
- If there is a pleural air leak, apply a dressing with your hand, but release it periodically or at any sign of respiratory distress, so pleural air can escape. Notify the doctor immediately and prepare for replacement of the tube.
- Do not clamp the chest tube during transport or ambulation unless specifically ordered by the doctor. Clamping the chest tube in patients with an air leak increases the chance for pneumothorax.

> Never clamp a chest tube during patient transport unless the chest drainage system becomes disrupted during patient movement, and then only if there is no air leak.

- A sudden (not gradual) cessation of drainage in the patient with mediastinal tubes can be caused by accumulated clotted blood occluding the tube. This can lead to life-threatening cardiac tamponade. To keep the tubes patent, or to dislodge clots, gently milk the tube.

PNEUMONIA

- An inflammation of the alveolar spaces of the lungs resulting in consolidation of the lung tissue as the alveoli fills with exudate.
- **Findings** include cough with greenish or rust colored sputum, rapid, shallow, respirations with expiratory grunt, nasal flaring, intercostals rib retraction, use of accessory muscles of respiration, dullness to flat upon percussion, pleural friction rub, high pitched bronchial breath sounds, rales or crackles, fever, chills, chest pain, weakness, tachycardia, cyanosis, profuse perspiration, abdominal distension, chest X-ray shows consolidation of the affected areas.
- **Treatment**
  - Antibiotics
  - Bronchodilators
  - Analgesics
  - Nebulization.

> Pneumonia is an inflammation of the alveolar spaces of the lungs resulting in consolidation of the lung tissue as the alveoli fills with exudate.

CANCER OF THE LARYNX

- Most common upper respiratory malignancy
- Most common type being squamous cell carcinoma.

- **Findings** include localized throat pain, burning while drinking hot fluids, dysphagia, dyspnea, weight loss, debility, cough, hemoptysis, muffled voice, progressive hoarseness, and enlarged cervical lymph nodes.
- **Treatment**
  - Chemotherapy
  - Radiotherapy
  - Surgery (partial/total laryngectomy) and total neck dissection.

> Squamous cell carcinoma of the larynx is the most common upper respiratory tract malignancy.

ORAL CANCER

- Oral cancer is part of a group of cancers called head and neck cancers. Oral cancer can develop in any part of the oral cavity or oropharynx.
- Most oral cancers begin in the tongue and in the floor of the mouth.

> Almost all oral cancers begin in the flat cells (squamous cells) that cover the surfaces of the mouth, tongue, and lips.

- When oral cancer spreads (metastasizes), it usually travels through the lymphatic system.
- Cancer cells can also spread to other parts of the neck, the lungs, and other parts of the body.
- **Risk factors for oral cancer**
  - **Tobacco:** Smoking in the form of cigarettes, cigars, or pipes; chewing tobacco; and dipping snuff are all linked to oral cancer. The risk is even higher for tobacco users who drink alcohol heavily.

> Three out of four oral cancers occur in people who use alcohol, tobacco, or both alcohol and tobacco.

  - **Alcohol:** People who drink alcohol are more likely to develop oral cancer than people who do not drink. The risk increases with the amount of alcohol that a person consumes. The risk increases even more if the person both drinks alcohol and uses tobacco.
  - **Sun:** Cancer of the lip can be caused by exposure to the sun. Using a lotion or lip balm that has a sunscreen can reduce the risk. The risk of cancer of the lip increases if the person also smokes.
  - **A personal history of head and neck cancer:** People who have had head and neck cancer are at increased risk of developing another primary head and neck cancer. Smoking increases this risk.
- **Symptoms**
  - Patches inside the mouth/lips that are white, a mixture of red and white, or red white patches (leukoplakia) are the most common.
  - Mixed red and white patches (erythroleukoplakia) are more likely than white patches to become malignant.
  - A sore on the lip or in the mouth that would not heal
  - Bleeding in the mouth
  - Loose teeth
  - Difficulty or pain when swallowing
  - Difficulty in wearing dentures
  - A lump in the neck
  - Earache.
- **Treatment**
  - Surgery
  - Chemotherapy
  - Radiotherapy
  - Combined effort of a team of specialist including dentist, speech pathologist, nutritionist and mental health counselor.
- Oral cancer prevention
  - Stopping tobacco and alcohol use
  - Minimize exposure to sun; use sunscreen whenever needed
  - Chemoprevention: Tobacco users who have had oral cancer often develop second cancers in the oral cavity or nearby areas, including the nose, throat, vocal cords, esophagus, and windpipe. Use of drugs, vitamins, or other agents can prevent or delay the growth of cancer or can keep it from coming back.

REVIEW QUESTIONS

1. **COPD comprises the following, except:**
   a. Bronchitis b. Emphysema
   c. Asthma d. Atelectasis
2. **Disorder characterized by destruction of the alveolar wall:**
   a. Asthma b. Emphysema
   c. Bronchitis d. Bronchiectasis
3. **Disease causing permanent abnormal dilatation and distortion of bronchi and bronchioles:**
   a. Bronchitis b. Bronchiectasis
   c. Emphysema d. Asthma
4. **Collapse of the lung tissue:**
   a. Emphysema b. Bronchitis
   c. Atelectasis d. Asthma

5. **Membrane covering the lung:**
   a. Pericardium b. Peritoneum
   c. Perimetrium d. Pleura

6. **Inflammation of the pleura:**
   a. Pleuritis b. Pleural effusion
   c. Empyema d. Emphysema

7. **Collection of pus in the lung tissue:**
   a. Emphysema b. Pneumonia
   c. Lung abscess d. Pneumothorax

8. **Air in the pleural space:**
   a. Pneumothorax b. Hemothorax
   c. Pleural effusion d. Pneumonia

9. **Fluid in the pleural space:**
   a. Pneumothorax b. Hemothorax
   c. Pleural effusion d. Pneumonia

10. **Blood in the pleural space:**
   a. Pneumothorax b. Hemothorax
   c. Pleural effusion d. Pneumonia

11. **Removal of a lobe of the lung:**
   a. Thoracotomy b. Wedge resection
   c. Segmental resection d. Lobectomy

12. **The respiratory center is situated in the:**
   a. Medulla b. Hypothalamus
   c. Cerebellum d. Cerebrum

13. **A potent respiratory center stimulant:**
   a. Oxygen b. Carbon dioxide
   c. Nitrous oxide d. Hypocalcemia

14. **Removal of entire lung tissue:**
   a. Thoracotomy b. Wedge resection
   c. Lobectomy d. Pneumonectomy

15. **Expectoration of blood stained sputum:**
   a. Hemostasis b. Hematemesis
   c. Hemoptysis d. Epistaxis

16. **Normal breathing is:**
   a. Eupnea b. Hyperpnea
   c. Apnea d. Dyspnea

17. **Total cessation of breathing:**
   a. Eupnea b. Hyperpnea
   c. Apnea d. Dyspnea

18. **Drugs that dilate bronchial tree:**
   a. Bronchodilators b. Antitussives
   c. Antibiotics d. Expectorants

19. **The drugs that inhibit cough reflex:**
   a. Bronchodilators b. Expectorants
   c. Antitussives d. Antibiotics

20. **Decreased amount of oxygen in the tissues:**
   a. Hypoxemia b. Hypoxia
   c. Hypercapnea d. Hypocapnea

21. **Decreased amount of oxygen in the blood:**
   a. Hypoxemia b. Hypoxia
   c. Hypercapnea d. Hypocapnea

22. **Decreased amount of carbon dioxide in the blood:**
   a. Hypoxemia b. Hypoxia
   c. Hypercapnea d. Hypocapnea

23. **Drugs that increase the bronchial secretions and aid in the expulsion of mucus are termed:**
   a. Expectorants b. Antitussives
   c. Bronchodilators d. Mucolytics

24. **Volume of air going in and out of the lungs in normal, quiet breathing:**
   a. Vital capacity b. Residual capacity
   c. Inspiratory capacity d. Tidal volume

25. **Average tidal volume:**
   a. 500 mL b. 1000 mL
   c. 1.5 L d. > 1.5 L

26. **Fracture of several ribs resulting in instability of the affected chest wall:**
   a. Fractured ribs b. Flail chest
   c. Pleural effusion d. Pneumothorax

27. **Barrel chest is a characteristic symptom in:**
   a. Emphysema b. Empyema
   c. Bronchiectasis d. Bronchial asthma

28. **Organism causing tuberculosis:**
   a. *Corynebacterium*
   b. *Streptococcus*
   c. *Staphylococcus*
   d. *Mycobacterium tuberculosis*

29. **Mantoux test is positive if the induration is:**
   a. > 5 mm b. > 10 mm
   c. > 15 mm d. > 20 mm

30. **Consolidation of lung tissue:**
a. Bronchitis b. Bronchiectasis
c. Pneumonia d. Bronchial asthma

31. **Sound that occurs as a result of air passing through fluid filled space:**
a. Rales b. Rhonchi
c. Consolidation d. Resonance

32. **Pigeon chest is a characteristic finding of:**
a. Bronchitis b. Rickets
c. Bronchial asthma d. Bronchopneumonia

33. **Bluish discoloration of skin and mucous membrane due to hypoxia:**
a. Spells b. Clubbing
c. Cyanosis d. Circum oral paresthesias

34. **Low pitched, hollow sounds heard over normal lung tissue:**
a. Resonance b. Fremitus
c. Wheeze d. Rhonchi

35. **Increase in the angle between nail plate and finger:**
a. Clubbing b. Polydactyly
c. Syndactyly d. Cyanosis

36. **Side effect of aminophylline:**
a. Hypertension b. Hypotension
c. Bradycardia d. Tachypnea

37. **Peritonsillar abscess is:**
a. Pleurisy b. Quincy
c. Cystic fibrosis d. Tonsillitis

38. **Most common malignant tumor of the larynx:**
a. Squamous cell carcinoma
b. Supraglottis cancer
c. Nonsquamous cell carcinoma
d. Small cell carcinoma

39. **Tracheostomy is done above:**
a. 3rd tracheal cartilage b. 5th tracheal cartilage
c. 2nd tracheal cartilage d. 6th tracheal cartilage

40. **The sound heard when there is sudden opening of small airways containing fluid:**
a. Wheeze b. Fremitus
c. Crackles d. Resonance

41. **Adam's apple is situated in:**
a. Cricoids cartilage b. Thyroid cartilage
c. Arytenoids cartilage d. Epiglottis

42. **Normal vital capacity of the lungs:**
a. 2 liters b. 3 liters
c. 4 liters d. 4.5 liters

43. **Common symptom of active tuberculosis:**
a. Marked weight loss b. Dyspnea on exertion
c. Mental status changes d. Constipation

44. **Hemoptysis is:**
a. Blood in urine b. Blood in vomitus
c. Blood in sputum d. Blood in feces

45. **Noninvasive monitoring of oxygen saturation:**
a. Capillary blood gas studies
b. Arterial blood gas studies
c. Venoclysis
d. Pulse oxymetry

46. **Normal residual volume of the lungs:**
a. 1000 mL b. 1100 mL
c. 1200 mL d. 1500 mL

47. **In an underwater seal drainage system, cessation of fluid fluctuation in the drainage tubes indicates:**
a. The lung has fully expanded
b. The lung has collapsed
c. Mediastinal space has decreased
d. Chest tube is in pleural space

48. **Indication for the use of an incentive spirometry:**
a. To strengthen abdominal muscles
b. To prepare for ambulation
c. To increase respiratory effectiveness
d. To stimulate circulation

49. **World no tobacco day is observed on:**
a. 31st May b. 7th April
c. 10th December d. 1st December

50. **Tuberculin test is known as:**
a. Schick test b. Mantoux test
c. VDRL d. ELISA

51. **The best time to collect a sputum specimen:**
a. After nebulization
b. After steam inhalation
c. After an antiseptic mouthwash
d. Before brushing the teeth in the morning

52. **Surgery done in chronic sinusitis:**
a. Shirodkar operation b. Caldwell-Luc operation
c. Mc-Donald operation d. Hypophysectomy

53. **Pus in the pleural cavity:**
a. Emphysema b. Pleural effusion
c. Empyema d. Pyorrhea

54. **The small division on a tuberculin syringe is equivalent to:**
a. 0.5 mL b. 0.1 mL
c. 1.0 mL d. 0.01 mL

55. **Right ventricular enlargement due to pulmonary problem:**
a. Corpulmonale b. Cardiac tamponade
c. Cardiomyopathy d. Emphysema

56. **Schick test is used to diagnose:**
a. Tuberculosis b. Diphtheria
c. Viral hepatitis d. Typhoid fever

57. **A harsh, vibrating, shrill sound produced during respiration and seen in laryngitis:**
a. Rale b. Wheeze
c. Stertorous d. Stridor

58. **The volume of air inhaled with normal quiet breathing:**
a. Vital capacity b. Inspiratory capacity
c. Tidal volume d. Lung capacity

59. **SARS is spread by:**
a. Bacteria b. Virus
c. Fungus d. Protozoa

60. **Important care after tracheostomy:**
a. Administration of antibiotics
b. Oxygen administration
c. Suctioning
d. Maintaining intake and output

61. **Tuberculosis of spine:**
a. Charcot's disease b. Pott's disease
c. Osteomalacia d. Rickets

62. **Pneumothorax is the condition in which there is:**
a. Water in the pleural space
b. Water in the visceral pleura
c. Air in the pleural space
d. Pus in the visceral space

63. **Best therapeutic measure for empyema:**
a. Chest drainage b. Postural drainage
c. Breathing exercise d. Fowler's position

64. **The position recommended for a patient with epistaxis:**
a. Supine
b. Sidelying
c. Prone
d. Sitting with head leaning forward

65. **Air-borne precautions for a patient with pulmonary tuberculosis has to be taken until:**
a. Tuberculin test is negative
b. No tubercle bacilli present in the sputum
c. Patient's temperature is normal
d. Patient had gained weight

66. **The vitamin administered with INH:**
a. Vitamin C b. Vitamin B_2
c. Vitamin B_{12} d. Vitamin A

67. **A reactive airway disease:**
a. Bronchitis b. Asthma
c. Emphysema d. Pleuricy

68. **A manifestation of hypoxia:**
a. Cyanosis b. Hemoptysis
c. Nasal flaring d. Tachycardia

69. **The most important risk factor for carcinoma lung:**
a. Alcohol intake b. Asthma
c. Betel chewing d. Smoking

70. **Dust disease is:**
a. Pneumonia b. Pneumoconiosis
c. Bronchitis d. Bronchial asthma

71. **Decrease in smell sensation:**
a. Anosmia b. Hyperresonance
c. Hyperosmia d. Hyposmia

72. **Thoracentesis is:**
a. Postural drainage
b. Drainage of air or fluid from the pleural space
c. Surgical removal of a portion of rib
d. Drainage of secretions from paranasal sinus

73. Opening made in trachea:
a. Thoracoplasty b. Stripping
c. Tracheostomy d. Thoracentesis

74. Adenoids are:
a. Pharyngeal tonsils
b. Peritonsillar abscess
c. Palatine tonsils
d. Submandibular salivary glands

75. Mucus secreting cells:
a. Alveolar cells
b. Goblet cells
c. Bronchopulmonary segments
d. Adenoids

76. The bronchus enter the lung through:
a. Antrum b. Transverse fissure
c. Hilum d. Oblique fissure

77. Nerve supplying diaphragm:
a. Vagus
b. Phrenic nerve
c. Glossopharyngeal nerve
d. Intercostals nerve

78. Hemoglobin bind with oxygen to form:
a. Carboxyhemoglobin
b. Oxyhemoglobin
c. Hemoxin
d. Saturated hemoglobin

79. Connection between the nasopharynx and middle ear:
a. Adenoids b. Eustachian tube
c. Antrum d. Cribriform plate

80. A sign in atelectasis:
a. Diminished breath sounds
b. Slow deep respirations
c. Fever
d. A dry cough

81. Heimlich maneuver is used:
a. To improve lung capacity
b. To improve circulation
c. To stimulate cardiovascular system
d. To expel foreign bodies in the respiratory tract

82. In hypoxia, muscle shows:
a. High levels of calcium
b. Low levels of lactic acid
c. High levels of glycogen
d. Low levels of ATP

83. Body system maintaining acid base balance:
a. Circulatory and nervous system
b. Respiratory and urinary system
c. Skeletal and cardiac system
d. Muscular and endocrine system

84. Acid fast bacilli is:
a. Influenza virus
b. *Bordetella pertussis*
c. Diphtheria bacillus
d. *Mycobacterium tuberculosis*

85. Oxygen and carbon dioxide are exchanged in the lungs by:
a. Osmosis b. Diffusion
c. Filtration d. Active transport

86. Sign of spontaneous pneumothorax include dyspnea and:
a. Increased chest movements
b. Unilateral chest pain
c. Hematemesis
d. Mediastinal shift towards the involved side

87. Before the removel of chest tubes, complete lung expansion is evaluated by:
a. Absence of drainage b. Decreased breath sounds
c. Normal tidal volume d. Chest X-ray

88. During PFT, the patient is asked to breathe normally to measure the:
a. Vital capacity b. Tidal volume
c. Inspiratory reserve d. Expiratory reserve

89. The position which facilitate maximum air exchange:
a. Fowler's position b. Semi-Fowler's position
c. Orthopneic position d. Supine position

90. In emphysema, hypoxia is due to:
a. Infectious obstructions
b. Respiratory muscle paralysis
c. Pleural effusion
d. Loss of aerating surface

91. In emphysema, oxygen should be given at a rate of:
a. 2 L/minute b. 4 L/minute
c. 4–6 L/minute d. 6–8 L/minute

92. The position given for a patient with dyspnea:
a. Trendelenburg b. Lithotomy position
c. Sim's position d. Orthopneic position

93. After thoracentesis, the patient should be observed for:
a. Increased breath sounds
b. Expectoration of blood
c. Periods of confusion
d. Decreased respiratory rate

94. Vomiting of blood is called:
a. Hematuria b. Hematemesis
c. Hematoma d. Hemoptysis

95. An important adverse effect of streptomycin:
a. Ototoxicity b. Nephrotoxicity
c. Gastritis d. Discoloration of urine

96. The drug that should not be given if a patient receiving anticoagulant:
a. Chlorpromazine b. Cefotaxime
c. Acetazolamide d. Aspirin

97. The patient on aspirin should be observed for:
a. Headache b. Epistaxis
c. Nausea d. Chest pain

98. Diuretic given in pulmonary edema:
a. Spironolactone b. Frusemide
c. Chlorothiazide d. Chlorpromazine

ANSWER KEY

1. d	2. b	3. b	4. c	5. d	6. a	7. c	8. a	9. c	10. b	11. d	12. a
13. b	14. d	15. c	16. a	17. c	18. a	19. c	20. b	21. a	22. d	23. a	24. d
25. a	26. b	27. a	28. d	29. b	30. c	31. a	32. b	33. c	34. a	35. a	36. d
37. b	38. a	39. a	40. c	41. b	42. c	43. a	44. c	45. d	46. b	47. a	48. c
49. a	50. b	51. d	52. b	53. c	54. d	55. a	56. b	57. d	58. c	59. b	60. b
61. b	62. c	63. a	64. d	65. b	66. c	67. b	68. a	69. d	70. b	71. d	72. b
73. c	74. c	75. b	76. c	77. b	78. b	79. b	80. a	81. d	82. d	83. b	84. d
85. b	86. d	87. d	88. b	89. c	90. d	91. a	92. d	93. d	94. b	95. a	96. d
97. b	98. b										

Diseases and Disorders of the Gastrointestinal System

REVIEW OF ANATOMY AND PHYSIOLOGY

The organs of the digestive system are grouped into the alimentary canal (GI tract) consisting of the mouth, esophagus, stomach small and large intestine and the accessory digestive organs including the liver, pancreas, gallbladder and ductal system. The primary functions of this system are movement of food, digestion, absorption, elimination and provision of a continuous supply of nutrients, electrolytes and water.

Mouth

Consists of the lips and the oral cavity, provides entrance and initial processing of nutrients and sensations such as taste, texture and temperature. Oral cavity contains the teeth, tongue, salivary glands and the pharynx. Saliva contains ptyalin for the digestion of starch. Pharynx aids in the swallowing function.

Esophagus

Muscular tube that receives food from the pharynx and propels it into the stomach by peristalsis.

Stomach

Stomach occupies hypochondriac, epigastric and umbilical regions. Stores and mixes food with gastric juices and mucus, producing chemical and mechanical changes in the bolus of food. After processing in the stomach, the food bolus called chime, is released into the small intestine through the duodenum. Stomach has two sphincters that control the rate of food passage viz. cardiac sphincter located at the opening between the esophagus and stomach and pyloric sphincter located between the stomach and duodenum. Secretions of the stomach include pepsinogen aids in protein digestion, hydrochloric acid (helps in protein digestion) intrinsic factor (secreted by parietal cells which promote absorption of vitamin B_{12}) and mucoid secretions (coats stomach wall and prevent autodigestion).

Small Intestine

Composed of the duodenum, jejunum and ileum. Extends from the pylorus to the ileocecal valve which regulates flow into the large intestine and prevents reflux into the small intestine. Major functions are digestion and absorption of the end-products of digestion. Structures of small intestine include villi (functional unit of the small intestine containing goblet cells secreting mucus and absorptive cells that absorbs digested food stuffs), crypts of Lieberkühn (produces secretions containing digestive enzymes) and Brunner's glands which secrete mucus.

Large Intestine

Large intestine is divided into the cecum, colon (ascending, transverse and descending), rectum and anus.

Serves as a reservoir for fecal material until defecation occurs; functions to absorb water and electrolytes.

Microorganisms present in the large intestine are responsible for a small amount of further breakdown and also makes some vitamins. Amino acids are deaminated by the bacteria, resulting on ammonia which is concerted to urea in the liver. Bacteria in the large intestine aid in the synthesis of vitamin K and some of the B vitamins. Feces leave the body via the rectum and anus. Anus contains internal sphincter (under involuntary control) and external sphincter (under voluntary control). Fecal matter is 75% water and 25% solid waste (roughage, dead bacteria, fat, protein and inorganic matter).

Liver

Largest internal organ, located in the right hypochondriac and epigastric regions of the abdomen. Liver lobules are functional units of the liver composed of hepatic cells. Hepatic sinusoids are lined with Kupffer cells which carry out phagocytosis. Portal circulation brings blood to liver from the stomach, spleen, pancreas and intestines. Functions of liver include metabolism of carbohydrate, fat and proteins, production of bile, conjugation and excretion of bilirubin, storage of vitamin A, D, B_{12} and iron, synthesis of coagulation factors, detoxification of many drugs and conjugation of sex hormones.

Biliary System

Biliary system consists of the gallbladder and associated ductal system. Gallbladder concentrates and stores bile; ductal system provides a route for the bile to reach the intestine. Bile is formed in the liver and excreted into the hepatic duct. Hepatic duct joins with the cystic duct to form the common bile duct. Bile enters the duodenum via the control of the sphincter of Oddi.

Pancreas

Located transversely in the upper abdominal cavity. Consists of a head, body and a tail along with a pancreatic duct which extends along the gland and enters the duodenum via the common bile duct. Has both exocrine and endocrine functions. Exocrine cells secrete trypsinogen and chymotrypsin for protein digestion; amylase to break down starch and lipase for fat digestion. Endocrine function is done by islets of Langerhans. Beta cells of the islets produce insulin and alpha cells produce glucagon.

PHYSIOLOGY OF DIGESTION AND ABSORPTION

Digestion is the physical and chemical breakdown of food into absorptive substances. Digestion is initiated in the mouth where food mixes with saliva and starch is broken down. Food then passes through the esophagus into the stomach. In the stomach, food is processed by gastric secretions into a substance called chyme. In the small intestine, carbohydrates are hydrolysed into monosaccharides; fats into glycerol and fatty acids and proteins to amino acids to complete the digestive process. When chime enters the duodenum, mucus is secreted to neutralize hydrochloric acid; in response to release of secretin, pancreas releases bicarbonates to neutralize acid chyme. Cholecystokinin and pancreozymin are also produced by the duodenal mucosa, stimulates contraction of the gallbladder along with the relaxation of the sphincter of Oddi to allow bile to flow into the duodenum and stimulate the release of the pancreatic enzymes.

DISEASES AND DISORDERS OF THE GASTROINTESTINAL SYSTEM

STOMATITIS

- Inflammation of the oral mucosa.
- Can occur as a complication of poor oral hygiene or as a result of chemotherapy or radiotherapy.
- Treated with mouthwashes and good oral hygiene.
- In severe cases, analgesics and antibiotics are given.

ORAL CANCER

- Can occur on the lips or within the mouth (tongue, floor of the mouth, buccal mucosa, palate, pharynx and tonsils).
- Most common type of oral tumor is squamous cell carcinoma.
- Caused by tobacco use, alcohol use, constant sun exposure and constant irritation from dental caries
- **Findings**
  - Ulcerations on the lip, tongue or buccal mucosa
  - Pain or soreness of the tongue upon eating hot or highly seasoned foods.
  - Leukoplakia, erythroplakia
  - Difficulty in chewing, speaking and dysphagia.
- **Treatment**
  - Radiation therapy
  - Chemotherapy
  - Surgery—mandibulectomy, hemiglossectomy, glossectomy or radical neck dissection
  - Combination therapy.

CANCER OF THE ESOPHAGUS

- Malignant tumor of the esophagus
- Usually appears as ulcerated lesions
- Occur most often in the middle and lower portions of the esophagus
- Cause unknown.
- **Contributing factors** include cigarette smoking, excessive alcohol intake, trauma, poor oral hygiene, achalasia and diverticula.
- **Findings**
  - Substernal burning after drinking hot fluids
  - Pain in the substernal and epigastric areas
  - Weight loss.
- **Treatment**
  - Radiation therapy
  - Chemotherapy; not found effective.
  - Surgery: Esophagectomy, esophagogastro-stomy, palliative gastrostomy in inoperable cases for feeding purpose.

ESOPHAGEAL VARICES

- Dilation of the veins of the esophagus
- Caused by portal hypertension; leads to blood to be shunted to the esophageal veins resulting in distention, hypertrophy and increased fragility.
- **Findings**
  - Anorexia, nausea, vomiting, hematemesis, fatigue, weakness
  - Splenomegaly, increased splenic dullness, ascites, caput medusa, peripheral edema and bruits.
  - Prolonged PT, reduced serum albumin, RBC, Hb and PCV
  - Increased LDH, SGOT, SGPT, BUN.
- **Treatment**
  - Fresh blood transfusion
  - Vitamin K therapy
  - Sengstaken-Blakemore tube insertion to control bleeding
  - Sclerotherapy

  - IV vasopressin
  - Surgery for portal hypertension: Ligation of esophageal and gastric veins; portacaval shunt, splenorenal shunt and mesocaval shunt.

HIATUS HERNIA

- Occurs when a portion of the stomach and vagus nerve slide upward into the thorax through an enlarged hiatus in the diaphragm.
- Causes reflux of gastric juices and inflammation of the lower portion of the esophagus
- May be caused by congenital weakness of the muscles in the diaphragm around the esophago-gastric opening, increased intra-abdominal pressure (obesity, pregnancy, ascites) and trauma.
- **Findings**
  - Heartburn especially after the meals, at night or with recumbent position
  - Dysphagia, regurgitation several hours after meals without vomiting.
- **Treatment**
  - **Drugs:** Antacids to reduce acidity and discomfort, cholinergic drugs
  - Avoid spicy foods and caffeine
  - **Surgery:** Reduction of hernia.

GASTRITIS

- An acute inflammatory condition that causes a breakdown of the normal gastric protective barriers with subsequent diffusion of hydrochloric acid into the gastric lumen resulting in hemorrhage, ulceration and adhesion of the gastric mucosa.
- **Caused by** excessive ingestion of certain drugs (salicylates, steroids, antibiotics), alcohol, food poisoning, large quantities of spicy, irritating foods in the diet.
- **Findings**
  - Anorexia, nausea, vomiting, hematemesis, epigastric fullness/discomfort, epigastric tenderness
  - Decreased Hb and PCV
  - Inflammation and ulceration of the gastric mucosa on endoscopy.
- **Treatment**
  - **Drugs:** Antacids, antiemetics
  - Bland diet, avoid irritants.

GASTRIC ULCERS

- Ulceration of the mucosal lining of the stomach
- Most commonly found in the antrum
- Gastric secretions and stomach emptying rate usually normal
- Rapid diffusion of gastric acid from the gastric lumen into gastric mucosa causes an inflammatory reaction with tissue breakdown.
- Also characterized by reflux into the stomach of bile containing duodenal contents.
- **Predisposing factors** include smoking, alcohol, emotional tension and drugs (salicylates, steroids).
- **Caused by** bacterial infection with *Helicobacter pylori.*
- **Findings**
  - Pain in left epigastrium with radiation to back, usually occurs 1 to 2 hours after meals
  - Weight loss
  - Decreased Hb and PCV.
- **Treatment**
  - **Supportive:** Rest, bland diet, stress management.
  - **Drugs:** Antacids, H_2 receptor antagonists (ranitidine, cimetidine, famotidine), anticholinergics, omeprazole and pantoprazole. Metronidazole and amoxicillin in ulcers caused by *H. pylori.*
  - **Surgery:** Gastric resection and anastomosis.

DUODENAL ULCER

- Ulceration of the mucosal lining of the duodenum
- Most commonly occurs in first 2 cm of the duodenum
- Characterized by gastric hyperacidity and a significant increased rate of gastric emptying
- **May be caused by** bacterial infection with *Helicobacter pylori*
- **Predisposing factors** include smoking, alcohol and emotional stress.
- **Findings**
  - Burning and cramping pain located in the mid-epigastrium and occurs 2 to 4 hours after the meals and is relieved by food.
- **Management:** Same for gastric ulcers.

GASTRIC SURGERY

A. **Vagotomy:** Severing of part of vagus nerve innervating the stomach to decrease gastric acid secretion.

B. **Antrectomy:** Removal of the antrum of the stomach to eliminate the gastric phase of digestion.

C. **Pyloroplasty:** Enlargement of the pyloric sphincter with acceleration of gastric emptying.

D. **Gastroduodenostomy (Billroth I):** Removal of the lower portion of the stomach with anastomosis of the remaining portion of the duodenum.

E. **Gastrojejunostomy (Billroth II):** Removal of antrum and distal portion of stomach and duodenum with anastomosis of the remaining portion of the stomach to the jejunum.

F. **Gastrectomy:** Removal of stomach.

G. **Esophagojejunostomy (Total gastrectomy):** Removal of entire stomach with a loop of jejunum anastomosed to the esophagus.

DUMPING SYNDROME

- A common complication of the gastric surgeries
- **Caused by** abrupt emptying of the stomach content to the intestine
- **Associated with** the presence of hyperosmolar chyme in the jejunum which draws fluid by osmosis from the ECF into the bowel
- Decreased plasma volume and distention of the bowel stimulates increased intestinal motility
- **Findings** include weakness, faintness, palpitations, diaphoresis, feeling of fullness/discomfort, nausea or occasionally diarrhea appear 15 to 30 minutes after meals and lasts for 20 to 60 minutes.
- **Management**
  - Avoid concentrated sweets
  - Small, frequent, dry meals
  - Avoid taking fluids with the meal
  - Assume recumbent position for half hour after meals.

CANCER OF THE STOMACH

- Most often develops in the distal third and spread through the walls of the stomach into the adjacent tissues, lymphatic, regional lymph nodes and other abdominal organs or through the blood stream to the lungs and bones.
- **Causes** are excessive intake of smoked/highly salted food, diet low in vegetables and fruits, atropic gastritis, achlorhydria and *H. pylori* infection.
- **Findings**
  - Fatigue, weakness, dizziness, shortness of breath, nausea and vomiting, hematemesis, weight loss, indigestion, epigastric fullness, feeling of early satiety when eating and late epigastric pain.
  - Pallor, lethargy, poor skin turgor and mobility, palpable epigastric mass.
  - Carcinoembryogenic antigen (CEA) positive.
- **Treatment**
  - Chemotherapy
  - Radiotherapy
  - **Surgery:** Subtotal gastrectomy (Billroth I or II); total gastrectomy
  - Treatment of anemia
  - Nutritional support.

ULCERATIVE COLITIS

- Inflammatory disorder of the bowel characterized by inflammation and ulceration that starts in the rectosigmoid area and spreads upwards
- The mucosa of the bowel become edematous, thickened with eventual scar formation.

The colon consequently loses its elasticity and absorptive capabilities

- **Cause** unknown.
- **Contributing factors** include autoimmune factors, viral infections, allergies, emotional stress and insecurity.
- **Findings**
  - Severe diarrhea (15–20 liquid stools per day containing blood, mucus and pus); severe tenesmus, weight loss, anorexia, weakness, crampy discomfort
  - Decreased skin turgor, dry mucous membrane.
  - Low grade fever, abdominal tenderness over the colon.
- **Treatment**
  - Low roughage food without milk.
  - **Drugs:** Antimicrobials, corticosteroids, anticholinergics, antidiarrheals, immune suppressive, hematinic agents.
  - **Bowel surgery:** Dissection and anastomosis of diseased portion of the bowel.

CANCER OF THE COLON/RECTUM

- Adenocarcinoma is the most common type of colon cancer
- May spread by direct extension through the walls of the intestine or through the lymphatics or circulatory system.
- Metastasis is most often to the liver
- **May be caused by** diverticulitis, chronic ulcerative colitis, and familial polyposis.
- **Findings**
  - Alternating diarrhea/constipation, lower abdominal cramps, abdominal distension, weakness, anorexia, weight loss, pallor, dyspnea
  - CEA is positive.

- **Treatment**
  - Chemotherapy
  - Radiation therapy
  - Bowel surgery.

BOWEL SURGERY

Type of surgery may vary depending upon the disease

1. **Abdominoperineal resection (APR):** Distal sigmoid colon, rectum and anus are removed through a perineal incision and a permanent colostomy is created. Surgery of choice for cancer of the colon/rectum.

> Abdominoperineal resection (APR) is the surgery of choice for cancer of the colon/rectum.

2. **Ileostomy:** Opening of the ileum on to the abdominal surface, most frequently done for ulcerative colitis.

> Ileostomy is the surgery commonly done for ulcerative colitis.

3. **Continent ileostomy (Kock's pouch):** An intra-abdominal reservoir with a nipple valve is formed from the distal ileum. The pouch acts as a reservoir for fecal material and is cleaned at regular intervals by insertion of a catheter.
4. **Cecostomy:** An opening between the cecum and the abdominal base; temporarily diverts the fecal flow to rest the distal portion of the colon after some types of surgery.
5. **Temporary colostomy:** Usually located in the ascending or transverse colon; most often done to rest the bowel.

> A temporary colostomy is usually done in the ascending or transverse colon.

6. **Double-Barrelled colostomy:** The colon is resected and both ends are brought through the abdominal wall creating two stomas, a proximal and a distal; done most often for an obstruction or tumor in the descending or transverse colon.
7. **Loop colostomy:** Often a temporary procedure whereby a loop of bowel is brought out above the skin surface and held in place by a glass and rod. There is one stoma but two openings, a proximal and a distal.
8. **Permanent colostomy:** Consists of a single stoma made when the distal portion of the bowel is removed; most often located in the sigmoid or descending colon.

> A permanent colostomy is usually done in the descending or sigmoid colon.

9. **Resection with anastomosis:** Diseased part of the bowel is removed and remaining portions anastomosed, allowing elimination through the rectum.

PERITONITIS

- Local or generalized inflammation of the part or all of the parietal and visceral surfaces of the abdominal cavity.
- **Caused** by trauma, inflammation (diverticulitis, ulcerative colitis), volvulus, intestinal ischemia or intestinal obstruction.
- **Findings**
  - Severe abdominal pain, rebound tenderness, muscle rigidity, absent bowel sounds, abdominal distention
  - Anorexia, nausea and vomiting
  - Shallow respirations, decreased urinary output, weak, rapid pulse and elevated temperature.
  - Elevated WBC and PCV.
- **Treatment**
  - NPO with fluid replacement
  - **Drugs:** Antibiotics for infection, analgesics for pain
  - **Surgery:** Laparotomy to determine the cause of peritonitis; depending on the cause, bowel resection may be necessary.

HEMORRHOIDS

- Congestion and dilation of the veins of the rectum and anus
- **Usually results** from impairment of blood flow through the venous plexus.
- May be internal or external
- **Predisposing conditions** include occupation requiring long periods of standing, increased intra-abdominal pressure caused by prolonged constipation, pregnancy, heavy lifting, obesity, straining at defecation and portal hypertension.
- **Findings**
  - Bleeding with defecation, hard stools with streaks of blood
  - Pain with defecation
  - Pain during sitting or walking
  - Protrusion of external hemorrhoids upon inspection
  - Decreased Hb and PCV if bleeding is severe and prolonged.
- **Management**
  - Stool softeners, local anesthetics or anti-inflammatory creams
  - High fiber diet with adequate fluids.
  - **Hemorrhoidectomy:** Surgical excision of hemorrhoids.

DISORDERS OF THE LIVER

HEPATITIS

- Widespread inflammation of the liver tissue with liver cell damage
- Caused by hepatic cell degeneration and necrosis
- Kupffer cells enlarged and proliferated
- Bile flow interrupted due to inflammation of the periportal areas.
- **Hepatitis A**
  - Transmitted by feco-oral route
  - Incubation period 15 to 45 days
  - Often occurs with crowded living with poor personal hygiene or from contaminated food milk or water.
- **Hepatitis B**
  - Transmitted by blood and body fluids; often from contaminated needles among IV drug abusers or by sexual contact.
  - Incubation period 50 to 180 days.
- **Hepatitis C**
  - Transmitted by parenteral route through blood and blood products, needles and syringes.
  - Incubation period 7 to 50 days.
- **Findings in Hepatitis**
  a. **Preicteric stage:** Anorexia, nausea and vomiting, fatigue, constipation or diarrhea, weight loss, right upper quadrant discomfort, hepatomegaly, splenomegaly, lymphadenopathy.
  b. **Icteric stage:** Fatigue, weight loss, light colored stools, dark urine, continued splenomegaly with tenderness, lymphadenopathy, jaundice, pruritis.
  c. **Posticteric stage:** Fatigue, but an increased sense of well-being, hepatomegaly gradually decreasing.
- **Diagnostic tests**
  - SGOT (AST), SGPT (ALT), alkaline phosphatase, bilirubin and ESR increased in all the three types in preicteric stage
  - WBC, lymphocytes, neutrophils all decreased in periicteric period
  - Hepatitis A virus (HAV) in stool before the onset of disease in hepatitis A
  - HBsAg positive; develops 4 to 12 weeks after infection in hepatitis B.
- **Treatment**
  - Nutrition with high carbohydrate foods
  - Steroids as indicated
  - Immune serum globulin (ISG) in hepatitis A and hepatitis B.

Cirrhosis of Liver

- Chronic progressive disease characterized by inflammation, fibrosis and degeneration of liver parenchymal cells
- Destroyed liver cells are replaced by scar tissue resulting in architectural changes and malfunctioning of the liver.
- **Types**
  1. Laënnec's cirrhosis: Associated with alcohol abuse and malnutrition; characterized by an accumulation of fat in the liver cells, progressing to widespread scar formation.
  2. Postnecrotic cirrhosis: Results in severe inflammation with massive necrosis as a complication of viral hepatitis.
  3. Cardiac cirrhosis: Occurs as a complication of right sided heart failure, manifested by hepatomegaly and some fibrosis.
  4. Biliary cirrhosis: Associated with biliary obstruction, usually in the common bile duct, results in chronic impairment of bile secretion.
- **Findings**
  - Fatigue, anorexia, nausea and vomiting, indigestion, weight loss, flatulence, irregular bowel habits.
  - **Hepatomegaly (early):** Pain located in the right, upper, quadrant, atrophy of liver (later); hard, nodular liver upon palpation, increased abdominal girth
  - Changes in mood, alertness and mental ability, sensory deficits, gynecomastia, decreased axillary and pubic hair in males, amenorrhea in young females
  - Jaundice of the skin, sclera and mucous membrane; pruritis
  - Easy bruising, spider angiomas, palmar erythema, muscle atrophy
  - SGOT (AST), SGPT (ALT), LDH, alkaline phophatase and serum bilirubin increased
  - Prolonged PT, decreased serum albumin, Hb and PCV.
- **Treatment**
  - Rest and supportive care
  - Prevent infection; avoid hepatotoxic drugs, diuretics as ordered.

ASCITES

- Accumulation of free fluid in the peritoneal cavity of the abdomen
- Most frequently caused by cirrhotic liver damage which produces hypoalbuminemia, increased portal venous pressure, hyperaldosteronism and congestive cardiac failure

- **Findings**
  - Anorexia, nausea, vomiting, fatigue, weakness, changes in mental functioning
  - Positive fluid wave and shifting dullness on percussion, flat or protruding umbilicus, abdominal distention/tautnes with striae and prominent veins, abdominal pain
  - Peripheral edema, shortness of breath
  - Decreased serum albumin and potassium, prolonged PT, increased SGOT (AST), SGPT (ALT), LDH, BUN and serum sodium.
- **Treatment**
  - **Supportive:** Diet and bed rest
  - Diuretic therapy
  - **Paracentesis:** Removal of peritoneal fluid by insertion of a needle into the peritoneal cavity
  - **Peritoneal-venous shunt (LeVeen shunt):** Used in chronic, unmanaged ascites; permits continuous reinfusion of ascitic fluid back into the venous system through a silicone catheter.

HEPATIC ENCEPHALOPATHY

- Terminal complication in liver disease
- Diseased liver unable to convert ammonia to urea, so that large quantities remain in the systemic circulation and cross the blood-brain barrier producing neurologic toxic symptoms
- Caused by cirrhosis, GI hemorrhage, hyperbilirubinemia, transfusions particularly with stored blood, thiazide diuretics, uremia, dehydration.
- **Findings**
  a. **Early symptoms:** Changes in the mental functioning (irritability), insomnia, slowed affect, slow, slurred speech, impaired judgment, slight tremor, Babinski's reflex, hyperactive reflexes.
  b. **Progressive disease:** Asterixis, disorientation, apraxia, tremors, fetor hepaticus, facial grimacing.
  c. **Late symptoms:** Coma, absent reflexes
  d. Serum ammonia increased, PT prolonged and Hb decreased.
- **Treatment**
  - Neuro-checks and supportive care
  - Protein restricted diet
  - Enema, cathartics, intestinal antibiotics and lactulose to reduce ammonia levels
  - Avoid hepatotoxic drugs.

DISORDERS OF THE GALLBLADDER

CHOLECYSTITIS

- Acute or chronic inflammation of the gallbladder
- Most commonly associated with gallstones
- Inflammation occurs within the walls of the gallbladder and creates a thickening accompanied by edema.
- There is impaired circulation, ischemia and eventually necrosis.

CHOLELITHIASIS

- Formation of gallstones, most common variety being cholesterol stones.
- **Findings**
  - Epigastric or right abdominal quadrant pain, precipitated by a heavy meal or occurring at night
  - Intolerance for fatty foods (nausea, vomiting, sensation of fullness)
  - Pruritis, easy bruising, jaundice, dark amber urine, steatorrhea
  - Cholecystogram positive for gallstones.
- **Treatment**
  - **Supportive:** NPO and nasogastric aspiration
  - Fat soluble vitamins supplementation.
  - **Narcotic analgesics:** Morphine is contraindicated because it causes spasms of the sphincter of Oddi
  - Antiemetics
  - **Surgery:** Cholecystectomy/choledocho-stomy.

> Cholecystectomy: Removal of the gallbladder with insertion of a "T" tube into the common bile duct. Can be performed laparoscopically also.
>
> Choledochostomy: Opening of CBD, removal of stone and insertion of a "T" tube.

DISORDERS OF THE PANCREAS

PANCREATITIS

- An inflammatory process with varying degrees of pancreatic edema, fat necrosis or hemorrhage
- Proteolytic and lipolytic pancreatic enzymes are activated in the pancreas rather than in the duodenum, resulting in tissue damage and auto-digestion of the pancreas.

- Caused by alcoholism, biliary tract disease, trauma, viral infection, penetrating duodenal ulcer, abscesses, drugs (steroids, thiazide diuretics and oral contraceptives), metabolic disorders such as hyperparathyroidism, hyperlipidemia.
- **Findings**
  - Pain in the left upper quadrant with radiation to back, flank or substernal area; may be accompanied by difficulty in breathing and is aggravated by eating.
  - Vomiting, shallow respiration with pain, tachycardia, decreased or absent bowel sounds, abdominal tenderness with muscle guarding, positive Grey Turner's spots (ecchymosis on flanks) and positive Cullen's sign (ecchymosis of periumbilical area).
  - Serum amylase, lipase, blood sugar and lipid level increased; serum calcium decreased.
- **Treatment**
  - **Drugs:** Analgesics and smooth muscle relaxants to relieve pain, anticholinergics (atropine) to decrease pancreatic stimulation, H_2 antagonists, vasodilators and calcium gluconate.
  - NPO and diet modification
  - Peritoneal lavage
  - Dialysis.

CANCER OF THE PANCREAS

- Majority of the tumors occurs in head of the pancreas and the most common type being adenocarcinoma.
- Tumor growth results in common bile duct obstruction and jaundice
- Contributing factors include carcinogens, smoking, high fat diet and diabetes mellitus.
- **Findings**
  - Anorexia, rapid, progressive weight loss, dull, abdominal pain located in the upper abdomen or left hypochondriacal region with radiation to the back
  - Pain related to eating
  - Jaundice
  - Serum lipase, bilirubin and amylase increased.
- **Treatment**
  - Radiation/chemotherapy
  - **Whipple's resection (pancreato-duodenectomy):** Resection of proximal pancreas, adjoining duodenum, distal portion of the stomach and distal segment of the common bile duct.
  - **Drugs:** Pancreatic enzymes, oral hypoglycemic agents or insulin, bile salts replacement after surgery.

REVIEW QUESTIONS

1. **A patient with ascites should take a diet which is:**
   a. Restricted potassium b. Increased potassium
   c. Increased fluids d. Restricted sodium
2. **A patient with liver failure will have:**
   a. Decreased serum creatinine
   b. Decreased sodium
   c. Increased ammonia
   d. Increased calcium
3. **An important clinical sign in massive GIT hemorrhage:**
   a. Bulging flanks b. Protruding umbilicus
   c. Cullen's sign d. Abdominal distention
4. **Enzyme present in saliva:**
   a. Ptyalin b. Lipase
   c. Amylase d. Pepsin
5. **The intrinsic factor is secreted by:**
   a. Beta cells of pancreas
   b. Parietal cells of stomach
   c. Alpha cells of pancreas
   d. Liver
6. **The secretion of stomach which help in protein digestion:**
   a. Trypsinogen b. Pepsinogen
   c. Ptyalin d. Protease
7. **In the small intestine, digestive enzymes are produced by:**
   a. Crypts of Lieberkühn b. Villi
   c. Brunner's glands d. Ileocecal junction
8. **In the small intestine, mucus is produced by:**
   a. Villi b. Ileocecal junction
   c. Brunner's glands d. Crypts of Lieberkühn
9. **In the liver phagocytosis is performed by:**
   a. Liver lobules
   b. Bile ducts
   c. Hepatic cells
   d. Kupffer cells
10. **The sphincter present in the duodenum at the opening of the bile duct:**
    a. External sphincter b. Internal sphincter
    c. Sphincter of Oddi d. Hepatic sphincter

11. **The organ responsible for concentration and storing of the bile:**
   a. Liver b. Gallbladder
   c. Spleen d. Pancreas

12. **Detoxification of drugs takes place in:**
   a. Pancreas b. Gallbladder
   c. Spleen d. Liver

13. **The enzyme secreted by the pancreas which aid in protein digestion:**
   a. Trypsinogen b. Amylase
   c. Lipase d. Ptyalin

14. **The largest gland in the human body:**
   a. Pancreas b. Liver
   c. Spleen d. Gallbladder

15. **The enzyme secreted by the pancreas which aid in fat digestion:**
   a. Trypsinogen b. Amylase
   c. Lipase d. Ptyalin

16. **Bile is secreted by:**
   a. Gallbladder b. Liver
   c. Spleen d. Pancreas

17. **Endoscopic visualization of the sigmoid colon:**
   a. Proctoscopy b. Colonoscopy
   c. Gastroscopy d. Sigmoidoscopy

18. **Radiological procedure done to evaluate the disorder of the gallbladder:**
   a. Renogram b. Cholecystogram
   c. Hepatogram d. Cystogram

19. **After liver biopsy, patient should be positioned in:**
   a. Right lateral b. Left lateral
   c. Fowler's position d. Semi-Fowler's position

20. **Endoscopic visualization of large intestine:**
   a. Sigmiodoscopy b. Colonoscopy
   c. Gastroscopy d. Cystoscopy

21. **An alternative method of feeding:**
   a. Gastrostomy b. Colostomy
   c. Ileostomy d. Ileal conduit

22. **Feeling of discomfort with a conscious desire to vomit:**
   a. Dyspepsia b. Pyrosis
   c. Malaise d. Nausea

23. **Persistent eating of substances such as paint, sand, etc.:**
   a. Anorexia nervosa b. Bulimia nervosa
   c. Pica d. Pyrosis

24. **The most common type of oral tumor:**
   a. Adenocarcinoma b. Hyperplasia of mucosa
   c. Lymphoma d. Squamous cell carcinoma

25. **A predisposing factor for oral cancer:**
   a. Tobacco use b. Taking hot fluids
   c. Taking cold fluids d. Taking spicy food

26. **Leukoplakia is the earliest sign of:**
   a. Liver cirrhosis b. Leukemia
   c. Lymphoma d. Oral cancer

27. **Vagotomy is performed to decrease:**
   a. Liver enzymes
   b. Intestinal secretions
   c. Gastric acid secretion
   d. Bile secretion

28. **Common complication after gastrectomy:**
   a. Bleeding b. Dumping syndrome
   c. Hypotension d. Infection

29. **Protrusion of a viscous from its normal cavity through a weakened area:**
   a. Polyp b. Hemorrhoid
   c. Diverticuli d. Hernia

30. **Inflammation and ulceration of the rectosigmoid area:**
   a. Peptic ulcer b. Ulcerative colitis
   c. Gastric ulcer d. Hemorrhoid

31. **A temporary colostomy is usually performed in:**
   a. Ascending colon b. Descending colon
   c. Sigmoid colon d. Rectosigmoid area

32. **Most common procedure done for ulcerative colitis which cannot be managed with drugs:**
   a. Ileostomy
   b. Colostomy
   c. Loop colostomy
   d. Abdominoperineal resection

33. **A permanent colostomy is usually performed in:**
   a. Ascending colon b. Descending colon
   c. Anus d. Transverse colon

34. Surgery of choice for cancer of the colon:
a. Colostomy
b. Ileostomy
c. Abdominoperineal resection
d. Cecostomy

35. Congestion and dilation of the veins of the rectum and anus:
a. Polyp b. Anal fissure
c. Hemorrhoids d. Diverticulitis

36. Out pouching of intestinal mucosa found in sigmoid colon:
a. Polyp b. Hemorrhoids
c. Anal fissure d. Diverticulitis

37. Abdominal muscle guard is present in:
a. Ascites b. Peritonitis
c. Hemorrhoids d. Peptic ulcer

38. Incubation period for hepatitis A:
a. 7–50 days b. 15–45 days
c. 50–180 days d. 50–100 days

39. Surface antigen present in the serum in hepatitis B:
a. HBeAG b. HBsAg
c. Anti-HBc d. Anti-HBe

40. Hepatitis B is transmitted by:
a. Faeco-oral route
b. Air-borne
c. Blood and body fluids
d. Contaminated food

41. The common type of cirrhosis associated with alcohol abuse:
a. Biliary cirrhosis b. Cardiac cirrhosis
c. Postnecrotic cirrhosis d. Laennec's cirrhosis

42. Hepatitis C is transmitted by:
a. Oral route b. Droplets
c. Parenteral route d. Contaminated food

43. Hepatitis A is transmitted by:
a. Contaminated air b. Feco-oral route
c. Parenteral route d. Sexual contact

44. Palmar erythema is a characteristic sign in:
a. Splenomegaly b. Pancreatitis
c. Cholecystitis d. Cirrhosis liver

45. Accumulation of fluid in the abdominal cavity:
a. Edema b. Ascites
c. Peritonitis d. Appendicitis

46. LeVeen shunt is done in:
a. Ascites b. Peritonitis
c. Cirrhosis d. Appendicitis

47. A clinical sign of portal hypertension:
a. Weakness b. Esophageal varices
c. Peritonitis d. Hepatitis

48. Life-threatening complication of cirrhosis liver:
a. Hepatitis b. Hepatic necrosis
c. Peritonitis d. Hepatic encephalopathy

49. Stone formation in the gallbladder:
a. Cholecystitis b. Cholelithiasis
c. Cholecystectomy d. Nephrolithiasis

50. Cholecystectomy is:
a. Removal of spleen b. Removal of liver
c. Removal of gallbladder d. Removal of pancreas

51. Acute or chronic inflammation of the gallbladder:
a. Cholecystitis b. Cholelithiasis
c. Choledochostomy d. Hepatitis

52. Rebound tenderness is a classical sign of:
a. Cholecystitis b. Hepatitis
c. Peritonitis d. Appendicitis

53. Ecchymosis of periumbilical area:
a. Rosuva's sign b. Cullen's sign
c. Grey Turner's spots d. Purpura

54. Ecchymosis on flanks:
a. Purpura b. Cullen's sign
c. Rosuva's sign d. Grey Turner's spots

55. Whipple's surgery is done in:
a. Ca liver b. Ca gallbladder
c. Ca cecum d. Ca pancreas

ANSWER KEY

1. d	2. c	3. c	4. a	5. b	6. b	7. a	8. c	9. d	10. c	11. b	12. d
13. a	14. b	15. c	16. b	17. d	18. b	19. a	20. b	21. a	22. d	23. c	24. d
25. a	26. d	27. c	28. b	29. d	30. b	31. a	32. a	33. b	34. c	35. c	36. d
37. b	38. b	39. b	40. c	41. d	42. c	43. b	44. d	45. b	46. a	47. b	48. d
49. b	50. c	51. a	52. d	53. b	54. d	55. d					

Diseases and Disorders of the Genitourinary System

REVIEW OF ANATOMY AND PHYSIOLOGY

The genitourinary system includes the kidneys, urethras, urinary bladder, urethra and the male and female genitalia.

URINARY SYSTEM

Kidneys

Two bean shaped organ that lie in the retroperitoneal space on either side of the vertebral column, adrenal glands are located on top of each kidney. Renal parenchyma consists of outer cortex and inner medulla. The functional unit of the kidney is nephrone which is divided into bowman's capsule proximal convoluted tubule and collecting duct.

Ureters

Two tubes approximately 25 to 35cm long extend from the renal pelvis to the pelvic cavity, where they enter the bladder convey urine from the kidneys to the bladder convey the urine from the kidneys to the bladder.

Bladder

Located behind the symphysis pubis, composed of muscular and elastic tissue that make it distensible, serves as reservor of urine capable of holding 1000–1800 mL. Internal and external urethral sphincters control of the flow of urine.

Urethra

A small tube extending from bladder to the exterior of the body. In the males urethra is approximately 20 cm long and in the females it is 3 to 5 cm long.

Regulatory Function of Kidney

Kidneys and urinary system play a major role in the maintenance of homeostatic control of the body. Kidneys remove nitrogenous wastes and regulate fluid and electrolyte balance. Urine is formed by the process like glomerular filtration, tubular reabsorption and secretion. Kidneys also regulate BP partly through maintenance of volume and by the renin-angiotensin system. When BP drops, kidneys release rennin which then activates angiotensin to cause vasoconstriction.

Male Reproductive System

Consist of the external structures penis, scrotum and testis and internal ductal system and testis and accessory glands.

Sperm is produced by testis and stored in the epididymis. Spermatic cord consists of vas deferens, arteries, veins, nerves and lymphatic vessels. Vas deferens joins with the duct of the seminal vesicles to become the ejaculatory duct.

Accessory glands include the prostate, cowpers glands which secrete lubricating fluid and seminal vesicles which contribute to nutrition and activation of the sperm.

DISORDERS OF THE URINARY TRACT

CYSTITIS

Inflammation of the bladder due to bacterial invasion, common in the females, predisposing factors include stagnation of urine, obstruction, sexual intercourses and high estrogen.

Findings

- Abdominal or flank pain/tenderness, frequency
- And urgency of urination, pain on voiding, nocturia
- Fever
- Diagnosed by urine culture and sensitivity.

Treatment

- Increase fluids (3 L/day)
- Antibacterial according to culture and sensitivity.

NEPHROLITHIASIS/UROLITHIASIS

Presence of stones anywhere in the urinary tract, calcium, oxalate and uric acid stones are common.

- Predisposing factors include diet containing large amounts of calcium and oxalate, increased uric acid levels, sedentary lifestyle, immobility, family history of gout or calculi, hyperparathyroidism.

Findings

- Abdominal or flank pain, renal colic
- Cool, moist skin
- Diagnosed by KUB.

Treatment

Surgery: Percutaneous nephrostomy, percutaneous nephrostolithotomy, extracorporeal shock wave lithotripsy.

GLOMERULONEPHRITIS

Immune complex disease resulting from an antigen antibody reaction, occur secondary to a beta-hemolytic streptococcal infection occurring elsewhere in the body, usually resolves in about 14 days, self-limiting.

Findings

- History of streptococcal infection (usually upper respiratory or impetigo)
- Edema, anorexia, lethargy
- Hematuria, dark colored urine, fever
- Hypertension.

Treatment

- Antibiotics for streptococcal infection
- Antihypertensive if BP is elevated
- Digitalis if circulatory overload
- Fluid restriction as per intake
- Peritoneal dialysis if severe renal or cardiopulmonary problems develop.

ACUTE RENAL FAILURE

Sudden inability of the kidneys to regulate fluid and electrolyte balance and remove toxic products from the body.

Causes

- Factors interfering with perfusion and resulting in decreased blood flow and glomerular filtrate, ischemia and diguria, include CHF, carcinogenic shock, acute vasoconstriction, hemorrhage, burns, septicemia hypertension, etc.
- Conditions that cause damage to the nephrones, include acute glomerulonepritis tumors blood transfusion reaction, hypercalcemia, nephrotoxins.
- Mechanical obstruction anywhere from the tubules to the urethra, include calculi, BPH, tumors strictures, blood clots, trauma and anatomical malformation.

Findings

a. Oliguric phase: Urine output less than 400 mL/24 hours, duration 1 to 2 weeks. Manifested by hypernatremia, hyperkalemia, hyperphosphatemia, hypocalcemia, hypomagnesemia and metabolic acidosis. BUN and creatinine elevated.
b. Diuritic phase: Diuresis may occur (output 3 to 5 liters per day), duration 2 to 3 weeks. Manifested by hyponatremia, hypokalemia and hypovolemia. BUN and creatinine elevated.
c. Recovery or convalescent phase: Over next 3 to 12 months.

Treatment

- Maintain fluid and electrolyte balance
- Drugs—diuretics, cardiac glycoside, antihypertensive
- Prevent infection.

CHRONIC RENAL FAILURE

Progressive irreversible destruction of the kidneys that continues until nephrones are replaced by scar tissue, gradual loss of renal function.

Predisposing factors include recurrent infection, exacerbations of nephritis, urinary tract obstruction, DM, HT.

Findings

a. Nausea, vomiting, diarrhea or constipation decreased urinary output, dyspnea
b. Stomatics, hypertension (early) hypertension (late) lethargy, convulsions, memory impairment, pericardial friction rib, CHF
c. WBC, protein and sodium elevated, platelets, specific gravity and calcium decreased.

Treatment

- Monitor and maintain serum electrolytes
- Prevent neurological complication
- Promote/maintain maximal cardiovascular function
- Dialysis renal transplantation
- Unmanaged cases.

SURGERY OF URINARY SYSTEM

a. Cystecomy removal of the urinary badder.
b. Urinary diversions
   1. Ureterosigmoidostomy: Ureters are excised from the bladder and implanted into sigmoid colon.
   2. Ileal conduit: Ureters are implanted into a segment of the ileum that has been resected from the intestinal tract with formation of an abdominal stoma; most common type of urinary diversion.
c. Cutaneous ureterostomy: Ureters are excised from the bladder and brought through abdominal wall with creation of the stone.
d. Nephrostomy: Insertion of a catheter into the renal pelvis via and invasion into the flank or by percutaneous catheter placement into the kidney.
e. Nephrectomy: Surgical removal of the entire kidney, indicated in renal tumor, massive trauma, removal for a donor and polycystic kidneys.

DISORDERS OF THE REPRODUCTIVE SYSTEM

EPIDIDYMITIS

Inflammation of the epididymis, one of the most common intrascrotal infections, may be sexually transmitted.

Findings

Sudden scrotal pain, scrotal edemas and tenderness over the spermatic cord.

Treatment

Antibiotics an analgesics bed rest, icepack to scrotal area.

PROSTATITIS

Inflammation of the prostate gland, may be bacterial, ascending infection from lower UTI can occur.

Findings

Fever, chills, dysuria, urethral discharge upon palpitation, in chronic cases backache, perineal pain, enlarged, firm and tender prostate upon palpitation may be seen.

Treatment

Antibiotics, analgesics and stool softeners.

BENIGN PROSTATIC HYPERTROPHY (BPH)

- Glandular enlargement, hyperplasia and overgrowth of the smooth muscles and connective tissues of the prostate.
- As prostate enlarges, it compresses the urethra resulting in urinary retention.

Findings

- Nocturia, frequency, decreased force and amount of urinary stream, hesitancy, hematuria and enlarged prostate upon palpitation.
- Prostate specific antigen (PSA) is elevated (normal is < 4 ng/mL).

Treatment

Antibiotics, drugs to relax bladder sphincter (e.g. terzosin), drugs to shrink enlarged prostate (e.g. finasteride).

PROSTATIC SURGERY

- Indicated BPH and prostatic cancer
- Types
- Transurethral resection of prostate (TURP): Insertion of a resectoscope into the urethra to excise prostatic tissue, most common type of surgery for BPH.
- Suprapublic prostatectomy: The prostate is excised by a low abdominal excision into the bladder to the anterior aspect of the prostate, alone for large tumors obstructing the urethra.
- Retropubic prostatectomy: To remove a large prostate mass high in the pelvic area.
- Perineal prostatectomy: Often used for prostatic cancer, the incision is made through the perineum which facilitates radical surgery if a malignancy is found.

DIALYSIS

- Removal by artificial mean of metabolic wastes, excess electrolytes and excess fluid from clients with renal failure.
- Principles involved are diffusion and osmosis
- Types: Hemodialysis and peritoneal dialysis.

Hemodialysis

Shunting of blood from the patient's vascular system through an artificial dialyzing system and return of dialyzed blood to the client's circulation. Dialysis will acts as the semipermeable membrane and the dialysate is a specially prepared solution. The access routes for dialysis are external AV shunt, AV fistula, femoral subclavian, graft, etc.

Peritoneal Dialysis

Introduction of a specially prepared dialysate solution into the abdominal cavity where the peritoneum act as a semipermeable membrane between the dialysate and blood in the abdominal vessels. The abdominal cavity where the peritoneum act as a semipermeable membrane between the dialysate and blood in the abdominal cavity is cannulated, the dialysate is allowed to flow unrestricted into peritoneal cavity, a dwell time is allowed for a prescribed period and the outflow is then allowed by gravity.

Continuous Ambulatory Peritoneal Dialysis (CAPD)

A continuous type of peritoneal dialysis, can be performed by the client at home.

Dialysate is delivered from flexible plastic containers through a permanent peritoneal catheter.

Following infusion of the dialysate, the bag is folded and tucked away during the dwell period after the dwell period, outflow is allowed.

OBJECTIVE QUESTIONS

1. **Functional unit of the kidney:**
   a. Neuron b. Nephron
   c. Bowman's capsule d. Loop of Henle
2. **Reabsorption of water and electrolytes in the kidney is controlled by the hormone:**
   a. Renin b. Angiotensin
   c. Aldosterone d. Antidiuretic hormone
3. **Hormon produced by the testes:**
   a. Testosterone b. TSH
   c. Andrones d. Cortisol
4. **Part of the ductal system that stores spermatogoa:**
   a. Testes b. Epididymis
   c. Vas deferens d. Spermatic cord
5. **Flouroscopic visualization of the urinary tract after injection with a radiopaque dye:**
   a. KUB b. IVP
   c. Cytoscopy d. Urethroscopy
6. **Movement of a particle from an area of high concentration to an area of low concentraction is termed as:**
   a. Osmosis
   b. Diffusion
   c. Active transport
   d. None of the above
7. **Outflow of the dialysate, during peritoneal dialysis will be brownish in the following condition:**
   a. Peritonitis b. Bowel perforation
   c. Peritoneal adhesions d. Bladder perforation
8. **The oliguric phase of the renal failure ranges from:**
   a. 1–2 days b. 3–7 days
   c. 3–4 days d. 1–2 days
9. **Presence of U wave in the ECG indicates:**
   a. Hyperkalemia b. Hypokalemia
   c. Hypernatremia d. Hyponatremia
10. **A normal finding in at atriovenous (AV) fistula created for dialysis:**
    a. Ecchymotic area b. Enlarged veins
    c. Pulselessness d. Redness
11. **Normal pH of urine:**
    a. 7.10 b. 7.42
    c. 5.5–6.5 d. 6.5–7.1
12. **Normal specific gravity of urine:**
    a. 1.010–1.020 b. 1.000–1.010
    c. 0.900–1.000 d. 1.020–1.050
13. **Normal glomerular filtration rate is:**
    a. 1000 mL/mt b. 125 mL/mt
    c. 150 mL/mt d. 180 mL/mt
14. **Burning sensation during micturition:**
    a. Oliguria b. Dysuria
    c. Anuria d. Cystis
15. **A characteristic red band that appears on nails in CRF patient is called:**
    a. Palmar erythema b. Spider nevi
    c. Cubbing d. Muehrcke's line
16. **A urinary diversion procedure:**
    a. Cystoscopy b. Cystectomy
    c. Ileal conduct d. Nephrectomy
17. **A characteristic feature of a functioning AV fistula:**
    a. Absence of pulsation
    b. Bruit on auscultation
    c. Color change of overlying skin
    d. Tenderness of the fistula arm
18. **Shohl's solution is:**
    a. Sodium citrate and citric acid
    b. Potassium citrate and citric acid
    c. Citric acid only
    d. Sodium citrate only
19. **Presence of stones in the urinary tract:**
    a. Cholelithiasis b. Cystis
    c. Urolithiasis d. Pylonephritis
20. **Collection of urine in the renal pelvis due to obstruction to outflow:**
    a. Hydrocele b. Urolithiasis
    c. Nephritis d. Hydronephrosis

21. **Immune complex disease affecting kidney:**
    a. Hydronephrosis b. Acuteglomerulonephritis
    c. Urolithiasis d. Pyelonephritis

22. **The organism responsible for acute glomerulonephritis:**
    a. Group A bete hemolytic streptococci
    b. *E. coli*
    c. Staphylococci
    d. *Neisseria gonorrhoeae*

23. **Autoimmune disease of the kidney leading to structural alternation of glomerular membrane:**
    a. Hydronephrosis b. Glomerulonephritis
    c. Nephrotic syndrome d. Pyelonephritis

24. **The syndrome presenting with proteinuria, edema and hyperlipidema is:**
    a. Nephrotic syndrome b. Hydronephritis
    c. Glomerulonephritis d. Pyelonephritis

25. **The inflammation of the renal pelvis and parenchyma causes by bacterial infection:**
    a. Hydronephritis b. Nephrotic syndrome
    c. Pyelonephritis d. Acute renal failure

26. **Prostate-specific antigen (PSA) is elevated in:**
    a. Acute renal failure
    b. Chronic renal failure
    c. Pyelonephritis
    d. Benign prostatic syndrome

27. **Most common type of surgery for BPH:**
    a. Suprapubic prostatectomy
    b. Perineal prostatectomy
    c. Transurethral resection
    d. Retropubic prostatectomy

28. **Treatment of kidney stones using sound waves:**
    a. Nephrectomy
    b. KUB
    c. Lithotrite
    d. Extracorporeal shock ware lithotripsy

29. **Daily loss of protein in urine in nephritic syndrome:**
    a. 2–3 gm/day b. > 3.5 gm/day
    c. 1–2 gm/day d. 2.5–3.5 gm/day

30. **Removal of bladder:**
    a. Cystostomy b. Cystotomy
    c. Cystectomy d. Cytoscopy

31. **Most common site of cancer of the urinary tract:**
    a. Ureter b. Bladder
    c. Kidney d. Urethra

32. **Removal of metabolic wastes by artificial mean:**
    a. Paracentesis b. Dialysis
    c. Ileal conduit d. None of the above

33. **The bladder dysfunction caused by the lesions of the central or peripheral nervous system:**
    a. Atrophy b. Cystocele
    c. Neurogenic bladder d. Nephrolithiasis

34. **Painless hematuria may be a sign of:**
    a. Renal stones b. Urolithiasis
    c. Cancer of bladder d. Acute renal failure

35. **Clinical signs of rejection after renal transplant include the following, except:**
    a. Fever
    b. Tenderness over transplant site
    c. Decreased urinary output
    d. Increased urinary output

ANSWER KEY

1. b	2. d	3. a	4. b	5. b	6. b	7. b	8. d	9. b	10. b	11. c	12. a
13. b	14. b	15. d	16. c	17. b	18. a	19. c	20. d	21. b	22. a	23. c	24. a
25. c	26. d	27. c	28. d	29. b	30. c	31. b	32. b	33. c	34. c	35. c	

Diseases and Disorders of the Musculoskeletal System

REVIEW OF ANATOMY AND PHYSIOLOGY

Bones

- Provide support to selected framework.
- Assist in the movement by acting as levers for muscles
- Protect vital organ and soft tissues
- Manufacture RBC in red bone marrow
- Provide site for storage of calcium and phosphorus
- Long bones, short bones, flat bones and irregular bones are there in the body.

Bones of the body

Part of body	Name of bone	Number
1. Axial skeleton		
a. Skull		
1. Cranium	• Frontal • Parietal • Temporal • Occipital • Sphenoid • Ethmoid	1 2 2 1 1 1
2. Face	• Nasal • Maxilla • Zygomatic • Mandible • Lacrimal • Palatine • Inferior conchae • Vomer	2 2 2 1 2 2 2 1
3. Ear ossicies	• Malleus (hammer) • Incus (anvil) • Stapes (stirrup)	2 2 2
b. Hyoid bone		
c. Vertebral column	• Cervical vertebrae • Thoracic vertebrae • Lumbar vertebrae • Sacrum • Coccyx	7 12 5 5 (fused) 4 (fused)
d. Ribs and sternum	• True ribs • False ribs • Sternum	7 pairs 5 pairs 1
2. Appendicular skeleton		
a. Upper extremities	• Clavicle • Scapula • Humerus • Radius • Ulna • Carpals • Metacarpals • Phalanges	2 2 2 2 2 16 10 28
b. Lower extremities	• Pelvic bone • Femur • Patella • Tibia • Fibula • Tarsals • Metatarsals • Phalanges	2 2 2 2 2 14 10 28
	TOTAL	**206**

Joints

- Articulation of bones occurs at joints, movable joint provide stabilization and permits a variety of movements.
- **Classification:**
  - Synarthroses: Immovable joints
  - Amphiarthroses: Partially movable
  - Diarthroses: Freely movable

Muscles

- Provide shape to the body, protect the bone, maintain posture and causes movement of body parts by contraction.

Types of Muscles

a. **Cardiac:** Involuntary, found in heart.
b. **Smooth:** Involuntary, found in the walls of hollow structures (e.g. intestine).
c. **Striated or skeletal:** Voluntary, have properties of contraction, extension as well as elasticity permitting isotonic and isometric movements.

Cartilage

- A form of connective tissue.
- Cushions bony prominences and offer protection where resiliency is required.

Major muscles and movements		
Parts of body moved	**Movement**	**Muscle**
Upper arm	Flexion	Pectoralis major
	Extension	Latissimus dorsi
	Abduction	Deltoid
	Adduction	Latissimus dorsi contracting with pectoralis major
Shoulder	Shrugging	Trapezius
	Elevating	Pectoralis minor
	Lowering	Serratus anterior
Lower arm flexion	With forearm supinated	Biceps brachii
	With forearm pronated	Brachialis
	With forearm semisupinated or semipronated	Brachioradialis
Lower arm	Extension	Triceps brachii
Thigh	Flexion	Iliopsoas (iliacus and psoas major) Rectus femoris
	Extension	Gluteus maximus
		Hamstring group
	Abduction	Gluteus medius and minimus
		Tensor fasciae latae
	Adduction	Adductor group
		(brevis, longus, magnus)
Lower leg	Flexion	Hamstring group (biceps femoris, semitendinosus, semimembranosus)
		Gastrocnemius
	Extension	Quadriceps femoris group
		(rectus femoris, vastus medialis, vastus intermedius)
Foot	Flexion (dorsiflexion) Extension (plantar flexion)	Tibialis anterior Gastrocnemius Soleus
Head	Flexion	Sternocleidomastoid
	Extension	Trapezius
Abdominal wall	Compress abdominal cavity therefore assists in straining, defecation, forced expiration, child-birth, posture, etc.	External oblique Internal oblique Transversus Rectus abdominis
Chest wall	Elevate ribs thereby enlarging antero-posterior and anterolateral dimensions of chest and causing inspiration Depress ribs pull floor of thorax downward, thereby enlarging vertical dimension of chest causing inspiration	Transversus Internal intercostals Diaphragm
Trunk	Flexion	Iliopsoas
	Extension	Sacrospinalis
		Quardratus lumborum

Tendons and Ligaments

- Composed of dense, fibrous connective tissue.
- Tendons attach muscles to bone and ligaments, attach bone-to-bone.

Rheumatoid Arthritis (RA)

- Chronic systemic disease characterized by inflammatory changes in joints and related structures.
- **Cause** unknown, may be an autoimmune process.
- Predisposing factors include fatigue, cold, emotional stress and infection.
- Joint distribution is symmetric, most commonly affects smaller peripheral joints of hands and also commonly involves wrists, elbows, shoulders, knees, hips, ankles and jaw.

Findings

Warm swollen, painful joints, limited in movements fatigue, weight loss, pyrexia and muscle weakness.

Treatment

a. Drugs: Aspirin, other NSAIDs and steroids.
b. Methotrexate and cytoxan may be given to suppress immune response.

Osteoarthritis

- Chronic, nonsystemic disorder of joints characterized by degeneration of articular cartilage.
- Cause unknown, predisposing factors include aging, obesity and joint trauma.
- Weightbearing joints (spine, knees and tips) and terminal interphalangeal joints of fingers are most commonly affected.

Findings :

a. Pain and stiffness of joints
b. Heberden's nodes: Bony overgrowths at terminal interphalangeal joints.
c. Decreased ROM, possible crepitations (grating sound when moving joints).

Treatment

a. Weight reduction
b. NSAIDs intra-articular injection of corticosteroids
c. Surgery: Joint replacement.

Gout

- A disorder of purine metabolism, causes high levels of uric acid in the blood and the precipitation of urate crystals in the joints.

Findings:

- Joint pain, redness, heat, swelling, joints of foot and ankles are most commonly affected
- Headache, anorexia and malaise
- Tachycardia, fever.

Treatment

- Drugs: Colchicine, NSAIDs (indomethacin, naproxen, and phenylbutazone).
- Uricosuric agents are used for the prevention of attacks, e.g. probenecid, sulfinpyrazone allopurinol.

Systemic Lupus Erythematosus (SLE)

- Chronic connective tissue disease involving multiple organ systems.
- Cause is thought to be immune, genetic or viral
- **Findings:**
  a. Fatigue, fever, anorexia, weight loss, malaise, history of remissions and exacerbations.
  b. Joint pain, morning stiffness
  c. Erythematous rash on face, neck or extremities, butterfly rash over bridge of the nose and cheeks, photosensitivity.
  d. Oral or nasopharyngeal ulcerations
  e. Alopecia
  f. Proteinuria, hematuria and renal failure.
  g. CNS involvement: Peripheral neuritis, seizures, organic brain syndrome, psychosis
  h. Pericarditis and pleurisy with cardiac involvement
  i. Increased susceptibility to infection
  j. ESR elevated, ANA positive.
- **Treatment**
  - Aspirin and NSAIDs for fever and arthritis
  - Corticosteroids
  - Immunosuppressive agents (Cyclophosphamide, azathioprine).
  - Plasmapheresis to remove circulating antibodies.

Fractures

- A break in the continuity of the bone, usually caused by trauma.
- Pathologic fractures may be found in osteoporosis, osteomyelitis, multiple myeloma and bone tumors.
- **Types**
  - **Complete:** Separation of bone into two parts.

- Incomplete: Only part of the bone is broken
- **Comminuted:** Bone in broken or splintered into pieces.
- **Closed or simple:** Bone is broken without break in skin.
- **Open or compound:** Break in skin with or without protrusion of bone.

Findings

- Pain aggravated by movement, tenderness
- Loss of motion, edema, crepitus, ecchymosis
- Fracture evident in X-ray.

Treatment:

- Traction
- Reduction: Closed or open reduction.
- Application or plaster cast.

OBJECTIVE QUESTIONS

1. **Total number of bones in human body:**
   a. 202 b. 204
   c. 206 d. 208
2. **The largest bone in human body:**
   a. Humerus b. Femur
   c. Tibia d. Fibula
3. **The radioisotope used in bone scan:**
   a. Lithium b. Technetium-99
   c. Cobalt d. Cesium
4. **Endoscopic examination of joints:**
   a. Arthroscopy b. Osteoscopy
   c. Cystoscopy d. Gastroscopy
5. **The longest muscle in human body:**
   a. Deltoid b. Sartorius
   c. Hamstring d. Vastus lateralis
6. **Instrument used to measure joint range of motion:**
   a. Goniometer b. Pelvimeter
   c. Perimeter d. Audiometer
7. **The most common type of arthritis:**
   a. Osteochrodrosis b. Osteoarthritis
   c. Osteomyelitis d. Rheumatoid arthritis
8. **A short bone:**
   a. Carpals b. Femur
   c. Humerus d. Tibia
9. **Immovable joints:**
   a. Sinovial joint b. Diarthroses
   c. Amphiarthroses d. Synarthroses
10. **Muscles found in heart:**
    a. Striated muscles b. Skeletal muscles
    c. Cardiac muscles d. Smooth muscles
11. **Connective tissues acting as cushions on bony prominences:**
    a. Cartilage b. Tendon
    c. Ligament d. Muscle
12. **Attachment of a muscle to a bone:**
    a. Ligament b. Tendon
    c. Cartilage d. Joint
13. **Aspiration of sinovial fluid from a joint:**
    a. Arthroscopy b. Arthrocentesis
    c. Bone scan d. Myelography
14. **Recording of activity of contracting muscles in response to electric stimulation:**
    a. ECG b. EMG
    c. NCV d. TENS
15. **Active exercise through contraction and relaxation of the muscle:**
    a. Isometric exercise b. Passive exercise
    c. Rom exercise d. Isotonic exercise
16. **Chronic, systemic disease characterized by inflammatory changes in joints:**
    a. Rheumatic fever b. Osteoarthritis
    c. Rheumatoid arthritis d. Osteoporosis
17. **Chronic, nonsystemic disorder of joints characterized by degeneration of articular cartilage:**
    a. Rheumatoid arthritis
    b. Osteoarthritis
    c. Gout
    d. Rheumatic fever
18. **A disease characterized by precipitation of uric acid crystals in articular tissue:**
    a. Rheumatoid arthritis b. Gout
    c. Osteoarthritis d. Rheumatic fever

19. Chronic, autoimmune connective tissue diseases.:
a. SLE b. Gout
c. Osteoarthritis d. Rheumatoid arthritis

20. Increase in the lumbar curve of the vertebral column:
a. Kyphosis b. Scoliosis
c. Lordosis d. Genu varum

21. First vertibra:
a. Axis b. Atlas
c. Maxilla d. Mandible

22. A pivot type of joint:
a. Knee joint b. Elbow joint
c. Wrist joint d. Atlantoaxial joint

23. Potts' fracture is fracture of:
a. Tibia b. Radius
c. Fibula d. Ulna

24. Fracture of radius:
a. Potts' fracture b. Greenstick fracture
c. Colle's fracture d. Open fracture

25. Only movable bone of skull:
a. Maxilla b. Mandible
c. Frontal bone d. Occipital bone

26. A lateral deformity of spine:
a. Scoliosis b. Kyphosis
c. Lordosis d. Genu varum

27. Exaggeration of thoracic curve:
a. Scoliosis b. Kyphosis
c. Lordosis d. None of the above

28. Horseshoe shaped bone flying in neck above larynx:
a. Vomer b. Thymus
c. Hyoid bone d. Cricoid

29. Bone disorder characterized by abnormal bone resorption and formation of one or more bones:
a. Rickets b. Osteoporosis
c. Osteopenia d. Pagets' disease

30. Moving arm away from body's midline:
a. Abduction b. Adduction
c. Flexion d. Extension

31. Fracture which occurs within last inch of distal radius:
a. Potts' fracture b. Colle's fracture
c. Greenstick fracture d. Comminuted fracture

32. Fracture of distal fibula is:
a. Potts' fracture b. Colles' fracture
c. Greenstick fracture d. Open fracture

33. Ligament injury resulting from overstress:
a. Strain b. Sprain
c. Dislocation d. Fracture

34. Break in the bone without break in the skin:
a. Closed fracture b. Complete fracture
c. Incomplete fracture d. Open fracture

35. Hematoma formation in bone heating comprises:
a. I stage of healing b. II stage of healing
c. III stage of healing d. IV stage of healing

36. A benign bone tumor:
a. Osteosarcoma b. Fibrosarcoma
c. Osteoblastoma d. Ewing's sarcoma

37. A malingnant bone tumor:
a. Osteoblastoma b. Osteoclastoma
c. Osteosarcoma d. Osteoporosis

38. Malingnant tumor of the cartilage:
a. Osteochoridroma b. Osteosarcoma
c. Chondrosarcoma d. Osteoporosis

39. Benign tumor of the cartilage:
a. Osteochondroma b. Osteoporosis
c. Osteosarcoma d. Chondrosarcoma

40. Fatal complication of femur fracture:
a. Infection b. Thrombophlebitis
c. Hemorrhage d. Fat embolism

ANSWER KEY

1. c	2. b	3. b	4. a	5. b	6. a	7. b	8. a	9. d	10. c	11. a	12. b
13. b	14. b	15. a	16. c	17. b	18. b	19. a	20. c	21. b	22. d	23. c	24. c
25. b	26. a	27. b	28. c	29. d	30. a	31. b	32. a	33. b	34. a	35. a	36. c
37. c	38. c	39. a	40. d								

Diseases and Disorders of the Endocrine System

REVIEW OF ANATOMY AND PHYSIOLOGY

The endocrine system is composed of an interrelated complex of glands that secrete a variety of hormones directly into the bloodstream. The endocrine glands are pituitary, hypothalamus, thyroid, parathyroid, adrenals, islets of Langerhans, ovaries and testes.

HORMONE REGULATION

Hormone

A chemical substance that act as messengers to target cells and organs.

Types

- Local: Hormones with specific effect in the area of secretion (e.g. secretion, cholecystokinin- pancreozymin).
- General: Hormones transported in the blood to distant sites where they exerts their effect (e.g. cortisol).
- Major means of regulating hormone levels is negative feedback mechanism, i.e. decreased concentration of a circulating hormone triggers production of a stimulating hormone from the pituitary gland, this hormone, in turn, stimulates its target organ to produce hormones.
- Some hormones are controlled by changing blood levels of specific substances, e.g. calcium, glucose.
- Certain hormones follow rhythmic patterns of secretion, e.g. female reproductive hormones.
- Hypothalamus controls release of hormones of the anterior pituitary gland through releasing and inhibiting factors that stimulate or inhibit hormone secretion.

Major Hormones	
Endocrine gland	**Hormones**
Anterior Pituitary	GH, TSH, ACTH, LH
	FSH, Prolactin
Posterior Pituitary	ADH, Oxytocin
Adrenal cortex	Mineralocorticoids
	(e.g. Aldosterone)
	Glucocorticoids
	(e.g. Cortisol, corticosterone)
	Sex hormones (Androgen, estrogen, progesterone)
Adrenal medulla	Epinephrine, norepinephrine
Thyroid	T3, T4, Thyrocalcitonin
Parathyroid	PTH
Islets of Langerhans of	Insulin, Glucogone
Pancreas	
Ovaries	Oestrogen, Progesterone
Testes	Testosterone

Hyper/Hypofunction effects		
Hormone	**Hyperfunction Effect**	**Hypofunction Effect**
Growth hormone	Gigantism	Dwarfism
Thyroid hormones	Hyperthy-roidism	Cretinism in children
		Myxedema in adults
Parathyroid hormone	Hypercalcemia	Hypocalcemia
Cortisol	Cushing's syndrome	Addison's disease
Aldosterone	Hypernatremia Hypokalemia	Hyponatremia, Hyperkalemia
ADH	Antidiuresis (Oliguria)	Diuresis (Diabetes insipidus)

OBJECTIVE QUESTIONS

1. **The gland that regulates the rate of oxygenation in all the body cells:**
   a. Pituitary gland b. Thyroid gland
   c. Adrenal gland d. Pancreas

2. **ADH is secreted by:**
   a. Anterior pituitary b. Adrenal cortex
   c. Adrenal medulla d. Posterior pituitary

3. **Glucocorticoids and mineralocorticoids are secreted by the:**
   a. Pancreas b. Adrenal gland
   c. Hypophysis d. Gonads

4. **Excessive thirst is called:**
   a. Polyphagia b. Polyuria
   c. Polydypsia d. Oliguria

5. **Adult hypothyroidism is called:**
   a. Myxedema b. Gigantism
   c. Cretinism d. Acromegaly

6. **Enlargement of the thyroid gland due to lack of iodine:**
   a. Cretinism b. Goiter
   c. Hyperthyroidism d. Graves disease

7. **Slowed body metabolism, decreased heat production and increased oxygen consumption by the tissues are features of:**
   a. Hypercalcemia b. Hypocalcemia
   c. Hyperthyrodism d. Hypothyrodism

8. **Hormone that regulates calcium metabolism:**
   a. Parathormone b. Thyroid hormone
   c. Adrenal hormone d. Androgen

9. **Inflammation of the thyroid gland:**
   a. Hypothyroidism b. Cretinism
   c. Thyroiditis d. Goiter

10. **Myxedema coma is a major complication of:**
    a. Hyperthyroidism b. Hypothyroidism
    c. Hyperpituitarism d. Hypopituitarism

11. **Drug of choice for thyroid replacement:**
    a. Thyroxine b. Insulin
    c. Glucagon d. Steroids

12. **Exophthalmos is a feature of:**
    a. Grave's disease b. Hypopituitarism
    c. Hypothyroidism d. Hyperpituitarism

13. **Abnormal projection of a eyeball:**
    a. Exophthalmos b. Keratitis
    c. Glaucoma d. Cataract

14. **Spasm of the facial muscles occurs in:**
    a. Hyperthyroidism b. Hypercalcemia
    c. Tetany d. Hyperkalemia

15. **Fatal acute episode of thyroid overactivity following thyroidectomy:**
    a. Grave's disease b. Thyroid storm
    c. Tetany d. Cretinism

16. **Hyposecretion of parathyroid gland leads to:**
    a. Hypokalemia b. Hyponatremia
    c. Hypercalcemia d. Hypocalcemia

17. **Idiopathic atrophy or destruction of adrenal gland by an autoimmune process:**
    a. Addison's disease b. Cushing's syndrome
    c. Cretinism d. Myxedema

18. **Hypersecretion of glucocorticoid:**
    a. Addison's disease b. Cushing's syndrome
    c. Cretinism d. Myxedema

19. **Buffalo hump is a feature of:**
    a. Gigantism b. Cretinism
    c. Myxedema d. Cushing's syndrome

20. **Most powerful mineralocorticoid:**
    a. Parathormone b. Thyroxine
    c. Cortisol d. Aldosterone

21. **A tumor of the adrenal medulla causing hyper- activity of the gland:**
    a. Pheochromocytoma b. Neroblastoma
    c. Addison's disease d. Wilson's disease

22. **Malignant tumor occurring in adrenal medulla:**
    a. Pheochromocytoma b. Wilson's disease
    c. Nephroblastoma d. Neuroblastoma

23. **The source of the glucose for maintaining normal levels when the blood glucose begins to fall:**
    a. Ingested food b. Intestinal hydrolysis
    c. Liver glycogen d. Gluconeogenesis

24. **Ketone bodies appear in the blood in the following condition:**
    a. Starvation
    b. Alcoholism
    c. Positive nitrogen balance
    d. Bone healing

25. **Oral hypoglycemic agents may be used for diabetic clients with:**
    a. Ketosis b. Some insulin production
    c. Type I diabetes d. Obesity

26. **Diabetic coma results from excessive accumulation of:**
    a. Nitrogen b. Ketones
    c. Glucose d. Sodium bicarbonate

27. **The most common cause of diabetic ketoacidosis is:**
    a. Increased insulin b. Inadequate food intake
    c. Emotional stress d. Infection

28. **Glucagon act by:**
a. Liberating glucose from the hepatic stores of glycogen
b. Blocking insulin's action at tissue sites
c. Providing a glucose substitute
d. Supplying glycogen to the brain and other vital organs

29. **Signs of hypokalemia include:**
a. Edema, bounding pulse, confusion
b. Apathy, weakness, abdominal distention
c. Sunken eyeballs, Kussmaul's breathing, thirst
d. Spasms, diarrhea, irregular pulse rate

30. **Hypotension associated with Addison's disease involves a disturbance in the production of:**
a. Glucocorticoids b. Androgens
c. Mineralocorticoid d. Estrogens

31. **Feature of Addison's disease:**
a. Emaciation, muscular weakness and fatigue
b. Apathy, weakness, abdominal distention
c. Spasms, diarrhea, irregular pulse rate
d. Edema, spasm, apathy

32. **Features of Addison's disease are due to disturbance in:**
a. Protein anabolism b. Electrolyte levels
c. Fluid balance d. Musculinizing effects

33. **A patient with diabetes insipidus will exhibit:**
a. Decreased serum osmolality
b. Increased blood glucose
c. Low urinary specific gravity
d. Elevation of BP

34. **The antidiuretic hormone important for maintaining fluid balance is released by the:**
a. Anterior pituitary b. Adrenal cortex
c. Adrenal medulla d. Posterior pituitary

35. **'Flight and fight' response made by the body in emergency situation is associated with the increased activity of:**
a. Adrenal gland b. Pituitary gland
c. Thyroid gland d. Pancreas

36. **Signs of hypoglycemia:**
a. Pallor, perspiration, tremors
b. Excessive thirst, dry hot skin
c. Anorexia, glycosuria
d. Fruity odor of breath

37. **Cushing's syndrome is:**
a. Deficiency of adrenocortical hormones
b. Insufficient ACTH production
c. Hyperplasia of the adrenal cortex
d. Pituitary hypoplasia

38. **Glucocorticoids and mineralocorticoids are secreted by the:**
a. Pancreas b. Hypophysis
c. Adrenal gland d. Gonads

39. **Features of Cushing's syndrome include:**
a. Buffalo hump and hypertension
b. Dehydration and menorrhagia
c. Pitting edema and frequent colds
d. Migrane headaches and dysmenorrhea

40. **Acromegaly is produced by oversecretion of:**
a. Growth hormone
b. Thyroid hormone
c. Thyroid stimulating hormone
d. Testosterone

41. **The hormone decreasing calcium concentration in the blood is:**
a. Aldosterone b. Thyrocalcitonin
c. Parathyroid hormone d. Thyroid hormone

42. **Under production of thyroxin produces:**
a. Myxedema b. Acromegaly
c. Cushing's syndrome d. Grave's disease

43. **A patient with low T3, T4, will have:**
a. Irritability b. Profuse diaphoresis
c. Tachycardia d. Cold intolerance

44. **Laryngeal nerve injury after thyroidectomy can be checked by assessing:**
a. Gag reflex
b. The ability to swallow
c. The ability to speak
d. The ability to turn the neck

45. **The action of glucagon:**
a. Provides more storage of glucose
b. Increases blood sugar levels
c. Stimulates release of insulin
d. Inhibits glycogenesis

46. The drug given in Cushing's syndrome:

a. Regular insulin
b. ACTH
c. Hydrocortisone
d. Pituitary extracts

47. A patient with excessive production of ADH will have:

a. Hyponatremia
b. Dehydration
c. Hyperglycemia
d. Polyuria

48. Cushing's syndrome will produce increased:

a. Urine output
b. Serum potassium
c. Glucose level
d. Immune response

49. A patient with hyperparathyroidism will exhibit:

a. Tetany
b. Seizure disorder
c. Bone destruction
d. Grave's disease

50. Accidental removal of parathyroid gland during thyroidectomy produce:

a. Tetany
b. Adrenocortical stimulation
c. Myxedema
d. Hypovolemia

51. Following hypophysectomy, the patient should be observed for:

a. Urinary retention
b. Bleeding at suture site
c. Increased intracranial pressure
d. Respiratory distress

ANSWER KEY

1. b	2. d	3. b	4. c	5. a	6. b	7. d	8. a	9. c	10. b	11. a	12. a
13. a	14. c	15. b	16. d	17. a	18. b	19. d	20. d	21. a	22. d	23. c	24. a
25. b	26. b	27. d	28. a	29. b	30. c	31. a	32. a	33. c	34. d	35. a	36. a
37. c	38. c	39. a	40. a	41. b	42. a	43. d	44. c	45. b	46. c	47. a	48. c
49. c	50. a	51. c									

Chapter 2 Nursing Foundations

NURSING

Nursing is to being the healthy and those who are suffering from disease to a condition for nature to act for preserving health, protecting disease and injury and to restore health and cure disease.

—**Florence Nightingale**

Nursing is assisting an individual sick or well in the performance of those action contributing to health or its recovery or to a peaceful death that he would perform unaided if he had the necessary strength, will or knowledge and to help him to be independent of such assistance as early as possible.

—**Virginia Henderson**

COMMUNICATION

- Communication is the basic component of human life.
- Communication is the interchange of thoughts or information conveyed to a person or persons in such a way that the meaning received is equivalent to those which the initiator of the message intended.

ESSENTIALS OF COMMUNICATION PROCESS

1. **Sender:** Person who convey a message.
2. **Message:** A piece of information passed from one person to another.
3. **Receiver:** The listener or the one who receives the message.
4. **Response:** The message that the receiver returns to the sender. It is also called the feedback.

Essentials of Good Communication

1. Sender and receiver express the ideas in common language and words.
2. Avoid abbreviations and technical words that are not in use.
3. There should be clarity in the expression of ideas.
4. Pay attention to the nonverbal messages.
5. Aware of both relevance and timing of communication.
6. There should be adaptability.
7. Sender should have a thorough knowledge about the subject.
8. Develop skills of effective communication like listening, problem solving and self-disclosure.

Barriers of Communication

1. **Emotional:** Fear, jealousy, anxiety, anger, lack of interest, etc.
2. **Physical:** Fatigue, illness, speech, defects, deafness and pain.
3. **Intellectual**: Low IQ, lack of knowledge, misinterpretation of words.
4. **Social factors:** Difference in culture language, race, professional and socioeconomic status.
5. **Environmental:** Noise, lack of privacy, uncomfortable accommodation, etc.

ETHICAL ASPECTS OF NURSING

- Ethics are the rules or principles that govern right conduct.
- Deal with what is good and what is bad and with moral duty and obligation.
- Designed to protect the rights of human beings
- International Council of Nursing (ICN) in 1973 adopted the code of ethics of nurses.

International Council of Nursing (ICN) in 1973 adopted the code of ethics of nurses.

NURSING PROCESS

- Series of steps that follow a logical sequence
- Gives a logical framework on which the nursing care is based
- Systematic problem solving approach for giving individualized comprehensive nursing care

- Steps: Assessment, nursing diagnosis, plan of action, implementation and evaluation.

Nursing process is a systematic problem solving approach for giving individualized comprehensive nursing care.

Assessment

- Logical collection of subjective and objective data that are helpful to identify and define problems
- **Subjective data or symptoms:** Client's feelings and statements about his or her health problems
- **Objective data or symptoms:** Observable, perceptible and measurable data
- **Primary source of data:** The patient himself
- **Secondary source of data:** Family members, health records, laboratory tests, diagnostic procedures, etc.

Nursing Diagnosis

- Identifying the clients problems
- Clinical judgment about individuals or community responses to actual or potential health problems/life processes.

Nursing diagnosis is a clinical judgment about individual's or community responses to actual or potential health problems/life processes.

Plan of Care

- Formulating and documenting measurable, realistic, client-focused goals
- Plan short-term and long-term goals
- Type of interventions include psychomotor, psychosocial, educational, maintenance, surveillance and sociocultural.

Implementation

- Action phase of nursing process
- Actual initiation of the plan and documenting of nursing actions

Evaluation

- Process of determining the extent up to which the goals of nursing care have been attained
- Ongoing and continuous process carried out throughout all phases of nursing process

MEDICAL AND SURGICAL ASEPSIS

Asepsis Freedom from infection or prevention of contact with microorganisms.

Medical asepsis refers to all practices used to protect the clients and his environment from the transmission of disease producing organisms.

Surgical asepsis refers to all procedures used to keep objects or areas sterile or completely free from all microorganisms

Sterilization of Articles

1. **Boiling:** Boiling for 10 minutes will kill most of the common pathogens and is a reliable method of disinfecting instruments. Sharp instruments cannot be put for boiling.
2. **Disinfection by disinfectants**
   - A chemical disinfectant act by coagulating the bacterial protein or by changing the composition of protein
   - Method used to sterilize the articles that are destroyed by heat and the metallic objects prone to corrosion
   - All disinfectants does not ensure sterilization.
3. **Fumigation**
   - Very effective if high concentration of gas is used
   - Destroy all vegetative forms of bacteria, viruses and most of the forms
   - Commonly used agents are formalin tablets and ethylene oxide liquids.
4. **Ultraviolet sterilization or radiation**
   - Effective for disinfecting working surfaces and air inside the rooms
   - Only the surfaces of an object in direct line with the light source are irradiated.
5. **Dry heat sterilization**
   - Method of choice for fine metal cannula and for glass syringes
   - Cannot be used for articles which are damaged by moisture.
6. **Steam under pressure or autoclaving**
   - Most widely used, economical and one of the most effective method of destroying microorganisms.
   - Uses high temperature, pressure and humidity to destroy bacteria.
   - For effective sterilization, the steam in the autoclave should be at 15 lbs/inch^2 (1.05kg/cm^2) pressure, at 121°C temperature, for 30 minutes.

For effective sterilization, the steam in the autoclave should be at 15 lbs/inch^2 (1.05kg/cm^2) pressure, at 121°C temperature, for 30 minutes.

Commonly used antiseptics and disinfectants		
Name	**Strength**	**Uses**
Savlon	1:100	Cleaning of wounds, preoperative skin preparation, swabbing and cleaning body parts before examination, as an antiseptic in the use of equipment
Savlon	1:30	Same as above Used in wet method of taking temperature
Dettol	1:40	Used in wet method of taking temperature
Hydrogen peroxide	Diluted form readily available	Cleaning of infected wounds and to remove slough, as a bleaching agent to remove blood stains
Spirit	70% alcohol	Preoperative skin preparation, cleaning of clear wounds, cleaning of skin before giving injections
Betadine	Readymade form available	Dressing of wounds, preoperative skin preparation
Glycerine magsulf	Readymade form available	used as hygroscopic solution to reduce edema
Cidex	Glutaraldehyde	Complete sterilization of instruments that cannot be autoclaved, quick action and is effective against spores

ASSESSMENT OF CLIENT

Physical Assessment

- Systematic collection of objective information that is directly observed or is elicited through examination techniques.
- Involves the use of one's senses to obtain information about the structure and function of an area being observed or manipulated.

Techniques of Physical Examination

1. **Inspection**
    - Systematic visual examination of the client
    - Involves observation of the color, shape, size, symmetry, position and movements.
    - Also uses the sense of smell to detect odors and uses the sense of hearing to detect sounds.

> Inspection is systematic visual examination of the client to observe size, shape, color, position, symmetry and movements of body parts.

2. **Palpation:**
    - Use of the hands and fingers to gather information through touch.
    - Feeling of the body or a part with hands to make the size and position of the organs.
    - The palmar surfaces of the fingers and finger pads are used to assess the texture, shape, size, fluid, consistency and pulsation.

> Palpation is the feeling of the body or a part with hands to gather information about the size and position of the organs through touch.

3. **Percussion**
    - Examination by tapping the fingers on the body to determine the condition of the internal organs by the sounds that are produced.
    - It provides the information about the nature of an underlying structure, outlines the size of an organ such as bladder or liver, and determines if the structure is air-filled, fluid-filled or solid.

> Percussion of the abdomen is tympanic, hyperinflated lung tissue is hyper-resonant, normal lung tissue is resonant, the liver is dull and the bone is flat.

4. **Auscultation**
    - Process of listening to sounds that are generated within the body.

- Done with the help of a stethoscope.
- When auscultating a part, that area should be exposed and the environment should be quiet.

Four characteristics of sound viz. pitch, loudness, quality and duration can be assessed by auscultation.

5. **Manipulation:** Moving of a part of the body to note its flexibility, limitation of movement, etc.
6. **Testing of reflexes:** Reflexes can be tested by percussion hammer, safety pin, wisp of cotton, hot or cold water.

SPECIMEN COLLECTION AND TESTING

Specimen

Small quantity of a substance or object which shows the kind and quality of the whole.

A specimen is a small quantity of a substance or object which shows the kind and quality of the whole.

Collection of Urine Specimen

- Usually morning specimens are collected.
- After cleaning the genital area, the mid- stream urine is collected directly into the specimen bottle.
- For collecting 24 hours urine specimen, start collecting urine at 6 am, discard the 6 am sample and continue collection till 6 am next morning, ask client to void at 6 am and include the 6 am urine also.
- While collecting urine specifies from a catheter especially for culture and sensitivity, clean the rubber tubing of the catheter and aspirate urine sample using a sterile syringe.

Examination of Urine

1. **Volume:** An amount of 1000 to 2000 mL of urine is excreted in 24 hours.

Abnormal increase in volume of urine is called polyuria and decrease is called oliguria.

2. **Color:** Normal urine is pale yellowish or amber in color.

When the quantity of urine is increased, the color becomes pale yellow and when the quantity of urine is decreased, the color becomes deep yellow.

3. **Appearance:** The normal urine is clear with no deposits.
4. **Odor:** The normal urine has aromatic-odor, when kept for sometimes, strong ammoniac smell comes due to the decomposition of urea.

Urine, when kept for sometimes, strong ammoniac smell comes due to the decomposition of urea.

Fruity odor of urine is due to the presence of ketone bodies and is seen in diabetic clients.

5. **Specific gravity:** The specific gravity of urine varies from 1.010 to 1.020 with normal fluid intake.

Urine specific gravity is measured using a urinometer, the more concentrated the urine, the higher the specific gravity.

6. **Urine pH**
   - Refers the kidneys ability to maintain a normal hydrogen ion concentration in plasma and extracellular fluid.
   - The normal pH of urine varies from 4.6 to 8.0, but usually averages below 6 (slightly acidic).

In cystitis, the reaction of urine may be alkaline.

7. **Constituents of urine:** The normal constituents of urine are water 96%, urea 2% and the remaining 2% consists of uric acid, urates, creatinine, chlorides, phosphates, sulphates and oxalates.

Albuminuria is seen kidney damage. Presence of sugar in the urine is called glycosuria and is seen in diabetic patients.

Examination of the Urine

1. **Physical examination**
   - Color
   - Appearance
   - Volume
   - Reaction
   - Specific gravity
   - Odor.
2. **Chemical examination**
   - Tests such as tests for albumin and sugar, acetone, bile salts and bile pigments.
3. **Microscopic examination**
   - Crystals
   - Pus cells
   - Casts
   - Epithelial cells
   - RBC
   - Bacteria.

Common tests of urine		
Constituents of urine	**Specific test**	**Reagent**
Albumin	Heat test	Acetic acid
Sugar	Benedict's test	Benedict's solution
Acetone	Rothera's test	Ammonium sulphate, sodium nitroprusside, liquor ammonia
Bile salts	Hay's test	Sulphur powder
Bile pigment	Smith's test	Iodine solution

Stool Specimens

Characteristics of normal stool

1. **Color:** Normally color is light to dark brown due to the presence of bile pigments.

Malena or black, tarry stools indicate bleeding in the upper GIT.

2. **Odor:** Normal stool has pungent smell, normally affected by the type of bacterial flora, food and medication ingested.

There will be foul smell of stool in malena and in dysentery.

3. **Frequency:** One or two per day and is usually painless.
4. **Quantity:** Depends upon the type and amount of food taken.
5. **Consistency and form:** In adult, the stool is well formed and semisolid.

Flattened, ribbon-like stool is found in intestinal obstruction.

"Rice water stools" are typical of cholera and "Pea-soup stools" are typical of typhoid fever.

Collecting Stool Specimen

- Waterproof disposable containers or wide mouthed containers are used.
- Client passes stool in a clean bed pan.
- A small amount of urine is collected with the help of a spatula and placed in the container.

Sputum Specimens

1. **Quantity:** Normally no sputum is expectorated, the amount of sputum coughed up in 24 hours varies with the diseases.
2. **Consistency:** May be serous, frothy, mucoid, purulent, seropurulent and hemorrhagic.

Spitting out of blood in sputum is called hemoptysis and is usually seen with pulmonary tuberculosis (TB).

Pink, froathy sputum is a characteristic sign of pulmonary edema.

3. **Odor:** Normally sputum is odorless. In lung diseases, the smell of sputum becomes foul.
4. **Color:** Mucoid sputum is colorless and translucent, when infected becomes yellowish.

Rusty color sputum is due to the altered hemoglobin as seen in pneumonia.

5. **Appearance:** Microscopic examination shows few WBC and epithelial cells.

Acid fast bacilli (AFB) staining of sputum reveals tubercle bacilli and is indicated in pulmonary TB.

Method of Collecting Sputum Specimen

- Wide-mouthed containers are used.
- Sputum should be collected in the morning before brushing the teeth and taking food.
- Do not rinse mouth with antiseptic solution before collecting the sputum.

Sputum sample should be collected in the morning before brushing the teeth and do not rinse mouth with antiseptic solution before collecting the sample.

Vaginal Discharge

- Abnormal excessive discharge or leukorrhea is found in inflammatory condition.
- In gonorrhea, the discharge may be purulent.
- Vaginal smears are taken with a cotton applicator or spatula and spread over a film, dry the slide and send to laboratory.

Blood Specimens

- Blood samples should be taken in appropriate containers with added fluoride or EDTA depending upon the test to be performed.
- The amount of blood needed for different tests may vary.

All specimens should be clearly labeled before sending to laboratory.

PERSONAL HYGIENE

Oral Hygiene

Provided to maintain integrity of clients teeth, guns, mucous membrane and lips.

Common Problems of Oral Cavity

A. Local Infections

1. Halitosis: It is the offensive odor of breath.
2. Dental caries: Destructive process causing decalcification of the enamels and dentin with resultant cavitations of the tooth.
3. Dental plaque: Soft thin film of food debris, mucin and dead epithelial cells that is deposited on the teeth and provides a medium for the growth of bacteria.
4. Calculus or tartar: When dental plaque remains on the teeth, it becomes hardened (calcified) and forms calculus or tartar. Tartar is an yellowish film of calcium phosphate, calcium carbonate, food particles and other organic matter deposited on the teeth by the salvia.
5. Bottle mouth syndrome: Infant's dental caries can be caused by allowing the infant to go to bed with a bottle feed.
6. Periodontal diseases or pyorrhea: It is the pus formation in the sockets of the teeth.
7. Sordes: Brown crusts which are formed on the teeth and lips. It is a collection of food, mucus and bacteria.
8. Cheilosis: It is the cracking or ulceration of the lips and angles of the mouth.
9. Bleeding gums: Occurs in vitamin C deficiency, pregnancy, bleeding disorders and with the use of hard and stiff brush.
10. Root abscess: It is pus formation in the root of the teeth.
11. Glossitis: It is an inflammation of the tongue.
12. Cancrum oris: It is gangrenous stomatitis.
13. Stomatitis: It is inflammation of the mucous membrane of the mouth.

B. Infection of the Neighboring Structures

Infection of the mouth can spread to neighboring structures leading to parotitis (inflammation of the parotid gland), sinusitis, otitis media (inflammation of the middle ear), adenitis (inflammation of the adenoids and lymph glands) and tonsillitis (inflammation of the tonsils).

Dentifrices Commonly Used for Oral Hygiene

- Toothpaste or tooth power
- Glycerin with lime juice
- Sodium bicarbonate paste
- Equal parts of sodium chloride, sodium bicarbonate and calcium carbonate
- Neem stick (natural dentifrice).

Emollients Used for Oral Hygiene

- Cream or butter
- Vaseline
- Glycerin
- Liquid paraffin
- Olive oil.

Bathing

- Bathing is an important intervention to promote hygiene.
- Choice of method depends upon clients' activity level.
- May be used for cleansing or for therapeutic measures related to some skin problems.

Temperature of Water for Bath

- For sponge bath: 110° to 115°F (43.3° to 46.1°C)
- For tub bath or bathroom bath: 90° to 100°F (32.2°–37.8°C).

PRESSURE SORE (BED SORE AND DECUBITUS ULCER)

- Pressure sores are ulcerated or sloughed area of tissue subjected to pressure from lying on mattress or sitting on a chair for a prolonged period time.
- Prolonged exposure to pressure result in slowing of circulation and death (necrosis) of tissues.

Common Sites of Pressure Sores

- Usually happens in bony prominences where there is no rich blood supply and has thin layer of skin.
- The common sites depend upon the position of the client in bed.
- In supine position: Back of heads (occiput), scapula, sacral region, elbows and heels.

Type of bath	Effect
Sits bath	Decrease pain and inflammation after perineal surgery or pain relief from hemorrhoids
Hot water bath	Relieve muscle spasm and muscle tension
Warm water bath	Relax and soothe
Cool water bath	Decrease fever and reduce muscle tension

- In sidelying position: Ears, acromion process of shoulder, ribs, greater trochanter of hip, medial and lateral condyles of the knee and malleolus of the ankle joint.
- In prone position: Ears, cheek, acromion process, breasts in females, genitalia in males, knees and toes.

Signs and Symptoms of Pressure Sores

- Early signs: Redness, tenderness, discomfort and smarting, area cold to touch and insensitive, local edema.
- Later signs: Area blue, purple or mottled, circulation is cut off, gangrene develops and affected area sloughs.

VITAL SIGNS

- Basic component of assessment of physiological and psychological health of client.
- Temperature, pulse, respiration and blood pressure are called vital signs.

Temperature

In a healthy individual, the body temperature may vary between 97°F and 99°F (36.1°–37.2°C with an average of 98.6°F (37°C).

Formula to convert Celsius and Fahrenheit scale
C=(F – 32) X 5/9
F=(C X 9/5) + 32

- The grading on the lotion thermometers are from the freezing point to the boiling point of water (0°–100°C or 32°–212°F).
- The grading on the clinical thermometer is from 35°–43.3°C or 95°–110°F.

The grading on the clinical thermometer is from 35°–43.3°C or 95°–110°F.

- The thermometers should be disinfected with a good disinfectant after use. The common solutions used are dettol, savlon and lysol.

Name of the disinfectant	Strength	Time
Dettol	1:40	5 minutes
Savlon	1:20	5 minutes
Lysol	1:40	3 minutes

- Electronic thermometers are available which provide reading in less than 60 seconds.
- Disposable paper thermometers, temperature sensitive strips and tympanic membrane thermometers are also available.
- The common sites for taking body temperature are mouth, axilla, groin, vagina and rectum, out of which axillary method is the most common.

FEVER

Fever is rise in body temperature above 99°F (37.2°C)

- The range in the body temperature within which the cells can function efficiently is between 34° and 41°C (94°–106°F).
- The CNS is extremely sensitive to the temperature variations.
- Irreversible changes may occur in the nervous system if the body temperature goes above 41°C or below 34°C.

Fever is rise in body temperature above 99°F (37.2°C). Irreversible changes may occur in the CNS if the body temperature goes above 41°C or below 34°C.

Types of Fever

Constant fever: Fever in which the temperature varies not more than two degrees between morning and evening and it does not reach normal for a period of days or weeks.

Remittent fever: Fever characterized by variations of more than two degrees between morning and evening but does not reach normal.

Intermittent fever: The temperature rises from normal or subnormal to high fever and back at regular intervals. Usually the temperature is higher in the evening than in the morning.

Inverse fever: Fever in which the highest range of temperature is recorded in the morning hours and the lowest in the evening.

Hectic swinging fever: Fever in which the difference between the high and low points is very great.

Relapsing fever: Fever in which there are brief febrile periods followed by one or more days of normal temperature.

Irregular fever: If the fever cannot be classified in the above categories, it is called irregular fever.

Ranges of Fever

Pyrexia	Range of temperature
Low pyrexia	Temperature between 99°–100°F
Moderate pyrexia	Temperature between 100°–103°F
High pyrexia	Temperature between 103°–105°F
Hyperpyrexia	Temperature above 105°F
Subnormal temperature	Temperature between 95°–97°F
Hypothermia	Temperature falls below 95°F

PULSE

- Alternate expansion and recoil of an artery as the wave of blood is forced through it during the contraction of the left ventricle.
- The pulse can be felt by the fingers on a point where an artery crosses bone close to the surface of the skin.

Common Pulse Sites

- Radial artery in front of the wrist
- Temporal artery over the temporal bone
- Carotid artery at the sides of the neck
- The brachial artery in the antecubital fossa
- Femoral artery in the groin
- Popliteal artery in the back of the knee
- The dorsalis pedis artery on the foot
- The posterior tibial artery behind the medial malleolus.

Characteristics of Pulse

The characteristics of pulse are rate, rhythm, volume and tension.

1. **Rate:** The number of pulse beats in a minute the normal rate in a testing adult is 60 to 100 per minute. A pulse rate above 100 per minute is called tachycardia and a pulse rate below 60 per minute is called bradycardia.

> A pulse rate above 100 per minute is tachycardia and a pulse rate below 60 per minute is bradycardia.

2. **Rhythm:** Refers to regularity of beats. When the interval between the beats varies, it is irregular.

> Dicrotic pulse: There is one heart beat and two arterial pulsations giving the sensation of a double beat.

3. **Volume:** Volume refers to the fullness of the artery. If the volume of the blood is decreased as in hemorrhage the pulse will be weak, feeble and rapid.

Abnormal Volume of Pulse

> **Water hammer pulse or Corrigan's pulse or collapsing pulse:** A full volume pulse but rapidly collapsing pulse occurring in aortic regurgitation or incompetence.
>
> **Bounding pulse:** Seen in increased stroke volume as in exercises, anxiety, anemia, hepatic failure and heart block.
>
> **Pulses alterans:** The rhythm is regular, but the volume has an alternative strong and weak character. Seen in LVF, heart block and digitalis toxicity.

Contd...

Contd...

> **Bigeminal pulse:** Irregular rhythm pulse in which there is a weak second or premature beat. Pulse deficit is also seen since the second beat is very weak. Seen in MI and digital is toxicity.
>
> **Weak, thready pulse:** A small weak pulse due to decreased stroke volume as seen in hemorrhage, loss of fluid from the body, etc.
>
> **Paradoxical pulse:** Force or strength of the pulse becomes weaker during inspiration. Can occur normally, if pronounced indicates cardiac damage.

4. **Tension:** Tension is the degree of compressibility of the artery.

RESPIRATION

Respiration is the act of breathing. It constitutes inspiration, expiration and pause. Respiration may be external or pulmonary respiration and internal or tissue respiration.

> The exchange of gases between the blood and the air in the lungs is external or pulmonary respiration. The exchange of gases between the blood and the tissue cells is called internal or tissue respiration.

Characteristics of Respiration

The characteristics of respiration are rate, depth, rhythm and easiness of respiration.

1. **Rate:** Rate is the number of full respiration in a minute. The normal rate of respiration in an adult is 16 to 20 breaths per minute.

> The normal rate of respiration is an adult is 16–20 breaths per minute.

> Increased respiratory rate over 24 breaths per minute is tachypnea and reduced respiratory rate below 10 breaths per minute is bradypnea.

2. **Depth of respiration**
   - The normal volume of air inhaled and exhaled during each respiration is about 500 mL (tidal volume).
   - If more than this quantity of air is inhaled, respiration is said to be deep.
   - Increase in the depth of respiration is called hyperpnea.

> Respiration is said to be deep if the quantity of air going in and out of lungs in each respiration exceeds the normal tidal volume of 500 mL.

3. **Rhythm:** Rhythm is the regularity of breathing. Critically ill patients and persons nearing death are found to have irregular respirations.

Cheyne-Stokes' respiration consists of a series of respiration that gradually become deeper and noisier until a peak, when a pause or aproea occurs and the entire cycle is repeated.

- **Stridor:** A harsh, vibrating, shrill sound during respiration as seen in laryngitis and in upper airway obstruction.
- **Rale:** An abnormal rattling or bubbling sound due to mucus in the air passages, seen in bronchitis and pneumonia.
- **Wheeze:** A high pitched, musical, whistling sound due to partial obstruction of smaller bronchi and bronchioles. Seen in asthma and emphysema.

BLOOD PRESSURE

- Blood pressure is the force exerted by the blood against the walls of the blood vessels as it flows through them.
- Systolic pressure is the highest degree of pressure exerted by the blood against the walls of the blood vessels during the ventricular systole when the left ventricle is forcing the blood into the aorta.
- Diastolic pressure is the lowest pressure that occurs when the heart is in its resting period just before the contraction of the left ventricle.
- Pulse pressure is the difference between the systolic and diastolic pressure and represent the volume output of the left ventricle.

Hypertension is condition in which there is abnormally high BP above 140/90 in at least two occasions of six hours apart.

The standard instrument used to measure the blood pressure is called sphygmomanometer.

Do not take the blood pressure reading on a client's arm if:

- The arm has an intravenous infusion on it.
- The arm is injured or diseased.
- The arm has a shunt or fistula for the renal dialysis.
- On the same side of the body where a female chest had a radical mastectomy.

BODY MECHANICS

- Body mechanics is the posture, alignment and balance in a coordinated effort to perform various activities such as lifting, bending and moving.
- Body mechanics uses the strongest and largest muscles of the body to perform work.

Body mechanics efficiently uses body as a machine and as a means of locomotion.

- Posture or body alignment is the way in which the body parts are aligned with one another.
- Posture in defined as the position in which the various parts of the body are held while sitting, standing, walking and lying down.

Center of gravity of human body lies in the area of pelvis, slightly anterior to the sacrum.

Abnormal Postures

- **Kyphosis:** It is an abnormal increased convexity in the thoracic spine.
- **Lordosis:** It is characterized by an exaggerated curvature of the lumbar spine.
- **Scoliosis:** It is the lateral deviation of the vertebral column.

Maintaining balance involves keeping the spine in vertical alignment, the feet positioned for a broad base of support and the body weight close to the center of gravity.

- Coordination of the movement is made possible by opposing voluntary muscle groups and neuromuscular reflexes.
- Use the stronger, larger and longer muscles of the body which include the shoulders, upper arms, thighs and hips to reduce muscle strain.
- While lifting, moving or carrying an object, keep it close to the body to prevent unnecessary strain on the muscle and to bring the center of gravity of the object close to the center of gravity of the body.

IMMOBILITY

Effect of Immobility on Musculoskeletal System

- Atrophy of the muscles
- Contractures
- Foot drop
- Wrist drop

Effect on Integumentay System

- Pressure ulcer
- Shear

- Excoriation
- Maceration

Effect on Cardiovascular System

- Orthostatic hypotension
- Deep vein thrombosis (DVT)
- Pulmonary embolism

Effect on Respiratory System

- Hypostatic pneumonia

Effect on GIT

- Anorexia
- Hypomotility and constipation

Effect on Genitourinary System

- Urinary tract infection (UTI)
- Renal calculi

EXERCISE

Exercise may be classified as:

1. Based on the source of energy—aerobic/anaerobic.
2. Based on the muscle tension required—isotonic/isometric/isokinetic.

Aerobic exercise: Increases the oxygen consumption thereby promoting cardiovascular conditioning and health of the lungs.

Anaerobic exercise: When the muscle cannot extract enough oxygen from the blood, anaerobic pathways are used to provide energy for a short time. All exercise can become anaerobic when oxygen sources are depleted.

Isotonic exercise: There is constant muscle tension, muscle contraction and active movement.

Isometric exercise: There is muscle contraction, but no movement of the muscle. Muscles are tightened and relaxed, pull or push against something that does not move.

Isokinetic exercise: Involves muscle contraction or tension against resistance.

COMFORT MEASURES

Different position and comfort devices are used to promote comfort of the client.

> Shearing of layers of skin occurs when the skin is dragged across a hard surface and leads to skin breakdown and ulceration. So lift not to drag client while changing the position.

Common Positions Used

1. Prone: Face down, lie on abdomen
2. Supine: Lying on back
3. High fowlers: Head of bed elevated to 90°
4. Semifowlers: Head of bed elevated to 45°
5. Low fowlers: Head of bed elevated to 30°
6. Dorsal recumbent: Supine with legs flexed in an elevated position.
7. Knee-chest: Rests on knees and chest.
8. Trendelenburg: Supine with head lower than the feet.
9. Lateral position: Side lying position.
10. Sim's position: Position between prone and side lying position.
11. Orthopneic position or cardiac position: Sitting position with backrest and pillows, client lean forward on an over bed table.
12. Lithotomy position: Supine position with hips flexed and calves and heels parallel to the floor.

ENEMA

Introduction of fluid into the lower bowel through the rectum for the purpose of clearing or to introduce medication or nourishment.

Classification of Enema

A. **Evacuant Enema**
   - Simple
   - Medicated (oil, purgative, astringent, anthelmintic, carminative enema)
   - Cold

B. **Retained enema:** Stimulant, nutrient, emollient, sedative, anesthetic enema.

Key Points

Size of the catheter: Adult 22 FS, children 14 to 18 FS, infant 12 FS.

Temperature: For evacuant enema temperature should be 105° to 110°F for adult and 100°F for children.

> Retained enema should be given at the body temperature.

Amount of solution: Depends upon the type of enema, age and size of the person. For evacuant enema 500 mL for adult, 250 to 500 mL for child, 250 mL or less for infant.

> For retained enema, do not give more than 100–150 mL at a time.

Position: Left lateral position

Insertion of tube: 3 to 4 inches for adult, 1 to 1.5 inches for children.

Height of the enema can: For cleansing enema, height should not be above 18 inches from the cot and for retention enema it should not be above 8 inches.

Solutions Used

Simple evacuant enema: Soap and water, normal saline

Oil enema: Olive oil, castor oil, gingelli oil

Purgative enema: Glycerin, glycerin and water, glycerin and castor oil.

HOT AND COLD APPLICATIONS

Hot Application

A. Local heat

Dry: Hot water bag, IR rays, heating lamps, electric heating pads

Moist: Hot fomentation, warm soaks, Sitz bath.

B. General

Dry: Sunbath, electric cradle, blanket bed

Moist: Steam bath, hot packs, immersion bath.

Therapeutic Uses of Hot Application

- Decreases pain
- Decreases muscle tone
- Promotes healing
- Promotes suppuration
- Relieves deep congestion
- Softens the exudates
- Provides warmth
- Stimulates peristalsis.

Contraindications

- Malignancies
- Serious kidney, heart and lung problems
- Acute inflammation
- Weak, paralyzed client
- Open wounds, bleeding, edema
- Patients who cannot communicate.

> While using hot water bottle, the temperature of the water should be between 120° and 149°F.

Recommended distance for heating lamps	
25 watt bulb	35 cm from body part
40 watt bulb	45 cm from body part
60 watt bulb	60–75 cm from body part

Cold Application

A. Local cold application

Dry: Ice bag, ice collar, ice pack

Moist: Cold compress, ice to suck.

B. General cold application

Dry: Hypothermia blanket

Moist: Cold sponging, cold bath, cold packs

Therapeutic Uses of Cold Application

- Relieves pain
- Prevents gangrene
- Reduce edema and inflammation
- Controls hemorrhage
- Checks growth of bacteria
- Reduces body temperature
- Anesthetic effect.

Contraindications

- Shock and collapse
- Clients with impaired sensation
- Muscle spasm
- Infected wound
- Low body temperature, shivering.

> While doing tepid sponging, the temperature of the water should be kept between 85 and 100°F.

ADMINISTRATION OF MEDICATIONS

Common drug preparations	
Aqueous	Drugs dissolved in water
Caplet	Tablet coated with gelatin
Capsule	Drug encased in a hard or soft outer case
Elixir	Drugs dissolved in water, alcohol solution, sweetening agent, etc.

Contd...

Contd...

Emulsion	Drug in which one liquid is spread by means of small droplet over another liquid or dispersions of fat globules in water
Enteric coated tablets	Tablets coated with substances that blocks absorption of drug until it reaches the small intestine
Liniments	Mixture of drugs with oil, soap, water or alcohol that is applied on the skin
Lotion	Drugs in liquid suspension intended for external use
Lozenges	Drugs in sweet base that is released as the base dissolves in mouth
Ointment	Drug in vaseline base that is applied to and absorbed by the skin
Poultice	Soft moist preparations that supply moist heat to the body
Suppository	Drug mixed in a firm base and shaped for insertion into the body cavities such as rectum, vagina, etc.
Suspension	Undissolved particles of drug placed in a liquid
Syrup	Drug dissolved in a solution containing water and sugar
Tincture	Alcoholic or hydroalcoholic solution prepared from drugs derived from plants

Abbreviations used regarding time of administration

Abbreviation	Meaning
ac	before meals
pc	after meals
am	before noon
pm	after noon
om	each morning
od	once a day
hs	at bedtime
cm	tomorrow morning
prn	when required
sos	in emergency
bd or bid	twice a day
tds or tid	thrice a day
qid	four times a day
stat	at once
q	every
h	hour

Routes of Drug Administration

1. **Oral administration:** Drug is administered orally.
2. **Sublingual administration:** Drug is placed under the tongue where it dissolves and get absorbed.
3. **Inhalation:** Client inhales fumes of volatile drugs.
4. **Inunctions:** Application of drug to the skin with friction.
5. **Instillation:** Putting a drug in the liquid form into the body cavity.
6. **Insertion:** Introducing solid forms of drug into the body orifices.
7. **Insufflation:** Administration of drug in the form of powder, vapor or air by using an insufflator.
8. **Implantation:** Putting in of solid drugs into the body tissues.
9. **Parenteral administration**
   a. Intramuscular
   b. Intradermal
   c. Subcutaneous
   d. Intravenous
   e. Intra-arterial
   f. Intracardiac
   g. Intrathecal—into the spinal cavity
   h. Intraosseous—into the bone
   i. Intraperitoneal—into the peritoneal cavity.

Preparation of Solution Using the Formula

Strength of a solution required =

$$\frac{\text{Desired strength}}{\text{Strength available}} \times \frac{\text{Quantity}}{\text{required}}$$

For example: Prepare 5000 mL of 2% solution from 10% solution

Ans: $\frac{2/100}{10/100} \times 5000 = 1000$ mL

Take 1000 mL of 10% solution and mix with 4000 mL of water to for 5000 mL of 2% solution.

Calculating Drops Per Minute

$$\frac{\text{Amount of solution} \times \text{Drop factor}}{\text{Time in minutes}}$$

Drop factor is 15 for ordinary drip set and 60 for micro drip set.

For example: 1000 mL of DNS should be given within 10 hours. Calculate the number of drops per minute.

Ans: $\frac{1000 \times 15}{10 \times 60} = 25$ drops/minute

Five Rights of Medicine Administration

- Right client
- Right drug
- Right dose
- Right time
- Right method.

Site of IM injection	Muscle used
Upper arm	Deltoid
Thigh	Vastus lateralis
	Rectus femoris
Buttocks	Gluteus

Route of administration	Size of needle in gauge
Intradermal	26 or 27
Subcutaneous	25
Intramuscular	21, 22, 23
Intravenous	18–21

Type of injection	Angle of insertion
Intramuscular	90°
Subcutaneous	45°
Intradermal	15°

OBJECTIVE QUESTIONS

1. **Sudden severe attack of shivering in which the body temperature rises rapidly**
   a. Stadium b. Fastigium
   c. Crisis d. Rigor
2. **Florence Nightingale was born on**
   a. 12th May b. 10th May
   c. 15th June d. 12th June
3. **Backflow of partly digested food into the mouth from the stomach is**
   a. Vomiting b. Nausea
   c. Regurgitation d. Dyspepsia
4. **Lack of oxygen in the blood stream is**
   a. Anoxemia b. Anoxia
   c. Asphyxia d. Hypoxia
5. **The most preferred site for IM injection for the children**
   a. Ventrogluteal site b. Vastuslateralis site
   c. Middeltoid site d. Dorsalgluteal site
6. **Acetone in urine is tested by**
   a. Smith's test b. Hey's test
   c. Rothera's test d. Benedict's test
7. **Substances used to counteract the effect of poison**
   a. Antidotes b. Antiseptics
   c. Antibiotics d. Antifungal
8. **One ounce is equal to**
   a. 60 mL b. 30 mL
   c. 15 mL d. 45 mL
9. **Hospital acquired infection is known as**
   a. Droplet infection b. Opportunistic infection
   c. Nosocomial infection d. Contamination
10. **Application of the drug to the skin by friction is called**
    a. Instillation b. Insertion
    c. Insufflation d. Inunction
11. **Bland diet is used for patients with**
    a. Diabetes mellitus
    b. Gastrointestinal disturbances
    c. Hypertension
    d. Cardiac disorders
12. **An increase in the depth of respiration**
    a. Orthopnea b. Apnea
    c. Hyperpnea d. Dyspnea
13. **The term stomatitis is**
    a. Inflammation of the stomach
    b. Inflammation of the mouth
    c. Inflammation of the lungs
    d. Inflammation of the gums
14. **The temperature for the sponge bath**
    a. 110°–115°F b. 100°–110°F
    c. 90°–100°F d. 120°–125°F

15. Disinfection means

a. Destroying all pathogenic microorganisms
b. Inhibiting growth of microorganisms
c. Killing only bacteria
d. Destroying all microorganisms

16. Sterilizing articles by means of steam under pressure is known as

a. Boiling b. Autoclaving
c. Pasteurization d. Incineration

17. Calculation of pediatric dosage of medicine is by using

a. Young's rule b. Clark's rule
c. Fried's rule d. All the above

18. Difficulty in getting off to sleep or in maintaining sleep is called

a. Amnesia b. Narcolepsy
c. Insomnia d. Hypersomnia

19. Moving a part of the body to note the flexibility

a. Percussion b. Palpation
c. Auscultation d. Manipulation

20. Primary effect of cold application

a. Vasodilation b. Violation
c. Ventilation d. Vasoconstriction

21. Tapping an area to elicit sound is termed as

a. Percussion b. Palpation
c. Observation d. Auscultation

22. Which of the following drug will soften, soothe and protect mucous membrane?

a. Emollient b. Caustics
c. Demulcents d. Astringent

23. Expectoration of blood stained sputum is termed

a. Hematuria b. Hematoma
c. Hemoptysis d. Hematemesis

24. Environmental barrier of communication is

a. Noise b. Deafness
c. Loss of concentration d. Loss of attention

25. Painful micturition is called

a. Dysuria b. Anuria
c. Glycosuria d. Oliguria

26. Complication of prolonged bed rest include

a. Fever b. Pain
c. Renal stone d. Jaundice

27. The administration of a medicine just below the skin is called

a. Intradermal b. Subcutaneous
c. Intramuscular d. Intrathecal

28. The best method of sterilizing gloves

a. Boiling b. Drying
c. Soaking d. Steam under pressure

29. Application of drug in liquid form into a body cavity

a. Inunction b. Instillation
c. Insertion d. Implantation

30. Pulse pressure is

a. Difference between systolic and diastolic pressure
b. Diastolic pressure
c. Aortic pressure
d. Systolic pressure

31. Device used to raise the head or foot end of bed

a. Bed cradle b. Bed block
c. Sand bag d. Foot rest

32. Which of the following bed is very useful to prevent bed sore

a. Fracture bed b. Blanket bed
c. Occupied bed d. Water bed

33. Rectal temperature is higher than the oral temperature:

a. 0.5°F b. 1.5°C
c. 1°C d. 1°F

34. Anorexia means

a. Indigestion b. Feeling of fullness
c. Loss of appetite d. Back flow of food

35. A patient is to receive 2000 mL of IV fluid in 12 hours. The drop factor is 10 drops per mL. The nurse should regulate the flow so the number of drops per minute is approximately

a. 27–29 b. 30–32
c. 40–42 d. 48–50

36. One tea spoon is equal to

a. 5 mL b. 1 mL
c. 0.5 mL d. 10 mL

37. The term bradycardia means

a. Grossly irregular heart beat
b. A heart rate over 90 per minute
c. A heart rate less than 60 per minute
d. A heart beat that has regular skipped beats

38. **How much salt must be added to one liter of water to make a solution of normal saline (0.9%)**
   a. 19 gm   b. 0.9 gm
   c. 9 gm   d. 90 gm

39. **The best time to collect sputum specimen**
   a. Before brushing teeth in the morning
   b. After an antiseptic mouthwash
   c. After nebulization
   d. After steam inhalation

40. **Reagent used for urine sugar test**
   a. Acetic acid   b. Benedict's solution
   c. Gentian violet   d. Methylene blue

41. **Nurse's day celebrated on**
   a. April 7th   b. August 15th
   c. May 12th   d. December 15th

42. **The process of destroying microorganisms including spores is**
   a. Disinfection   b. Sterilization
   c. Infection control   d. Isolation

43. **The term used for generalized edema is**
   a. Anasarca   b. Pitting edema
   c. Periorbital edema   d. Septicemia

44. **The pH of fresh urine is about**
   a. 7.1   b. 5.0
   c. 8.4   d. 9.9

45. **Sand bags are used to prevent**
   a. Foot drop
   b. Wrist drop
   c. Internal rotation of thigh
   d. All of them

46. **Temperature of water for preparing hot water bag is**
   a. 60°–65°C   b. 65°–70°C
   c. 70°–75°C   d. 90°–100°C

47. **The chemical agent used for testing albumin in urine**
   a. Iodine   b. Sulphur powder
   c. Sodium nitroprusside   d. Acetic acid

48. **Temperature, pulse, respiration and BP are called**
   a. Vital statistics   b. Vital functions
   c. Vital signs   d. Vital symptoms

49. **Glycerine enema is an example of**
   a. Astringent enema   b. Purgative enema
   c. Emolient enema   d. Retention enema

50. **Cracking or ulceration of lips and angles of mouth**
   a. Halitosis   b. Glossitis
   c. Stomatitis   d. Cheilosis

51. **For administering 3000 mL of fluid for 24 hours, the flow rate is**
   a. 31 drops/mt   b. 15 drops/mt
   c. 45 drops/mt   d. 52 drops/mt

52. **Separation of an infected person from noninfected persons**
   a. Incubation   b. Isolation
   c. Inoculation   d. Immunization

53. **The best method of refuse disposal in a hospital is**
   a. Dumping   b. Controlled tipping
   c. Incineration   d. Composting

54. **Gastric lavage is contraindicated after ingestion of which of the following**
   a. Aspirin
   b. Organophosphorus compound
   c. Corrosive alkali
   d. Odolum

55. **Abbreviation of 'od' denotes**
   a. Once a day   b. At bed time
   c. Whenever necessary   d. After meals

56. **One teaspoon is approximately**
   a. 50 drops   b. 75 drops
   c. 100 drops   d. 120 drops

57. **Exercises that a patient does for himself**
   a. Passive exercises   b. Isotonic exercise
   c. Isometric exercises   d. Active exercises

58. **Pyorrhea is**
   a. Foul smelling breath   b. Bleeding gums
   c. Pus in the sockets of teethd.Brown crusts on the teeth

59. **Nature's toothbrush**
   a. Coal   b. Neem stick
   c. Drum stick   d. Food

60. **Antibiotics are the drugs used to treat**
   a. Infection   b. Inflammation
   c. Pain   d. Itching

61. **A harsh, vibrating, shrill sound produced during respiration seen in laryngitis is**
   a. Rale   b. Wheeze
   c. Stertorous   d. Stridor

62. Step of nursing process that includes the statement of the client's actual or potential health problems

a. Assessment b. Nursing diagnoses
c. Planning d. Implementation

63. Implementation of the nursing process involves

a. Data collection
b. Formulating nursing problems
c. Giving actual nursing care
d. Evaluation of care given

64. Examination with the help of stethoscope

a. Inspection b. Percussion
c. Palpation d. Auscultation

65. Isotonic saline means saline having a concentration of

a. 0.45 % b. 0.5 %
c. 0.1 % d. 0.9 %

66. Presence of sugar in urine

a. Oliguria b. Glycosuria
c. Hematuria d. Pyuria

67. The year in which Florence Nightingale was born

a. 1620 b. 1720
c. 1820 d. 1920

68. Position used for taking rectal temperature

a. Supine b. Right lateral
c. Left lateral d. Prone

69. Immediate disinfection of all contaminated articles during the course of a disease

a. Sterilization b. Fumigation
c. Concurrent disinfection d. Terminal disinfection

70. Oral medication cannot be given to a client having

a. Vomiting b. Diarrhea
c. Abdominal distention d. Abdominal pain

71. For effective sterilization in the autoclave, the temperature should be

a. 115°F b. 115°C
c. 121°F d. 121°C

72. In hyperpyrexia, the body temperature is

a. Between 99°–100°F b. Between 100°–103°F
c. Above 103°F d. Above 105°F

73. The sudden fall of temperature to normal is called

a. Crisis b. Lysis
c. Fastigium d. Stadium

74. When the body temperature falls below 95°F, it is called

a. Hyperthermia b. Hypothermia
c. Subnormal temperature d. High pyrexia

75. Total cessation of breathing

a. Eupnea b. Apnea
c. Hyperpnea d. Tachypnea

76. A condition in which bacterial growth is checked

a. Bacteriostasis b. Asepsis
c. Bacteriocide d. Antiseptic

77. Destruction of all microorganisms, both pathogenic and nonpathogenic

a. Disinfection b. Sterilization
c. Immunization d. Bacteriostasis

78. Gas sterilization is

a. Disinfection b. Autoclaving
c. Sterilization d. Fumigation

79. Hey's test is used for testing

a. Sugar b. Albumin
c. Acetone d. Bile salts

80. Smith's test is used for

a. Sugar b. Albumin
c. Bile salts d. Bile pigments

81. Brown crusts which are formed on the teeth and lips are called

a. Calculus b. Sordes
c. Enamel d. Dentin

82. A sensation to vomit

a. Heartburn b. Regurgitation
c. Nausea d. Pyrosis

83. Pus in urine

a. Hematuria b. Pyuria
c. Dysuria d. Polyuria

84. The angle of insertion for IM injection

a. 15° b. 25°
c. 45° d. 90°

85. Cone shaped fusible medicated mass

a. Carminative b. Pills
c. Lozenges d. Suppository

86. Visual examination of the body

a. Inspection b. Palpation
c. Percussion d. Auscultation

87. Gradual decline of body temperature

a. True crisis b. False crisis
c. Lysis d. Fastigium

88. Small quantity of a substance or object which shows the kind and quality of the whole

a. Model b. Specimen
c. Poultice d. Emulsion

89. Drugs in sweet base that is released as the base dissolves in mouth

a. Emulsion b. Lotion
c. Lozenges d. Tincture

90. prn means

a. When required b. One daily
c. Before food d. After food

91. Introduction of fluid into the lower bowel through the rectum

a. Gastric lavage b. Gastric gavage
c. Enema d. Purgative

92. Abnormal increased convexity in the thoracic spine

a. Lordosis b. Scoliosis
c. Kyphosis d. Atrophy

93. A high pitched, musical, whistling sound due to partial obstruction of smaller bronchi and bronchioles

a. Rale
b. Wheeze
c. Stridor
d. Cheyne-Stokes respiration

94. The normal rate of respiration is an adult

a. 10–12 breaths per minute
b. 16–20 breaths per minute
c. 20–24 breaths per minute
d. > 24 breaths per minute

95. Irregular rhythm pulse in which there is a weak second or premature beat

a. Paradoxical pulse b. Bigeminal pulse
c. Pulsus alternans d. Dicrotic pulse

96. A pulse in which force or strength of the pulse becomes weaker during inspiration

a. Paradoxical pulse b. Bigeminal pulse
c. Pulsus alternans d. Dicrotic pulse

97. Yellowish film of calcium phosphate, calcium carbonate, food particles and other organic matter deposited on the teeth

a. Calculus b. Tartar
c. Sordes d. Cheilosis

98. The specific gravity of urine is

a. 1.000 to 1.010 b. 1.010 to 1.020
c. 1.020 to 1.030 d. 1.030 to 1.040

99. Cidex is

a. Formaldehyde b. Dettol
c. Savlon d. Glutaraldehyde

100. Observable, perceptible and measurable data

a. Subjective data b. Objective data
c. Primary data d. Secondary data

ANSWER KEY

1. d	2. a	3. c	4. a	5. b	6. c	7. a	8. b	9. c	10. d	11. b	12. c
13. b	14. b	15. d	16. b	17. d	18. c	19. d	20. d	21. a	22. a	23. c	24. a
25. a	26. c	27. b	28. d	29. b	30. a	31. b	32. d	33. d	34. c	35. b	36. a
37. c	38. c	39. a	40. b	41. c	42. b	43. a	44. b	45. a	46. b	47. d	48. c
49. c	50. d	51. a	52. b	53. c	54. c	55. a	56. b	57. d	58. c	59. b	60. a
61. d	62. b	63. c	64. d	65. d	66. b	67. c	68. c	69. c	70. a	71. d	72. d
73. a	74. b	75. b	76. a	77. b	78. d	79. d	80. d	81. b	82. c	83. b	84. d
85. d	86. a	87. c	88. b	89. c	90. a	91. c	92. c	93. b	94. b	95. b	96. a
97. a	98. b	99. d	100. b								

Chapter 3

Mental Health Nursing

PERSONALITY

- Sum of all traits that differentiate one individual from another.
- Total behavior pattern of an individual through which the inner interests are expressed.
- The individual's unique and distinctive way of behaving and relating with others.
- Constellation of defense mechanism for dealing with inner and outer pressures.

> Personality is the sum of all traits that differentiate one individual from another.

Factors Involved in Personality Development

a. Behavior develops as a result of part experiences.

b. These past experiences are organized in the psyche on three different levels viz. conscious, subconscious, unconscious.

Conscious: Core composed of past experiences that are easily recalled, that creates little trauma if any emotional discomfort and tend to be somewhat pleasant.

Subconscious: Core composed of materials that has been deliberately pushed out of conscious but can be recalled with some effort.

Unconscious: Contains the largest body of material and cannot bring into awareness, since it is usually unacceptable and painful to the individual.

c. **According to Sigmund Freud**, the personality consists of three parts: id, ego and superego.

Id: Contains the instincts, impulses and urges, is totally self centered and conscious.

Ego: Is the conscious self, deals with reality, the part of the personality that is shown to the environment.

Superego: Controls, inhibits and regulates impulses and instructs whose uncontrolled expression would endanger the emotional well being of the individual and stability of the society.

> According to Sigmund Freud, the personality consists of three parts viz. id, ego and superego.

ANXIETY AND BEHAVIOR

Anxiety is a state of apprehension, tension or uneasiness; is the internal phenomenon aroused by impulses; occurs when ego is threatened; may arise from known, unknown or recognized sources.

> Anxiety is a state of apprehension, tension or uneasiness.

Levels of Anxiety

- **Alertness level:** Automatic response of the central nervous system (CNS) that prepares the body for danger by regulating internal processes.
- **Apprehension level:** Response to anticipation of short-term danger that prepares the individual for efficient performance and creates some conscious awareness of discomfort.
- **Free-floating level:** Response to generalized anxiety that creates a feeling of impending doom and produces on acute feeling of discomfort.
- **Panic level:** Total response to anxiety characterized by uncontrolled, unrealistic behavior that lessens the perception of the environment to protect the ego from awareness.

Behavioral Defenses Against Anxiety

- **Conscious:** These are the first line defenses against anxiety, used by all people in times of stress, comprise the individual's deliberate effort to maintain, control, reduce tension and limit anxiety.
- **Unconscious:** These include the second, third and fourth line defenses against anxiety, may be used by all people in extremely stressful situation, but if used constantly, indicate that the individual is emotionally ill.

DEFENSE MECHANISMS

- Defense mechanisms provide initial protection for the personality.
- Although all individuals may, in times of severe emotional stress, use many of the behaviors, defense mechanism is the repetitive use of these behaviors.
- Identifiable patterns of response begin to from when individuals respond to most situations they encounter with the same type of behavior.
- Commonly used defense mechanism that help an individual to deal with reality are:
  a. **Identification:** The individual internalizes the characteristics of an idealized person.
  b. **Substitution**: The individual replaces one goal for another.
  c. **Compensation:** The individual makes up for a perceived lack in one area by emphasizing capabilities in another.
  d. **Sublimation:** A socially acceptable behavior is substituted for an acceptable instinct; this is used when the expression of these instincts would prove a threat to the self.
  e. **Compromise:** Reciprocal give and take; necessary in many relationships to salvage some part of the situation or the goal.
  f. **Rationalization:** The individual make acceptable excuses for behavior and feelings, attempts to explain behavior by logical reasoning.
  g. **Conversion:** Emotional conflict is consciously changed into physical symptom that into expressed openly and without anxiety.
  h. **Denial:** Emotional conflict is blocked from the conscious mind and the individual refuses to recognize its existence.
  i. **Displacement:** Emotions related to an emotionally changed situation or objects are shifted to a relatively safe substitute situation or object.
  j. **Fantasy:** Conscious distortion of unconscious wishes and needs to obtain gratification and satisfaction.
  k. **Projection:** Unconscious denial of unacceptable feelings and emotions in oneself while attributing turn to other.
  l. **Reaction formation:** The individual unconsciously reverses inacceptable feelings and behaves in the exact opposite manner.
  m. **Regression:** Return to an earlier stage of behavior when stress creates problems at the present stage.
  n. **Repression:** Involuntary exclusion from consciousness of those ideas, feelings and situation that are creating conflict and causing discomfort.
  o. **Suppression:** Voluntary exclusion from unconsciousness of those ideas, feelings and situation that are creating conflict and causing discomfort.
  p. **Transference:** Positive or negative feelings and emotions that were previously present toward important figures are applied and attributed to another person in the present.
  q. **Intellectualization:** Use of thinking ideas, or intellect to avoid emotions.
  r. **Introjections:** Complete acceptance of another opinions and values as one's own.

DEVIANT PATTERNS OF BEHAVIOR

a. **Withdrawn Behavior:** Pathologic retreat from, or an avoidance of people and the world of reality.
b. **Projective Behavior:** Pathologic denial of one's own feelings, faults, failures and emotions while continually attributing them to other.
c. **Aggressive Behavior:** Pathologic anger and hostility that are turned outward onto others or inward on oneself.
d. **Neurotic Behavior:** Includes anxiety reactions, conversion reactions, phobic reactions and obsessive compulsive reactions.
e. **Socially Aggressive Behavior:** Maladjustive response resulting from a defect in the development of the personality that is characterized by peculiar actions or misbehavior.
f. **Addictive Behavior:** Repeated or chronic use of alcohol or drugs with a resulting dependency on these substances.
g. **Self Destructive Behavior:** Chronically indulging in self destructive behavior, by non-compromise with medical regimens habitually abusing food, drugs, alcohol, or cigarettes or engaging in high-risk activities.

BASIC PRINCIPLES IN PSYCHIATRIC NURSING

- Accept and respect people as individuals regardless of their behavior.
- Limit or reject the individuals in appropriate behavior without rejecting the individual.
- Recognize that all behavior has meaning and is meeting the needs of the performer regardless of appears to others.
- Accept the dependency heads of the individuals while supporting and encouraging more towards independence.
- Help individuals to express their feeling in an atmosphere free of reprisal or judgment.

- Recognize that individuals need to use defenses until other defenses can be substituted.
- Recognize how feelings affect behavior and influence relationship.
- Recognize that individuals frequently respond to the behavioral expectation of others viz. family, peers and coworkers.
- Recognize that all individuals have a potential for movement toward higher levels of emotional health.

THERAPEUTIC NURSE-PATIENT RELATIONSHIP

Phases of Relationship

1. **Orientation or introductory phase:** The nurse establishes a trusting relationship with the client; charts are never pushed to discuss areas of concern that are upsetting to them.
2. **Working phase:** The nurse and client discuss areas of concern and the client is helped to plan, implement and evaluated a nurse of action.
3. **Termination phase:** End of the therapeutic relationship between the nurse and the client, the time parameters should be set early in the relationship with meetings spaced further and further apart near the end.

DRUGS IN EMOTIONAL DISORDERS

Minor Tranquilizers

- Used to produce sedation and relieve anxiety without producing sleep.
- **Acts by** dose related CNS depression with inhibition of limbic and reticular activation system of the brain, many also exerts skeletal muscle relaxation and anticonvulsant effects.
- **Available as** oral and parenteral preparations.
- **Used** when the individual has difficulty in coping with environment stress and accomplishing daily activation.
- **Different drugs available are:**
  - Chlordiazepoxide hydrochloride (Librium)
  - Clorazepate dipotassium (Tranxene)
  - Diazepam (Valium)
  - Hydroxyzine hydrochloride (Atarax)
  - Oxazepam
  - Alprazolam
  - Meprobamate
- **Adverse Effects:** drowsiness, hypotension, muscle relaxation, decreased ability to concentrate, hypersensitivity reaction.

> Minor tranquilizers are used to produce sedation and relieve anxiety without producing sleep.

Major Tranquilizers

- **Used** to alter the symptoms of individuals experiencing detachment, from reality and having the potential for manifesting destructive behavior.
- **Act by** blocking dopamine receptors in the CNS and sympathetic nervous system activity, some also exert antiemetic, anticholinergic, antihistaminic effects.
- **Available** in oral and parental form.
- **Used** when the individual is incapable of coping with environmental stress and accomplishing daily activities.
- Major tranquilizers control behavior when the clients controlled action are destructive to self, others and the environment.
- **Drugs available are**
  - Chlorpromezine hydrochloride
  - Fluphenazine hydrochloride
  - Perphenazine
  - Prochlorperazine
  - Thioridazine
  - Trifluoperazine
  - Fluphenzine decanoate injection
  - Haloperidol
  - Chlorprothixene
  - Thiothixene
- **Adverse effects:** Agranulocytosis, jaundice, signs of extrapyramidal tract irritation, drowsiness, orthostatic hypotension, constipation, urinary retention, anorexic, hypersensitivity reactions, photo-allergic reaction, cessation of ovulation and menstruation, impotence, cardiac toxicity.

Extrapyramidal symptom: Acute dystonic reactions, pseudoparkinsonism, akinesis (weakness of arms and legs), akathesia (motor restlessness), tardive dyskinesia (involuntary movement of face, jaw and tongue). Antiparkinsonian drugs are used to treat extrapyramidal symptom, e.g. benztropine, diphenhydramine and trihexyphenidyl.

> Major tranquilizers are used to alter the symptoms of individuals experiencing detachment from reality and having the potential for manifesting destructive behavior.

Antidepressants

- Used to improve the general behavior and mood of clients experiencing depressive episodes.
- Antidepressant drugs increase the level of norepinephrine at subcortical neuroeffector sites.
- Available in oral and parenteral form.
- Norepinephrine blockers provide elevated levels of the neurohormone by preventing reuptake and storage at the axon (tricyclic compounds).
- Monoamine oxidase inhibitors (MAO inhibitors) elevate norepinephrine levels in brain tissues by interfering with the enzyme MAO, act as psychic energizers.
- Fluoxetine hydrochloride promoters the uptake of serotonin in the CNS.

Types

1. Norepinephrine blockers

- Amitriptyline hydrochloride
- Doxepin hydrochloride
- Imipramine hydrochloride
- Nortriptyline hydrochloride

2. MAO inhibitors

- Isocarboxazid
- Phenelzine sulfate
- Tranyl cypromine sulfate

3. Fluoxetine hydrochloride

Adverse effects of norepinephrine blockers: Orthostatic hypertension, skin rash, drowsiness, dry mouth, blurred vision, constipation, urinary retention, tachycardia, CNS stimulation, nightmares, delusion, disorientation and insomnia.

Adverse effects of MAO inhibitors: Orthostatic hypotension, skin rash, drowsiness, dry mouth, blurred vision, constipation, urinary retention, tachycardia, sexual dysfunction, nightmares, delusions, disorientation, insomnia.

Adverse effects of Fluoxetine: Insomnia, headache, flu like syndrome, dry mouth and sexual dysfunction.

Lithium

- Used to control the manic episode of mood disorders.
- Acts by reducing adrenergic neurotransmitter levels in cerebral tissue through alteration of sodium transport.
- Available in tablets, capsules, liquid preparation.
- Improves productivity by decreasing psychomotor activity or response to environment stimuli.
- Norepinephrine uptake accelerator that alters sodium transport in nerve and muscle cells and affects a shift in intraneural metabolism of norepinephrine.
- **Adverse effects of Lithium:** Excess voiding and extreme thirst caused by drug suppression of antidiuretic hormone (ADH) function, which causes dehydration; slurred speech, disorientation, confusion, cogwheel rigidity, ataxia, renal failure, respiratory depression, and coma are toxic side effects.
- Therapeutic blood level of lithium—0.6–1.2 mEq/L.

> Diarrhea, vomiting, tremors, drowsiness, muscle weakness and ataxia are signs and symptoms of lithium toxicity.

> A patient on lithium therapy should maintain a fluid intake of 2500–3000 mL per day to promote adequate lithium excretion.

> Therapeutic blood level of lithium is 0.6–1.2 mEq/L.

Drugs that Produce Sedation and Sleep

- Sedation and hypnotics can be used in addition to tranquilizers for psychiatric and other clients.
- CNS depressants have antianxiety effects in low dosages, produce sleep in high doses and general anesthetic like states in very high dosages.
- All hypnotic drugs probably alter either the character or the duration of REM sleep.

Types

- **Trichloroacetic acid:** Produces natural sleep, e.g. chloral betaine, chloral hydrate.

Adverse effects: Gastric irritation causing diarrhea.

- **Paraldehyde:** Used primarily to diminish hyperactivity in alcoholics or to control convulsions.
- **Phenothiazine derivates:** Act like antihistamines; used for induction of sleep in anxious clients, e.g. methotrimeprazine hydrochloride, promazine hydrochloride.

Adverse effects: Hypotension, dizziness, dry mouth, palpitations, jaundice, extrapyramidal symptoms and agranulocytosis.

- **Barbiturate sedatives:** Most frequently used hypnotics, e.g. hexobarbital, pentobarbital, butabarbital, phenobarbital.

Adverse Effects: Hypersensitivity reactions, morning drowsiness, respiratory depression and hypotension.

- **Other sedatives and hypnotics,** e.g. ethchlorvynol, ethinamate, flurazepam, sodium bromide, glutethimide.

MENTAL RETARDATION

Usually defined as low 1Q (70 or below).

Causes

1. **Prenatal:** Heredity, Down's syndrome, severe malnutrition, rubella, maternal drug use including alcohol.
2. **Natal:** Kernicterus, intracranial hemorrhage, anoxia, physical injury.
3. **Postnatal:** Meningitis, encephalitis, neoplasm, recurrent convulsions.
4. **Metabolic imbalance** in essential nutrients, metabolic or endocrine disorders such as hypothyroidism.

Classification

1. Normal : 1Q 90–110
2. Borderline : 1Q 71–89
3. Mild : 1Q 50–70
4. Moderate : 1Q 35–50
5. Severe : 1Q 20–35
6. Profound : 1Q below 20

Mild MR	:	IQ 50–70
Moderate MR	:	IQ 35–50
Severe MR	:	IQ 20–35
Profound MR	:	IQ below 20

Findings

1. Delayed milestones.
2. Mental abilities limited, cannot learn from errors, cannot carry out complex instructions.
3. Does not relate with peers, more secure with adults, comforted by physical touch.
4. Short attention span, but usually attracted to music.

Major signs of mental retardation include 5 Ds
- Decreased cognitive and intellectual functioning
- Deficits in psychomotor skills
- Difficulties in performing self care activities
- Degrees of neurological impairment

Treatment

- Prevent causes that damage the brain cell.
- Minimize long-term consequence: Treatment of associated problems, infect stimulation, parent education.

PERVASIVE DEVELOPMENTAL DISORDERS

Autistic Disorder

- Failure to develop satisfactory relationships with significant adults, regardless of the cause, appears to be an underlying problem.

Findings

1. An alienation or withdrawal from reality.
2. A severe disturbance in the child's feeling of self identity.
3. Inability to differentiate between self and environment.
4. Confusion in self boundaries frequently characterized by speaking of self only in the third person.
5. A defect in ego formation or an inadequately functioning ego system.
6. A conflict between self and reality.
7. Defect in the adaptive, inhibitory, and steering mechanism of the personality.
8. Child appears to be mentally retarded.
9. Lack of meaningful relationships with outside world.
10. Turning to inanimate objects and self centered activity for security.

Treatment

1. Pychotherapy directed toward the developmental level of the child: Play, group or individual therapy.
2. Medications: Tranquilizers and amphetamines provide some reduction in symptoms.
3. Removal from the home situation, day school situations provide some relief.

DISRUPTIVE BEHAVIOR DISORDERS

Attention Defect Hyperactivity Disorder

- Evident before 7 years of age, testing at least 6 months; behavior reflecting impulsiveness and in alteration, child easily distracted by extraneous stimuli.
- Findings: Inappropriate inattentiveness, excessive impulsiveness, short attention span, squiring and fidgeting, hyperactivity may or may not present.

Children with attention defect hyperactivity disorder (ADHD) may seem disorganized because of their impulsiveness and distractibility. Few have psychotic symptoms such as delusions, hallucinations or thought disorders.

Treatment

1. Structure situation to provide less stimulation.
2. Provide firm and consistent discipline.
3. Psychological counseling.
4. Drugs: Methylphenidate or dextroamphitamine sulfate.

Conduct Disorders

- The child may be socialized or under socialized, may be aggressive or non-aggressive.
- Behavior is destructive to the child's non general aims.

Findings

1. Behavior is repeated despite rational arguments to the contrary and despite punishment
2. Behavior leads to getting caught and punished.
3. Behavior includes stealing, arguency, running away, excessive rebelliousness and physical cruelty to others and animals.
4. Conduct involves discharge of affects stemming from unconscious conflicts.

Treatment

1. Psychological counseling.
2. Milieu therapy.

EATING DISORDERS

Anorexia Nervosa

- Anorexia of food due to excessive concern about obesity, more seen in adolescent girls.

People with eating disorders are preoccupied with their weight and shape.

- Apparent failure to separate from mother and become autonomous, unconscious fear of grouping up.
- Usually triggered by an adolescent crisis.

Findings

1. Weight loss than 85% of expected weight
2. Distorted self image: Appear fat to themselves even when emaciated.
3. Instance fear of becoming fat.
4. Very manipulative, high academic achievers.
5. Frequent disorder in family relationships, especially with mother.
6. Amenorrhea in females.
7. Fatigue, nausea, constipation, emaciation, hypotension, low blood glucose, anemia, low BMR.

Malnutrition may lead to edema and hypokalemia which eventually results in ventricular arrhythmias.

Treatment

1. Behavior modification techniques that focus on client's responsibility for weight gain.
2. Nasogastric and IV fluids if weight loss in severe and if features of malnutrition and fluid electrolyte imbalance present.
3. Psychotherapy, group therapy, family therapy.

Bulimia Nervosa

- Obsession with food results from a morbid fear of obesity and the pathologic need to binge, cannon in adolescent females.

Findings

1. Compulsive eating binges characterized by rapid consumption of excessive amounts of high calorie foods in brief periods followed by induced purging.
2. Periods of severe dieting or fasting between binges.
3. Sporadic vigorness exercising between binges.
4. Weight may be within normal range with frequent fluctuations.
5. Depression and self deprecating thoughts follow binges.
6. Impulsive, extroverted, intermittent substance abuse seen.
7. Treatment same as anorexia nervosa.

Bulimia nervosa is marked by episodes of binge eating followed by feelings of guilt, humiliation, depression and self condemnation.

GENDER DENTITY DISORDERS

1. Persistent discomfort with one's assigned gender and a feeling that it is inappropriate or in accurate.
2. Persistent repudiation of current gender anatomy.
3. Preoccupation with activities and clothing of opposite gender.

Findings

Prepubescent gender identity disorder has intense discomfort with own gender and desires to be the opposite sex or believes that he or she is the opposite sex:

1. Rejects anatomical structures associated with own gender.
2. Cross-dresses and participates in activities associated with opposite sex.
3. Has not reached puberty.

Transsexualism

1. Has intense desire to exchange own sexual characteristics for those of the opposite sex.
2. Complaints of discomfort wearing clothing of assigned sexual role.
3. Has anxiety and depression related to conformity with assigned sexual role.
4. Has reached puberty.
5. Can be asexual, homosexual or heterosexual.

Non-transsexual Type

1. Has no intense desire to acquire sexual characteristics of opposite sex, yet a persistent feeling of discomfort with one's assigned gender.
2. Cross-dressing is practiced but without the purpose of sexual excitement.
3. Anxiety and depression are usually decreases when the person in cross-dressing.
4. Has reached puberty.
5. Can be asexual, homosexual or heterosexual.

Treatment

- Individual or group psychotherapy.
- Anti anxiety drugs needed.

TIC DISORDERS

Classified as gross motor movement disorder

Types

1. Tramient tic disorder.
2. Chronic motor tic disorder.
3. Tourettes' disorder: thought to be familial or genetic.

Findings

1. Involuntary, uncontrolled, multiple, rapid movements of muscles such as eye blinking, twitching and head shaking that occur in bouts throughout the day.
2. Involuntary production of sounds such as throat clearing, grunting, barking, or the utterance of socially unacceptable words is usually associated with Tourtte's disorder.
3. Can often be controlled for short direction, not present during sleep, increased during times of stress.
4. Starts in early childhood.
5. More common in boys than girls.

Treatment

1. Treat any precipitating factor such as head injury, psychoactive substance intoxication, or infection.
2. Supportive individual or group counseling.
3. Medication such as sedation or phenytion may be prescribed although they are not shown to be effective with these disorders.

ELIMINATION DISORDERS

1. Functional encopresis: Involuntary or intentional defecation in inappropriate places, including clothing after the age years 4.
2. More common in boys then girls.

Findings

1. No identifiable physical problems are present.
2. Can occur before toilet training has been accomplished (primary) or after a period of controlled continence (secondary).
3. Nocturnal bedwetting is most frequent; child may or may not be aware of voiding or recall a dream about the act of wine ting.
4. Academic difficulties, loss of self-esteem, rejection by peers and severe anxiety.

Treatment

1. Rule out structural or organic causes.
2. Psychotherapy.
3. Medication such as antidepressants, have been found to be effective with some clients.

SPEECH DISORDERS

- Inability to begin or interruption in normal pattern of speech in the absence of physiological causes.

Types

1. Cluttering: Abnormally rapid, erratic, dysrhythmic, speech pattern that make communication very difficult to follow.
2. Stuttering: Frequent repetition of sounds or syllables impairing speech fluency although child has normal laryngeal skill, usually occurring at the beginning of a word or phrase.

Findings

1. Presence of faulty speech patterns that are persistent and increased by stress.
2. Anxiety, avoidance of social situation, loss of self-esteem.

Treatment

1. Speech therapy.
2. Counseling to reduce anxiety.

ORGANIC MENTAL SYNDROMES AND DISORDERS

- Progressive cerebral impairment and neurological losses, aphasia, apathy and/or withdrawal from others.
- Change in usual communication patters, inability to meet role expectations, inability to meet basic needs, alteration in social participation, high incidence of accidents.
- Sensory perceptual alteration (visual, auditory, kinesthetic, gustatory, tactile, olfactory) related to progressive cerebral impairment and progressive neurological losses.
- Progressive inability to carry out activities of daily living, altered nutrition due to confusion, depression and anorexia.
- Inability to handle situation or events and difficulty making decisions.

Treatment

1. Treat baseline causes.
2. Continually orient the client to time, date and place.
3. Quiet environment to be provided, reduce stimuli.
4. Maintain nutrition.
5. Provide diversional activities.
6. Maintain nonjudgmental attitude.

Delirium

- Syndromes from which client normally recovers since the changes are often reversible and temporary.
- Stressors like infection of CNS, systemic, toxic infection, trauma to the head, circulating impairment, metabolic disorders, ingestion of psychoactive substances or the accumulative CNS effect of prescribed medication, etc. all will precipitate an attack.

Findings

1. Delirium and its accompanying confusion, hallucinations and delusions.
2. Disorientation and confusion to time, place, identity.
3. Memory defects for both recent and remove events and facts.
4. Slurring of speech may occur along with an indistinct pronunciation or use of words.
5. Tremors, in coordination, imbalance and incontinence.
6. Physical symptoms such as depressed respiration, cardiac irregularities and gastrointestinal changes.

Treatment

1. Reduce caustic agent.
2. Prevent further damage.
3. Provide diet high in calories, protein and vitamins.
4. Provide mild sedative if needed.

Dementia

- Syndromes from which the client does not reader, since the damage is irreversible or permanent.
- May be some improvement with treatment of the underlying cause, but disturbances in memory and judgment will remain.

Stressors

Prenatal injury or malformation

1. Infection, trauma of brain.
2. Circulatory disturbances causing anoxia and permanent brain damage (e.g. cerebral arteriosclerosis CVA).
3. Nutritional deprivation of brain cells.
4. Damage may result from generalized diseases (hepatolenticular disease, Parkinson's disease, AIDS).
5. Damage resulting from pressure of braintumors.
6. Toxins.

Findings

1. Disorientation
2. Restlessness
3. Agitation
4. Memory loss
5. Impaired judgment
6. Decreased attention span
7. Inappropriate social behavior
8. Decreased cognitive functioning
9. Resistance to change.

> In vascular dementia, blockage of small blood vessels leads to brain damage and ultimately a gradual mental decline.

Treatment

Same as those for delirium with great emphasis on further damage.

ALZHEIMER'S DISEASE AND DEMENTA OF THE ALZHEIMERS TYPE

- Primary degenerative dementia, senile onset: Occurs after 65 years.
- Primary degenerative dementia presenile onset: Occurs before 65 years.
- **Characteristics**
  1. Atrophy of brain accompanied by widened cortical sulci and enlarges cerebral ventricles.
  2. Microscopic brain damages include senile plaques and a granulo vacuolar degeneration of neurons.
  3. Believed to be related to the brain's inability to produce sufficient neurotransmitters that transmit messages through the brain.
  4. Stressors:
     a. Higher than normal amounts of aluminum deposits found in the brain of clients with Alzheimer's disease.
     b. Immunological defect suspected because of higher titers of antibodies in clients with Alzheimer's disease.
     c. Possible chromosomal defect linked to Down's syndrome.
     d. Previous severe head injury.

Findings

- More common in females.
- Differs from normal changes associated with ageing.
- Dementia has an insidious onset with symptoms following a progressively downhill course; changes are unrelated to any other specific cause.
- Progression moves from mild forgetfulness for recent events to mutism, inability to carry out any activities of daily living, and incontinence, degeneration usually ends in a vegetative state and coma, disease is 100% fatal and death usually occur within 5 years.

Treatment

1. Rule out causes such as electrolyte imbalances, vitamin deficiencies, excessive mediation, and exogenous poisons or metabolic disorders.
2. Provide supportive care including good nutrition and vitamin supplements.

PSYCHOACTIVE SUBSTANCE-INDUCED ORGANIC MENTAL DISORDERS

- CNS directly affected by substances taken nonmedically viz. alcohol, opiates, barbiturates, cocaine, etc. to alter mood and behavior.
- Usually occur in individuals with substance abuse disorders.
- Behavioral changes may be related to a vitamin deficiency, especially in long-term alcohol abuse such as Korsakoffs' syndrome.

Findings

1. Specific neuralgic and psychologic signs and maladaptive behavior such as euphoria, dysphasia, apathy, psychomotor agitation, excitement or depression, hypervigilance, fighting or violent behavior.
2. Symptoms of demerit or delirium may be present depending upon the substance used.
3. Physical symptoms such as depressed respiration, cardiac irregularities and gastrointestinal changes may occur.

Treatment Same as delirium.

PSYCHOACTIVE SUBSTANCE USE DISORDERS

Alcohol Abuse

- Alcohol intake that interferes with normal functioning or is necessary as a prerequisite to normal functioning.
- Premorbid personality utilizes the compensatory mechanisms of the addictive pattern of behavior.

> Alcohol intoxication can be fatal if the blood alcohol level exceeds 400 mg/dL.

Findings

1. **Intoxication:** State in which coordination or speech is impaired and behavior is altered.
2. **Episode excessive drinking:** Becoming intoxicated as infrequently as four times a year; episode may vary in length from hours to days or weeks.
3. **Habitual Excessive drinking:** Becoming intoxicated more than 12 times a year or being recognizably under the influence of alcohol more than once a week even though not considered intoxicated.
4. **Alcohol addictions:** Direct or strong presumptive evidence of dependence on alcohol, demonstrated by withdrawal symptoms or by the inability to so far a dry without drinking; when there is a history of heavy drinking for 3 or more months, the individual is considered addicted to alcohol.
5. **Early symptoms of alcoholism:** Frequent drinking sprees, increased intake, drinking alone or in the early morning, occurrence of blackouts.

Alcohol withdrawal symptoms may include anorexia, nausea, anxiety, fever, insomnia, diaphoresis, agitation, tremor progressing to severe tremulousness and possibly hallucinations and violent behavior. Major motor seizures may occur.

Treatment

1. Should be a multifaceted approach: Social and medical involving group therapy, family therapy, individual therapy.
2. Self help groups such as alcoholics anonymous (AA).
3. Negative conditioning with disulfiram (antabuse), but never without client's consent.
4. Relaxation therapy.

Substance abuse is the repeated use of alcohol or other psychoactive drugs that leads to problems – but not to compulsive use or addiction.

Substance dependence refers to the persistent use of alcohol or other psychoactive drugs despite problems caused by such use.

Drug Dependence

- Misuse of drugs, usually by self-administration, in such a way as to bring about physical, emotional or behavioral changes.
- Stressors include premorbid personality, utilizing compensatory mechanism of the addictive pattern of behavior.
- **Addiction:** Habituation and tolerance of drugs other than alcohol, tobacco and ordinary caffeine containing beverages, medically prescribed drugs are excluded, if they are taken under medical direction; addiction can occur simultaneously to two or more drugs or to alcohol and drugs (poly substance abuse) , lately combined addiction to a multiplicity of drugs has become more common.
- **Habitation:** It may be both physical and psychologic dependency.
- **Tolerance:** Physical dependency to a drug in which the presence of the drug in increasingly higher dosage is needed to achieve the same effect, tolerance can exceed the usual lethal limits of a drug.
- **Potentiation:** Two or more substances interact in the body to produce an effect greater than the sum of the effects of each substance taken alone.
- **Antagonism:** Two or more substances interact in the body to produce an effect less than the sum of the effects of each substance taken along.
- **Withdrawal:** Characteristic pattern of reaction and behavior that occur when the used substance is abruptly stopped or amount taken significantly reduces, withdrawal symptom varies with the specific substance, the amount being used and the length of time the substance has been used and the individual taking the substance.

Tolerence: Decreased response to a drug that comes with repeated use.

Physical dependence: An adaptive state that occurs as a normal physiologic response to repeated drug exposure.

Withdrawal: An uncomfortable syndrome that occurs when tissue and blood levels of the abused substance decrease in a person who has used that substance heavily over a prolonged period.

Intoxication: A reversible substance specific syndrome caused by ingestion of or exposure to that substance.

Findings

1. Needle marks on limbs along the path of a vein.
2. Addicted individuals may laid to wear long sleeved shirts, even in warm weather to mask the needle pricks.
3. Yawning, lacrimation, rhinorrhea and perspiration appear 10–15 hours the last opiate injection, unrealistic high, pronounced depression.
4. Severe abdominal cramps if too much time has elapsed between injections.
5. Physical examination may reveal an underweight, malnourished individual with multiple dental caries and depressed CNS functioning.
6. Job or academic failure, marital conflicts, poor reality test of, personality change.
7. History of violent acting out with total disregard for human life or suffering.
8. History of sterling to support habits.
9. Nasal discharge with possible destruction of nasal septum if cocaine snorting has been practiced.
10. Inability to maintain activities of daily living or fulfill role obligation.
11. Marked tolerance with a progressive need for higher closes to achieve desired effects.
12. Marked let down with a progression to severe depression after cocaine use.
13. Hallucinations, hypervigilance and paranoid ideation with cocaine use.

Treatment

1. Drug over dosage may be treated with narcotic antagonists the nalorphine, naloxone, etc. Nalorphine will increase

respiratory depression if barbiturates have also been used, so naloxone is preferred when in doubt about the substance used. These antagonists completely or partially reverse narcotic depression and may produce an acute withdrawal syndrome by blocking the euphoric and physiologic effects of the narcotic.

2. Treatment for withdrawal symptoms.
3. Antidepressants to block the 'high' from stimulant abuse and diminish the craving for the substance.
4. Clonildine suppresses the narcotic withdrawal symptom and decreases adrenergic excess while opiate receptors return to normal levels. Clonidine should not be used in those addicted individuals who also abuse alcohol or those who have unstable psychiatric or cardiovascular conditions.
5. Decreasing amounts of tranquilizers are often administered to reduce psychologic and psychologic discomfort of withdrawal.
6. High calorie, high protein, high vitamin diet because of poor eating habits.
7. Psychotherapy, family therapy.
8. Vocational counseling.

Schizophrenic Disorders

Schizophrenia refers to a group of severe, disabling psychiatric disorders marked by withdrawal from realty, illogical thanking, possible delusions and hallucinations, and other emotional, behavioral or intellectual disturbances.

Five Subtypes: Catatonic, Paranoid, Disorganizes, Residual and Undifferentiated

1. **Catatonic type:** Picture of withdrawal and distortions in reality testing, accompanied by total ambivalence, which is frequently exhibited in rather unpredictable motor activity, the ambivalence can render movement and decision making impossible, since the individual is unable to decide how or where to move, may literally be frozen in position, akinetic (stuporous)—or forced into aimless hyperkinetic fugue (excited) movements.
2. **Paranoid type:** Uses withdrawal compensatory mechanism to distort intricate delusional system by using the projective pattern of behavior, is secretive and suspicious, uses ideas of reference, finally develop delusion of grandeur.
3. **Disorganized type:** Picture of severe and pronounced mental capacity; great mental and emotional deterioration occurs, behavior is retards, with sexual preoccupations, emotional dulling and infantile silliness, onset is usually between 12 and 25 years of age.
4. **Residual type:** Continues to use many of the compensatory mechanism common to this disorder in the absence of prominent delusions, hallucinations, incoherence, or grossly disorganized behavior.
5. **Undifferentiated type:** Demonstrates the primary thought, affect, and withdrawal defects of schizophrenia but cannot be classified under a specific type because of mixed symptoms.

Findings

1. Alterations in feeling, thinking and relating to the external world.
2. Association defects occur, and association links weaken, the individual appears inherent, bizarre and unpredictable.
3. Distortions interfere with attention, perception, concentration and memory.
4. Affect and emotional expression are flattened.
5. Ambivalence is common and frequently so exaggerated that any actions and decisions become impossible.
6. Detachment from reality results in autistic thinking and serves to further distort reality.
7. Disturbance occurs in body image since the undeveloped ego has few strength and no boundaries, the individual frequently refers to self in the second or third person instead of using the first person.
8. Secondary symptoms such as hallucinations, delusions, confusion, stupor and catatonia may or may not be present.

Patients with schizophrenia have trouble distinguishing reality from fantasy.

Treatment

1. Psychotherapy (individual, family and group counseling).
2. Motivational therapy.
3. Occupational and vocational therapy.
4. Drugs: Antipsychotic drugs (major tranquilizers).

Patients who experience positive symptoms of schizophrenia may have both hallucinations and delusions—especially delusions of paranoia and persecution.

Mood Disorders

- Characterized by a disturbance of mood, encompassing to emotional extreme, individual demonstrates the vehement energy of main, the despair and lethargy of depression or both.

- Bipolar disorders: Presence of one or more manic or hypomanic episodes in a client with a history of depressive episodes; usually a response to a loss, change in life events or role change, biochemical changes occur in the body specifically a disturbance in biogenic amines, cyclic, periodic episodes of acute self-limiting mood swings; can be all manic, all depressed or mixed manic and depressed.

Depressive episode-clinical findings:

1. Triad of symptom with lowering of the mood tone, dejection, slowing of thinking and speech, decrease in psychomotor activity.
2. Insomnia-difficulty in falling asleep and staying asleep, tending to wake early.
3. Decreased appetite.
4. Feelings of guilt and worthlessness.
5. Difficulty in performing daily tasks.
6. Tearful with suicidal ruminations.
7. Speaking slowly using monosyllabic words.
8. Orientation and logic unaffected.
9. Sex drive decreased.
10. Constipation and urinary retention may occur.

Treatment of Depressive Episode

1. Electroconvulsive therapy: Succinylcholine hydrochloride, a depolarizing muscle relaxant causing paralysis, is used to reduce the intensity of muscle contractions during the convulsive state, used most of time for client with recurrent depressions, delusions, suicidal ideations and those who are resisted to drug therapy.
2. High protein, high carbohydrate diet.
3. Psychotherapy.
4. Antidepressant drugs: Increase the level of norepinephrine at subcortical neuroeffector sites.

Manic Episode-Clinical Findings

1. Begin suddenly with rapid acceleration of symptoms.
2. Excessive involvement in pleasurable activities that may have painful consequences.
3. Marked impairment of occupational functioning, social activities or relationships.
4. Mood is elevated, expansive or irritable.
5. Psychomotor agitation.
6. Flight of ideas.
7. Easy distractibility.
8. Difficulty sleeping, decreased need for sleep.
9. Extremely active, always in a hurry.
10. Humor good, although remarks can be caustic, euphoric.
11. Monopolizing conversations, irritability only superficially covered.
12. Orientations clear, but judgment poor.
13. Always planning and scheming.
14. Increased sex drive.
15. Inflated self-esteem, grandiosity.
16. Excessive spending of money.

Treatment of Manic Episode

1. High calorie, high carbohydrate, high protein diet.
2. Psychotherapy.
3. Antmanic drugs.

Major Depression

- No organic factors identified; psychosocial stresses play a role.
- Usually occurs in late twenties but may occur at any age, including infancy.
- **Clinical findings:**
  - Diminished interest or pleasure in all activities.
  - Decreased appetite with weight loss.
  - Psychomotor retardation.
  - Anxiety and tearfulness.
  - Insomnia or hypersomnia.
  - Feelings of worthlessness.
  - In appropriate suits.
  - Interruption in thinking and concentration that may interfere with occupational and social functioning.
  - Recurrent thoughts of death, suicidal ideation with or without a specific plan to carry it out.

> The major signs and symptoms of depression in children and adolescents include SWAP:
> S – School problems
> W – Withdrawal
> A – Alteration in sleep, appetite and energy levels
> P – Physical health problems

Treatment: Same as depressive episode of bipolar disorder

Phobic Disorders

- Uses the compensatory mechanism of the psychoneurotic pattern of behavior.
- Development of phobia usually permits some measure of social adjustment.
- Early life rigid and orderly, begins in early twenties as a result of environmental factors in childhood.

- Pressures of decision making regarding life-style that occur in the early adult years seem to act as precipitating factors.
- Anxiety unconsciously transferred to an inanimate object or situation, which then symbolically represents the conflict and can be avoided.

Findings

1. Anxiety appears when client find themselves in places that threaten their sense of security.
2. Attempts are made to avoid these distressing situations.
3. Depending on the phobic object, the individuals' lifestyle is often greatly hunted.
4. Fear of being trapped, embarrasses or humiliated in social situations.

Types

1. Agoraphobia: Fear of being alone or in public places where help would not be immediately available if necessary; includes tunnels, bridges, crowds, buses and trains.
2. Social phobia: Fear of public speaking or situations in which public scrutiny may occur.
3. Simple phobia: Fear of specific objects, animals or situations.

Treatment

1. Psychotherapy.
2. Family therapy.
3. Group therapy.
4. Behavior modification with exposure to phobic object or situation in controlled doses to provide desensitization.

Obsessive Compulsive Disorder (OCD)

- Uses the compensatory mechanism of the psychoneurotic pattern of behavior.
- Development of the ritual usually permits some measure of social adjustment.
- Commonly begin in early twenty's as a result of environmental factors in childhood.
- Pressures of decision making regarding lifestyle that occur in the early adult years seem to act as precipitating factor.
- Unconscious control of anxiety by the use of rituals and thoughts.

Findings

1. Thoughts persist and become repetitive and obsessive.
2. Thoughts may be turned into compulsions that are repetitive acts of irrational behavior that the individual is emotionally forced to carry out although they serve no rational purpose.
3. Client is indecisive and demonstrates a striving for perfection and superiority.
4. Intellectual and verbal defenses are used.
5. Anxiety and depression may be present in various degrees, particularly if rituals are prevented.

Treatment

1. Individual therapy.
2. Group therapy.
3. Family therapy.
4. Behavior modification to attempt to limit the length and/or the frequency of the ritual.

Post-traumatic Stress Disorder

- Follows a devastating event that is outside the range of usual human experience (e.g. rape, assault, military combat, hostage situations).
- The traumatic event is persistently re-experiences as flash backs, distressing dreams, sense of reliving the experience, or exposure to situations that foster recall of the event.

Findings

1. Feeling of isolation.
2. Difficulty sleeping.
3. Violent outbursts of anger.
4. Depression.
5. Interrupted concentration.
6. Hyper vigilance.

Treatment

1. Individual therapy, group therapy and family therapy.
2. Behavior modification to provide controlled exposure to recall of the event.

Generalized Anxiety Disorder

- Uses the compensatory mechanisms of the psychoneurotic pattern of behavior.
- Development of the anxiety usually permits some measure of social adjustment.
- Commonly begin in early 20s as a result of environmental factors in childhood.
- Pressures of decision making regarding life- style that occur early adult years seem to act as precipitating factors.

- Excessive anxiety and worry about at least two of life situations.

Findings

- Pervasive continuous feeling of free floating anxiety, tension and apprehension.
- Episodes of dyspnea, palpitations, irritability, dizziness, insomnia fainting, weakness, chest pain, trembling and headaches.
- Symptoms usually appear in relation to stress situations such as crowded room, public gatherings, pregnancy and military service.

Treatment

1. Individual therapy.
2. Group therapy.
3. Behavior modification techniques.

Conversion Disorder

- Anxiety unconsciously converted to physical symptoms that are not under voluntary control, these symptoms permit the individual to avoid some unacceptable activity.
- Development of symptoms usually permits some measure of social adjustment.
- Generally begins before 30 years of age.
- Early life often rigid and orderly; physical illness frequently used by the family as an excuse for problems.
- Pressure of decision making regarding lifestyle in early adult years seem to be precipitating factors.

Findings

1. History of lost motor or sensory function without any adequate physical cause (e.g. paralysis, blindness, deafness).
2. Noticeable lack of concern has been labeled 'Labelle indifference'.
3. Impairment may vary over different episodes and does not follow an automatic structure, paralysis or numbness may circle the foot and arm instead of beginning at the joint and is known as 'stocking and glove anesthesia'.
4. The individual appears relieved by symptoms and demonstrates little anxiety when observed.

Treatment

1. Complete medical workup to reassure the individual and rule out medical problems.
2. Psychotherapy, family therapy and group therapy.
3. Sedatives and minor tranquilizers if necessary.
4. Anti-anxiety drugs (minor tranquilizers) used when the individual is incapable of coping with environmental stresses and accomplishing daily activities.

Body Dysmorphic Disorder

- Preoccupation with imagined defect in a normal appearing person (not of delusional intensity).
- Generally begin in early adolescence and lasts several years.
- No predisposing factor in early life or family patterns has been identified.
- A minor defect is grossly exaggerates.

Findings

1. History of multiple visits to plastic surgeons to correct imagined defects.
2. Avoidance of social situation because of anxiety over minor defects.
3. Often exhibits symptom of depression or obsessive compulsive personality traits.

Treatment

Same as conversion disorders.

Hypochondriasis

- Preoccupation with the belief that one has a serious illness because of how physical symptoms are interpreted.
- A positive medical evaluation does not allay their fears.
- Knowledge of symptoms associated with gives disease aids in the clients'.
- Developing a similar set of symptom, leading them to conclude that they have the disease.
- Psychosocial stresses are believed to lead to development of this disorder.
- Usually begins between 20 and 30 years of age.

Findings

1. Misinterpretation and exaggeration of physical symptoms.
2. Inability to accept reassurance even after exhaustive testing and therapy, leads to "doctor-shopping".
3. History of repeated absence from work.
4. Adoption of sick role and invalid lifestyle.

Treatment

Same as conversion disorders.

Sexual Disorders

- Abnormal sexual activities that are directed toward anything or other than consenting adults or are performed under unusual circumstances.
- Fundamental principles in cering for clients with sexual disorders.
    1. Accept the individual as a person in emotional pain.
    2. Avoid punitive remarks/responses.
    3. Protect the individual from others.
    4. Set limits on the individuals' sexual acting out.
    5. Provide diversional activities.

Paraphilias

- Sexual urges or fantasies that are directed toward non-human objects, the pain to self or partner, or children and other no consenting individuals.
- Diagnosis is made when the individual has acted on urges or is extremely distressed by the urges.
- Sexual arousal accompanies paraphiliac fantasies or stimuli.
- Person may or may not be able to function sexually without the paraphiliac fantasy or stimuli.
- May be symptomatic of other personality or psychiatric disorders or may occur as a behavior aberration or a distorted personality.

Types

1. **Fetishism:** Substitution of an inanimate object for the gavials.
2. **Transvestism:** Wearing clothes of the opposite sex to achieve sexual pleasure.
3. **Exhibitionism:** Sexual pleasure obtained by exposing the genitals.
4. **Pedophilia:** Attraction to children as sex objects.
5. **Voyeurism:** Sexual gratification obtained by watching the sexual play of others.
6. **Sadism:** Sexual gratification obtained from cruelty to others.
7. **Masochism:** Sexual gratification obtained from self-suffering.
8. **Frotteurism:** Sexual pleasure obtained by touching or rubbing against a non-consenting person, usually occurs in crowds or in public transportation.
9. **Necrophilia:** Sexual gratification obtained from sexual relationship with a corpse.
10. **Telephone scatologia:** Sexual gratification from or during lewdness on the telephone.

Treatment

1. Rather unsuccessful with these individuals unless they really want to change.
2. If change is desired by the individual, psychotherapy may be effective.

Personality Disorders

- Borderline states characterized by defects in the development of the personality or by pathologic trends in its structure.
- Habitual attitudes and reaction patterns in human relationships develop early in life and form the character structure of the individual.
- In most instances, these behaviors create little discomfort or stress.
- Personality disturbances are, in reality, the selection and utilization of specific defense mechanism that are used so often that they form a life-long pattern of action that, although not normal, is neither neurotic nor psychotic.

Types

1. Paranoid personality disorder
    - Frequent use of projective mechanism.
    - Suspiciousness, fear, irritability, and stubbornness.
    - Reality testing not generally impaired.
2. Schizoid personality disorder
    - Avoidance of meaningful interpersonal relationships.
    - Use of autistic thinking, emotional detachment and daydreaming.
    - Introverted since childhood but maintaining fair contact with reality.
3. Schizotypal personality disorder
    - Unattached, withdrawn.
    - Affectively and intellectually diminished
    - Frequently part of transient groups of society.
4. Antisocial personality disorder
    - Chronic lifelong disturbances that conflict with society's' laws and customs.
    - Unable to postpone gratification.
    - Randomly act out their aggressive egocentric impulses on society.
    - Do not profit from past experience or punishment, live only for the movement.
    - Have the ability to ingratiate themselves but "do not wear well".
    - Are in contact with realty but do not seem to care about it.

5. Borderline personality disorder
   - Unstable and intense interpersonal relationships.
   - Impulsive unpredictable behavior that is potentially self-destructive.
   - Marked mood shifts.
   - Identity disturbances.
   - Chromic feeling of emptiness.
6. Histrionic personality disorder
   - Emotional instability and hyperexcitability.
   - Extroverted and directed toward gaining attention.
   - Vain and deliberately manipulative.
7. Narcissistic personality disorder
   - Over blown sense of importance.
   - Strong need for attention and admiration.
   - Relationships marked by ambivalence.
   - Preoccupation with appearance.
8. Avoidant personality disorder
   - Social discomfort and timidity.
   - Loner, unwilling to get involved with other people.
   - Fear of negative evaluation from others.
9. Department personality disorder
   - Unable to make decisions.
   - Lack of self-confidence.
   - Dependent and submissive.
   - Induces others to assume responsibility.
10. Obsessive compulsive personality disorder
    - Rigidity, over conscientiousness, inordinate capacity for work.
    - Driven by obsessive concerns.
    - Behavior contains many rituals.
11. Passive aggressive personality disorder
    - Rather helpless and indecisive, demonstrating passive obstructionism while clinging and pouting.
    - Frequent outbursts and temper tantrums when frustrated.
    - Often create problems for others.

Treatment

1. Individual therapy.
2. Group and family therapy.
3. Crisis intervention when necessary.
4. Vocational and occupational therapy.

REVIEW QUESTIONS

1. The currently used system for classifying and diagnosing mental disorders was established by the

a. American Nurses Association
b. American Psychiatric Association
c. American Medical Association
d. State Board of Nursing

2. Over the course of a day, the patient may exhibit changes in

a. Orientation b. Affect
c. Mood d. Consciousness.

3. The mental status examination (MSE) investigates all of the following except the patient's

a. Mood, affect and perceptions
b. ADL
c. LOC
d. Medication effects

4. A preoccupation that is acted out is called

a. A compulsion b. An obsession
c. A hallucination d. A delusion

5. The test for assessing patient's orientation and recall

a. Beck Depression Inventory
b. Mini Mental Status Examination
c. Thematic Apperception Test
d. Millon Clinical Multiaxial Inventory III

6. Signs and symptoms of ADHD include the following except

a. Inattention b. Impulsivenmess
c. Hyperactivity d. Good concentration

7. In a child with conduct disorder, aggressive behavior is

a. Caused by anxiety
b. Masking low self-esteem
c. Caused by temporary changes in relationships
d. Caused by heredity

8. An important point to monitor in a child who is getting methylphenidate

a. Blood glucose level b. Growth and development
c. Intelligence by IQ test d. Test for hearing

9. **Signs and symptoms of oppositional defiant disorder (ODD) include**
   a. Anxiety b. Compulsive behavior
   c. Testing of limits d. Hallucinations
10. **Priority area while caring for a child with depression**
   a. Developing strength and improving self-esteem
   b. Addressing ways to learn to complete tasks
   c. Determining strategies to help handle fear
   d. Developing communication skills
11. **A child with Tourette syndrome is most likely to experience**
   a. Academic difficulties b. Poor social skills
   c. Speech impediment d. Peer teasing
12. **Major side effect of haloperidol**
   a. Drowsiness
   b. Dry mouth
   c. Extrapyramidal reactions
   d. Anorexia
13. **Neurobehavioral disorder characterized by sudden, involuntary, muscle movements (motor tics) and vocalizations**
   a. Tourette syndrome b. ADHD
   c. ODD d. Depression
14. **A drug for treating depression**
   a. Methylphenidate b. Premoline
   c. Fluoxetine d. Benztropine
15. **Drug given to reduce extrapyramidal reactions**
   a. Pimozide b. Benztropine
   c. Methylphenidate d. Pemoline
16. **Intelligence quotient (IQ) in mild mental retardation**
   a. < 50 b. 50–70
   c. 70–80 d. 80–90
17. **Gradually occurring global impairment of cognitive functioning, memory and personality**
   a. Dyskinesia
   b. Age related cognitive decline
   c. Alzheimer's type dementia
   d. Vascular dementia
18. **Age related cognitive decline may grow more significant by about age**
   a. 60 b. 65
   c. 70 d. 75
19. **A drug used to treat Alzheimer's disease is**
   a. Aspirin b. Chlorpromazine
   c. Tacrine d. Sertraline
20. **An appropriate way to teach an elderly patient is to use**
   a. Audiotapes
   b. Pictures and simple wording
   c. Television programmes
   d. Musical recordings
21. **Flattening of emotions refers to**
   a. Anhedonia b. Associality
   c. Blunted affect d. Regression
22. **Imaginary perceptions are called**
   a. Delusions b. Hallucinations
   c. Illusions d. Magical thinking
23. **A schizophrenic patient exhibits jerking movements of the neck and mouth one week after taking haloperidol. The signs may be**
   a. Dystonia b. Psychosis
   c. Akathisia d. Parkinsonism
24. **False ideas or beliefs that the patient accepts as real are called**
   a. Delusions b. Hallucinations
   c. Illusions d. Magical thinking
25. **A positive symptom of schizophrenia is**
   a. Hallucination b. Blunted affect
   c. Anhedonia d. Associality
26. **A tricyclic antidepressant include all the following except**
   a. Amitriptyline b. Clomipramine
   c. Imipramine d. Methylphenidate
27. **A side effect of Amitriptyline**
   a. Vertigo b. Agranulocytosis
   c. Muscle twitching d. Skin rash
28. **Severe pathological mood swings, from hyperactivity and euphoria to sadness and depression occur in**
   a. Dysthymic disorder b. Cyclothymic disorder
   c. Depressive disorder d. Bipolar disorder
29. **A bipolar episode may be triggered by**
   a. Hyperthyroidism b. Anti-seizure drugs
   c. Hypothyroidism d. Anti-manic drugs

30. Rapid cycling refers to bipolar disorder with

a. One or more episodes of depression or mania in one year
b. Two or more episodes of depression or mania in one year
c. Four or more episodes of depression or mania in one year
d. No episodes of depression

31. A patient on lithium should

a. Maintain minimum amount of fluids
b. Maintain a high fluid intake
c. Restrict sodium intake
d. Exercise in hot weather

32. Electroconvulsive therapy (ECT) may be used to treat

a. Dysthymic disorder b. Major depressive disorder
c. Cyclothymic disorder d. Bipolar I disorder

33. Signs and symptoms of acute stress disorder may occur

a. Immediately after a trauma
b. As early as 2 days after a trauma
c. About one month after a trauma
d. Several months after a trauma

34. Fear of situations or places that may be difficult or embarrassing to leave describes

a. Social phobia
b. Panic disorder
c. Agoraphobia
d. Generalized anxiety disorder

35. Unresolved conflicts, a tendency to misinterpret events, and avoidance of new situations may be risk factors for

a. Panic disorder
b. Generalized anxiety disorder
c. Social phobia
d. Cacophobia

36. A fear of losing one's mind or having a heart attack is most likely to occur in

a. Social phobia
b. Generalized anxiety disorder
c. Panic disorder
d. Myctophobia

37. Flashbacks of an unpleasant, terrifying, or painful experience may occur in

a. PTSD b. Panic disorder
c. Agoraphobia d. OCD

38. A patient with panic disorder most likely fears

a. Loss of maturity b. Loss of control
c. Loss of memory d. Loss of identity

39. Fear of embarrassing oneself in public characterizes

a. Generalized anxiety disorder
b. Panic disorder
c. Specific phobia
d. Social phobia

40. The defense mechanism most often used to block traumatic experiences in patients with dissociative disorders

a. Passive aggression b. Reaction formation
c. Denial d. Repression

41. Feeling of a dream like state or of being a detached observer typically occur in

a. Dissociative fugue
b. Dissociative amnesia
c. Depersonalization disorder
d. Dissociative identity disorder

42. Multiple personality disorder is also known as

a. Dissociative fugue
b. Dissociative amnesia
c. Depersonalization disorder
d. Dissociative identity disorder (DID)

43. Factors that may contribute to dissociative identity disorder (DID) include all of these except

a. History of seizures
b. Emotional, physical or sexual abuse
c. Genetic predisposition
d. Extreme stress and trauma

44. Signs and symptoms of dissociative fugue are most pronounced

a. Weeks before the fugue episode
b. During the fugue episode
c. After the fugue episode
d. Hours before the fugue episode

45. The personality disorder that is characterized primarily by mistrust is
a. Paranoid personality disorder
b. Antisocial personality disorder
c. Dependent personality disorder
d. Schizotypal personality disorder

46. For patients with most personality disorders, the treatment of choice is
a. Group therapy
b. Individual psychotherapy
c. Selfhelp support groups
d. Inpatient therapy

47. Ideas of reference and magical thinking may occur in
a. Schizotypal personality disorder
b. Borderline personality disorder
c. Schizoid personality disorder
d. Histrionic personality disorder

48. The hallmark of borderline personality disorder is
a. Irresponsibility
b. Reckless disregard for others
c. Impulsivity
d. Unlawful behavior

49. If a patient with dependant personality disorder reports physical complaints, then
a. Overlook the symptoms
b. Encourage patient to talk about the symptoms
c. Disregard symptoms until emotional issues have been explored
d. Explore symptoms in a matter of fact way

50. A patient who is preoccupied with details and lists is most likely to have
a. Histrionic personality disorder
b. Obsessive compulsive personality disorder
c. Schizotypal personality disorder
d. Narcissistic personality disorder

51. To qualify for the diagnosis of anorexia nervosa, the patient's weight must drop below
a. 75% of ideal body weight
b. 80% of ideal body weight
c. 85% of ideal body weight
d. 90% of ideal body weight

52. The most serious complication of anorexia nervosa
a. High-risk of mortality
b. Coexisting depression
c. Poor family relationships
d. Social isolation

53. Purging behavior is usually triggered by
a. Sensation of fullness or bloating
b. Guilt, humiliation, and self-condemnation
c. Fear of being discovered as a binge eater
d. Feeling of nausea

54. Medications to treat bulimia nervosa include the following except
a. Paroxetine b. Amitriptyline
c. Diazepam d. Imipramine

55. Expected effects of Disulfiram reaction include
a. Chest pain, chills and hypertension
b. Slow pulse, chills and excitation
c. Slow pulse, slow respiratory rate and hypertension
d. Chest pain, headache and hypotension

56. A patient admits taking 'crystal', which is a
a. Depressant b. Stimulant
c. Hallucinogen d. Antidepressant

57. The assessment finding that strongly suggests IV drug abuse is
a. Skin lesions b. Gastritis
c. Tachycardia d. Tachypnea

58. The drug use to treat tachycardia induced by cocaine
a. Buprenorphine b. Digoxin
c. Propranolol d. Lidocaine

59. The effects of LSD typically lasts
a. 4–6 hours b. 6–8 hours
c. 8–12 hours d. 14–16 hours

60. An antagonist that is administered for narcotic overdose is
a. Disulfiram b. Naloxone
c. Diazepam d. Bupropion

61. Chronotherapy is
a. Manipulating patient's sleep schedule
b. Manipulating patient's environment
c. Adjusting to stimuli
d. Adjusting working hours

62. Use of bright light to manipulate the circadian rhythm
a. Chronotherapy b. Luminotherapy
c. Milieu therapy d. Group therapy

63. The treatment used in circadian rhythm sleep disorder include the following except
a. Chronotherapy
b. Luminotherapy
c. Chronopharmacotherapy
d. Group therapy

64. Sudden uncontrollable attack of deep sleep even during eating and lasting up to 20 minutes

a. Narcolepsy b. Hypnopompia
c. Hypnologic d. Cataplexy

65. Kleine-Levin syndrome is

a. Recurrent episodes of vomiting
b. Recurrent episodes of hypersomnia
c. Recurrent episodes of insomnia
d. Recurrent episodes of forgetfulness

66. Repid eye movement (REM) sleep is characterized by

a. Light sleep
b. Paralysis of the muscles
c. Restricted eye movements
d. Non-vivid dreams

67. Non-rapid eye movement (NREM) sleep is regulated by the

a. Pons b. Hypothalamus
c. Basal forebrain d. Amygdala

68. Cataplexy is a symptom of

a. REM sleep b. Primary hypersomnia
c. OSAS d. Narcolepsy

69. A classic feature of OSAS is

a. Snoring
b. Sneezing
c. Early morning awakening
d. Bursts of energy

70. Sleep drunkenness is a common finding in patients with

a. Primary insomnia b. Primary hypersomnia
c. Narcolepsy d. Alcoholism

71. Information typically gathered in asleep dairy includes

a. Usual bedtime
b. Foods consumed before the bedtime
c. Daily weights
d. Fluid consumption

72. Complex psychosexual disorder marked by sexual fantasies centered on inanimate objects

a. Pedophilia b. Paraphilia
c. Voyuerism d. Flirting

73. The phase of sexual response cycle involving fantasy and expectation is the

a. Desire phase b. Excitement phase
c. Orgasm phase d. Resolution phase

74. Cause/contributing factor sexual dysfunction

a. Drug abuse
b. Dissociative disorders
c. Supplemental vitamin use
d. Exercise

75. A persistent urge to show one's private parts to a stranger occurs in

a. Fetishism b. Pedophilia
c. Exhibitionalism d. Transsexualism

76. Treatments commonly recommended for a female with orgasmic disorder is

a. Taking soothing bubble baths
b. Touching her partner
c. Having sexual intercourse more often
d. Increasing the degree of sexual arousal

77. A non-living object may replace a human partner in a patient with

a. Fetishism b. Gender identity disorder
c. Transsexualism d. Sexual desire disorder

78. Gender identity disorder should be suspected if the patient

a. Has the strong desire to be of the same sex
b. Insists that he or she is of the opposite sex
c. Prefers the opposite sex
d. Engages in games with the same sex

79. Distorted or invented words that have meaning only for the patient

a. Neologism b. Obsessions
c. Projection d. Regression

80. Displacement of negative feelings onto another person

a. Introjection b. Displacement
c. Projection d. Reaction formation

81. Sexual attraction to children is termed

a. Pedophilia b. Sadism
c. Necrophilia d. Exhibitionism

82. An irrational or disproportionate fear of objects or situations

a. Obsession b. Phobia
c. Negativism d. Sublimation

83. Hiding a weakness by stressing too strongly the desirable strength

a. Reaction formation b. Rationalization
c. Sublimation d. Compensation

84. A diminished capacity to experience pleasure
a. Ambivalence b. Associality
c. Anhedonia d. Avoidance

85. Meaningless repetition of words or phrases
a. Echopraxia b. Echolalia
c. Extinction d. Flooding

86. Involuntary repetition of body movements of others
a. Echolalia b. Echopraxia
c. Extinction d. Flooding

87. False sensory perceptions that has no base in reality
a. Delusions b. Illusions
c. Hallucinations d. Fantasy

88. Provides a reward when the patient imitates the desired behavior
a. Focusing b. Modeling
c. Rewarding d. Reference

89. Extreme distrust of others
a. Paraphilia b. Paranoia
c. Obsessions d. Delusions

90. Return to earlier developmental stage
a. Regression b. Projection
c. Rationalization d. Introjection

91. Transforming unacceptable needs into acceptable ambitions
a. Projection b. Rationalization
c. Introjection d. Sublimation

92. An increased need for a substance to achieve an effect
a. Rationalization b. Withdrawal
c. Tolerance d. Withdrawal

93. Creation of unrealistic images to escape from daily pressures and responsibilities
a. Withdrawal b. Rationalization
c. Extinction d. Fantasy

94. Rapid succession of incomplete and poorly connected ideas
a. Flight of ideas b. Flat affect
c. Derailment d. Flooding

95. Unconscious filling of gaps in the memory with fabricated facts and experiences
a. Hallucination b. Delusion
c. Confabulation d. Fantasy

96. Speech that vacillates from one subject to another
a. Flat affect b. Flight of ideas
c. Flooding d. Derailment

97. Redirecting attention toward something specific
a. Focusing b. Flooding
c. Concept formation d. Reaction formation

98. A lack of interest in relationships
a. Ambivalence b. Asociality
c. Aversion d. Anhedonia

99. Coexisting strong positive and negative feelings
a. Aversion b. Ambivalence
c. Anhedonia d. Dissociation

100. Words that rhyme or sound alike used in an illogical manner
a. Clang association b. Clanging
c. Cognitive impairment d. Avoidance

101. The level of mental experience which best portrays one's attitudes, feelings and desires
a. Fore conscious b. Preconscious
c. Unconscious d. Conscious

102. The level of anxiety that best enhances the individual's power of perception
a. Mild b. Moderate
c. Severe d. Panic

103. Sublimation helps the individual
a. Act out in reverse something already done or thought
b. Channel unacceptable sexual desires into socially approved behavior
c. Return to an earlier less mature stage of development
d. Exclude from the conscious things that are psychologically disturbing

104. Displacement means
a. Ignoring unpleasant aspects of reality
b. Imaginative activity to escape reality
c. Pent up emotions directed to other than the primary source
d. Resisting any demands made by others

105. Personality reflects the individual's
a. Genetic back ground and placement in the family
b. Biologic constitution, and psychological development
c. Childhood experiences and intellectual capacity
d. Race and socioeconomic status

106. Individual protect and enhance the ego by
a. Ritualistic behavior b. Withdrawal patterns
c. Defense mechanisms d. Affective reactions

107. Another term for superego
a. Self b. Ideal self
c. Narcissism d. Conscience

108. The extreme important relationship in the development of personality
a. Sibling b. Parent – child
c. Peer d. Heterosexual

109. Fight or flight reaction is the function of
a. Central nervous system
b. Peripheral nervous system
c. Parasympathetic nervous system
d. Sympathetic nervous system

110. Communication ties people to their
a. Environmental surroundings
b. Social surroundings
c. Physical surroundings
d. Materialistic surroundings

111. The primary emergence of the personality is demonstrated by the age of
a. 6 months b. 9 months
c. 2 years d. 6 years

112. Dependence versus independence is the developmental task of
a. Infancy b. Toddler
c. Preschooler d. Schooler

113. The basic emotional task for the toddler is
a. Trust b. Independence
c. Identification d. Industry

114. The basic emotional task for the infant is
a. Industry b. Independence
c. Trust d. Identification

115. The problem of separation anxiety initially occur at the
a. Oral stage b. Anal stage
c. Phallic stage d. Latency stage

116. Surgery should be delayed if possible, because of the effects on personality development during the
a. Oral stage b. Anal stage
c. Oedipal stage d. Latency stage

117. Play for the preschool age child is necessary for the emotional development of
a. Projection b. Competition
c. Introjection d. Independence

118. During the oedipal stage of growth and development, the child
a. Loves the parent of the same sex
b. Loves both parents
c. Loves and hates both parents
d. Loves the parent of the opposite sex

119. The stage of growth and development which is concerned with role identification
a. Oral stage b. Oedipal stage
c. Latency stage d. Genital stage

120. The defense mechanism in which emotional conflicts are expressed through motor, sensory or somatic disability is
a. Dissociation b. Psychosomatic
c. Compensation d. Conversion

121. A person perceives a design in the wall as an animal, this is
a. Delusion b. Illusion
c. Idea of reference d. Hallucination

122. The ability to tolerate frustration is the function of
a. Unconscious b. Id
c. Ego d. Superego

123. The superego is that part of the psyche which
a. Is the source of creative energy
b. Develops from internalizing the concepts of parents and significant others
c. Contains the instinctual drives
d. Operates on the pleasure principle

124. Evidence of the existence of the unconscious is best demonstrated by
a. De ja vu experiences b. Slips of the tongue
c. The ease of the recall d. Free floating anxiety

125. The most important characteristic of emotionally disturbed children
a. Respond to any stimuli
b. Are totally involved with the environment
c. Respond to little external stimulus
d. Seems unresponsive to the environment

126. Autistic child shows

a. Not wanting to eat
b. Crying for attention
c. Catatonic like rigidity
d. Enjoying being with the people

127. Hyperkinesis children is usually treated with

a. Chlorpromazine hydrochloride
b. Haloperidol
c. Methocarbamol
d. Methylphenidate hydrochloride

128. Projection, rationalization, denial and distortion by hallucinations are examples of disturbance in

a. Association b. Logic
c. The thought process d. Reality testing

129. The patient fears that somebody is trying to kill him, this is an example of

a. Delusion of persecution
b. Error in judgment
c. Hallucination
d. Self accusatory delusion

130. The affect most commonly found in a patient with schizophrenia

a. Apathy and flatness b. Sadness and depression
c. Happiness and elation d. Anger and hostility

131. Functional mental illnesses are mainly the result of

a. Genetic endowment
b. Infection and inflammation
c. Deterioration of brain tissue
d. Social environment

132. The phobic reaction will never occur unless the person

a. Thinks about the feared object
b. Absolves the guilt of the feared object
c. Comes into contact with the feared object
d. Introjects the feared object into the body

133. The elderly confused person with socially aggressive behavior needs an environment that

a. Can be manipulated
b. Allows freedom of expression
c. Is mainly group oriented
d. Provides control by setting limits

134. An extrapyramidal symptom that is a potentially irreversible side effect of antipsychotic drugs are

a. Tardive dyskinesia b. Occulogyric crisis
c. pseudoparkinsonism d. Torticollis

135. Lithium is the drug of choice for

a. Acute agitation of schizophrenia
b. Paranoid state
c. Modification of depressive phase
d. Control of manic episode of bipolar disorder

136. Common manageable side effect of the major tranquilizers is

a. Jaundice b. Unintentional tremors
c. Ptosis d. Melanocytosis

137. The client should be warned about the following while taking MAO inhibitors

a. Ingesting wines and aged cheeses
b. Engaging in active physical exercise
c. Prolonged exposure to the sun
d. Use of drug with a cough formula

138. Photosensitization is a side effect of

a. Chlorpromazine hydrochloride
b. Thioridazine hydrochloride
c. Methylphenydate hydrochloride
d. Lithium carbonate

139. The major tranquilizers are the drug of choice in

a. Psychosis b. Depression
c. Hyperkinesis d. Narcotic withdrawal

140. Drugs like Trihexyphenidyl and benztropine are prescribed with

a. Barbiturates b. Antidepressants
c. Major tranquilizers d. Minor tranquilizers

141. Group therapy can help those clients who

a. Have no one to listen to them
b. Are emotionally ill
c. Are dependent on othersd. Feel they have a problem

142. In group therapy, focus is on

a. Behavior of individual members
b. Personal feelings affecting behavior
c. Jointly experienced stress
d. Confrontation between members

143. The type of speech in which words and phrases of others are repeated

a. Neologism b. Echolalia
c. Autism d. Echopraxia

144. A depressed client should be provided with

a. To make major decisions
b. A simple daily schedule
c. Many varied activities
d. A great deal of stimuli

145. Drug abuse is

a. A physiologic need for a drug
b. A psychological dependence on a drug
c. A compulsion to take a drug
d. An excessive drug use inconsistent with acceptable medical practice

146. Hard drugs easily cause dependence because of their ability to

a. Ease pain b. Clear sensorium
c. Blur reality d. Decrease motor activity

147. Alcoholics anonymous (AA) is a self-help group for

a. Patients with bipolar disorders
b. Drug users
c. Alcoholics
d. Maniacs

148. The primary rehabilitator of an alcoholic is

a. The physician b. The patient himself
c. Family members d. The nurse

149. An organic mental disorder is characterized by

a. Hypoxia of selected areas of brain tissue
b. Areas of brain destruction called senile plaques
c. Periodic remissions and exacerbations
d. Aggressive acting out behavior

150. A mentally healthy person is one who

a. Has insight into his or her own problems
b. Is not exhibiting pathologic symptoms
c. Is able to meet his or her own basic needs
d. Is free from both physical and emotional problems

151. Abrupt withdrawal from barbiturates can cause

a. Diarrhea b. Urticaria
c. Ataxia d. Convulsions

152. Making stories to fill up gaps in memory is termed as

a. Lying b. Rationalizing
c. Denial d. Confabulation

153. A somatoform disorder is

a. A psychosomatic reaction to stress
b. A psychologic defense against stress
c. An unconscious means to control conflict
d. A conscious defense against anxiety

154. A person who is exhibiting physical symptoms during anxiety is using a defense mechanism

a. Psychosomatic b. Psychoneurotic
c. Regressive d. Projective

ANSWER KEY

1. b	2. c	3. d	4. a	5. b	6. d	7. b	8. a	9. c	10. a	11. d	12. c
13. a	14. c	15. b	16. b	17. c	18. d	19. c	20. b	21. c	22. b	23. d	24. a
25. a	26. d	27. b	28. d	29. c	30. c	31. b	32. b	33. b	34. c	35. b	36. c
37. a	38. b	39. d	40. d	41. c	42. d	43. a	44. c	45. a	46. b	47. a	48. c
49. d	50. b	51. c	52. a	53. b	54. c	55. d	56. b	57. a	58. c	59. c	60. b
61. a	62. b	63. d	64. a	65. b	66. b	67. c	68. d	69. a	70. b	71. a	72. b
73. a	74. a	75. c	76. b	77. a	78. b	79. a	80. b	81. a	82. b	83. d	84. c
85. b	86. b	87. c	88. b	89. b	90. a	91. d	92. c	93. d	94. a	95. c	96. d
97. a	98. b	99. b	100. a	101. c	102. a	103. b	104. c	105. b	106. c	107. d	108. b
109. d	110. b	111. c	112. b	113. b	114. c	115. a	116. c	117. c	118. d	119. b	120. d
121. b	122. c	123. b	124. b	125. d	126. a	127. d	128. d	129. a	130. a	131. d	132. c
133. d	134. a	135. d	136. a	137. a	138. a	139. a	140. c	141. d	142. b	143. b	144. b
145. d	146. c	147. c	148. b	149. b	150. c	151. d	152. d	153. c	154. b		

HISTORY OF PSYCHIATRIC NURSING

1. **Indian Mental Health Act was passed in the year**
   a. 1980 b. 1985
   c. 1987 d. 1990
2. **The term hallucination was coined by**
   a. D. Goldman b. Jean-Etienne Esquirol
   c. Eugin Bleuler d. Emil Kraepelin
3. **First psychiatric nursing text book was written by**
   a. Schneider b. Harriet Baily
   c. Hildegard E. Peplau d. Linda Richards
4. **The first use of convulsive therapy for the treatment of a psychiatric disorder in modern times is attributed to**
   a. AE Bennett b. Kurt Schneider
   c. Ladislaus von Meduna d. Egas Moniz
5. **Psychodrama was introduced by**
   a. Maxwell Jones b. Joseph Wolpe
   c. Joseph Pratt d. Jacob Moreno
6. **Freud used the case of "Little Hans", a 5-years-old boy to explain**
   a. Oedipus complex b. Inferiority complex
   c. Electra complex d. Behavior problems
7. **The first therapeutic use of electrically induced seizures in the treatment of mental disorders is related to**
   a. Karl Jaspers
   b. Harold Sackeim
   c. Holmberg and S. Thesieff G
   d. Cerletti and Bini
8. **The York Retreat was founded by**
   a. John Conolly b. William Tuke
   c. Benjamin Rush d. Linda Richards
9. **Existential philosophy was proposed by**
   a. Schneider b. Heidegger
   c. Jaspers d. Immanuel Kant
10. **Who authored the book "Interpersonal Relations in Nursing"?**
    a. Hildegard E. Peplau b. John Hopkins
    c. Linda Richards d. AE Bennett
11. **Mourning and Melancholia, (1917) was written by**
    a. Emil Kraepelin b. Sigmond Freud
    c. Phillippe Pinel d. Immanuel Kant
12. **Alcoholics Anonymous was founded in 1935 in Akron, Ohio, by**
    a. Bill Wilson b. Immanuel Kant
    c. Phillippe Pinel d. Alois Alzheimer
13. **The Indian Lunacy Act was passed in the year**
    a. 1912 b. 1921
    c. 1935 d. 1980
14. **The term catatonia was first explained by:**
    a. Carl Rogers b. Kahlbaum
    c. Sigmund Freud d. Dorothea Dix
15. **Which law in India has deemed the attempt to commit suicide is a punishable offence?**
    a. Section 309 of the IPC
    b. Section 114 (b) of the IPC
    c. Mental Health Act
    d. Sections 328–339 of the IPC
16. **In 1935 Leo Kanner first explained about a condition in child psychiatry, which is known as**
    a. Childhood autism
    b. Gilles de la Tourette syndrome
    c. Dyslexia
    d. Asperger's syndrome
17. **The Narcotic Drugs and Psychotropic Substances Act (NDPSA) was passed in the year**
    a. 1980 b. 1985
    c. 1990 d. 1995
18. **Minnesota Multi-phasic Personality Inventory, was developed by**
    a. David Wechsler
    b. Binet
    c. Herman Rorschach
    d. SR Hathaway and JC McKinley
19. **A Mind That Found Itself (1909) was written by**
    a. Hildeguard Peplau b. Sigmund Freud
    c. Cliford Bears d. Carl Rogers
20. **Imbalance of four essential humors-phlegm, yellow bile, black bile, and blood as the causes of mental illness was explained by**
    a. Plato b. Aristotle
    c. Hippocrates d. Galen

21. The theory of operant conditioning was proposed by

a. Watson b. Ian Pavlov
c. Harry Stock Sullivan d. Frederick Skinner

22. A projective test using 10 inkblot cards for revealing psychodynamics was first proposed by

a. Herman Rorschach b. Sigmund Freud
c. Manfred Sakel d. Cerletti

23. The term dementia praecox was coined by

a. Eugin Bleuler b. Sigmund Freud
c. Leon Festinger d. Emil Kraepelin

24. Psychosurgery was first introduced by

a. Egaz Moniz b. Ladislas Meduna
c. Jacob Moreno d. Eugin Bleuler

25. Jacob Levi Moreno, who introduced

a. Electroconvulsive therapy
b. Psychodrama
c. Psychosurgery
d. Therapeutic community

26. In 1933 Jacob Kasanin coined the term

a. Autism b. Schizophrenia
c. Catatonia d. Melanholia

27. Anatomy of Melancholy was written by

a. Manfred Sakel b. Sigmond Freud
c. Erik Erickson d. Richard Burton

ANSWER KEY

1. c	2. b	3. b	4. c	5. d	6. a	7. d	8. b	9. b	10. a	11. b	12. a
13. a	14. b	15. a	16. a	17. b	18. d	19. c	20. c	21. d	22. a	23. d	24. a
25. b	26. c	27. d									

PSYCHIATRIC DISEASES

1. **As per the current evidence, which statement is *not* correct**
   a. Bilateral ECT is superior in efficacy to unilateral ECT
   b. Unilateral ECT is more likely to cause cognitive deficits
   c. Brief-pulse ECT delivery is asscoiated with decreased cognitive deficits
   d. Unilateral ECT is administered to the non-dominant hemisphere
2. **Negativism, waxy flexibility, mutism, posturing and stupor are characteristics of**
   a. Paranoid schizophrenia
   b. Disorganized schizophrenia
   c. Catatonic schizophrenia
   d. Undifferentiated schizophrenia
3. **What is the best accepted placement of electrodes in unilateral ECT**
   a. Bifrontotemporal b. Parietotemporal
   c. Occipital d. D'Elia position
4. **An unconscious defense mechanism in which unacceptable mental contents are banished or kept out of consciousness is**
   a. Sublimation b. Suppression
   c. Rationalization d. Repression
5. **Factors predisposing to postictal confusional state include, all *except***
   a. High-dose ECT b. Existing CNS disease
   c. Multiple ECT d. A younger age group
6. **Psychopathological repeating of words or phrases of one person by another; tends to be repetitive and persistent is termed as**
   a. Echopraxia b. Echolalia
   c. Verbigeration d. Mannerism
7. **The best unit for quantification of ECT stimuli is**
   a. Millicoulombs (mC) b. Joules
   c. Watts d. Volt
8. **Characteristics of OCD include all the following, *except***
   a. Obsessive thoughts
   b. Compulsive acts
   c. Considerable degree of anxiety
   d. Ordered flight of ideas
9. **An elimination disorder in which the patient suffers from incontinence of urine during sleep is termed as**
   a. Enuresis b. Encopresis
   c. Dyspareunia d. Pseudocyesis
10. **Obsessional personality disorder is also called**
    a. Anankastic personality disorder
    b. Schizoid personality disorder
    c. Histrionic personality disorder
    d. Paranoid personality disorder
11. **The most persistent adverse effect of ECT is**
    a. Retrograde amnesia b. Fractures
    c. Seizures d. Hypertension
12. **Symptoms such as sleep disturbance (especially early morning awakening), decreased appetite, constipation, weight loss, and loss of sexual response usually observed in depression are collectively called**
    a. Negative signs b. Vegetative signs
    c. Positive signs d. Cardinal signs
13. **Most effective in OCD management**
    a. Psychodynamic psychotherapy
    b. Interpersonal psychotherapy
    c. Cognitive behavior therapy
    d. Supportive psychotherapy
14. **Which of the following is *not* a recommended preparation for ECT procedure?**
    a. Informed consent in writing
    b. Morning bath, cleaning the oil from the head, overnight fast
    c. Premedication with an anticholinergic agent
    d. Administration of an anticonvulsant 30 minutes before ECT
15. **Folie à deux is also called as**
    a. Shared psychotic disorder
    b. Formal thought disorder
    c. Labile affect
    d. La belle indifference
16. **The most common indication of ECT**
    a. Schizophrenia
    b. Generalized anxiety disorder
    c. Manic episodes
    d. Major depression

17. **The antidepressant which is contraindicated in a patient with seizure disorder**
a. Nefazodone b. Fluoxetine
c. Venlafaxine d. Mirtazapine

18. **Feigning disease to achieve a specific goal, for example, to avoid an unpleasant responsibility is**
a. Malingering b. Factitious disorder
c. Amnestic disorder d. Conversion disorder

19. **Recurrent, intrusive, senseless ideas, thoughts, and images that are ego-dystonic and involuntary**
a. Obsessions b. Compulsions
c. Hypochondreasis d. Obstrusiveness

20. **The antidepressant most selective for inhibition of neuronal reuptake of serotonin**
a. Mirtazapine b. Venlafaxine
c. Bupropion d. Sertraline

21. **Craving and eating of non-food substances, such as paint and clay observed in some mental illness**
a. Binge eating b. Verbigeration
c. Polyphagia d. Pica

22. **The rTMS is found to have antidepressant properties when applied to**
a. Temporal-parietal regions of the cortex
b. Dorsolateral prefrontal cortex (DLPFC)
c. Occipital cortex
d. Parieto-occipital cortex

23. **A kind of delusion in which the patient believes one's thoughts are being removed from one's mind by other people or forces**
a. Delusional perception b. Thought broadcasting
c. Thought blocking d. Thought withdrawal

24. **The most acceptable etiologic hypothesis in OCD**
a. Dopamine hypothesis
b. Serotonin hypothesis
c. Acetylcholine hypothesis
d. Glutamate hypothesis

25. **The condition associated with long-term use of lithium in mood disorders**
a. Hypothyroidism b. Hyperprolactinemia
c. Hypoglycemia d. Hypertension

26. **A state of uncritical compliance with influence or of uncritical acceptance of an idea, belief, or attitude; commonly observed among persons with hysterical traits**
a. Sublimation b. Mannerism
c. Suggestibility d. Paranoid ideation

27. **The antidepressants requiring therapeutic blood monitoring for safe use**
a. Paroxetine b. Phenelzine
c. Nortriptyline d. Venlafaxine

28. **Unconscious defense mechanism in which a person undergoes a partial or total return to earlier patterns of adaptation**
a. Sublimation b. Displacement
c. Regression d. Repression

29. **Which is *not* included in the OCD spectrum disorders?**
a. Trichotillomania b. Tourette's disorder
c. Kleptomania d. Schizotypal disorders

30. **Combining MAOIs with SSRIs may cause**
a. Serotonin Syndrome
b. Extrapyramidal symptoms (EPS)
c. Neroleptic malignant syndrome (NMS)
d. Agranulocytosis

31. **Hallucination with content that is consistent with either a depressed or manic mood**
a. Elementary hallucination
b. Mood-congruent hallucination
c. Mood-incongruent hallucination
d. Partial hallucination

32. **Penile priapism is known to be associated with use of**
a. Buproprion b. Venlafaxine
c. Escitalopram d. Trazadone

33. **The area of brain known to be associated with OCD**
a. Reticular system b. Nigrostraital pathway
c. Basal ganglia d. Corpus callosum

34. **A clinical term used to explain a major depressive disorder superimposed on an underlying dysthymia**
a. Agitated depression b. Double depression
c. Secondary depression d. Neurotic depression

35. **Hallucination primarily involving taste**
   a. Gustatory hallucination b. Tactile hallucination
   c. Haptic hallucination d. Olfactory hallucination

36. **A dissociative disorder characterized by a period of almost complete amnesia, during which a person actually flees from an immediate life situation and begins a different life pattern**
   a. Neurasthenia b. Dissociative amnesia
   c. Dissociative fugue d. Trance

37. **Eugen Bleuler renamed dementia precox as**
   a. Autism
   b. Schizophrenia
   c. Bipolar affective disorder
   d. Melancholia

38. **The drugs is associated with lower seizure thresholds when administering ECT**
   a. Lithium b. Anticonvulsants
   c. Benzodiazepines d. Barbiturates

39. **As per DSM-IV-TR classification, antisocial personality disorders is classified under**
   a. Cluster-A b. Cluster-B
   c. Cluster-C d. Cluster-D

40. **First rank symptoms of schizophrenia (FRSS) include all the following, *except***
   a. Third person/running commetary auditory hallucinations
   b. Thought alienation phenomena
   c. Passivity phenomenon
   d. Mood disturbances

41. **What is the minimum seizure duration required for effectiveness of ECT**
   a. 1–3 seconds b. 5–10 seconds
   c. 30–90 seconds d. 180–200 seconds

42. **Eugen Bleuler's characteristic symptoms (fundamental symtoms) of schizophrenia include all the following, *except*:**
   a. Ambivalance b. Autism
   c. Affective disturbances d. Apraxia

43. **Morbid, insatiable sexual need or desire in a male**
   a. satyriasis b. nymphomania
   c. pseudocyesis d. gynecomastia

44. **The first effective antipsychotic drug**
   a. Chlorpromazine b. Thioridazine
   c. Haloperidol d. Trifluperazine

45. **Which is *not* a positive sign seen in schizophrenia?**
   a. hallucinations b. delusions
   c. thought disorder d. flat affect

46. **What is considered as the gold standard for confirmation of seizure in ECT**
   a. Cuff method
   b. Electroencephalography (EEG)
   c. Electromyogram (EMG)
   d. Galvanic skin response (GSR)

47. **A kind of aphasia characterized by difficulty in giving the correct name of an object**
   a. Nominal aphasia b. Amnestic aphasia
   c. Sensory aphasia d. Receptive aphasia

48. **Which is *not* a negative sign seen in schizophrenia**
   a. Flat affect b. Alogia
   c. Hallucination d. Apathy

49. **What is the average mortality rate with ECT**
   a. 3–4 per 100,000 b. 10–25 per 100,000
   c. 10–20 per 10,000 d. 50–60 per 100,000

50. **Unconscious defense mechanism by which the emotional component of an unacceptable idea or object is transferred to a more acceptable one**
   a. Dissociation b. Denial
   c. Displacement d. Devaluation

51. **Highest rates of sexual dysfunction is reported with**
   a. Bupropion b. Mirtazapine
   c. Citalopram d. Paroxetine

52. **Haptic hallucination is**
   a. Hallucination of touch b. Hallucination of smell
   c. Hallucination of taste d. Hallucination of sound

53. **Sedation associated with use of antidepressants is attributed to the**
   a. Blockade of histamine H1 receptor
   b. Blockade of muscarinic acetylcholine receptors
   c. Blockade of alpha-1-receptors
   d. Antagonism of 5-HT2 receptors

54. **Which is *not* a characteristic of schizotypal personality disorder?**
   a. Inappropriate, inconsistant affect
   b. Odd eccentric appearance/behavior
   c. Odd beliefs or magical thinking
   d. Excessive sensitiveness to set backs and rebuffs

55. **Pathological fire-setting is also called**
a. Pyromania b. Kleptomania
c. Trichotillomania d. Dipsomania

56. **A clinician-rated scale for monitoring outcome of depression treatment**
a. Beck Depression Inventory (BDI)
b. Zung Depression Scale
c. Geriatric Depression Scale (GDS)
d. Hamilton Depression Rating Scale (HAM-D)

57. **A drug found to be effective in intermittent explosive disorders**
a. Fluoxetine b. Topiramate
c. Fluoxamine d. Carbamazepine

58. **Therapeutic options for refractory depression include all, *except***
a. Thyroid hormone supplementation
b. Stimulant augmentation
c. Transcranial magnetic stimulation
d. Glucocorticoid therapy

59. **As per DSM-IV-TR classification, personality disorders with odd and eccentric behaviors are classified under**
a. Cluster—A b. Cluster—B
c. Cluster—C d. Cluster—E

60. **Which of the following is *not* associated with use of Tricyclic Antidepressants (TCA)?**
a. Dry mouth b. Constipation
c. Blurred vision d. Urinary Incontinence

61. **The following condition is not classified under personality disorders in ICD-10 classification**
a. Paranoid b. Schizoid
c. Schizotypal d. Dissocial

62. **The recommended dose of duloxetine for major depressive disorder**
a. 40–60 mg/day b. 75–150 mg/day
c. 300–600 mg/day d. 37.5–75 mg/day

63. **Therapeutic blood level of lithium**
a. 11–20 mg/dL b. 1.5–2 mEq/L
c. 0.8–1.2 mEq/L d. 150–200 mg/dL

64. **Prefrontal lobotomy was proposed as a treatment for serious mental illnesses by**
a. Ugo Cerletti b. Walter Cannon
c. Egas Moniz d. Adolph Meyer

65. **Narcissistic personality disorder is characterised by**
a. Callous unconcern for feelings of others
b. Self-dramatization, theatericality
c. Ideas of grandiosity and inflated sense of self-importance
d. Significant and persistant disturbances of identity of self.

66. **Which of the following is known to have least cardiovascular side effects?**
a. Amitriptyline b. Imipramine
c. Citalopram d. Clomipramine

67. **Clozapine is associated with a higher risk of the following than other antipsychotics**
a. Extrapyramidal symptoms
b. Seizures
c. Neuroleptic malignant syndrome
d. Anticholinergic side effects

68. **Incapacity to experience guilt and to profit from experience, particularly punishment is seen in**
a. Antisocial personality disorder
b. Schizotypal personality disorder
c. Schizoid personality disorders
d. Dependent personality disorder

69. **The usual therapeutic dose range of lithium carbonate in the treatment of bipolar disorders**
a. 30–60 mg/day b. 900–1500 mg/day
c. 2000–3000 mg/day d. 15–30 mg/day

70. **The most safe drug in pregnant patients with acute schizophrenia**
a. Haloperidol b. Chlorpromazine
c. Trifluperazine d. Thioridazine

71. **A common adverse effect of venlafaxine**
a. Increase in blood pressure
b. Decrese in blood pressure
c. Hypersalivation
d. Bradycardia

72. **The instrument related to assessment of personality trait**
a. B. PANSS b. C. MMSE
c. D. AIMS d. E. MMPI

73. **An important expressed emotion (EE) affecting the course of schizophrenia**
a. Over involvement
b. Hostility
c. Criticism
d. Non-sequential communication

74. Behaviorism, "the science of behavior" was proposed by

a. Sigmond Freud b. Erik Erickson
c. JB Watson d. Ivan Pavlov

75. The antidepressant having relatively short biological half-life

a. Mirtazapine b. Fluoxetine
c. Trazodone d. Citalopram

76. Trichotillomania refers to

a. Pathological fire-setting
b. Pathological-stealing
c. Compulsive-hair pulling
d. Compulsive-drinking

77. Who among the following would be *least* likely to talk about unconscious mind and conflicts.

a. Wundt b. James
c. Watson d. Wertheimer

78. The antidepressant approved by FDA for Smoking cessation

a. Fluvoxamine b. Bupropion
c. Paroxetine d. Venlafaxine

79. Behavior means

a. Outward or overt action and reactions
b. Mental processes
c. Internal covert process
d. Meaningful thoughts

80. Experessive aphasia is also called

a. Nominal aphasia b. Global aphasia
c. Broca's aphasia d. Cortical sensory aphasia

81. Operant conditioning was proposed by

a. Ivan pavlov b. BF Skinner
c. Sigmond Freud d. Abraham Maslow

82. A reversible inhibitor of monoamine (RIMA) — reversible inhibitor of monoamine oxidase group of antidepressant

a. Phenelzine b. Isocarboxazid
c. Tranylcypromine d. Moclobemide

83. Filling up of memory spaces with a detailed false description of an event

a. Confabulation b. Neologism
c. Circumstantiality d. Tangentiality

84. Which theory views that people have free-will and potential for self-actualization?

a. Behaviorism b. Psychodynamic theory
c. Cognitive theory d. Humanism

85. Antipsychotic known to elevate serum prolactin levels

a. Quetiapine b. Clozapine
c. Aripiprazole d. Amisulpride

86. Confabulation is commonly observed in patients with

a. Obsessive-compulsive disorders
b. Delusional disorders
c. Personality disorders
d. Amnesic syndrome

87. Indian Psychoanalytic Society was established by

a. Prof S. M Mohisin
b. Dr NN Sengupta
c. Prof Girindra Sehkhar Bose
d. H.P Maiti

88. Drugs associated with neuroleptic malignant syndrome

a. Antidepressants b. Anticholinergics
c. Antipsychotics d. Mood stabilizers

89. A condition in which some patients assert that some or all the people whom they met are doubles of real people

a. Capgras syndrome b. Conard syndrome
c. Ganser syndrome d. Tourette syndrome

90. Specialization in psychology deals with diagnosis and treatment of mental disorders

a. Clinical b. Developmental
c. Experimental d. Personality

91. Tetrabenazine is effective in controlling

a. Neuroleptic-induced parkinsonism
b. Neuroleptic-induced tardive dyskinesia
c. Weight gain
d. Hyperprolactemia

92. Gestalt is a German term meaning

a. Self-reliance b. Good form
c. Internal conflicts d. Meaning

93. A liability to outbursts or as a state of poor control over aggressive impulses directed toward others, more frequently to those nearest and dearest

a. Anxiety b. Irritability
c. Assertiveness d. Homicide

94. **A term used to explain "seeking sexual pleasure from wearing the clothes of the opposite sex"**
   a. Bestiality b. Transvestism
   c. Fetishism d. Sadism

95. **Cognitive dissonance as a Theory of the Self was proposed by**
   a. Leon Festinger b. Abraham Maslow
   c. Sigmund Freud d. Eroc Burne

96. **Perceptual abnormality**
   a. Delusion b. Attention
   c. Hallucination d. Orientation

97. **One of the child psychiatric patient sign**
   a. Dancing b. Happiness
   c. Body Rocking d. Smiling

98. **A neuroleptic agent that has the lowest likelihood of producing tardive dyskinesia**
   a. Imipramine b. Chlorpromazine
   c. Clozapine d. Fluoxetine

99. **A neurologic condition in which hallucinations of taste or smell is experienced**
   a. Huntington's disease b. Parkinson's disease
   c. Epilepsy d. SSPE

100. **In standard form of modified ECT, short-acting muscle relaxant used is**
   a. Pancronium bromide b. Succinyl choline
   c. Thiopentone d. Atropine

101. **Absence of speech and activities**
   a. Autism b. Mutism
   c. Aphasia d. Cretinism

102. **Drug useful in the management of the neuroleptic malignant syndrome, although it can worsen the symptoms of schizophrenia**
   a. Risperidone b. Thiothixene
   c. Haloperidol d. Bromocriptine

103. **Systematic desensitization is introduced by**
   a. John Hickley b. Albert Ellis
   c. Wolpe d. Aaron Beck

104. **Antagonism of which dopaminergic pathway is attributed to be the cause of therapeutic actions of antipsychotic drugs**
   a. Nigrostriatal system
   b. Mesolimbic-mesocortical system
   c. Tuberoinfundibular pathway
   d. Reticular activating system

105. **A technique producing unpleasant sensation in the patient in association with stimulus is**
   a. Aversion b. Modeling
   c. Flooding d. Abreaction

106. **A phenothiazine**
   a. Chlorpromazine b. Clozapine
   c. Olanzapine d. Risperidone

107. **A condition in which the person seeks sexual excitement by giving pain to the partner**
   a. Masochism b. Fetishism
   c. Sadism d. Transvestism

108. **Multiple referrals between psychiatrists and other professionals is**
   a. Steering b. Ping Ponging
   c. Ganging d. Touting

109. **Mechanism for the cause of extrapyramidal reactions**
   a. Alpha-adrenoceptor blockade
   b. D2-receptor blockade
   c. H1 histamine receptor blockade
   d. D2-receptor up-regulation

110. **The drug having pharmacological actions characterized by high antipsychotic potency and high potential for extrapyramidal toxicity**
   a. Thioridazine b. Haloperidol
   c. Flumazenil d. Clozapine

111. **Voluntary agreement, compliance or permission**
   a. Competence b. Preamble
   c. Confidentiality d. Consent

112. **The systematic study of abnormal experiences, cognition and behavior**
   a. Epidemiology b. Ethnology
   c. Psychopathology d. Pathophysiology

113. **Common side effect of ECT is impairment of**
   a. Judgement b. Speech
   c. Thought d. Memory

114. **Tardive dyskinesia after long-term antipsychotic administration is thought to be due to**
   a. A decrease in dopamine synthesis
   b. Enhanced stimulation of D2 dopamine autoreceptors
   c. Loss of cholinergic neurons in striatum
   d. Up-regulation of striated dopamine receptors

115. **Study of subjective experiences**
   a. Phenomenology b. Ethnography
   c. Psychoanalysis d. Behaviorism

116. Chlorpromazine (100 mg) equivalent oral dose of haloperidol

a. 2 mg b. 10 mg
c. 30 mg d. 100 mg

117. Sleep walking is termed as

a. Sleep terror
b. Somnabulism
c. Pickwickian syndrome
d. Bruxism

118. Manifestations is *not* caused by blockade of muscarinic cholinoreceptor

a. Blurred vision b. Urinary retention
c. Constipation d. Amenorrhea

119. A technique used in hypnosis

a. Flooding b. Socratic questioning
c. Suggestion d. Desensitization

120. A butyrophenone

a. Pimozide b. Haloperidol
c. Fluphenazine d. Trifluoperazine

121. Which of the following terms is *not* related to memory as per information processing model?

a. Retention b. Retrieval
c. Recall d. Replication

122. The phase of sleep cycle characterized by sleep spindles and K-complexes

a. REM Sleep b. Stage 1 NREM sleep
c. Stage 2 NREM sleep d. Stage 3 NREM sleep

123. A condition in which the defect is predominantly in the retrieval of recently acquired information

a. Capgras syndrome b. Pseudologica fantastica
c. Jamais vu d. Korsakov's syndrome

124. A circadian rhythm disorder

a. Somnabulism b. Nightmares
c. Narcolepsy d. Jet-lag

125. The response that was appropriate to a first stimulus being given inappropriately to a second different stimulus

a. Conditioning b. Confabulation
c. Circumstantiality d. Perseveration

126. Investigation specifically related to sleep disorders

a. BEAM
b. Galvanic skin response (GSR)
c. Dexamethasone suppression test (DST)
d. Polysomnography

127. Perceptual disturbances of visceral, olfactory, gustatory and visual modality are common in

a. Temporal lobe disorder b. Schizophrenia
c. Parkinson's disease d. Mental retardation

128. REM sleep is also called as

a. Orthodox sleep b. Paradoxical sleep
c. Slow wave sleep (SWS) d. EEG synchronized sleep

129. Which of the following is *not* a feature of Gnaser's syndrome?

a. Approximate answers b. Clouding of conciousness
c. Pesecutory delusions d. Pseudohallucinations

130. A condition characterized by sudden, brief loss of muscle tone, in the waking state usually triggered by emotional arousal (laughing, anger, surprise), normally occurring during REM sleep

a. Dyssomnia
b. Circadian rhythm sleep disorders
c. Cataplexy
d. Sleep bruxism

131. Lilliputian hallucinations are typical of

a. Delusional disorders b. Delirium tremens
c. Tourette syndrome d. Lithium toxicity

132. An EEG wave characterized by an initial brief, low-amplitude component, followed by a high-amplitude, long-lasting component and is a characteristic of stage 2 sleep

a. Alpha wave b. Delta wave
c. K-complex d. Vertex sharp transients

133. A stimulant

a. Alcohol b. Diazepam
c. PCP d. Barbiturates

134. Flight of ideas is typical of

a. Schizophrenia b. Mania
c. OCD d. Autism

135. Somnabulism refers to

a. Sleep-talking b. Sleep-walking
c. Sleep-related enuresis d. Sleep-terrer

136. A synthetically produced substance

a. Nicotine b. Amphetamine
c. Caffeine d. Cocaine

137. Klien-Levin syndrome is characterized by

a. Hypersomnia b. Hyperphagia
c. Hypersexuality d. Hyperesthesia

138. A drug used as deterrent agent in the treatment of alcohol dependence syndrome

a. Acamprosate b. Naltrexone
c. Disulfiram d. Buproprion

139. Pickwickian syndrome refers to

a. Obstructive sleep apnea seen in obese and elderly
b. Sleep disorder caused by rapid change in time zones
c. A type of periodic leg movement disorder
d. Restless leg syndrome

140. LSD is taken from

a. Fungus b. Lichen
c. Algae d. Bacterium

141. The tetrad of symptoms-sleep attacks, catelepsy, hypnagogic hallucinations and sleep paralysis are characteristics of

a. Narcolepsy
b. Somnambulism
c. Circadian rhythm sleep disorders
d. Klein-Levin syndrome

142. An opiate narcotic

a. Bhang b. Charas
c. Heroin d. Nicotine

143. Delta sleep refers to

a. REM sleep
b. NREM stage 1 sleep
c. NREM stage 2 sleep
d. NREM stage 3 and stage 4 sleep

144. Zolpidem is a

a. Benzodiazepine b. Imidazopyridine
c. Barbiturate d. Antipsychotic

145. A CNS depressant drug

a. Amphetamine b. Caffeine
c. Opium d. Cocaine

146. The area of brain associated with generation and maintenance of waking states or arousal

a. Corpus callosum
b. Reticular activating system
c. Limbic system
d. Hypothalamus

147. A hallucinogen

a. LSD b. Heroin
c. Cocaine d. Morphine

148. A characteristic feature of depression

a. Short REM latency and decreased delta sleep
b. Long REM latency and increased delta sleep
c. Periodic leg movement
d. Sleep attacks, visual hallucinations, cataplexy and sleep paralysis

149. Slow respiration, slow pulse and constriction of pupil occurs due to

a. Morphine and opium b. Cocaine and heroin
c. Alcohol and thalidomide d. Nicotine and caffeine

150. The drug least likely to cause sexual dysfunction

a. Imipramine b. Thioridazine
c. Captopril d. Mirtazapine

151. Stimulant cocaine is obtained from

a. Rauwolfia b. Erythroxylon
c. Papaver d. Eucalyptus

152. A sexual pain disorder reported in females

a. Anorgasmia b. Vaginismus
c. Peyronie's disease d. Impotence

153. A delusion in which the patient denies the existence of his body, mind, his loved ones, and the world around him is

a. Persecutory delusion b. Nihilistic delusion
c. Extracampine delusion d. Delusion of reference

154. Ordered flight of ideas is called

a. Circumstantiality b. Tangentiality
c. Proilixity d. Thought withdrawal

155. Priapism is a sexual dysfunction seen in treatment with

a. Chlorpromazine b. Trazadone
c. Clozapine d. Lithium

156. Synthetic drugs structurally related to adrenaline

a. Amphetamines b. Barbiturates
c. Hallucinogens d. Analgesics

157. Excessive sexual desire in women

a. Satyriasis b. Frigidity
c. Vaginismus d. Nymphomania

158. Diacetylmorphine is

a. Morphine b. Heroin
c. Cocaine d. Hashish

159. Sildenafil citrate is administered in

a. Impotence b. Erectile dysfunction
c. Paraphilias d. Premature ejaculation

160. The drug used for reducing male hypersexuality

a. Papaverine b. Cyproterone
c. Sildenafil d. Alprostadil

161. Brown sugar is

a. Diacetylmorphine hydrochloride
b. Theophylline
c. Lorazepam
d. Metherdine

162. Which of the following is *not* a characteristic of schizotypal personality disorder?

a. Inappropriate, inconsistent affect
b. Odd eccentric appearance/behavior
c. Odd beliefs or magical thinking
d. Excessive sensitiveness to set backs and rebuffs

163. The drug having the highest potential for physical dependence

a. Opioids b. Cannabis
c. Cocaine d. LSD

164. Narcissistic personality disorder is characterized by

a. Callous unconcern for feelings of others
b. Self-dramatization, theatricality
c. Ideas of grandiosity and inflated sense of self-importance
d. Significant and persistent disturbances of identity of self

165. The drug of choice in the management of alcohol withdrawal

a. Barbiturates b. Benzodiazepines
c. Disulfiram d. Acamprosate

166. Incapacity to experience guilt and to profit from experience, particularly punishment is seen in

a. Antisocial personality disorder
b. Schizotypal personality disorder
c. Schizoid personality disorders
d. Dependent personality disorder

167. The most dependence-producing derivative of opium is

a. Meperidine b. Diphenoxylate
c. Methadone d. Heroin

168. The instrument related to assessment of personality traits

a. B. PANSS b. C. MMSE
c. D. AIMS d. MMPI

169. Disulfiram-ethanol like reaction is caused by

a. Propranolol b. Haloperidol
c. Ciprofloxacin d. Metronidazole

170. Elevated mean corpuscular volume (MCV) value is an indicator of

a. Thiamine deficiency b. Nicotine dependence
c. Alcohol dependence d. Opium dependence

171. Recurrent, intrusive, senseless ideas, thoughts, and images that are ego-dystonic and involuntary are termed as

a. Obsessions b. Compulsions
c. Hypochondriasis d. Obtrusiveness

172. Mood-congruent psychotic features in depressed patients include all, *except*

a. Nihilistic delusions b. Delusion of guilt
c. Delusion of poverty d. Delusion of love

173. The investigation related to diagnosis of alcohol dependence

a. MCV b. Serum CPK-MB
c. Serum prolactin levels d. VDRL

174. The most common obsession is

a. Fear of contamination b. Pathological doubt
c. Need for symmetry d. Aggressive obsessions

175. Instrument used for alcohol dependence screening

a. SANS b. HDRS
c. T-BOCS d. MAST

176. Obsessive-compulsive symptoms are intimately linked with

a. Bipolar disorders b. Autistic disorders
c. Tourette's disorder d. ADHD

177. GGT (gamma-glutyl transaminase) is elevated in

a. Cannabis dependence b. Nicotine dependence
c. Heroin dependence d. Alcohol dependence

178. An indication for ECT

a. Severe depression b. Hypomania
c. Autistic disorders d. Tourette syndrome

179. The common defense mechanism with OCD

a. Sublimation b. Projection
c. Denial d. Undoing

180. Characteristic features of manic episode include the following, *except*

a. Elevated, expansive, irritable mood
b. Increased psychomotor activity
c. Thought echo, thought insertion or thought withdrawal
d. Flight of ideas

181. **Compulsory-drinking**
  a. Dipsomania b. Pyromania
  c. Trichotillomania d. Dyslexia

182. **A tricyclic antidepressant**
  a. Fluoxamine b. Fluoxetine
  c. Escitalopram d. Clomipramine

183. **Wernicke's encephalopathy is attributed to**
  a. Severe riboflavin deficiency
  b. Excessive blood alcohol content
  c. Severe thiamine deficiency
  d. Excessive GGT levels

184. **Which of the following is *not* a contraindication for use of disulfiram**
  a. Recent CAD b. History of psychosis
  c. Seizure disorder d. Nicotine dependence

185. **A poor prognostic factor in mood disorders**
  a. Acute or abrupt onset of illness
  b. Typical clinical features
  c. Well-adjusted premorbid personality
  d. Co-morbid personality disorders

186. **The therapeutic blood level of sodium valproate in mood disorders**
  a. 0.8–1.2 mEq/L b. 10–20 mEq/L
  c. 20–40 mcg/mL d. 45 and 100 mcg/mL

187. **The antidepressant having high anticholinergic side effects**
  a. Mirtazapine b. Sertraline
  c. Amitriptyline d. Fluoxetine

188. **A tricyclic antidepressant drug**
  a. Escitalopram b. Imipramine
  c. Paroxetine d. Fluoxetine

189. **Inability to recognize objects by touch is known as**
  a. Adiadochokinesia b. Anosognosia
  c. Apraxia d. Astereognosis

190. **Feeling of sadness and irritability is termed as**
  a. Dysphoria b. Anhedonia
  c. Depression d. Apathy

191. **Omega sign is noticed in patients with**
  a. Dementia b. Schizophrenia
  c. Depression d. OCD

192. **Which is not a negative symptom of schizophrenia**
  a. Asociality b. Anhedonia,
  c. Avolition d. Delusion

193. **A kind of hallucination which is experienced by the subject when falling asleep is called**
  a. Hypnopompic hallucination
  b. Hypnogogic hallucination
  c. Hypnotic hallucination
  d. Pseudo hallucination

ANSWER KEY

1. b	2. c	3. d	4. d	5. d	6. b	7. a	8. d	9. a	10. a	11. a	12. b
13. c	14. d	15. a	16. d	17. a	18. a	19. a	20. d	21. d	22. b	23. d	24. b
25. a	26. c	27. c	28. c	29. d	30. a	31. b	32. d	33. c	34. b	35. a	36. c
37. b	38. a	39. a	40. d	41. c	42. d	43. a	44. a	45. d	46. b	47. a	48. c
49. a	50. c	51. b	52. a	53. a	54. d	55. a	56. d	57. d	58. d	59. a	60. d
61. c	62. a	63. c	64. c	65. c	66. b	67. b	68. a	69. b	70. a	71. a	72. d
73. a	74. c	75. c	76. c	77. c	78. b	79. a	80. c	81. b	82. d	83. a	84. d
85. d	86. d	87. c	88. c	89. a	90. a	91. b	92. b	93. b	94. b	95. a	96. c
97. c	98. c	99. c	100. b	101. b	102. d	103. c	104. b	105. a	106. a	107. c	108. b
109. b	110. b	111. d	112. c	113. d	114. d	115. a	116. a	117. b	118. d	119. c	120. b
121. d	122. c	123. d	124. d	125. d	126. d	127. a	128. b	129. d	130. c	131. b	132. c
133. c	134. b	135. b	136. b	137. d	138. b	139. a	140. a	141. a	142. c	143. d	144. b
145. c	146. b	147. a	148. a	149. a	150. d	151. b	152. b	153. b	154. c	155. b	156. a
157. d	158. b	159. b	160. d	161. d	162. d	163. a	164. c	165. b	166. a	167. d	168. d
169. d	170. c	171. a	172. d	173. a	174. a	175. d	176. c	177. d	178. a	179. d	180. c
181. a	182. d	183. c	184. d	185. d	186. d	187. c	188. b	189. d	190. a	191. c	192. d
193. b											

Chapter 4

Child Health Nursing

THE NEWBORN

Adaptation to Extrauterine Life

A. Immediate needs at the time of delivery

a. Aspiration of mucous to open up the airway.
b. APGAR score at 1 minute and 5 minutes.
c. Maintain body temperature to prevent acidosis.
d. Cord care, eye care.

B. Changes in the newborn during the first week of life

1. **Circulatory:**
   - Closure of the foramen ovale and ductus arteriosus and obliteration of the umbilical arteries produce an adult like circulation within one hour after birth.
   - Heart rate regular 120–160/mt, but variable depending, soft heart murmur common for first month of life. Clotting mechanism poor because of low prothrombin concentration, injection vitamin K is necessary.
   - Liver large but immature, cannot destroy excessive RBC in the newborn, resulting in physcological jaundice by 3rd day.
   - Hb level 14–20 gm% and WBC count 6,000–22,000 cells/cubic mm.
2. **Respiratory:** Respirations diaphragmatic, irregular, abdominal, 30–50 per minute, quiet with periods of apnea.
3. **Excretory**
   - Kidneys immature: Newborn should void within first 24 hours; albumin and urates (brick red staining on diaper) common during first week because of dehydration.
   - Stools: First stool, black green and tenacious (meconium), by third day becomes mixed with highest yellow (transitional).
4. **Integumentary**
   - Lanugo: Fine downy hair growths over the entire body.
   - Milia: Small, whitish, pinpoint spots over the nose caused by retained sebaceous recreations.
   - Mongolian spots: Blue black discoloration on back, buttocks, and sacral region that disappear by first year.
5. **Digestive:** Has stores of nutrients from intrauterine life, needs only very little nourishment for first few days, roots and sucks when anything is brought to mouth; digests simple carbohydrates, fats and proteins, cardiac sphincter of stomach not well developed; so chance of regurgitation if overfull, needs to be burped frequently to get rid of air in the stomach.
6. **Endocrine**
   - *Metabolic:* All newborns normally lose 10% of their body weight by first week of life.
   - *Hormonal:* Enlargement of breasts in boys (gynecomastia) and girls is normal, pseudo-menstruation in girls may also be present.
7. **Neural:** CNS and brain not well developed infant need constant supply of oxygen; breathing, sucking and crying are early neural activities.
8. **Sleep:** Sleep lowers body metabolism, newborns sleep for 20–22 hours and this helps restore and assimilate energy for growth.

PRETERM (PREMATURE) OR LOW BIRTH WEIGHT INFANT

- An infant born before term (37 weeks) is called preterm or premature.
- A low birth weight infant is one who weighs 2500 g or less.
- Full term infants may be low birth weight, premature infant need not be.

Characteristics of Preterm Infants

1. Has less subcutaneous fat, skin wrinkled, blood vessels and bony structures visible, lanugo present over face, eyebrows absent and ears are poorly supported by cartilage.
2. Head circumference is quite large in comparison with the chest, the fontanels are small and bones are soft.

3. Skin color changes when the preterm infant is moved, upper half of body pale and lower half red (harlequin color change).
4. Posture is of complete relaxation with marked flexion and abduction of the thighs.
5. Heat loss rapid due to poor CNS development, large skin surface area, slower circulation and poor oxygenation; insufficient heat production caused by inadequate metabolism.
6. Respirations weak due to muscular weakness of lungs and rib cage, retraction at xiphoid is evidence of air hunger.
7. Greater tendency due to capillary fragility and intracranial hemorrhage, RBC and WBC counts low with resulting anemia.
8. Nutrition is difficult to maintain due to reflexes, small capacity of the stomach, low gastric acidity, and slow emptying area of the stomach.

Management

- Open up airway after delivery
- Intubation if needed
- Maintain temperature
- Manage in a newborn ICU.

SPECIAL CONDITIONS IN THE NEONATE

ASPHYXIA NEONATORUM OR NEONATAL RESPIRATORY DISTRESS

Asphyxia neonatorum occurs when respirations are not well established within 60 seconds after birth as a result of cerebral damage, anoxia or narcosis.

Findings

1. Asphyxia livida: Persistent generalized cyanosis and good muscle tone.
2. Asphyxia pallida: Marked pallor, poor muscle tone.

Major Findings

Include respiratory rate over 60/minutes, retraction, grunting, cyanosis, nasal flaring and chin lag; increased apical pulse, hypothermia, decreased activity level, elevated levels of CO_2 and metabolic acidosis.

Treatment

- Maintain temperature, nutrition.
- O_2 therapy, CPAP and PEEP ventilation may also be used.
- Monitor infants blood gases, provide chest physiotherapy and postural drainage if needed.
- Surfactant administration via endotracheal tube for if facility newborns available.
- Sequelae of asphyxia include
  a. **Hyperbilirubinemia.**
  b. **Retrolental fibroplasias:** Retinal changes, visual impairment and eventually blindness, resulting from too high oxygen levels during treatment.
  c. **Bronchopulmonary dysplasia (BPD):** Change to the alveolar epithelium of the lungs related to high oxygen concentrations and positive pressure ventilation.
  d. **Necrotizing enterocolitis.**

HYPERBILIRUBINEMIA

- Elevated serum bilirubis in the newborn resulting in jaundice.
- In physiologic, average increase from 2 mg/dL in cord blood to 6 mg/dL by 72 hours, not exceeding 12 mg/dL.
- May result from immaturity of liver; Rh or ABO incompatibility, infection, birth maternal diabetes, hypothermia, medications. (Brain damage caused by high levels of unconjugated bilirubin)

Findings

1. Pathologic jaundice usually appear early, up to 24 hours after birth, represents a process ongoing before birth.
2. Unusual pattern of progression is from head to foot, blanch skin over bony area or look at conjunctiva and buccal membranes in dark skinned infants.
3. Pallor, dark, concentrated urine, behavior changes (irritability, lethargy).
4. Pdycythemia, increased serum bilirubin.

Treatment

1. Identify and treat condition contributing to hyperbilirubinemia.
2. Prevent progression or complications.
3. Prevent condition that contribute to development of hyperbilirubinemia (e.g. cold stress, hypoxia, acidosis, hypoglycemia, dehydration, infection).
4. Phototherapy.
5. Exchange transfusion.

HEMOLYTIC DISEASE OF THE NEWBORN (ERYTHRO BLASTOSIS FOETALIS)

- **Characterized by** RBC destruction in the newborn, with resultant anemia and hyperbilirubinemia.
- **Possibly caused by** Rh or ABO incompatibility between may be sensitized in Ist pregnancy in RH incompatibility, the sub-segment fetuses may be affected if they are Rh +ve.

- First born may be affected in ABO incompatibility because 'O' mother may have anti A and anti B antibodies even before pregnancy; but reaction are tens severe than Rh incompatibility.

Findings

- Jaundice and pallor within first 24-36 hours
- Anemia
- Erythropoiesis
- Enlarged Placenta
- Edema and ascites.

Treatment

1. Determine blood type and Rh early in pregnancy.
2. Determine results of indirect comb's test early and at 28–32 weeks in pregnancy.
3. Determine results of direct comb's test in cord blood.
4. Administer RhoGam (Rh-D immuneglobulin) to the mother.
5. Phototherapy and exchange transfusion in needed cases.

NEONATAL SEPSIS

- **Associated with** the presence of pathogenic microorganism in the blood especially gramnegative organism (*E coli*, *Klebsiella* and *Proteus*) and grampositive Group B beta hemolytic streptococci.
- **Contributing factors** include prolonged rupture of membranes more than 24 hours, prolonged or difficult labor, maternal infection, infection in hospital personnel and aspiration at birth or later.

Findings

a. Behavioral changes: Lethargy, irritability, poor feeding.
b. Frequent periods of apnea.
c. Jaundice, low grade fever.
d. Vomiting, diarrhea.

Treatment

1. Antibiotics as per culture and sensitivity.
2. Maintain body temperature, oxygen if needed.
3. Monitor vital signs and maintain hydration.

HYPOGLYCEMIA

- Common in infants of diabetic mothers, these infants are usually macrosomic (large for gestational age) due to high maternal glucose levels that have crossed placenta, stimulating fetal pancreas to secrete more insulin which then act as a growth hormone.
- At birth, with loss of supply of maternal glucose, newborn may become hypoglycemic.
- Large size may have caused traumatic vaginal birth or may have necessitated cesarean birth.
- Hypoglycemia can also occur in infants who are full term, SGA, postterm, septic or with any condition that subject the infant to stress.

Findings

1. May be born prematurely due to complications.
2. Infants of diabetic mothers may be immature/dysmature, higher incidence of congenital anomalies in IDMs (infant of diabetic mother).
3. Puffy body, enlarged organs, tremors, feeding difficulty, irregular respirations, lethargy, hyper-bilirubinemia, hypothermia and hypoglycemia and respiratory distress.
4. Blood glucose levels below 40 mg/dL (20 mg/dL in premature infant).

Treatment

1. Care of prematurity.
2. Monitor blood glucose level frequently and give frequent feedings.
3. Nasogastric/IV fluids if baby has poor sucking reflex.

GROWTH AND DEVELOPMENT

Growth: Physical Maturation

1. **Heart rate:** Decreases with increasing age, infancy 120 bpm, one year 80–120 bpm, childhood 70–110 bpm, adolescence and adulthood 55–90 bpm.
2. **BP** increases with age: 65/40 in newborn, increases about 2–3 mm of Hg per year beginning at 7 years of age.
3. **Hb:** Highest at neonates (17–20 gm%), decreases to 10–15 gm % by one year; gradual increase in Hb level to 14.5 gm% between one to 12 years of age.
4. **Respiratory rate:** Decrease with increase in age, infancy 30–40 per minute, childhood 20–24 per minute, adolescence and adulthood 16–18 per minute, gradual increase of vital capacity throughout childhood.
5. Basal metabolism high in newborn, decreases with increases in age.
6. Glomerular filtration rate greatly increased by 6 months of age, GFR reaches adult values between 1 and 2 years of age.

7. Stomach size small at birth, rapidly increases during infancy and childhood; peristaltic activity decreases with advancing age, blood sugar levels gradually rise from 75–80 mg% in infancy to 95–100 mg% during adolescence. Premature infants have lower blood sugar levels than do full term infants; secretions of hydrochloric acid and salivary enzymes increases with age until adolescence.
8. Brain reaches 90% of total size by 2 years of age, all brain cells are present by the end of the first years, maturation of brain cell and spinal cord follows cephalocaudal and proximodistal laws.
9. Pediatric doses of drugs differ from adults due to immature liver function, immature kidney function, decreased gastric function and decreased plasma protein concentration, dose calculated based on body surface area.
10. Play needs changes with age; infancy (solitary play), toddler period (parallel play), preschool age (co-operative play).

CHILD WITH CHROMOSOMAL ABNORMALITIES

Down's Syndrome (Trisomy 21)

Small rounded skill with flat occiput, inner epicanthal folds and oblique palpebral fissures, specking of the iris (Brush field's spots), small nose with depressed bridge (saddle nose) protruding tongue, low-set ears, short, thick neck, hypotonic musculature (protruding abdomen, umbilical hernia), hyperflexible and laxed joints, simian line (transverse crease on the palmer side of the hand), broad hands and feet, delayed incomplete sexual development.

Trisomy 18

Several physical anomalies of the head, ears, mandible, hands, feet, heart and kidneys.

Turner's Syndrome (Gonadal Dysgenesis)

XO karyotype in females, short stature, webbed neck, infantile genitalia, developmental failure of secondary sexual characteristic at puberty, usually intelligence is normal.

Klinefelters' Syndrome

XXY in males, tall, skinny, long, legs and arms, small firm testes, gynecomastia and poorly developed secondary sex characteristics at puberty, behavioral disorders and mental defects.

DISORDERS OF GASTROINTESTINAL SYSTEM

CLEFT LIP

Failure of union of embryonic structure of face, fusion of maxillary and premaxillary processes occurs between 5 and 8 weeks of fetal life; may be bilateral or unilateral.

Findings

Difficulty feeding; increased swallowed air due to mouth breathing leading to distended abdomen, mucous membrane of the oropharynx become dried and cracked with increased rise of infection.

Treatment

Surgical correction, performed soon after birth, may be repeated for further modifications.

CLEFT PALATE

Failure of union of palatal structures, normal fusion normally occurs between 9 and 12 weeks; may involve the soft or head palate and may extend into the nose, forming an oronasal passage way.

Findings

Infection usually aspiration pneumonia, defective speech, excessive dental caries, malocclusion from displacement of the maxillary arch; hearing problem due to recurrent otitis media.

Treatment

Surgical correction between 6 months and 3 years before speech is developed.

TRACHEOESOPHAGEAL ANOMALIES

May be absence of the esophagus, atresia of the esophagus without a tracheal fistula, and tracheoesophageal fistula.

Findings

Excessive drooling, excessive mucus in the nasopharynx causing cyanosis; chocking, sneezing and coughing during feeding with regurgitation of feeds through the mouth and nose inability to pass a catheter into the stomach.

Treatment

Surgical repair.

INTESTINAL OBSTRUCTION

- Congenital, life-threatening obstruction of the intestines may be mechanical (constricted or narrowed lumens) or muscular (interfere with normal muscular contraction).
- As a result of an obstruction, there is an increased peristalsis, distension by the fluids and gas and increased bacterial growth proximal to the obstruction. Intestinal secretions are increased and bowels absorptive capacity is reduced.

Findings

1. Pain
2. Fever
3. Vomiting may be the early sign of obstruction in the higher tract and later sign in the obstruction of the lower tract.
4. Dehydration due to loss of fluids and electrolytes.
5. Absence of passing the flatus or stools.
6. Patient may be drowsy.
7. In severe cases, respiratory difficulty results due to the upward pressure on the diaphragm.

Treatment

1. Mechanical causes are treated with surgery.
2. Specific treatment—if obstruction is due to worm infestation.

PYLORIC STENOSIS

Hypertrophy (thickening) of the pyloric sphincter causing stenosis and obstruction.

Findings

1. Olive sized bulge under right ribcage.
2. Vomiting as obstruction increases, vomiting becomes more forceful and projectile.
3. Peristaltic waves during and after feeding (look like rolling balls under abdominal wall).
4. Failure to thrive.
5. Dehydration: Sunken fontanels, poor skin turgor, decreased urinary output.

Treatment

Surgery: Pyloromyotomy (Fredet-Ramstedt surgery): Longitudinal splitting of the hypertrophic circular muscles down to the submucosa allowing the pylorus to expand so that fluid may pass.

INTUSSUSCEPTION

Telescoping of bowel into itself (usually at the ileocecal valve) causing edeme, obstruction and possible necrosis of the bowel.

Findings

1. Piercing cry
2. Severe abdominal pain (pulls legs up)
3. Vomiting
4. Bloody mucus in stool
5. Current—jelly stool.

Treatment

1. Barium enema to reduce telescoping by hydrostatic pressure.
2. Surgery if barium enema is unsuccessful or if signs of peritonitis.

OMPHALOCELE (EXOMPHALUS)

- Herniation of abdominal organs into the umbilical cord with evisceration into the sac; an embryonic mid-gut grows and elongates and project abdominal products into the base of the umbilical cord.
- The sac of omphalocele may rapture and cause adhesions.

Treatment

- Antibiotics to prevent injection.
- Surgical reduction of evisceration.

HIRSCHSPRUNG'S DISEASE (Congenital Aganglionic Megacolon)

- Absence of automatic parasympathetic ganglion cells in a portion of the large colon; usually occurs 4–25 cm proximally from anus.
- Defect results in decreased motility in that portion of the colon and signs of functional obstruction.
- When stool enters the affected part of the colon, lack of peristalsis causes it to remain there until additional stool pushes it through, colon dilates as stool is impacted.

Findings

1. Failure or delay in passing meconium.
2. Abdominal distention, failure to pass stool.
3. Temporary relief following digital rectal examination.
4. Loose stools, only liquid can get around impaction (may also be a ribbon like stool).

5. Nausea, anorexia, lethargy.
6. Bile stained or fecal vomiting.
7. Loss of weight, failure to grow.
8. Volvulus (bowel twits upon itself, causing obstruction and necrosis) and entero-colitis due to fecal stagnation.

Treatment

1. Drugs: Stool softners.
2. Isotonic enemas.
3. Low residue diet.
4. Surgery.

a. Palliative: Loop or double barrel colostomy.
b. Corrective: Abdominal perineal pull through (Duhamel's surgery), bowel containing ganglia is pulled down and anastomosed to the rectum.

APPENDICITIS

- Inflammation of the appendix that prevents mucus from passing into the cecum.
- If untreated, ischemia, gangrene, rupture and peritonitis occur.
- May be caused by mechanical obstruction (fecaliths, intestinal parasites) or anatomic defect; may be related to decreased fiber in diet.

Findings

a. Diffuse pain, localized in lower right quadrant.
b. Nausea/vomiting.
c. Guarding of abdomen, rebound tenderness, walks stoops over.
d. Decreased bowel sounds.
e. Fever.

Treatment

1. Antipyretics, antibiotics.
2. Prevent perforation of appendix, do not give enemas, do not do forceful, vigorous abdominal palpations.
3. Surgery: Appendicectomy.

IMPERFORATE ANUS

- Congenital malformation caused by abnormal fetal development.
- Often associated with fistula formation to the rectum or vagina other congenital anomalies.

Findings

1. No stool passage within 24 hours of birth.
2. Meconium stool from inappropriate orifice if fistula present.
3. Inability to insert thermometer.

Treatment

1. If suspected, do not take rectal temperature because of the risk of perforation causing peritonitis.
2. Perform manual dilatation as ordered.
3. Surgical correction.

DISORDERS OF THE NEUROSENSORY SYSTEM

INCREASED ICP

- Increased amount of CSF within the ventricles the brain.
- May be caused by obstruction of CSF flow or by overproduction or inadequate reabsorption of CSF.
- May result from congenital malformation or be secondary to injury, infection or tumor.

Types

- **Non-communicating:** Flow of CSF from ventricles to subarachnoid space is obstructed.
- **Communicating:** Flow is not obstructed, but CSF is inadequately reabsorbed in subarachnoid space.

Findings

Depend on age of onset and amount of CSF in the brain

1. **Infant to 2 years:** Enlarging head size, bulging, non-pulsating fontanels, downward rotation of the eyes (sunset appearance), separation of cranial sutures, poor feeding, vomiting, lethargy, irritability, high pitched cry and abnormal muscle tone.
2. **Older children:** Changes in head size less common, signs of increased ICP (ataxia, vomiting, headache), alteration in consciousness and papilledema (late signs).

Treatment

1. **Shunts:** Insertion of a flexible tube into the lateral ventricle of the brain, catheter is threaded under the skin and distal end positioned in the peritoneum (ventriculoperitoneal shunt) or in the right atrium (ventriculoatrial shunt).
2. Antibiotics to prevent infection in the postoperative period.

SPINA BIFIDA (MYELODYSPLASIA)

- Failure of posterior vertebral arches to fuse during embryologic development.
- Radiation, viral and environmental factors have been suggested as causative.
- Approximately 85% of the defects in the spine involve the lower thoracic, lumber or sacral area.

Types

1. **Spina bifida occulta:** Spinal cord and meninges remain in the normal anatomical position, defect may not be visible, or may be identified by a dimple or a tuft of hair on the spine; child is asymptomatic or may have slight neuromuscular deficit; no treatment needed if asymptomatic, otherwise treatment aimed at specific symptoms.
2. **Meningocele:** Sac filled with spinal fluid protrudes through opening in the spinal canal, sac is covered with thin skin, and no nerve in sac; so there is no motor or sensory loss, good prognosis after surgery.
3. **Meningomyelocele:** Same as meningocele except there are spinal nerves in the sac, child will have sensory and motor deficit below the site of the lesion.

Treatment

1. **Surgery:** Closure of sac, shunt procedure if accompanying hydrocephalus, orthopedic surgery to correct associated defects of lip, knees or feet.
2. **Drugs:** Antibiotics to treat infection, anti-cholinergic drugs to increase bladder capacity and lower intravascular pressure.

REYES SYNDROME

- An acute encephalopathy with fatty degeneration of the liver.
- Cerebral completion may reach an irreversible state.
- Increased ICP secondary to cerebral edema is a major factor contributing to morbidity and mortality.

Findings

1. Child appears to be recovering from viral illness such as influenza or chickenpox, during which salicylates have appear that follow a definite pattern, which has led to clinical staging

   Stage I: Sudden onset of persistent vomiting, fatigue and listlessness.

   Stage II: Personality and behavior changes, disorientation, confusion hyper-reflexia.

   Stage III: Coma, decorticate posturing.

   Stage IV: Deeper coma, decerebrate rigidity.

   Stage V: Absent DTR (deep tendon reflex), seizures, respiratory depression, flaccid paralysis.
2. **Pathophysiologic changes** include increased free fatty acid level, hyperammonemia due to reduction of enzyme that converts ammonia, impaired liver function, structural changes in mitochondria in muscle and brain tissue, significant swelling of the brain.

Treatment

Depend upon staging, supportive care depending upon the level of ammonia and coma.

SEIZURE DISORDERS

- Seizures: Recurrent, sudden changes in consciousness, behavior, sensations, and or muscular activities beyond voluntary control that are produced by excess neuronal discharge.
- Epilepsy: Chronic recurrent seizures. Seizures may be symptomatic or acquired, caused by tumors, subdural hematomas, metabolic abnormalities like hypoglycemia, hypocalcemia and hyponatremia, meningitis, encephalitis, encephalopathy, hydrocephalus, intracranial hemorrhage, etc.

Classification

1. **Generalized seizures or grand-mal seizures:** May be preceded by aura, has tonic and clonic phases.

   Tonic phase is characterized by contraction and stiffness of limbs, pupils dilate and eyes roll on to one side, glottis closes causing noise on exhalation, may be incontinent, occurs as same time as loss of consciousness. Clonic phase has repetitive movements and increased mucus production. Tonic phase lasts for 20–40 seconds and clonic phase slowly tapers.

   Seizure ends with postictal period of confusion and drowsiness.
2. **Absence seizure:** (Petitmal seizure): Usually non-organic brain damage present, sudden onset, with twitching or rolling of eyes, lasts a few second.
3. **Myoclonic seizures:** Associated with brain damage, may be precipitated by tactile or visual sensations.
4. **Akinetic seizures:** Related to organic brain lesions and there is temporary loss of consciousness.
5. **Febile seizures:** Commonly present in under fives than adults, seizure occurs only when fever is rising.
6. **Status epilepticus:** Generalized grand-mal seizure, seizure is prolonged, or there are repeated seizures without regaining consciousness, can result in decreased oxygen supply and possible cardiac arrest.

Findings

Clinical findings vary according to type of seizure.

Treatment

1. Protect from injury
2. Keep airway open
3. Observe and record seizure
4. Antiepileptics.

CEREBRAL PALSY

- Neuromuscular disorder resulting from damage to or altered structures of the part of the brain responsible for controlling motor function.
- May be caused by a variety of factors resulting in damage to the CNS like:
  1. **Prenatal causes:** Genetic, altered neurological development or trauma or anoxia to mother.
  2. **Intranatal causes:** During the birth process (drugs at delivery, precipitate delivery, fetal distress, breech deliveries with delay).
  3. **Postnatal causes:** Kernicterus or head trauma.

Findings

Disease itself does not progress once established, but the progressive complications cause changes in signs and symptoms.

1. **Spasticity:** Exaggerated hyperactive reflexes (increased muscle tone, increase in stretch reflex, scissoring of legs, poorly coordinated body movements for voluntary activities.
2. **Athetosis:** Constant involuntary, purposeless, slow, writhing movements, occurs with extra-pyramidal tract lesions, athetosis disappears during sleep, therefore contractures do not develop, movements increase with increase in physical or emotional stress, also affects facial muscles.
3. **Ataxia:** Disturbance in equilibrium, diminished writing reflex (lack of balance, poor coordination, dizziness, hypotonia) occurs with cerebellar lesions, muscles and reflexes are normal.
4. **Tremors:** Repetitive rhythmic involuntary contractions of flexor and extensor muscles.
5. **Rigidity:** Resistance to flexion and extension resulting from simultaneous contraction of both agonist and antagonist muscle group, occurs with basal ganglia lesions, diminished or absent reflexes, potential for severe contractures.
6. **Associated problems:** Mental retardation, hearing loss, defective speech, dental anomalies, orthopedic problems from contractures, visual disabilities, disturbance in body image, touch, perception.

Treatment

1. **Drugs:** Antianxiety drugs, skeletal muscle relaxants, local nerve blocks.
2. Physiotherapy, occupational therapy.
3. Speech therapy.
4. **Surgery:** Muscle and tendon releasing procedures.

DISORDERS OF THE EYE

BLINDNESS

- May result from genetic disorders, maternal infection during pregnancy, prematurity, retrolental fibroplaisa, trauma, childhood infection, etc.

Findings

1. Vacant stare, obvious failure to look at things.
2. Rubbing eyes, tilting head, examining objects very close to eyes.
3. Does not reach for objects if the baby is over 4 months.
4. Does not smile when mother smiles (over 3 months), but does smile in response to mother's voice.
5. Crawls or walks into furniture.
6. Does not respond to the motion of others.
7. No concept of the look of an object, no concept of color or reflection of self.
8. Other senses become keenly developed to compensate.
9. Unable to copy the movements of others.

Treatment

1. Treatment of cause.
2. Use multisensory stimulation.
3. Speak to child before touching and always tell what you are going to do.
4. Ensure safety.

CONJUNCTIVITIS

Infection and inflammation of the membrane covering the anterior surface of the eye globe and inner surface of the eye globe and inner surface of the eyelid (conjunctiva).

May be due to viral, bacterial and allergic factors.

Findings

1. Weeping eye
2. Reddened conjunctiva
3. Sensitivity to light
4. Eyelid stuck shut with exudates.

Treatment

1. Ophthalmic antibiotics-gentamycin eye drops, ciplox eye drops.
2. Steroids.

DISORDERS OF THE EAR

DEAFNESS

- Hearing impairment may be total or partial

Causes

1. *Conductive:* Interference in transmission from outer to middle ear from chronic otitis media, foreign bodies.
2. *Sensory neural:* Dysfunction of the inner ear, damage to cranial nerve VIII from rubella, meningitis, drugs, etc.

Findings

1. Infant fails to react to loud noises (does have a moro reflex; but not to noise).
2. Makes no attempt to locate the sound.
3. Remains in babbling stage or cases to babble.
4. Fails to develop speech.
5. Startled by sudden appearances.
6. Responds only when speakers lips are visible.
7. Cannot concentrate for long on visual images.
8. Always puzzled or withdrawn, or strain to hear.
9. Use high volume on TV/radio.
10. Hearing deficit on audiologic tests.

Treatment

1. Treat the causative factor if any.
2. Speech therapy.
3. Hearing aids.
4. Surgery depending on the cause.

OTITIS MEDIA

- Infection of middle ear due to bacterial or viral cause.
- More common infants and preschoolers as the ear canal is shorter and more horizontal than in older children.
- Common in children with cleft lip and palate.
- Blockage of eustachian tube causes lymphedema and accumulation of fluid in the middle ear.

Findings

1. Dysfunction of eustachian tube.
2. Ear infection usually related to respiratory infection.
3. Increased middle ear pressure, bulging tympanic membrane.
4. Pain, infant pulls or touches ear frequently.
5. Irritability; cough, nasal congestion.
6. Causative organism revealed in culture and sensitivity.

Treatment

1. Systemic and otic antibiotics.
2. Analgesics.
3. Antipyretics.
4. Nasal decongestants.
5. Myringotomy and drainage of pus collection.

DISEASES AND DISORDERS OF THE CARDIOVASCULAR SYSTEM

NORMAL CHANGES IN FETAL CIRCULATION AFTER BIRTH

1. When the umbilical cord is clamped and severed, the blood supply from the placenta is cut off and oxygenation must than take place in the newborns' lungs.
2. As the lungs expand with air, the pulmonary artery pressure decreases and circulation to lung increases.
3. **Ductus venosum:** After the umbilical cord is severed, flow through the ductus venosum decreases and certainly cases, it constricts within 3–7 days after birth and eventually becomes ligamentum venosum.
4. **Foramen ovale:** Functional closure of foramen ovale (opening between right left atria) occurs when the pressure in the left atrium exceeds pressure in the right. Expansion of the pulmonary artery causes a drop in pulmonary artery pressure and in right a trial and ventricular pressure. At the same time there is increased pulmonary blood flow to the left atrium and increased aortic pressure from clamping of the umbilical cord which in turn raises left ventricular and left a trial pressure.

   Anatomical closure of foramen ovale occurs within the first week after birth with the deposit of fibrin.

5. **Ductus arteriosus**
    - Increase in aortic blood flow increases aortic pressure and decreases right to left shunt through the ductus arteriosus, shunt become bi-directional.
    - Increased pulmonary blood flow increases arterial oxygen, causing vasoconstriction of ductus arteriosus within hours of birth.
    - Functional closure occurs when this constriction causes cessation of blood flow, usually 24 hours after birth.
    - Anatomic closure occurs when there is growth of fibrous tissue in the tubes of the ductus arteriosus, i.e. by 1–3 weeks.

CONGESTIVE CARDIAC FAILURE

- A symptom complex reflecting the hearts' inability to meet the metabolic demands of the body.
- Usually due to a surgically correctable structural abnormality of the heart that result in increased blood volume and pressure.

Findings

1. Tachycardia, gallop rhythm, cardiomegaly, decreased peripheral pulses and mottling of the extremities.
2. Tachypnea, retractions, grunting, nasal flaring, cough, cyanosis, orthopnea.
3. Hepatomegaly, edema, distended neck veins and peripheral veins, decreased urine output.
4. Failure to thrive, decrease exercise tolerance.

Treatment

1. Goal is to improve cardiac function and to conserve energy.
2. Drugs
    a. Digitalis to improve myocardial contractility and to slow the heart rate.
    b. Diuretics to decrease the total body water and to increase urinary output.
    c. Potassium supplement if diuretic is potassium depleting.
    d. Antihypertensive drugs.

CONGENITAL HEART DEFECTS

A. Acyanotic Heart Defects

a. Oxygenated blood is shunted from the systematic to pulmonary circulation (left to right shunt) and blood leaving the aorta is completely oxygenated.

b. Increased blood volume on right side of heart results in hypertrophy of right ventricle.

c. Eventually most cyanotic heart defects will result in CHF.

B. Cyanotic Heart Defects

a. Unoxygenated blood is shunted from the right to the left side of the heart where it mixes with oxygenated blood.

b. The blood pumped to the peripheral tissues has much lower oxygen contest than normal, causing cyanosis.

ACYANOTIC HEART DEFECTS

1. **Atrial Septal Defect**
    - Abnormal opening in the septum between left and right atria, causing a left-to-right shunt.
    - Symptoms include decreased exercise tolerance, dyspnea and systolic ejection murmur heard best in the upper left sternal border.
    - Surgical correction performed between 2 and 4 years of age.
2. **Ventricular Septal Defect (VSD)**
    - Opening in the septum between ventricles, causing a left to right shunt.
    - Symptoms depend on size of the defect, child's age and degree of pulmonary vascular resistance.
    - Small VSDs may be asymptomatic, larger defects may result in hypertrophy, potential failure of the right ventricle and CHF.
    - Symptom include tachycardia, increased respiratory effort, dyspnea, fatigue, frequent respiratory infections, systolic murmur at lower left sternal border, CHF.
    - Surgical correction indicated if medical management fails to diminish symptoms or if the child continues to have a persistent shunt by 3–4 years of age.
3. **Patent Ductus Arteriosus (PDA)**
    - Failure to close ductus arteriosus at birth.
    - Allows oxygenated blood pumped into the aorta from the left ventricle to return to the lungs.
    - A small PDA may be asymptomatic, larger PDA cause excess blood in the lungs and volume overload, leading to CHF.
    - Machinery type murmur best heard at middle to upper left sternal border.
    - In premature infants treatment with indomethacin (prostaglandin inhibitor) sometimes cause closure.
    - Definitive surgery is legation of PDA.

4. **Coarctation of Aorta**
   - Narrowing of the aorta usually just beyond the left subclavian artery.
   - Causes a significant reduction in blood flow to abdomen and legs with majority of blood shunted to head and arms.
   - Clinical manifestations may depend on degree of narrowing and include blood and pulse pressure higher in arms then legs, high pulse pressure in carotid and radial pulses, low pulse pressure in femoral pulses, warm upper body and cool lower body, nose bleeds and headaches.
   - Predisposition to stroke.
   - Surgical treatment depend on location of coarctation.
5. **Pulmonary Stenosis**
   - Abnormally narrowed valvular orifice.
   - If stenosis is mild to moderate, children may be asymptomatic and require no treatment.
   - More severe pulmonic value stenosis can result in right ventricular hypertrophy and even hepatomegaly.
   - Severe stenosis require valvotomy.
6. **Aortic stenosis**
   - Abnormally small aortic value orifice, value may be bicuspid rather than tricuspid.
   - Mild to moderate stenosis may not produce symptoms; more severe stenosis produces left ventricular hypertrophy, left heart failure, and decreased cardiac output.
   - Valvotomy is preferred treatment for children, but valve replacement may be necessary later.

CYANOTIC HEART DEFECTS

1. **Tetralogy of Fallot**
   - Most common cyanotic heart defect.
   - **Four diseases:** Pulmonary artery stenosis, VSR, over riding of aorta and ventricular hypertrophy.
   - Symptoms depend on degree of pulmonary stenosis.
   - Aorta sits near core of heart over the VSD and therefore receives blood from both ventricles.
   - Decreased blood flow to the lungs, mixture of unoxygenated blood going to aorta causes cyanosis and dyspnea.
   - Symptoms also include activity intolerance, irritability, failure to thrive, polycythemia, harsh systolic murmur best heard along the left sternal border and TET spells.
   - **TET spells**: Hypoxic episodes caused by transient increase in the obstruction of the right ventricular outflow tract, symptoms include cyanosis, tachypnea, flaccidity, altered level of consciousness, may progress to seizures, CVA and death, episodes may be precipitated by crying, feeling or defection, treatment includes positioning in a knee-chest position, oxygen, propranolol and morphine.
   - Surgical correction: Surgical intervention indicated when infant or child becomes symptomatic, Blalock-Tausig shunt is a palliative procedure which produces anastomosis of the right of left subclavian artery to the pulmonary artery, total correction of stenosis may be needed.
   - Life long antibiotic prophylaxis to prevent endocarditis for certain procedures like dental procedures.
2. **Transposition of the Great Vessels (TGA)**
   - Aorta arises from right ventricle and pulmonary artery arises from left ventricle.
   - Oxygenated blood therefore circulates through left side of heart to lungs and back to left side unoxygenated blood enters right atrium from body, goes to left ventricle and back out to the body without being oxygenated.
   - Child cannot live without a communication between atria or ventricles.
   - Foramen oval remains open for short while as pressure in heart is not sufficient to close it.
   - Poor oxygenation makes these children cyanotic.
   - Treatment includes surgical incision or balloon septoplasty to create an ASD-(rash kind procedure).
   - When the child is old enough, defect will be corrected surgically (Mustard procedure) to redirect blood flow.
   - An arterial switch is performed when associated with a VSD.
3. **Truncus Arteriosus**
   - Only one vessel exits heart from both ventricles, always associated with a large VSD.
   - As there is no septum to divide aorta and pulmonary trunk, oxygenated and unoxygenated blood mixes causing cyanosis.
   - Drugs: Digitalis and diuretics, if growth failure occurs despite treatment, surgical correction is done.
   - Pulmonary banding or complete intra-cardiac repair may be done.
4. **Hypoplastic Left Heart Syndrome**
   - Concomitant presence of aortic valve atresia, mitral atresia or stenosis, diminutive or absent left ventricle, severe hypoplasia of ascending aorta and aortic arch.
   - Usually fatal, no satisfactory treatment, surgical correction has limited success.

Tetralogy of Fallot consists of four defects viz. pulmonary artery sterosis, VSD, overriding of aorta and right ventricular hypertrophy.

RHEUMATIC FEVER

- An inflammatory disorder that may involve the heart, joints, connective tissue and the CNS.
- Thought to be an autoimmune disorder preceded by an infection of Group A beta hemolytic streptococcus (usually a streptococcal sore throat).
- Antigenic markers for streptococcal toxin closely resemble markers for cardiac valves; this resemblance causes antibodies made against the streptococcus to also attack heart valves.
- Prognosis depends upon the degree of heart damage.

Findings

1. Major symptom (Jones' criteria)

a. **Carditis**
   - Seen in 50% of chests.
   - Aschoff nodules (areas of inflammation and degeneration around heart valves, pericardium and myocardium).
   - Valvular inefficiency of mitral and aortic valve.
   - Cardiomegaly.
   - Shortness of breath, hepatomegaly, edema.

b. **Polyarthritis**
   - Migratory, therefore no contractures develop.
   - Most common in large joints, which become red, swollen and painful.
   - Sterile sinovial fluid.
   - No arthralgia.
   - Sydenhams' chorea (St. vitus dance).
   - CNS disorder characterized by abrupt, purposeless involuntary muscular movements.
   - Mostly seen in prepubertal girls; gradual, insidious onset, start with personality change or clumsiness.
   - May appear months after streptococcal infection and lasts 1–3 months.

c. **Subcutaneous nodules**
   - Usually a sign of severe disease.
   - Occur with active carditis.
   - Firm, nontender nodes on bony prominences of joints.
   - Tests for weeks.

d. **Erythema marginatum**
   - Transient, nonpruritic rash starting with central red patches, that expand, results in series of irregular patches, with raised margins and pale centers (resemble giragge spots).

2. Minor Symptoms

a. History of fever
b. Recent history of streptococcal infection
c. ESR and ASO titer increased, changes seen in ECG.

Treatment

Drug: Penicillin, salicylates, steroids.

DISEASES AND DISORDERS OF THE HEMATOLOGIC SYSTEM

ANEMIAS

Iron Deficiency Anemia

Due to deficiency of iron in the diet.

Findings

- Pallor, fatigue, irritability, diet deficient in iron, normocytic, normochronmic anemia.
- Treated with iron rich foods and iron supplements.

Sickle Cell Anemia

- Inherited disorder (autosomal recessive inheritance).
- Structure of Hb changed; sixth ring of the beta chain changes glutamine for valine.
- RBC crescent shaped, rigid and inflexible.
- Sickles RBC live for 6–20 days instead of 120 days.
- Death usually occur due to infection or occlusion.

Crescent shaped RBC is seen in sickle cell anemia, sickled RBCs live for 6–20 days instead of 120 days.

Findings

a. First sign may be 'colic' due to abdominal pain (abdominal infarct).
b. Infants may have dactylitis (hand-foot syndrome), symmetrical painful soft tissue swelling of hands and feet in the absence of trauma.
c. Splenomegaly: Initially due to hemolysis or phagocytosis; later due to fibrosis from repeat infarct to spleen.

d. Weak bones or spiral defects due to hyperplasia of narrow and osteoporosis.
e. Frequent infections.
f. Leg ulcers due to blockage of blood supply.
g. Delayed growth and development.
h. CVA due to infarct in CNS.
i. Heart failure due to hemosiderosis.
j. Renal failure due to renal infarcts.
k. Priapism: May result in impotence.
l. Pain wherever vaso occlusive crisis occurs.
m. Sickle cell crisis: Vasoocclusive crisis due to blockage of blood vessels results from agglutination of RBC.

> Anoxia and dehydration precipitate sickle cell crisis.

Treatment

- Analgesics and narcotics to control pain.
- Antibiotics to combat infection.
- Exchange transfusion.
- Hydration Splenectomy.

> Avoid aspirin in patients with sickle cell disease because aspirin enhances acidosis which promotes sickling.

IDIOPATHIC THROMPOCYTOPENIC PURPURA (ITP)

- Platelet count less than 1,00000/mm^3 due to increased destruction of platelets.
- Exact cause unknown, thought to be due to auto immune mechanism.

Findings

1. Petechiae: Spider web appearance of bleeding under the skin due to small size of platelets.
2. Ecchymosis.
3. Blood in any body secretions, bleeding from mucous membranes, nose bleeds.

Treatment

1. Steroids and immunosuppressive agents.
2. Platelet transfusion.
3. Splenectomy.

> As far as possible, avoid in injection in a patient with Idiopathic Thrombocytopenic Purpura.

HEMOPHILIA

- Group of bleeding disorder due to deficiency of one of several factors needed for blood clotting
- Sex-linked inherited disorder.

> Classic form of hemophilia affects males only.

Types

1. **Hemophilia A:** Due to factor VIII deficiency (75% of all hemophilia).
2. **Hemophilia B** (Christmas disease): Due to factor IX deficiency.
3. **Hemophilia C:** Factor XI deficiency, autosomal recessive, affects both sexes.

Findings

1. Prolonged bleeding after minor injury.
2. Bruising and hematomas but no petechiae.
3. Peripheral neuropathies (due to bleeding near peripheral nerves).
4. Hemarthrosis: Bleeding into joints.

Treatment

1. Control bleeding episodes.
2. Avoid sutures, cauterization and aspirin: All exacerbate bleeding.
3. Hemostatic agents.
4. Factor VIII transfusion.

> Infuse factor VIII immediately when thawed, because factor VIII deteriorates at room temperature.

DISEASES AND DISORDERS OF THE RESPIRATORY SYSTEM

> **Variations from the Adult**
> - Infants are obligatory nose breathers and diaphragmatic breathers.
> - Number and size of alveoli continue to increase until 8 years of age.
> - Until 5 years, structures of the respiratory tract have a narrow lumen and children are more susceptible to obstruction/distress from inflammation.

TONSILLITIS

- Inflammation of tonsils often as a result of a viral or bacterial pharyngitis.
- If caused by Group A beta hemolytic streptococci, it can lead to carditis.

Findings

1. Enlarged red tonsils, fever.
2. Sore throat, difficulty swallowing, mouth breathing, snoring.
3. White patches of exudates on tonsillar pillars, enlarged cervical lymph nodes.

Treatment

1. Symptomatic treatment.
2. Antibiotics.
3. Surgery: Tonsillectomy if recurrent tonsillitis present or there is peritonsillar abscess and airway obstruction due to enlarged tonsils.

> Increased swallowing could be a sign of hemorrhage after tonsillectomy.

ACUTE SPASMODIC LARYNGITIS (CROUP)

- Respiratory distress characterized by paroxysmal attacks of laryngeal obstruction.
- Attacks occur mostly at night, onset sudden and usually preceded by a mild upper respiratory tract infection.
- Respiratory symptoms last several hours, may occur in a milder form on a few subsequent nights.

Findings

1. Inspiratory stridor, hoarseness, barking cough, anxiety, retractions.
2. A febrile, skin cool.

Treatment

1. Usually self-limiting, steam vapors provide some relief.
2. If spasm continues, take child to the causality.

BRONCHIAL ASTHMA

- Obstructive disease of the lower respiratory tract
- Often caused by an allergic reaction to an environmental allergen, may be seasonal.
- Immunologic/allergic reaction results in histamine release which produces edema of the mucous membranes, spasm of the smooth muscles of bronchi and bronchioles and accumulation of tenacious secretions.

Findings

Respiratory distress: Shortness of breath, inspiratory wheeze, prolonged expiratory phase, air trapping, use of accessory muscles of respiration, irritability and diaphoresis.

Treatment

- Positioning–High fowlers' position.
- Oxygen inhalation.
- Drugs bronchodilators, steroids, antibiotics.
- Breathing exercises, chest percussions.
- Hyposensitization.

> Chronic asthmatic patients will have barrel chest.

DISEASES AND DISORDERS OF THE GENITOURINARY SYSTEM

Variation from the Adult

- Glomesular filtration rate is 30% below adult levels at birth, reaches normal level by 2 years.
- Tubular function is immature at night; tubular absorption and secretion reach adult levels by 2 years.
- Urethra is shorter in children and more prone to ascending infection, also urethra is closer to anus as a source of contamination.

URINARY TRACT INFECTION (UTI)

- Bacterial invasion of the bladder and urinary tract.
- Usually caused by *E. coli*
- Predisposing factors include poor hygiene and urinary reflux.

Findings

1. Abdominal pain.
2. Enuresis, pain/burning on urination, frequency, hematuria.
3. Low to high grade fever.

Treatment

1. Antibiotics.
2. Increase fluid intake.
3. Perineal hygiene.

VESICOURETERAL REFLUX

- Regurgitation of urine from the bladder into the ureters due to faulty valve mechanism at the vesico ureteral junction.
- Reflux leads to UTIs, pyelonephritis and hydronephrosis.

Findings

Same as that of UTI.

Treatment

Surgery.

UNDESCENDED TESTS (CRYPTORCHIDISM)

- Unilateral or bilateral absence of testes in the scrotum.
- 75% descend spontaneously by 1 year of age.

> Testes normally descends at 8 months of gestation, so may be undecided in babies born before 8 months.

Findings

Absence of testes in scrotal sac.

Treatment

Orchipexy: Surgical procedure to correct cryptorchidism, usually performed between 1–3 years of age.

> If testes are undescended and remain in the abdomen for longer periods, it may predispose to sterility due to increased body temperature.

HYPOSPADIAS

- Urethral opening located anywhere along the ventral surface of the penis.
- Ventral curvature of the penis (chordee) is often associated, causing construction.

Findings

- Urinary meatus in the ventral surface.
- Inability to make straight stream of urine.

Treatment

Surgery.

> Neonatal circumcision is not usually performed in infants with hypospadias since tissue may be needed for corrective repair of the defect.

ACUTE GLOMERULONEPHRITIS

- Immune complex disease resulting from an antigen-antibody reaction.
- Inflammation occurs secondary to the infection by Group A beta hemolytic streptococci elsewhere in the body.
- Self-limiting, resolves by about 14 days.

Findings

- History of streptococcal infection, usually upper respiratory tract infection or skin infection.
- Edema, anorexia, lethargy.
- Hematuria or dark colored urine, fever.
- Hypertension.

> Cola colored urine is a classical sign of acute glomeruls nephritis.

Treatment

1. Antibiotics for streptococcal infection.
2. Antihypertensives.
3. Digitalis if circulatory overload present.
4. Fluid restriction if renal impairment present.
5. In severe renal and cardiopulmonary symptoms, dialysis is recommended.

NEPHROTIC SYNDROME (NEPHROSIS)

- Autoimmune process leading to structural alteration of glomerular membrane that results in increased permeability to plasma protein particularly albumin.
- Protein shift causes altered oncotic pressure and lowered plasma volume.
- Hypovolemia triggers renin-angiotensin-aldosterone mehcanism which lead to sodium and water retention.
- Lower BP also stimulates release of ADH, increasing the edema.

Findings

1. Proteinuria, hypoproteinemia, hyperlipidemia.
2. Dependent body edema—puffiness around eyes in the morning, as cites, scrotal edema, ankle edema.
3. Anorexia, vomiting and diarrhea.
4. Malnutrition.
5. Pallor, lethargy.
6. Hepatomegaly.

Treatment

1. Antibiotic for infection.
2. Corticosteroids to resolve edema.
3. Thiazide diuretics if edema present.
4. High protein, low sodium diet.

> Avoid IM injection in child with nephrotic syndrome since medication is not well absorbed due to tissue edema.

HYDRONEPHROSIS

- Collection of urine in the renal pelvis due to obstruction to outflow.
- Obstruction most common at ureteropelvic junction, but may also be caused by adhesions, ureterocele, calculi or congenital malformations.
- Constriction leads to increased pressure in the renal pelvis, decreased circulation, atrophy of the kidney leading to renal insufficiency.
- May be unilateral or bilateral.

Findings

1. Recurrent UTIs.
2. Failure to thrive.
3. Abdominal pain.
4. Fever.
5. Fluctuating mass in the region of kidney.

Treatment

1. Prognosis good if treated early.
2. Symptomatic treatment.
3. Surgery.

DISEASES AND DISORDERS OF THE MUSCULOSKELETAL SYSTEM

Variations from the Adult

Bones

A. Linear growth results from skeletal development

1. Centers of Ossification
    a. Primary centers in diaphyses.
    b. Secondary centers in epiphyses.
    c. Used in the assessment of bone age; number of ossification centers in the wrist equals age in years plus 1.
2. Metaphysis
    a. Cartilaginous plate between diaphysis and epiphysis.
    b. Disappears over time with bony fusion of epiphysis and diaphysis.
    c. Linear growth ends with epiphyseal fusion.

B. Bone circumference: Growth occurs as new bone tissue is formed beneath the periosteum.

C. Skeletal maturity is reached by 17 years of age in boys and 2 years after menarche in girls.

D. Certain characteristics of bone in children affect injury and healing, bones are more prone to injury and injury results from relatively minor accidents.

> Bone growth in children is affected by Wolffs' law: Bone will grow in the direction in which stress is placed on it.

CONGENITAL DISLOCATION OF THE HIP (CDH)

- Displacement of the head of the femur from acetabulum, present at birth and not usually diagnosed at birth.
- May be associated with spina bifida.
- Cause unknown, may be fetal position in utero (breach delivery), genetic predisposition or laxity of ligaments.
- The acetabulum is shallow and the head of the femur cartilaginous at birth, contributing to the dislodgement.

Findings

1. May be unilateral or bilateral, partial or complete.
2. Limitation of abduction (cannot separate legs to change diaper).
3. Ortolani's sign: With infant in spine position, bend knees and place thumbs on bent knees, fingers at hip joint. Bring femur 90° to hip, then abduct. With dislocation, there is a palpable click where those head of the femur snaps over edge of the acetabulum.
4. Barlow's sign: With infant on back, bend knees. Affected knees will be lower because the head of the femur dislocates toward bed by gravity (telescoping of limb).
5. Additional skin folds with knees bent, from telescoping.
6. When lying on abdomen, buttocks of affected side will be flatter because head of femur fall toward bed from gravity.
7. Trendelenburg test (used if child is old enough to walk): Have child stand on affected leg only, pelvis will dip on normal side as child attempts to stay erect.

Treatment

1. Hip spica to maintain hip in abduction with the head of the femur in acetabulum.
2. Surgical correction.

> Ortolani's click and positive Barlow's test are indicative of congenital dislocation of hip.

> Dislocation of the lip one side causes asymmetry of skin folds near buttocks and thighs.

CLUBFOOT (TALIPES)

- Abnormal rotation of foot at angle.
- Varieties of talipes
  1. Varus (inward rotation): Child would walk on ankles with bottoms of feet face each other.
  2. Valgus (outward rotation): Child would walk on inner ankles.
  3. Calcaneous (upward rotation): Child would walk on heels.
  4. Equinas (downward rotation): Child would walk on toes.
- 95% of the deformity is talipes equinovarus.
- Usually unilateral and congenital.
- Cause unknown.

Findings

Foot cannot be manipulated by passive exercises into correct position.

Treatment

1. Exercises.
2. Casting (cast is changed periodically to change angle of foot).
3. Bar shoes: Metal bar with shoes attached to the bar at specific angle.
4. Surgery and casting for several months.

OSTEOGENESIS IMPERFECTA

An inherited disorder affecting collages formation resulting in pathologic fractures.

Types

1. Osteogenesis imperfecta congenita: Autosomal recessive disorder.
2. Osteogenesis imperfecta tarda: Autosomal dominant, involvement of varying degrees.

Findings

1. Osteogenesis imperfecta congentia
   a. Multiple fractures at birth.
   b. Possible skeletal deformity due to intrauterine fracture.
   c. Bones of skill soft.
   d. Occasional intracranial hemorrhage.
2. Osteogenesis imperfecta tarda
   a. Delayed walking, fractures and structural scoliosis as child grows.
   b. Lower limbs more frequently affected.
   c. Hypermobility of joints.
   d. Prone for dental caries.

Treatment

1. Reduction and immobilization of fractures.
2. Magnesium oxide supplementation.

> Symptoms of ostegenesis imperfecta decrease at puberty due to hormone production and child's ability to prevent injury.

SCOLIOSIS

- Lateral curvature of the spine.
- Commonly seen in adolescent girls.
- Disorder may be associated with other neuromuscular disorder.
- Cause may be idiopathic; other causes can be congenital abnormality of vertebral, neuromuscular disorders and trauma.

Types

1. Nonstructural or functional: 'C' curve of spine, due to posture, can be corrected voluntarily and disappears when lying down; not progressive, can be treated with posture exercises.
2. Structural or progressive: 'S' curve of spine, structural change of spine does not disappear with position changes; more aggressive intervention needed.

Findings (Structural Scoliosis)

1. Failure of curve to straighten when child bends forward with knees straight and arms hanging down to feet (curve disappears with functional scoliosis).
2. Uneven bra strap marks
3. Uneven hips
4. Uneven shoulders
5. Asymmetry of rib cage
6. X-ray reveals curvature.

Treatment

1. Stretching exercise of the spine for nonstructural changes.
2. Brace worn for 23 hours, day
3. Plaster jacket cast
4. Spinal fusion with insertion of Harrington rod.

DISEASES AND DISORDERS OF THE ENDOCRINE SYSTEM

Variation from the Adult

A. Adenohypophysis (anterior lobe of pituitary gland)

1. Growth hormone
   a. Does not affect prenatal growth.
   b. Main effect on liver growth is through increase of cells in skeletal bones.
   c. Maintain rate of synthesis of body protein.
2. Thyroid stimulating hormone (TSH) important for normal development of bones, teeth and brain.
   a. Secretion decreases throughout childhood, then increase at puberty.
3. Adrenocorticotropic hormone (ACTH)
   a. Little is produced throughout childhood.
   b. Becomes active in adolescence.
   c. Stimulates adrenals to secrete sex hormones.
   d. Influences production of gonadotropic hormone by hypothalamus; gonadotropic hormones activate gonads and gonads secrete estrogen or testosterone which stimulate development of secondary sex characteristics.
4. Estrogen has inhibitory effect on epiphyseal growth.

DIABETES MELLITUS

- Children typically develop Type I insulin dependent diabetes mellitus.
- Treatment needs to vary based on rapid growth rate in children.
- Risk of complication is high due to dietary facts and varying growth rate; most commonly include retinopathy, neuropathy, nephropathy, skin changes and predisposition to injection.

Findings

1. Polyuria, polyphagia, Polydipsia, weight loss and fatigue.
2. Ketoacidosis.
3. Dry, flushed skin with hyperglycemia.

Treatment

1. Insulin.
2. Dietary modification.
3. Exercise.
4. Prevention of complication.

CONGENITAL HYPOTHYROIDISM (CRETINISM)

- Disorder due to non-functioning or absent thyroid.
- Newborns are supplied with maternal thyroid hormones that last upto 3 months.

Findings

1. Altered body proportion; short statue with legs shorter than they should be in proportion to trunk.
2. Tongue is enlarged and protrudes from mouth, may result, is breathing and feeding difficulties.
3. Hypothermia with cool extremities.
4. Short thick neck, delayed dentition.
5. Hypotonia.
6. Low levels of T3 and T4.

Treatment

1. Prevention may be achieved with neonatal screening blood test.
2. Thyroid hormone replacement (oral thyroxin).

> Uncreated cretinism will lead to mental retardation and development delay in children.

HYPOPITUITARISM (PITUITARY DWARFISM)

- Hyposecretion of growth hormone by the anterior lobe of the pituitary gland.
- Cause unknown, may be due to craniopharyngioma.

Findings

1. Newborn is of normal size, but child falls below the third percentile by one year.
2. Child is well proportioned, but may be overweight for height.
3. Underdeveloped jaw, abnormal position of teeth, high voice, delayed puberty.
4. Delayed closing of epiphyseal plates of long bones in X-ray.
5. IQ may be normal.

Treatment

Growth hormone administration is the definitive treatment, but difficult to procure since got from human cadavers.

> Underdeveloped jaw, normal IQ and size and delayed closing of epiphyseal plates of long bones in children are indicative of hypopituitarism.

HYPERPITUITARISM (GIGANTISM)

- Hypersecretion of growth hormone.
- May be related to a tumor of the anterior lobe of pituitary.
- Changes noticeable at puberty.

Findings

1. Height beyond maximum upper percentile.
2. Proportional weight and muscle growth.
3. Coarse facial features.
4. Signs of increased ICP if caused by a tumor.
5. Enlarged bones of head, hands and feet and overgrowth of long bones.

Treatment

1. Surgery to remove tumor.
2. Radiation therapy if there is no tumor.

> The syndrome of diabetes mellitus, diabetes insipidus, optic atrophy and deafness comprise Wolfram syndrome.

REVIEW QUESTIONS

1. The type of play during infancy
a. Solitary play b. Parallel play
c. Associative play d. Cooperative play

2. Child between 12 months and 15 months learns to
a. Say simple words b. Use a spoon
c. Walk erect d. Climb stairs

3. A viral disease that begins with respiratory symptoms and skin rash and may result in grave complication
a. Rubeola b. Dengue fever
c. Yellow fever d. Chickenpox

4. Immunity by antibody formation during the course of a disease
a. Active natural immunity
b. Active artificial immunity
c. Passive natural immunity
d. Passive artificial immunity

5. The type of immunity developed after giving antitoxin
a. Active natural immunity
b. Active artificial immunity
c. Passive natural immunity
d. Passive artificial immunity

6. A viral infection characterized by rashes and Koplik's spots in the mouth
a. Rubeola b. Rubella
c. Chickenpox d. Mumps

7. The virus causing chickenpox can also produce
a. Athlete's foot b. Infectious hepatitis
c. Herpes zoster d. German measles

8. An injection consisting of bacterial cells that have been modified
a. A vaccine b. An antitoxin
c. A toxoid d. A toxin

9. A viral disease caused by one of the smallest human viruses that infect the motor cells of the anterior horn of a spinal cord
a. Rubeola b. Rubella
c. Chickenpox d. Poliomyelitis

10. A streptococcal infection characterized by swollen joints, fever and the possibility of endocarditis and death is
a. Whooping cough b. Tetanus
c. Rheumatic fever d. Measles

11. Encephalitis can be a complication of
a. Chickenpox b. Pertussis
c. Poliomyelitis d. Rubella

12. Gingival hyperplasia is a complication of
a. Phenobarbitone b. Phenytoin
c. Diazepam d. Amoxycillin

13. A child is getting 5% Dextrose 1000 mL IV in 24 hours, The minidropper delivers 60 drops / mL. The rate of flow will be
a. 30 drops per minute b. 32 drops per minute
c. 38 drops per minute d. 42 drops per minute

14. A child with a Wilm's tumor should not be subjected to
a. An IVP b. A renal biopsy
c. A nephrectomy d. An abdominal CT scan

15. The child is getting injection morphine 20 mg and the vial contains 50 mg/mL. The amount to be given to get the ordered dose
a. 0.6 mL b. 0.4 mL
c. 0.8 mL d. 1.0 mL

16. The serious side effect of vincristine
a. Neurotoxicity b. Irreversible alopecia
c. Fever and anemia d. GIT symptoms

17. Drug of choice to treat leukemia

a. Prednisolone b. Methotrexate
c. Vincristine d. Vinblastine

18. Chickenpox can be fatal if the child is receiving

a. Antibiotics b. Steroids
c. Anticonvulsants d. Insulin

19. Most important complication of mumps in adolescent boys

a. Hypothyroidism b. Hypopituitarism
c. Sterility d. Cachexia

20. Oral thrush is caused by

a. Neisseria gonorrhea b. Entamoeba
c. Candida albicans d. Varicella

21. Name of the oral polio vaccine

a. BCG b. TAB
c. Salk d. Sabin

22. Mode of transmission of pertussis

a. Vector transmission
b. Through contaminated water
c. Droplet infection
d. Faeco oral

23. Tripple Antigen denotes

a. DPT b. BCG
c. TAB d. OPV

24. Time required to measure the Mantoux test

a. 24–48 hours b. 48–72 hours
c. 10–12 hours d. 2–4 hours

25. Causative organism of diphtheria

a. Mycobacteria
b. Streptococcus
c. Coryne bacterium diphtheria
d. Staphylococcus

26. Average weight of a newborn baby

a. 2 kg b. 4 kg
c. 3 kg d. 5 kg

27. Discoloration of teeth is a side effect of

a. Streptomycin b. Neomycin
c. Tetracycline d. Penicillin

28. The birth weight of the baby doubles at the age of

a. 3 months b. 6 months
c. 9 months d. 12 months

29. The signs of dehydration in child are the following except

a. Sunken tearless eyes
b. Koss of skin elasticity
c. Diuresis
d. Depressed fintenelle

30. Eruption of teeth starts at the age of

a. 4 months b. 6 months
c. 8 months d. 10 months

31. The most common site for internal bleeding in children with hemophilia

a. Gums b. Cerebrum
c. Joints d. Intestines

32. A child with uncontrolled vomiting can develop

a. Tetany b. Metabolic alkalosis
c. Metabolic acidosis d. Hyperactivity

33. Digoxin should not be given if the 5-year-old child's apical pulse rate is below

a. 60 beats per minute b. 80 beats per minute
c. 90 beats per minute d. 100 beats per minute

34. A 2-year-old child with cyanotic heart disease will have

a. Edema in the extrimities
b. An elevated PCV
c. Absence of pedal pulse
d. Orthopnea

35. A child with tracheoesophageal fistula will have

a. Excessive drooling of saliva
b. Tachycardia
c. Hypotension
d. Hypertension

36. Speech development may be delayed in a child with

a. Congenital heart disease
b. Cleft palate
c. Mumps
d. Oral thrush

37. Trisomy 21 is

a. Klinefelters syndrome b. Gonadal agenesis
c. Turner's syndrome d. Down's syndrome

38. Simian crease is a characteristic feature of

a. Klinefelters syndrome b. Gonadal agenesis
c. Turner's syndrome d. Down's syndrome

39. Small, whitish pinpoint spots found in infant's nose

a. Vernix b. Mangolian spot
c. Milia d. Pustule

40. The most important parameter of APGAR score is

a. Heart rate b. Respiratory rate
c. Grimace d. Reflex

41. Protein deficiency leads to

a. Kwashiorkor b. Marasmus
c. Pellagra d. Beriberi

42. Energy deficiency leads to

a. Kwashiorkor b. Marasmus
c. Pellagra d. Beriberi

43. Immunoglobulin present in human milk

a. Ig G b. Ig M
c. Ig E d. Ig A

44. Xerophthalmia is caused by

a. Vitamin B b. Vitamin C
c. Vitamin A d. Vitamin D

45. The first stool of newborn

a. Transitional stools b. Meconium
c. Breast milk stools d. Watery stools

46. Bitot's spots are due to the deficiency of

a. Vitamin A b. Vitamin B_2
c. Vitamin C d. Vitamin K

47. Deficiency of Vitamin C leads to

a. Xerophthalmia b. Scurvy
c. Night blindness d. Beriberi

48. Universal immunization program was launched in the year

a. 1975 b. 1985
c. 1971 d. 1965

49. Thiamine deficiency leads to

a. Xerophthalmia b. Scurvy
c. Night blindness d. Beriberi

50. Deficiency of vitamin D leads to

a. Scurvey b. Rickets
c. Beriberi d. Pellagra

51. Cyanocobalamin is

a. Vitamin B_1 b. Vitamin B_2
c. Vitamin B_6 d. Vitamin B_{12}

52. Route of administration of BCG vaccine

a. Intradermal b. Intravenous
c. Intramuscular d. Subcutaneous

53. Bedwetting during night

a. Enuresis b. Nocturnal enuresis
c. Encopresis d. Insomnia

54. Ophthalmia neonatorum is caused by

a. *Neisseria gonorrhea* b. Cytomegalovirus
c. Herpes virus d. Human papiloma virus

55. Color of urine in glomerulonephritis

a. Brown colored b. Green colored
c. Yellow colored d. Dark, cola colored

56. Highly malignant tumor of kidney

a. Retinoblastoma b. Ewing's sarcoma
c. Wilm's tumor d. Osteosarcoma

57. Causative organism of Ascariasis

a. *Neisseria gonorrhea* b. Ascaris lumbricoids
c. Rubeola virus d. Pediculus capitus

58. Congenital, aganglionic, megacolon is

a. Pyloric stenosis b. Volvulus
c. Hirschsprungs disease d. GERD

59. Characteristics of stool in Hirschsprungs disease

a. Ribbon shaped stool b. Rice water stool
c. Loose stools d. Clay colored stools

60. Boot shaped heart in X-ray is seen in

a. Overriding of aorta
b. Tetralogy of Fallot
c. Right ventricular hypertrophy
d. Aortic stenosis

61. Physiological jaundice appears

a. On 2nd and 3rd day b. Within 24 hours of birth
c. After 7 days of birth d. On 6th day

62. Life-threatening complication of hyperbilirubinemia in newborn

a. Liver failure b. Renal failure
c. Carditis d. Kernicterus

63. When the forehead is tapped gently in new born, eyes will blink. This reflex is

a. Moro reflex b. Rooting reflex
c. Glabellar reflex d. Blink reflex

64. Moro reflex disappear by

a. One month b. Three months
c. Six months d. Eight months

65. Hemolytic disease in newborn is due to

a. Neonatal jaundice b. Rh incompatibility
c. Anemia d. Sepsis

66. Newborns routinely need the following

a. Vitamin A injection b. Vitamin K injection
c. Vitamin D injection d. Vitamin E injection

67. APGAR score of a newborn baby born with severe respiratory depression

a. < 3 b. 3–5
c. 5–7 d. > 9

68. Folic acid deficiency in pregnancy predisposes to

a. Cardiac defects b. Cataract
c. Neural tube defects d. Limb abnormalities

69. Pernicious anemia is

a. Vitamin B_6 deficiency b. Vitamin B_2 deficiency
c. Vitamin B_{12} deficiency d. Vitamin B_1 deficiency

70. Folic acid deficiency leads to

a. Pernicious anemia b. Iron deficiency anemia
c. Magaloblastic anemia d. Normocytic anemia

71. The vitamin which is activated by sunlight

a. Vitamin A b. Vitamin D
c. Vitamin E d. Vitamin K

72. A fat soluble vitamin

a. Vitamin A b. Vitamin B_1
c. Vitamin C d. Vitamin B_{12}

73. A water soluble vitamin

a. Vitamin A b. Vitamin D
c. Vitamin K d. Vitamin C

74. Injectable polio vaccine is

a. Salk vaccine b. Sabin vaccine
c. Triple vaccine d. OPV

75. Oral polio vaccine is

a. Salk vaccine b. Sabin vaccine
c. Triple vaccine d. IPV

76. Normal heart rate in the newborn

a. 80–100 beats per minute
b. 100–110 beats per minute
c. 100–140 beats per minute
d. More than 160 beats per minute

77. Normal respiratory rate in the newborn

a. 20–40 breaths per minute
b. 30–60 breaths per minute
c. 60–80 breaths per minute
d. More than 70 breaths per minute

78. World breastfeeding week is celebrated on

a. August 1st week b. August 2nd week
c. May 1st week d. May 2nd week

79. Baby Friendly Hospital Initiative (BFHI) was launched in the year

a. 1990 b. 1992
c. 1994 d. 1996

80. Children with prolonged diarrhea are prone for

a. Metabolic alkalosis b. Metabolic acidosis
c. Respiratory alkalosis d. Respiratory acidosis

81. Common complication that can occur while feeding a baby with cleft lip and palate

a. Drooling b. Regurgitation
c. Aspiration d. Vomiting

82. Abnormal opening between trachea and esophagus

a. Tetralogy of Fallot
b. Tracheostomy
c. Esophageal atresia
d. Tracheoesophageal fistula

83. Telescoping of one part of bowel to another part is

a. Megacolon b. Intussusception
c. Pyloric stenosis d. Intestinal obstruction

84. Bile stained vomiting is a typical feature of

a. Megacolon b. Pyloric stenosis
c. Worm infestation d. Intussusception

85. Herniation of abdominal organs into the umbilical cord with evisceration into sac

a. Omphalocele b. Exophthalmos
c. Omphalitis d. Diaphragmatic hernia

86. Ramsted's surgery is done for

a. Megacolon b. Pyloric stenosis
c. Worm infestation d. Intussusception

87. Congenitral absence of ganglion cells in the intestine leading to dilatation of colon is

a. Megacolon b. Hirschsprung's disease
c. Worm infestation d. Intussusception

88. Duhamel's surgery is done for
a. Megacolon b. Worm infestation
c. Intussusception d. Hirschsprung's disease

89. Accumulation of air in the pleural space
a. Pneumothorax b. Hemothorax
c. Pyothorax d. Tamponade

90. Croup is
a. Laryngo tracheal bronchitis
b. Tracheoesophageal fistula
c. Tracheal fistula
d. Esophagitis

91. Airway obstruction due to spasm of bronchial smooth muscles
a. Bronchospasm b. Emphysema
c. Asthma d. Empyema

92. Inspiratory stridor is a characteristic feature of
a. Emphysema b. Hemothorax
c. Epiglotitis d. Pneumothorax

93. Collection of pus in the pleural cavity
a. Bronchospasm b. Emphysema
c. Asthma d. Empyema

94. Collection of blood in the thoracic cavity
a. Hemothorax b. Pneumothorax
c. Pyopneumothorax d. Empyema

95. Hyaline membrane disease is
a. Respiratory infection
b. Respiratory distress syndrome
c. Respiratory paralysis
d. Ulcerative colitis

96. Waiter's tip position is seen in
a. Bell's palsy
b. Facial Palsy
c. Erb's palsy
d. Congenital dislocation of hip

97. Abnormal opening between right and left atrium
a. ASD b. VSD
c. TOF d. RVH

98. Drug used in infants with PDA
a. Aspirin b. Indomethacin
c. Inderal d. Allopurinol

99. BT shunt is done for children with
a. ASD b. VSD
c. TOF d. RVH

100. An inflammatory autoimmune disease that affects the connective tissue of the heart and joints is
a. Rheumatic fever b. Rheumatoid arthritis
c. Osteoarthritis d. Osteochondritis

101. Aschoff's nodules are seen in
a. Rheumatoid arthritis b. Osteoarthritis
c. Rheumatic fever d. Osteochondritis

102. Patau syndrome is
a. Trisomy 18 b. Trisomy 21
c. Trisomy 13 d. Down's syndrome

103. Cloudy CSF is a feature of
a. Meningitis b. Meningioma
c. Meningocele d. Meningomyelocele

104. CSF protein level will increase in
a. Meningioma b. Meningitis
c. Meningocele d. Meningomyelocele

105. Flattened nasal bridge is a feature of
a. Trisomy 18 b. Trisomy 21
c. Trisomy 13 d. Down's syndrome

106. Sun setting eyes are found in
a. Down's syndrome b. Hydrocephalus
c. Encephalitis d. Meningitis

107. Cracked pot resonance of head is a diagnostic feature of
a. Down's syndrome b. Encephalitis
c. Meningitis d. Hydrocephalus

108. Opisthotonus posture is seen in
a. Down's syndrome b. Encephalitis
c. Meningitis d. Cerebral palsy

109. Polydactyly is seen in
a. Down's syndrome b. Encephalitis
c. Meningitis d. Cerebral palsy

110. Undescended testis is called
a. Cryptorchidism b. Inguinal hernia
c. Unbilical hernia d. Hydrocele

111. The management of persistent pulmonary hypertension of the newborn includes all of the following except
a. Correction of acidosis
b. Ventillation with 100% oxygen
c. Pulmonary vasodilators
d. Indomethacin

112. The major function of surfactant is to

a. Increase pulmonary compliance
b. Lubricate the alveoli
c. Increase alveolar surface tension
d. Decrease the work of breathing

113. The commonest cause of congestive heart failure in a 24-hour-old baby born to a diabetic mother is

a. PDA b. Diabetic cardiomyopathy
c. TGA d. RDS

114. Immunization against DPT should be administered via

a. Oral route b. Intra muscular route
c. Subcutaneous route d. Intradermal route

115. The most common feature in tracheoesophageal fistula without atresia is

a. Excessive secretions at birth
b. Abdominal distention
c. Recurrent aspiration pneumonia
d. Regurgitation of food

116. Susceptibility to bilirubin toxicity is increased in

a. Cold stress b. Starvation
c. Hemolysis d. Acidosis

117. Acceptable rate of increase in head circumference of a healthy term infant in the first 2 months of life

a. 0–5 cm/month b. 1–2 cm/month
c. 2–3 cm/month d. 1–5 cm/month

118. Left ventricular hypertrophy during the neonatal period is associated with all the following conditions except

a. Aortic stenosis
b. Pulmonary atresia
c. Transposition of great vessels
d. Tricuspid atresia

119. Abnormal calcification in abdominal radiography is seen in all of the following except

a. Neuroblastoma b. Teratoma
c. Hepatoblastoma d. Hydronephrosis

120. Drug of choice for respiratory depression in a newborn whose mother received morphine during labor

a. Naloxone b. Digoxin
c. Lidocaine d. Adrenaline

121. Which of the following combination of blood types is most likely to produce hemolytic disease of the newborn

a. Negative mother and positive father
b. Positive mother and negative father
c. Negative mother and negative father
d. Positive mother and positive father

122. Compared to mature breast milk, human colostrums has all the following except

a. Higher specific gravity
b. Higher concentration of immunoglobulins
c. Higher fat content
d. Lower fat content

123. Poliomyelitis is transmitted through

a. Water b. Air
c. Blood d. Vectors

124. Edema over the dorsum of the feet is present in

a. SIADH
b. Turner's syndrome
c. Congenital adrenal hyperplasia
d. Down's syndrome

125. Rickets is due to deficiency of

a. Vitamin D b. Vitamin A
c. Vitamin B d. Vitamin C

126. MCH service includes

a. Prenatal and postnatal care
b. Under fives care
c. Family planning service
d. All of the above

127. Koplik's spot is seen in

a. Chickenbox b. Measles
c. Mumps d. Variola

128. An example of a congenital cyanotic heart disease is

a. Rheumatic heart disease b. Ventricular septal defect
c. Aortic stenosis d. Tetralogy of Fallot

129. Which of the following is a typical sign of trachea esophageal fistula?

a. Continuous drooling
b. Diaphragmatic breathing
c. Slow response to stimuli
d. Passage of frothy meconium

130. A 4-year-old child having a weight of 7.8 kg belongs to

a. Grade I PEM b. Grade II PEM
c. Grade III PEM d. Grade IV PEM

131. Expected time of closure of anterior fontanel is

a. 4–6 weeks b. 6–8 months
c. 9–12 months d. 16–18 months

132. Absence of ganglion cells in colon is a feature of

a. Ulcerative colitis
b. Hirschsprung's disease
c. Anorectal malformation
d. Reye's syndrome

133. Birth injury due to damage of brachial plexus

a. Facial palsy b. Erb's palsy
c. Cephal hematoma d. Subdural hematoma

134. Weaning starts at

a. 6th month b. 9th month
c. 12th month d. 15th month

135. Oral polio vaccine is

a. Live attenuated vaccine
b. Killed vaccine
c. Toxoid
d. Combined vaccine

136. Best and cheapest investment in the health of children

a. Nutrition b. Immunization
c. Breastfeeding d. Growth cards

137. Causative agent of diphtheria

a. *Mycobacterium* b. *Bordetella pertussis*
c. *Corynebacterium* d. *Salmonella*

138. Frequent cyanotic spells occurs in

a. VSD b. Coarctation of aorta
c. PDA d. Tetralogy of Fallot

139. Best method of oxygen administration in a 2-month-old baby is via

a. Oxyhood b. Oxygen mask
c. Nasal canula d. Nasal prongs

140. Urethral meatus on the penile dorsal surface is seen in

a. Paraphimosis b. Epispadias
c. Phimosis d. Hypospadias

141. Presence of alpha fetoprotein (AFP) in amniotic fluid indicates

a. Hydrocephalus
b. Tetralogy of Fallot
c. Tracheoesophageal fistula
d. Spina bifida

142. A killed vaccine

a. BCG b. Measles
c. Typhoid d. Yellow fever

143. Ribbon like stool is a feature of

a. Intussusception b. Hirschsprung's desease
c. Ulcerative colitis d. Diverticulitis

144. Sudden jarring causing sudden extension and abduction of extremities and fanning of fingers in a newborn is called

a. Moro reflex b. Sucking reflex
c. Tonic neck reflex d. Rooting reflex

145. Which of the following is true for Cephal hematoma

a. Swelling appears immediately after birth
b. Pitting on pressure
c. Scalp is movable
d. It does not cross a suture

146. Ophthalmia neonatorum is caused by

a. *Candida albicans* b. *E. coli*
c. *Staphylococcus* d. Gonococci

147. Developmental task during the toddler period is

a. Trust Vs mistrust
b. Autonomy Vs shame and doubt
c. Initiative Vs guilt
d. Industry Vs role confusion

148. Ramstad's operation is done for

a. Hiatus hernia b. Pyloristenosis
c. Congenital megacolon d. Repair of cleft lip

149. The most common cause of apnea in a preterm baby is

a. Pulmonary surfactant deficiency
b. Pneumonia
c. Aspiration
d. Hypoglycemia

150. Common type of fracture in children

a. Simple fracture b. Colles fracture
c. Greenstick fracture d. Complicated fracture

151. Dr Salk discovered a vaccine for the prevention of

a. Measles b. Poliomyelitis
c. Smallpox d. Tetanus

152. The bilirubin encephalopathy due to high concentration of indirect bilirubin on brain and basal ganglia in the neonatal period is

a. Status epileptics b. Kernig's sign
c. Kernicterus d. Jaundice

153. A congenital hemolytic disease caused by Rh incompatibility is

a. Sickle cell anemia b. Erythroblastosis fetalis
c. Megaloblastic anemia d. Jaundice

154. The most common type of jaundice in newborn

a. Hemolytic b. Physiological
c. Obstructive d. Hepatogenic

155. Chorioretinitis is present in babies with the following infections

a. Congenital toxoplasmosis
b. Cytomegalovirus infection
c. Congenital rubella
d. Congenital syphilis

156. The important clinical parameter for assessing the degree of hypoxia at birth

a. Respiratory rate b. Color of skin
c. Heart rate d. Muscle tone

157. Most effective factor that leads to absorption of lung fluid at birth

a. Negative pressure of the first breath
b. Vaginal delivery
c. Optimal lung maturity
d. Osmolality of the lung fluid

158. Which of the following does not resolve spontaneously

a. Erythema toxicum b. Portwine stains
c. Capillary hemangioma d. Cephalhematoma

159. Auditory brainstem evoked response (BERA) should be tested in the following babies except

a. Neonatal seizures
b. Aminoglycoside therapy
c. Hyperbilirubinemia
d. Infant of a mother with thyrotoxicosis

160. Which of the following condition is associated with neonatal hypoglycemia

a. Nesidioblastosis
b. Congenital hypothyroidism
c. Infant of a mother with thyrotoxicosis
d. Lucy Driscoll syndrome

161. Hypertrophy and hyperplasia of the Langerhans is seen in

a. Erythroblastosis fetalis b. Congenital toxoplasmosis
c. Down's syndrome d. Adrenogenital syndrome

162. Total body water in a newborn is

a. 50–55% of body weight
b. 55–60% of body weight
c. 65–70% of body weight
d. 70–75% of body weight

163. Congenital rubella syndrome has the following except

a. IUGR b. Neonatal hepatitis
c. Hydrocephalus d. Congenital cataract

164. Which statement is incorrect about hydrops fetalis

a. Has hypoproteinemia
b. Is always due to Rh hemolytic disease
c. May have congestive cardiac failure
d. Usually accompanied by ascites

165. Neonatal period means

a. From birth to one week
b. From birth to two weeks
c. From birth to four weeks
d. From birth to one year

166. Infancy means a period

a. From birth to one week
b. From birth to two weeks
c. From birth to four weeks
d. From birth to one year

167. Period from one year to three years of age is called

a. Infancy b. Toddler
c. Preschooler d. Schooler

168. Newborn baby recognize his mother at

a. One month b. Three months
c. Six months d. One year

169. An infant can sit without support at

a. Two months b. Three months
c. Four months d. Six months

170. Developmental task during the infancy is

a. Trust Vs mistrust
b. Autonomy Vs shame and doubt
c. Initiative Vs guilt
d. Industry Vs role confusion

171. The head circumference becomes equal to chest circumference at

a. One year b. Two years
c. Three years d. Four years

172. Developmental task during the school age is

a. Trust Vs mistrust
b. Autonomy Vs shame and doubt
c. Initiative Vs guilt
d. Industry Vs inferiority

173. Yellow, thick secretion from the breasts in the first three days of the delivery

a. Colostrum b. Transitional milk
c. Mature milk d. Fatty milk

174. A killed vaccine

a. OPV b. BCG
c. Tetanus d. Cholera

175. MMR vaccine gives protection against the following except

a. Measles b. Mumps
c. Rubella d. Rubeola

176. A toxoid

a. Diphtheria b. BCG
c. MMR d. OPV

177. Bilirubin encephalopathy is termed as

a. Kernig's sign b. Portal hypertension
c. Kernicterus d. Phenylketonuria

178. The drug given in hyperbilirubinemia

a. Phenobarbitone b. Phenytoin
c. Diazepam d. Bromocryptine

179. Infection of the eye of newborn due to gonococci

a. Lymphogranuloma venereum
b. Ophthalmia neonatorum
c. Kernicterus
d. Moniliasis

180. Oral thrush is caused by

a. Gonococci b. *E. coli*
c. *Candida albicans* d. *Staphylococcus*

181. Opisthotonus posture is seen in

a. Oral thrush
b. Kernicterus
c. Ophthalmia neonatorum
d. Tetanus

182. A high pitched cry is seen in

a. Hunger b. Anger
c. Maternal deprivation d. Intracranial tension

183. Old man's appearance is seen in

a. Fever b. Marasmus
c. Jaundice d. Encephalopathy

184. Visible peristalsis may be seen in

a. Congenital megacolon b. Constipation
c. Pyloric stenosis d. Peritonitis

185. The Mantoux test is read at

a. 24–48 hours b. 48–72 hours
c. < 24 hours d. > 72 hours

186. The Mantoux test is positive if induration is

a. More than 10 mm b. More than 15 mm
c. 5–10 mm d. < 5 mm

187. The following are antituberculosis drugs except

a. INH b. Rifampicin
c. Ethambutol d. Vancomycin

188. Chickenpox is caused by

a. Variola virus b. Vericella virus
c. Rubeola virus d. Rota virus

189. The incubation period of chickenpox

a. 7–14 days b. 14–21 days
c. > 21 days d. 1–2 months

190. A complication of chickenpox

a. Encephalitis b. Carditis
c. Nephritis d. Urethritis

191. Measles is spread by

a. Feco oral route b. Parenteral route
c. Blood borne d. Droplet infection

192. Poliomyelitis is transmitted through

a. Water b. Air
c. Blood d. Vectors

193. The vein which will most likely be used to give exchange transfusion in the newborn

a. Jugular vein b. Femoral vein
c. Temporal vein d. Umbilical vein

194. Vaccines and toxoids produce

a. Natural immunity b. Active immunity
c. Passive immunity d. Acquired immunity

195. Which of the following vitamin deficiency results in scurvy?

a. Vitamin C b. Vitamin B
c. Vitamin D d. Vitamin A

196. Drug of choice for respiratory depression in a newborn whose mother received morphine during labor

a. Naloxone b. Digoxin
c. Lidocaine d. Adrenaline

197. Immunization against DPT should be administered via

a. Oral route b. Intramuscular route
c. Subcutaneous route d. Intradermal route

198. The ability of the body to recognize, destroy and eliminate antigenic material

a. Energy b. Immunity
c. Adaptation d. Resistance

199. Separation of an infected person from noninfected persons

a. Incubation b. Isolation
c. Inoculation d. Immunization

200. The best indicator of infant nutrition

a. Height b. Weight
c. Vital signs d. Vital statistics

201. Dryness of the eye due to vitamin A deficiency

a. Bitot's spot b. Night blindness
c. Xerophthalmia d. Keratomalacia

202. One ounce is

a. 5 mL b. 15 mL
c. 30 mL d. 50 mL

203. Change in the shape of fetal head when it passes through the birth canal

a. Koulding b. Casting
c. Shaping d. Spalding

204. Tuberculin test is commonly known as

a. Shick test b. Mantoux test
c. VDRL d. ELISA

205. Regional enteritis is also called

a. Ulcerative colitis
b. Conn's disease
c. Irritable bowel syndrome
d. Crohn's disease

206. Spalding sign in X-ray indicates

a. IUGR b. Preterm pregnancy
c. Intrauterine death d. Postterm pregnancy

207. Causative agent of diphtheria

a. *Corynebacterium* b. *Bordetella*
c. *Klebsiella* d. *Salmonella*

208. Anterior fontanelle is also called

a. Bregma b. Lambda
c. Vertex d. Glabella

209. Urethral meatus is on the penile dorsal surface in

a. Paraphimosis b. Epispadias
c. Phimosis d. Hypospadias

210. Dose of vitamin A in vitamin A prophylaxis program

a. 1,00,000 IU b. 1,50,000 IU
c. 2,00,000 IU d. 2,50,000 IU

211. APGAR score for color done at 5 minutes after birth is recorded as 2. It indicates.

a. Pallor
b. Body pink, extremities blue
c. Cyanosed
d. Pink

212. Sudden jarring causes sudden extension and abduction of extremities and fanning of fingers in a newborn is called

a. Mororeflex b. Startle reflex
c. Tonic neck reflex d. Rooting reflex

213. Wilms tumor is affecting the

a. Liver b. Kidney
c. Bone d. Skin

214. Which of the following vaccination should be taken for a 10-year-old child as per the national immunization schedule?

a. Tetanus toxoid b. TAB
c. DT d. Hepatitis B

215. Braun's splint is used for

a. Fracture of the arms
b. Fracture of pelvis
c. Fracture of the lower limbs
d. Fracture of collar bone

216. Tuberculosis of the spine is also called
a. Osteomalacia b. Charcot's disease
c. Erving's disease d. Pott's disease

217. Trismus is a characteristic feature of
a. Measles b. Poliomyelitis
c. Smallpox d. Tetanus

218. Risus sardonicus is seen in
a. Measles b. Poliomyelitis
c. Smallpox d. Tetanus

219. Clinical sign seen in tetanus
a. Koplik's spots b. Pseudomembrane
c. Opisthotonus d. Hydrophobia

220. Typhoid fever is transmitted by
a. Feco oral route b. Contaminated air
c. Fomites d. Parenteral route

221. Incubation period of typhoid
a. 2–7 days b. 5–10 days
c. 7–21 days d. 15–30 days

222. Hepatitis A is transmitted through
a. Blood b. GIT
c. Respiratory tract d. Sexual contact

223. AIDS is caused by
a. Human papilloma virus
b. Human immunodeficiency virus
c. Rota virus
d. Toga virus

224. Characteristic feature of marasmus
a. Buffalo hump b. Barlow's sign
c. Scleroderma d. Old man appearance

225. PEM is otherwise called
a. Marasmus b. Kwashiorkor
c. Down's syndrome d. Mongolism

226. Keratomalacia is due to the deficiency of
a. Vitamin A b. Vitamin B_2
c. Vitamin B_6 d. Vitamin D

227. The vitamin needed for carbohydrate metabolism
a. Vitamin A b. Vitamin B
c. Vitamin C d. Vitamin D

228. Glossitis occurs due to deficiency of
a. Folic acid b. Vitamin A
c. Vitamin D d. Vitamin E

229. Ascorbic acid is
a. Vitamin A b. Vitamin B
c. Vitamin C d. Vitamin D

230. A parasitic infection
a. Pellagra b. Megacolon
c. Ascites d. Ascariasis

231. Hookworm infestation is
a. Ancylostomiasis b. Leischmaniasis
c. Oxyurias d. Ascariasis

232. Obstruction of larynx leads to
a. Pharyngitis b. Otitis
c. Croup d. RDS

233. Collapse of the lungs
a. Bronchitis b. Bronchiectasis
c. Atelectasis d. Bronchial asthma

234. Distention of the alveoli due to loss of elasticity of the lungs
a. Bronchial asthma b. Bronchiectasis
c. Atelectasis d. Emphysema

235. Pus in the pleural cavity
a. Empyema b. Bronchiectasis
c. Atelectasis d. Bronchitis

236. Loud, harsh, pansystolic murmur is observed in
a. VSD b. ASD
c. RVH d. TGA

237. Condition in which the foreskin is narrowed and cannot be retracted
a. Hypospadias b. Epispadias
c. Phimosis d. Cryptorchidism

238. Cooley's anemia is
a. Sickle cell anemia b. Thalassemia
c. Iron deficiency anemia d. SLE

239. Common form of childhood cancer
a. Neuroblastoma b. Wilm's tumor
c. Leukemia d. Nephroblastoma

240. Strabismus is
a. Cataract b. Squint
c. Glaucoma d. Trachoma

241. Preferred site for IM injection in children
a. Rectus femoris b. Ventrogluteal
c. Dorsogluteal d. Vastus lateralis

242. A common type of fracture in children
- a. Simple fracture
- b. Compound fracture
- c. Greenstick fracture
- d. Colli's fracture

243. Antipellagra vitamin is
- a. Niacin
- b. Thiamin
- c. Pyridoxine
- d. Riboflavin

244. Allergen causes
- a. Bronchitis
- b. Asthma
- c. Bronchiectasis
- d. Pneumonia

245. The disease transferred through contact is called
- a. Communicable disease
- b. Infectious disease
- c. Epidemic disease
- d. Contagious disease

246. A bath which is taken in a sitting position is
- a. Bed bath
- b. Partial bath
- c. Sitz bath
- d. Tepid sponge

ANSWER KEY

1. a 2. c 3. a 4. a 5. d 6. a 7. c 8. a 9. d 10. c 11. a 12. b
13. d 14. b 15. b 16. a 17. c 18. b 19. c 20. c 21. d 22. c 23. a 24. a
25. c 26. c 27. c 28. b 29. c 30. b 31. c 32. b 33. b 34. b 35. a 36. b
37. d 38. d 39. c 40. a 41. a 42. b 43. d 44. c 45. b 46. a 47. b 48. b
49. d 50. b 51. d 52. a 53. b 54. a 55. d 56. c 57. b 58. c 59. a 60. b
61. a 62. d 63. c 64. b 65. b 66. b 67. a 68. c 69. c 70. c 71. b 72. a
73. d 74. a 75. b 76. c 77. b 78. a 79. b 80. b 81. c 82. d 83. b 84. d
85. a 86. b 87. b 88. d 89. a 90. a 91. c 92. c 93. d 94. a 95. b 96. c
97. a 98. b 99. c 100. a 101. c 102. c 103. a 104. b 105. d 106. b 107. d 108. d
109. a 110. a 111. d 112. d 113. b 114. b 115. c 116. d 117. c 118. c 119. d 120. a
121. a 122. c 123. a 124. b 125. a 126. d 127. b 128. d 129. a 130. b 131. d 132. b
133. b 134. a 135. a 136. c 137. c 138. d 139. a 140. b 141. d 142. c 143. b 144. a
145. d 146. d 147. b 148. b 149. a 150. c 151. b 152. c 153. b 154. b 155. a 156. c
157. a 158. b 159. d 160. a 161. a 162. d 163. c 164. b 165. c 166. d 167. b 168. b
169. d 170. a 171. b 172. d 173. a 174. d 175. d 176. a 177. c 178. a 179. b 180. c
181. d 182. d 183. b 184. c 185. b 186. a 187. d 188. b 189. b 190. a 191. d 192. a
193. d 194. d 195. a 196. a 197. b 198. b 199. b 200. b 201. c 202. c 203. a 204. b
205. d 206. c 207. a 208. a 209. b 210. c 211. b 212. a 213. b 214. a 215. c 216. d
217. d 218. d 219. c 220. a 221. c 222. b 223. b 224. d 225. b 226. a 227. b 228. a
229. c 230. d 231. a 232. c 233. c 234. d 235. a 236. a 237. c 238. b 239. c 240. b
241. d 242. c 243. a 244. b 245. d 246. c

Chapter 5 Community Health Nursing

PRIMARY HEALTH CARE

Primary health care is the key to achieve the goal "Health for all by the year 2000" has been defined by the "attainment of a lead of health that will enable every individual to lead a socially and economically productive life".

Summary of Goals Include

- Reduction of infant mortality rate from 125 to below 60 by the year 2000 AD.
- To raise the expectation of life at birth from 52 years to 64 by the year 2000 AD.
- To reduce the crude birth rate from 32 per 1000 population to 21 per 1000 by the year 2000 AD.
- To reduce the crude death rate from 12 per 1000 population to 9 by the year 2000 AD.
- To achieve a net reproduction rate of one by the year 2000 AD.

Definition

Primary health care is defined as the essential health care made universally accessible to individuals and acceptable to then, through their full participation and at a cost that the community and country can afford.

Elements

- Education of the people about preventing health problem and methods of preventing and controlling them.
- Promotion of food supply and proper nutrition.
- Adequate supply of safe water and basic sanitation.
- Maternal and child health care and family planning.
- Immunization against major infectious diseases.
- Prevention and control of locally endemic diseases.
- Appropriate treatment of common diseases and injuries.
- Production of essential drugs.

Principles

1. Equitable distribution
2. Community involvement
3. Appropriate technology
4. Focus on prevention
5. Multisectoral approach.

Principles of Community Health Nursing

1. Meet the community
2. Identification of health problems and needs
3. Setting priorities among health problem
4. Planning and problem solving
5. Interventions or implementation
6. Evaluation.

MATERNAL AND CHILD HEALTH

- Mothers and children make up the majority of the population in almost all the countries.
- Mothers and children constitute a special risk or valuable group in terms of illness and deaths, connected with pregnancy and child birth in the case of mothers and growth and development in the case of children.
- By improving the health of mothers and children, health of the family and community can be improved.
- Ensuring child survival is a further investment for the family and community.

Objectives of MCH Care

1. Reduction in maternal, perinatal, infant and child mortality and morbidity.
2. Promotion of reproductive health.
3. Promotion of physical and psychological development of the child and adolescent within the family.

HEALTH PROBLEMS OF INDIA

1. Communicable diseases problem:
   - Malaria
   - Tuberculosis
   - Diarrheal diseases
   - Acute respiratory infection
   - Leprosy
   - Filaria
   - STD
   - AIDS
   - Others: Helmenthiasis, enteric fever, meningitis, etc.
2. Nutritional problems:
   - Protein calorie malnutrition
   - Endemic goitre
   - Vitamin deficiencies
   - Anemia
   - Lathyrism: Crippling disease as a result of eating the kesari dal.
   - Fluorosis
3. Environmental sanitation problem
4. Population problems.

HEALTH PROGRAMS OF INDIA

1. **National Anti-Malaria Program:**
   Originally known as National Malaria Control Program (1953) and later in 1958, changed into National Malaria Eradication Program. In 1994, Malaria Action Program evolved with the following objectives:
   - Management of serious and complicated Malaria cases
   - Prevention of mortality with particular reference to high-risk groups
   - Control of outbreaks and epidemics
   - Reduction and morbidity
   - Reduction of *Plasmodium falciparum* incidence and containment of drug resistant malaria
   - Maintenance of low incidence status
2. **National Filaria Control Program:** Launched in 1955, the main activities are:
   - Anti-mosquito and anti-larval measures in endemic areas
   - Establishment of filaria clinics for the detection and treatment of positive microfilaria cases
   - Provision of underground drainage in hyperendemic cities and towns.
3. **National TB Control Program**
   Centrally sponsored program and the activities include:
   - Early detection and domiciliary treatment of TB cases
   - BCG vaccination of infants and children
   - Isolation facilities especially for those who require surgery or emergency treatment
   - Research.

> Revised National TB Control Program (RNTCP) has been introduced in the country as a pilot project since 1993.

4. **National Leprosy Eradication Program**
   The main objective of the program is early detection of leprosy cases and their treatment with multidrug therapy to control the spread of leprosy.
   The modified leprosy eradication campaign was started in 1997.
5. **National AIDS Control Program**
   This program was launched in the year 1987. The aim of the program is to prevent further transmission of HIV, to decrease the morbidity and mortality associated with HIV infection and to minimize the socioeconomic impact resulting from HIV infection. The national strategy has the following components:
   - Establishment of surveillance centers to cover the whole community
   - Identification of high-risk groups and their screening
   - Issuing specific guidelines for management of detected cases and their follow-up
   - Formulating guidelines for blood bank, blood product manufactures, blood donors and dialysis units.
   - Information, education and communication activities by involving mass media and research for reduction of personal and social impact of the diseases
   - Control of sexually transmitted diseases
   - Condom program.
6. **Reproductive and Child Health Program (RCH)**
   This program aims at improving the health status of young women and children. RCH program incorporates the components relating to child survival and safe motherhood (CSSM) and includes two additional components, one relating to sexually transmitted disease and other relating to reproductive tract infections.
   The CSSM program envisage the following maternal care:
   a. Immunization during pregnancy
   b. Antenatal check-up

c. Prevention and treatment of anemia
d. Early identification of maternal complication
e. Promotion of institutional deliveries
f. Management of obstetric emergencies
g. Birth spacing
h. Diagnosis and treatment of RTIs and STDs.

The package of services for children are:

a. Essential newborn care
b. Immunization
c. Appropriate management of diarrhea
d. Appropriate management of ARI
e. Vitamin A prophylaxis.

7. **National Program for Prevention of Blindness**

   The Government of India had launched this program in 1976. Under this program, children between 1 to 5 years are being given an oral dose of 2,00,000 IU of Vitamin A once in every six months. The National Trachoma Control Program which was launched in 1963, for the control of blindness due to trachoma has been integrated with the national program for prevention of blindness.

8. **Universal Immunization Program**

   UIP was taken up in the year 1985 to 86, the program became operational by the year 1989 to 90 and became part of CSSN program in 1992 and RCH program in 1997. Under the immunization program vaccination to infants are given to control of vaccine preventable diseases namely, diphtheria, pertussis, tuberculosis, poliomyelitis, measles and neonatal tetanus and to pregnant women against tetanus. As a supplement to UIP, the pulse polio immunization (PPI) campaign has been taken up in 1995 for eradication of poliomyelitis.

9. **National Family Welfare Program**

   Launched officially on 1952 by the Union Ministry of Health and Family Welfare, Government of India. During the first and second five years plan (1951–1961), the program was taken up in a modest way with a clinical approach, with emphasis on four components—education, service, training and research. During 1992, different welfare programs for the mother and the children were integrated under child survival safe motherhood program (CSSM). The process of integration of related programs initiated a new step further in 1994 when the reproductive and Child Health Program (RCA Program) is being implemented.

ENVIRONMENTAL HEALTH

- Environment means all the external factors, living and non-living, material and non-material which surround man.
- Components of environment:
  1. **Physical:** Water, air, soil, housing, wastes, radiation, etc.
  2. **Biologic:** Plant and animal life including bacteria, viruses, insects, rodents and animals.
  3. **Social:** Customs, culture, habits, income, occupation, religion, etc.

Environmental Sanitation

The science of safeguarding health. According to WHO, "The control of all those factors in the man's physical environment which exercise or may exercise a deleterious effect on his physical development, health and survival".

The term environmental sanitation is now being replaced by the term environmental health.

WATER

Safe and wholesome water is a basic health need. The WHO (World Health Organization) has coined the slogan "Safe water for all by the year 1990" as part of its activities to advise health for all by 2000.

> The 1980s were dedicated as the "Decade of water" by international agencies.

Safe and Wholesome Water

- Free from pathogenic agents
- Free from harmful chemical substances
- Pleasant to the taste
- Portable or made for domestic purposes.

Sources of Water

1. Rain
2. Surface water
   a. Artificial lakes
   b. Rivers stream
   c. Ponds and tanks
3. Ground water
   a. Shallow well
   b. Deep well
   c. Springs.

> Rain is the prime source of water and is the purest water in nature.

Importance of Water

A. **Dissolved impurities**
   1. Inorganic:
      a. Gases; H_2S, CQ_2, NH_3, N_2
      b. Salts: Salts of calcium, magnesium, sodium, iron, lead, manganese.

2. Organic: Albuminoid, ammonia.

B. **Suspended impurities**
   1. Inorganic: Particles of sand, clay, silt.
   2. Organic:
      a. Plant organ: Dead leaves, algae, peat.
      b. Animal origin: Bacteria, viruses, ova, cysts, insects.

Water Pollution

The sources of pollution are:

1. **Sewage:** Contain decomposable organic matter and pathologic agents.
2. **Industrial wastes:** Toxic agents from industries pollute water and are a growing problem in many countries.
3. **Agriculture:** During water sources may be polluted by fertilizers or pesticides used in agricultural practice.

Water Related Diseases:

Includes the classical waterborne diseases, the heaviest being diarrheal diseases:

A. Biological (Waterborne diseases)

1. Those caused by the presence of an infective agent
   a. Viral: Viral hepatitis A, hepatitis E, poliomyelitis, rotavirus diarrhea
   b. Bacterial: Typhoid and paratyphoid fever, bacillary dysentery, *E. coli* diarrhea, cholera
   c. Protozoal: Amebiasis, giardiasis
   d. Helminthic: Roundworm, threadworm hydatid disease
   e. Leptospiral: Weil's disease.
2. Those due to the presence of an aquatic host
   a. Snail: Schistosomiasis
   b. Cyclops: Guinea worm, fish tape worm.

B. Chemical

Chemical pollutants produce their acute toxic effects or long-term effects which are often non-specific and difficult to detect.

Hardness of Water

A hard water is one in which will not readily form leather with soap. Temporary and permanent hardness in there.

Causes of Hardness

1. Bicarbonates of calcium and magnesium
2. Sulphates and chlorides of calcium and magnesium
3. Salt of iron, zinc and silica.

> Temporary hardness in due to the presence of bicarbonates of calcium and magnesium. Temporary hardness is removed by boiling.

> Permanent hardness is not removed by boiling and it is due to sulphates, chlorides and nitrates of calcium and magnesium.

Measurement of Hardness

- Hardness is expressed as mg of calcium carbonate per liter of water. Water with hardness less than 100 mg/liter is regarded as soft. Water with a hardness of more than 300 mg/liter is regarded as hard.

> Drinking water should have hardness in the range 100–150 mg/liter as calcium carbonate.

Disadvantage of Hardness

- Wastage of soap
- Greater fuel consumption
- Scaling of boilers
- Cooking takes long time
- Fabric tend to have shorter life
- Unsuited for industries.

Removal of Hardness

Temporary hardness:

a. Boiling
b. Addition of lime
c. Addition of sodium carbonate
d. Permutit process.

Permanent Hardness

a. Addition of sodium carbonate
b. Base exchange process or Permutit process.

Purification of Water

a. Purification of water on a large scale

Based on a system of water purification which contains storage, filtration and disinfection.

> Chlorine act best as a germicide when the pH of water is around 7.

b. Purification of water on a small scale

1. **Household methods:** Boiling, chemicals, domestic filters.
2. **Disinfection of wells:** Using bleaching powder.

> 2.5 gm of good quality bleaching powder is needed for disinfecting 1,000 liters of water.

AIR

Air is part of man's environment. It is the basis of all form of life. It is a mixture of gases viz. nitrogen, oxygen and carbon dioxide.

Nitrogen constitutes 78.1% of external air.

Factors which maintain air composition:

a. Wind
b. Sunlight
c. Rain
d. Plant life.

Air Pollution

Air pollution is one when there is an excessive concentration of foreign matter in the outdoor atmosphere, which is harmful to man.

Sources of air pollution are:

a. **Domestic sources:** Burning of coal, wood, oil
b. **Industrial sources:** From factories and industries
c. **Automobiles:** Motor vehicles, roadways
d. **Others:** Nuclear explosion.

Air Pollutants

The substances that pollute air are called air contaminants.

The important one are—carbon dioxide, carbon monoxide, sulphur dioxide, hydrogen sulphate, fluorine compounds, cancer producing substances, dust, smoke, etc.

To decrease the nuisance of air pollution, the Government of India have enacted "The Prevention and Control of Air Pollution Act" in 1981.

Effective room temperature which offers comfort is 25–27°C.

VENTILATION

- Exchange of air between outdoors and indoors.
- Implies control of air temperature, humidity, velocity and purity.
- Types of ventilation.
  a. Natural
  b. Mechanical or artificial.

Door and windows facing each other provide "Cross ventilation".

LIGHTING

- Essential for proper vision.
- Light is usually measured in term of 'foot candles'.
- Recommended light intensity for casual reading is 6 to 10 foot candles.

NOICE

- Wrong sound in the wrong place at the wrong time.
- Sources: Domestic, automobile, factories and industries, air craft.
- Noise is measured in units called decibels.

The recommended maximum noise level is 85 decibels. The extreme limit of human noise tolerance is 140 decibels.

REFUSE

- Refuse is discarded waste matter
- Methods of refuse disposal
  - Burning
  - Dumping
  - Controlled tipping
  - Composting.

Incineration is the best way to dispose majority of hospital wastes.

MOSQUITO BORNE DISEASES

1. **Anopheles mosquito:** Malaria
2. **Culex mosquito:** Filaria, Encephalitis
3. **Aedes:** Yellow fever, Dengue fever, hemorrhagic fever
4. **Mansonoids:** Filaria.

Method of control of mosquito by eliminating the breeding places is known as "Source reduction".

EPIDEMIOLOGY OF DISEASE

Epidemiology is concerned with the patterns of disease occurrence in human populations and of the factors that influence these patterns.

Factors responsible for the spread of communicable diseases.

- Agent
- Host
- Environment.

1. **Agent factors**
   a. **Biological agents:** Living agents, e.g. viruses, bacteria, fungi, protozoa, etc. These are found in the reservoir of infection (e.g. man, animal, insect, soil).
   b. **Nutrient agents:** Protein, fats, carbohydrates, vitamins, minerals and water. An excess or deficiency of nutrients may lead to nutritional diseases.
   c. **Physical agents:** Heat, cold, pressure, radiation and electricity.
   d. **Chemical agents:** These may be metals (e.g. lead) fumes, dusts, gases, etc.
   e. **Mechanical agents:** Chronic friction and other mechanical forces may cause trauma, injuries and fractures.
2. **Host factors**
   a. **Age:** Certain diseases are more frequent in certain age groups than in others, e.g. measles in childhood and atherosclerosis in old age.
   b. **Sex:** There are sex differences in disease occurrence.
   c. **Heredity:** Harmful genes in the constitution may give rise to disease, e.g. hemophilia, color blindness, albinism, etc.
   d. **Nutrition:** Poor nutrition is frequently associated with nutritional deficiency diseases, e.g. anemia, kwashiorkor.
   e. **Occupation:** The occupation of the host may predispose him to certain occupational diseases, e.g. silicosis, bagassosis, accidents.
   f. **Customs and habits:** Certain customs are prejudicial to health smoking is related to oral and lung cancer.
   g. **Human behavior:** Lack of physical exercise, indulgence in alcohol and certain drugs are known to effect health adversely.
3. **Environmental factors**
   a. **Physical environment:** Much of the ill health in India is due to poor environment—unsafe water, contaminated soil, poor housing, lack of disposal facilities for human excreta and solid wastes.
   b. **Biological environment:** The causes of disease may be found in the biological environment, e.g. animals, insects, rodents, etc.
   c. **Social environment:** The customs, habits, culture, education, standard of living are all implicated in disease occurrence directly or indirectly.

DISEASE CYCLE

The course of most communicable diseases are marked by certain stages.

These are:
1. **Incubation period:** Time interval between the entry of the disease agent in the body and the manifestation of clinical signs and symptom.
2. **Prodromal period:** Short period ranging from 1 to 4 days and is marked by vague sign and symptom.
3. **Fastigium:** This represents the height of the disease. Sign and symptoms are clear cut.
4. **Defervescence:** Patient begins to feel better, the body defenses begin to respond.
5. **Convalescence:** The patients recovery is established; he is improving fast.
6. **Defection:** The patient recovers from illness.

LEVELS OF PREVENTION

1. **Primary Prevention**
   - Actions taken prior to the onset of disease, which removes the possibility that a disease will ever occur.
   - Interventions include health promotion and specific protection.
   - Health promotion: Includes adequate nutrition, provision of safe water supply, facilities for the safe disposal of human excreta and other human wastes, personal hygiene, health education, physical education, periodic health screening and improving the quality of life of the people.
   - Specific protection: Preventing specific diseases by specific measures, e.g. immunization against TB, diphtheria, etc, vitamin A prophylaxis to prevent xerophthalmia, etc.
2. **Secondary Prevention**
   - Actions which halt the progress of a disease at its incipient stage and prevents complications. The specific interventions include early diagnosis and treatment.
   - **Early diagnosis:** Screening tests, case finding programs.
   - Adequate treatment prevents complication associated with a particular disease.
3. **Tertiary Prevention**

All measures available to reduce or limit impairments and disabilities, minimize suffering caused by existing departures from good health and to promote the patient's adjustment to irremediable condition. The specific interventions are disability limitation and rehabilitation.

TERMINOLOGY RELATED TO EPIDEMIOLOGY

1. **Infection:** The entry and development or multiplication of a disease producing agent in the body of man or animal.

2. **Epidemic:** An outbreak of disease in a community in excess of normal expectation.
3. **Endemic:** The constant presence of disease within a geographic area, or the usual prevalence of a given disease in a particular area.
4. **Sporadic:** The incidence at intervals of single, scattered cases of disease. A sporadic may be the starting point of an epidemic.
5. **Pandemic:** An epidemic which spreads from country to country or over the whole world.
6. **Zoonosis:** Diseases or infections which are naturally transmitted between vertebrate animals and man.
7. **Communicable disease:** An illness due to a specific infectious agent or its toxic products which under certain condition, tends to spread among individuals in a community.
8. **Noncommunicable disease:** Term applies to diseases such as cancer, cardiovascular diseases and diabetes which are not communicated from person to person.
9. **Incubation period:** Time interval between the entry of the disease agent into the body and the appearance of the first sign or symptom of the disease.
10. **Isolation:** The separation of a person with infections disease from contact with other human beings for the period of communicability.
11. **Quarantine:** Isolation of well persons who have come in contact with infectious diseases for a period of time equal to the largest incubation period of that disease.
12. **Carrier:** A person who harbors the infection agent without having any outward sign and symptoms of that disease. A temporary carrier is one who excretes the diseases agent only for short periods, e.g. cholera, diphtheria, dysentery. A chronic carrier is one who sheds the disease agent for indefinite periods, e.g. typhoid fever, amebiasis.
13. **Antiserum:** Serum containing specific antibody, e.g. ATS (Anti tetanus serum).
14. **Fomites:** Inanimate articles other than food or water contaminated by the infectious discharges from a patient, and capable of harboring and transferring the infection agent to a healthy person, e.g. handkerchief, toys, utensils, etc.
15. **Vector:** Usually an arthropod (e.g. mosquito) which transfers an infectious agent from an infected person to a healthy host.
16. **Virulence:** Measure of the severity of the disease.
17. **Pathogenicity:** Ability to cause disease.

DISEASE TRANSMISSION

Disease is spread in many different ways from the source or reservoir of infection to a susceptible human host.

1. **Source of infection**

   The source of infection in most cases, is man himself, who has the disease. He may be a case or carrier. Sometimes the source of infection may be an infected animal (zoonosis, e.g. rabies).
2. **Modes of transmission**

A. Direct transmission
   a. Direct contact, e.g. sexually transmitted disease, leprosy, scabies.
   b. Droplet infection, e.g. tuberculosis, measles, diphtheria.
   c. Contact with infected soil, e.g. tetanus, hookworm.
   d. Inoculation into skin or mucosa, e.g. rabies, hepatitis B.
   e. Transplacetal or vertical transmission, e.g. acquired immunodeficiency syndrome, toxoplasmosis, syphilis.

B. Indirect transmission
   a. Vehicle-borne transmission, e.g. enteric fever, cholera.
   b. Vector-borne transmission, e.g. malaria, filaria, kala-azar.
   c. Air-borne transmission, e.g. tuberculosis, pneumonia, influenza.
   d. Fomite-borne transmission, e.g. respiratory infections, influenza, measles.

IMMUNITY

Ability of the body to recognize, destroy and eliminate the antigenic material viz. bacteria, viruses and foreign protein.

- Antigen is a substance that stimulates the formation of an antibody.
- Antibodies are proteins that are formed in response to an antigen and react specifically with the antigen that provoked their production. Antibodies are produced in the body by B lymphocytes, a type of white blood cells.
- Humoral immunity is based on the production of antibodies. These antibodies are specific and they react with the same antigen which stimulated their production.
- Cellular immunity is more complex and based on T cells. The T cells are active against some pathogenic agents which are intracellular and escape the bactericidal action of leukocytes, such as *salmonella typhi* and *mycobacterium leprae*.

Classification of Immunity

1. Natural immunity
2. Acquired immunity

1. **Natural Immunity:** Natural immunity or inherited immunity is that immunity which the individual inherits or possesses by virtue of his genetic makeup.

2. **Aquired Immunity:** Can be active or passive immunity.
   a. Active immunity: It is the immunity that a person develops as a result of infection by pathogenic organism or their toxic products. The body produces its own antibodies (immunoglobulins) to fight the infection. Active immunity may be acquired by:
      i. An attack of disease, e.g. measles, chickenpox.
      ii. Subclinical infections, e.g. polio, diphtheria.
   b. Passive immunity: When antibodies produced in one person are transferred to another to give protection against a disease, it is called passive immunity. The body does not produce its own antibodies, but depend upon readymade antibodies. Passive immunity is short lived and declines in a few days or weeks and disappears. Passive immunity may be acquired in the following ways.
      i. Injection of antisera, e.g. diphtheria antitoxins to protect against diphtheria.
      ii. Injection of gamma globulin obtained from immune persons, e.g. measles, hepatitis A.
      iii. Maternal antibodies transferred to fetus across the placenta or through breast milk. These passively acquired antibodies protect the infant during the first few month of life against certain communicable diseases such as measles, polio, mumps, chickenpox, etc.

Human gammaglobulin: The human gamma-globulin or immunoglobulin preparations are of two types viz. human normal immunoglobulin prepared from human plasma of multiple donors and human specific immunoglobulin prepared from donors who have been immune against or have recovered fromspecific infectious diseases.

Antisera or antitoxins: These are prepared from animal sources such as horses, used against tetanus, diphtheria, botulism, gas gangrene and snakebite. There is risk of anaphylactic shock while administering antisera.

Hypersensitivity: Hypersensitivity or allergy refers to the reaction that occurs who a foreign substance is introduced into the body. There are two main forms of hypersensitivity reaction—immediate and delayed. Immediate is antibody mediated and delayed is cell mediated type. The clinical example of the immediate reaction is anaphylactic reaction. The clinical examples of delayed type of hypersensitivity reaction are tuberculin hypersensitivity, allergy to fungi, skin graft rejection, etc.

IMMUNIZING AGENTS

Immunizing agents may be classified as vaccines, immunoglobulins and antisera.

Vaccines

Vaccine is a preparation of disease agent or its toxic products which when administered stimulates specific antibody formation. Administration of a vaccine induces active immunity.

Vaccine are Prepared from

1. Live attenuated organism, e.g. polio vaccine
2. Killed organism, e.g. cholera and typhoid vaccine
3. Toxiods, e.g. diphtheria and tetanus vaccines
4. A combination of the above.

Common vaccines	
Live Attenuated Vaccines	BCG Oral Polio, Measles, Yellow fever
Killed Vaccines	Typhoid, Cholera Whooing cough, Cerebro-spinal meningitis, Plague, Polio (SalkType), Rabies, Influenza
Toxoids	Diphtheria, Tetanus

Combined (Mixed) Vaccines

Combined vaccines simplify administration, reduce costs and minimize the number of injections. The common examples are:

i. DPT: Which protects against diphtheria, whooping cough (pertussis) and tetanus.
ii. DT: Which protects against diphtheria and tetanus.
iii. Typhoid (bivalent): Which protects against typhoid and paratyphoid A.

NATIONAL IMMUNIZATION SCHEDULE

Immunization against preventable diseases is essential for child survival and child development. The major vaccine preventable diseases are Poliomyelitis, Pertussis (whooping cough), Tetanus, Measles, Diphtheria and Tuberculosis.

It is important to give the vaccination to the children at the recommended age. If for some reason a child misses a dose, it should be given as soon as possible after the scheduled date. The immunization can be given if the child is having mild illnesses like fever, diarrhea, vomiting or respiratory infection.

National immunization schedule		
a.	For infants	schedule
	At birth	BCG and OPV 0 dose
	At 6 weeks	DPT-1 OPV-1
	At 10 weeks	DPT-2 OPV-2
	At 14 weeks	DPT-3 OPV-3
	At 9 months	Measles
b.	At 16–24 months	DPT & OPV
c.	At 5–6 years	DT
d.	At 10 years and 16 years	TT
e.	For pregnant women	TT 2 doses at one month interval

COLD CHAIN

Vaccines must be stored at the proper temperature in order to be effective. It exposed to heat, they will lose their potency. The cold chain is a system of transporting and storing vaccines at the recommended temperatures. The equipments used are walk in coolers, ice-lined refrigerators, cold boxes, vaccine carriers and day carriers, refrigerated vans, etc. All vaccines can be stored for few months at 2 to 8°C. DPT and tetanus toxoid should not be frozen.

PORTALS OF EXIT

The disease agent may find its way out of the body in order that it may reach a new lost.

The main portals of exit are:

1. **Nose and throat secretions:** For example, diphtheria bacilli, tubercle bacilli, viruses of common cold, mumps, measles and influenza.
2. **Faces:** Some organisms are excreted in faces, e.g. salmonella, shigella, poliovirus, hepatitis A virus, cholera, eggs and cysts of intestinal parasites such as roundworm and hookworm.
3. **Urine:** Some organisms are excreted in urine, e.g. *S. typhi.*
4. **Skin:** The organisms exit by means of wounds and discharges, etc. e.g. lepra bacilli, agents of STD, scabies, skin infections, etc.

GENERAL MEASURES FOR THE CONTROL OF INFECTIOUS DISEASES

The measures of control can be classified broadly as:

1. Controlling the source or reservoir of infection.
2. Blocking the channels of transmission.
3. Protecting the susceptible population.

1. Controlling the source or reservoir of infection
   a. Early diagnosis of cases and carriers.
   b. Notification to the higher authorities to enable further action to control the spread of infection.
   c. Isolation: Hospital or home isolation can be done up to the infectious period of the disease.
   d. Treatment: Cut short the duration of illness, prevents the development of secondary cases.
   e. Surveillance: Prompt field investigation of all cases to find out the sources of infection and institution of prompt control measures.
   f. Disinfection: Destruction of infectious against in the excretions of the patient and the articles (fomites) contaminated by the patient.
2. Blocking the channels of transmission
   a. Disinfection of water supplies.
   b. Safe disposal of human excreta and solid wastes.
   c. Control of insects and rodents.
   d. Improving the standards of food, hygiene, etc.

Which method is to be enforced will depend upon the organism involved and its portal of exit.

3. Protecting the susceptible population
   a. Immunization before the onset of disease.
   b. Health education to the community.

DISINFECTION

Related Terminology

1. **Disinfectant:** A disinfectant or germicide is an agent which kills infections against (not usually spores) outside the body by direct exposure to physical or chemical agents. They are usually used on inanimate surfaces.
2. **Antiseptic:** An antiseptic is an agent which destroys or inhibits the growth of infections agents and which can be applied to living tissues, e.g. alcohol, dettol. A disinfectant in low concentration acts as an antiseptic.
3. **Deodorant:** An agent which suppresses bad odors, e.g. lime, bleaching powder.
4. **Detergent:** A surface cleaning agent which acts by lowering surface tension, e.g. soap which removes bacteria with dirt.
5. **Disinfection:** Killing of infectious agent outside the human body by direct exposure to physical or chemical agents.
6. **Disinfestation:** Any physical or chemical process serving to destroy arthropods or rodents present on the person, the clothing, or in the environment of an individual or in domestic animals (e.g. delousing).
7. **Sterilization:** Destruction of all microorganism and their spores.

Types of Disinfection

1. **Concurrent disinfection:** The application of disinfective measures as soon as possible after the discharge of infectious material from the body of an infected person, e.g. (urine, stool) or after the soiling of articles (e.g. contaminated lines) with such infections discharges.
2. **Terminal disinfection:** The application of disinfective measures after a patient has been died or has been removed to a hospital or has caused to be a source of infection.
3. **Prophylactic disinfection:** Boiling of water, pasteurization of milk, washing hands with soap and water are examples of prophylactic or pre- disinfection.

Classification of Disinfectants

Natural	Sunlight Air
Physical	
a. Dry heat	Burning, hot dry air
b. Moist heat	Boiling, pasteurization, Steam under pressure
c. Radiation	
Chemical	
a. Liquids	Phenol, cresol, alcohol, chlorhexidine, savlon
b. Solids	Bleaching powder, lime, potassium permanganate
c. Gases	Ethylene oxide, formalin, chlorine

COMMUNICABLE DISEASES

SMALLPOX (VARIOLA)

- Acute, highly infectious disease caused by variola virus.
- Characterized by sudden onset of fever, headache and body ache. On the third day of fever, typical ache or eruption appears. The reach passion through the stages of macule, papule, vesicle, pustule and scar. The crests fall off in about 3 week leaving behind permanent pock marks.
- World Health Organization in 1967 began intensified programs to eradicate smallpox.
- India was declared smallpox free in July 1975.
- World Health Assembly in May 1980 confirmed the global eradication of smallpox.

> India was declared smallpox free in July 1975. World Health Assembly in May 1980 confirmed the global eradication of smallpox.

CHICKENPOX (VARICELLA)

- An acute, infectious disease caused by varicella zoster virus. Now termed as human (alpha) herpes virus 3.
- Characterized by fever, malaria, aches and appearance of a vesicular rash within 24 hours.
- Occurs in both epidemic and endemic forms.
- Source of infection is a case of chickenpox. The virus is present in the nose and throat secretions and lesions of the skin, mucous membranes and blood. Unlike smallpox, the scabs of chickenpox are not infective.
- The case is infection for a period of about one week, commencing 1 to 2 days before the appearance of rash and 4 to 5 days thereafter.
- Spread mainly by droplet infection.
- Incubation period in 14 to 17 days.

Chickenpox	
Causative agent	: Varicella zoster (Human alpha herpes virus 3)
Incubation period	: 14 to 17 days
Period of infectivity	: One week, 1 to 2 days before appearance of rash and 4 to 5 days thereafter.
Mode of transmission	: Droplet infection

- The main clinical features are fever and rash. The first lesion to be noticed are fluid filled vesicles with rapid evolution of rash and completed within five days.
- Prevention and control
  1. Isolation for one week
  2. Disinfection of articles used by the patient.

MEASLES (RUBEOLA)

- Primarily a disease of children.
- Highly infectious disease caused by a virus.
- Characterized by fever, coughing, sneezing, running nose followed by a typical rash.
- Source of infection: A case of measles.
- Period of infectivity: Four days before and five days after the appearance of the rash.
- An attack of measles gives lifelong immunity.
- Mode of transmission: Droplet transmission, which spread by means of articles such as spoons and cups recently contaminated by the patient.
- Incubation period is 10 to 14 days.

Measles	
Causative agent	: Virus (RNA paramyxovirus)
Incubation period	: 10–14 days
Period of infectivity	: 4 days before and 5 days after the appearance of rash
Mode of transmission	: Droplets, fomites

Clinical Features

a. **Pre-eruptive stage:** The early symptoms may be similar to common cold viz. fever, running nose, watery and red eyes and sneezing. Small bluish white spots on a red base (Kopliks' spots) occur on the inner surface of the cheek during the prodromal period and are diagnostic. Prodromal symptoms last for 3 to 4 days.

b. **Eruptive stage:** About the 4th day of illness, a typical, dusky—red, macular rash appears, first on the face and neck, behind the ears and then spreads down the body taking 2 to 3 days to progress to the lower limbs. The eruption lasts for about 5 to 6 days and gradually fades leaving a dark pigmentation of the skin.

Complications

- Measles can be fatal in children especially who are malnourished due to deficiency of protein, calories and vitamins. Complications include bronchitis, pressure, diarrhea and encephalitis.
- Prevention: By measles vaccination at the age of 9 to 12 month. Measles immunoglobulin if given within three days of contact found to be effective.
- Control:
  - Isolation of child.
  - Disinfection of nose and throat discharges.
  - Immunization of susceptible children.

GERMAN MEASLES (RUBELLA)

- Viral infection occurring primarily in childhood, causative agent being toga virus characterized by mild prodromal symptoms and a typical eruption.
- Source of infection is a case of rubella.
- Nose and throat secretion are infectious.
- Spread by droplet infection. Congenital transmission result in birth defects.
- Incubation period: 2 to 3 weeks.

German Measles (Rubella)	
Causative agent	: Toga virus
Incubation period	: 2–3 weeks
Mode of transmission	: Droplet infection, transplacental transmission

- Signs and symptoms of rubella consist of mild fever, cough and sore throat. A discrete, pinkish, macular rash appears in 1 to 2 days, first on the face, then on the other parts of the body. The rash disappears by 2nd or 3rd day. In many instances, the infection is subclinical without any rash, so clinical diagnosis requires serological confirmation.
- Live vaccine available; given to school going girls, widely practiced in western countries.

MUMPS

- Acute infection disease caused by paramyxovirus.
- Characterized by swelling and tenderness of one or both the parotid glands.
- Source of infection: Patients suffering from mumps and subclinical cases.
- Period of infection: Six days before the onset of symptoms until the swelling of parotid glands subsides.
- Mode of spread is through saliva and respiratory droplets.
- Immunity is usually lifelong after infection; rarely second attacks occur.
- Incubation period : 2 to 3 weeks.

Mumps	
Causative agent	: Paramyxovirus
Incubation period	: 2–3 weeks
Period of infectivity	: 6 days before the onset of symptoms until the swelling of parotid gland subsides
Mode of transmission	: Saliva and respiratory droplets

- Clinical features include non-suppurative swelling of the parotid glands with pain and stiffness on opening the mouth. Fever and headache may be present in severe cases. Swelling subsides slowly over 1 to 2 weeks.
- Prevention: By live vaccine given as combination with measles and rubella (MMR vaccine), given at 15 months of age.

DIPHTHERIA

- Acute infectious disease caused by the exotoxin of *Corynebacterium diphtheriae*.
- Affects throat, tonsils, larynx or nose where it produces a grayish white membrane which spreads into the air passages.
- Source of infection may be a patient or a carrier.
- Infective material is nose and throat secretions.
- Period of infection varies between 14 to 28 days from the onset of disease.

- Spreads by droplet infection, fomites and contaminated articles such as toys, clothes, etc.
- Incubation period: 2 to 5 days

Diphtheria	
Causative agent	: *Corynebacterium diphtheriae*
Incubation period	: 2–5 days
Period of infectivity	: 14–28 days from the onset of disease
Mode of transmission	: Droplets, fomites

- **Signs and symptoms** include sore throat, dysphagia and formation of membrane over tonsils and throat, fever and edema of neck in severe cases. Laryngeal diphtheria causes strider and asphyxia.
- **Treatment**
  1. Antibiotics
  2. Diphtheria antitoxins.
- **Schick test:** Intradermal test to find out those who are immune to diphtheria.
- **Prevention:** By DPT immunization or diphtheria vaccine.
- **Control**

1. Disinfection of all articles used by child.
2. Diphtheria antitoxin to all who are not previously immunized.

WHOOPING COUGH

- Highly infectious disease of the respiratory tract caused by the bacilli *Bordetella pertussis*.
- Characterized by severe attacks of irritating cough which becomes paroxysmal producing the typical whoop.
- Source of infection: Nose and throat secretion of a case. A carrier state does not exist.
- Highly infectious during the later part of the incubation period and before the appearance of typical cough; may extend from a week after exposure to about three weeks after the onset of the paroxysmal stage.
- Incubation period is 7 to 14 days.
- One attack of pertussis gives lifelong immunity.
- Spreads directly by droplet infection or by fomites.

Pertussis (Whooping Cough)	
Causative agent	: *Bordetella pertussis*
Incubation period	: 7–14 days
Mode of transmission	: Droplets, fomites
Period of infectivity	: One week after exposure to about 3 weeks after the onset of the paroxysmal stage

- Clinical features: Fever, running nose, irritating cough that gradually becomes paroxysmal within 1 to 2 weeks.
- Control is by early diagnosis, isolation and disinfection of discharges from nose and throat.
- Prevention by DPT immunization as per National Immunization Schedule.

SEVERE ACUTE RESPIRATORY SYNDROME (SARS)

- Communicable viral disease caused by a new strain of corona virus.
- Typical symptoms include fever, malaise, chills, headache, myalgia, dizziness, cough, sore throat and running nose. In some cases acute respiratory distress requiring ventilator support develops.
- CXR findings begin with a small, unilateral, patchy shadowing and progress over 1 to 2 days to become bilateral and generalized with interstitial infiltration.
- Incubation period is 2 to 7 days.
- Transmitted through droplets and fomites.
- Prevention and control: Early case detection, isolation, disinfection of secretions from nose and throat, screening of international travelers.

Severe Acute Respiratory Syndrome (SARS)	
Causative agent	: Corona virus
Incubation period	: 2–7 days
Mode of transmission	: Droplets, fomites

TUBERCULOSIS (TB)

- Chronic infectious disease caused by tubercle bacilli (*Mycobacterium tuberculosis*).
- Primarily affects lungs.
- Can also affect intestine, meninges, bones and joints, lymph glands, skin and other tissues of the body.
- Can affect animals such as cattle (bovine tuberculosis).
- Human source and bovine source is there. Infected sputum of human beings and infected milk and milk products are sources of infection.
- More likely to occur in malnourished persons and persons who are living in overcrowded places where standards of living are poor.
- Spread mainly by droplets, also by inhalation of infected dust.
- Incubation period may be weeks to months.
- Commonest signs and symptoms include chronic cough, continuous low grade fever, chest pain, hemoptysis and loss of weight.

- Mantoux test: To find out infected persons. Carried out by injecting intradermally one tuberculin unit of purified protein derivative (PPD) into the forearm. Test is read on 3rd day (72 hours). Test is positive if there is swelling of at least 10 mm diameter of the site of injection. Reactions less than five mm are negative and those between six and nine are considered doubtful. Those who are negative should be given BCG vaccine.
- Control by early diagnosis, drug therapy, BCG vaccination and health education.
- Early case finding is by sputum examination; sputum must be examined for any patients presenting one or more of the following symptoms of respiratory disease.
  - i. Cough lasting more than 2 weeks
  - ii. Continuous fever
  - iii. Chest pain
  - iv. Hemoptysis.
- Chemotherapy is based on multidrug therapy.
- Short course chemotherapy: Treat with rifampicin, streptomycin, INH and pyrazinamide for 6 to 8 months.
- DOTS (Direct Observed Treatment, Short course): DOTS is the recommended strategy for global tuberculosis control. During the intensive phase of chemotherapy, all the drugs are administered under direct supervision. DOTS will be given under the supervision by peripheral health workers and voluntary health workers.
- Revised National Tuberculosis Control Program (RNTCP) is introduced in 1993 with the objective to achieve at least 85 percent cure rate of infection cases through DOTS.
- BCG Vaccine is a live attenuated. The vaccine is given intradermal using a tuberculin syringe. The usual site of injection is just above the insertion of the deltoid muscle of the left arm.

> The usual site of injection of BCG vaccination is just above the insertion of the deltoid muscle of the left arm.

MENINGOCOCCAL MENINGITIS

- Meningococcal meningitis or cerebrospinal fever is an acute communicable disease caused by *Neisseria meningitidis*.
- Usually begin with intense headache, vomiting and stiff neck and progresses to coma within a few hours.
- Man is the only known natural host; carriers are the most important source of infection.
- Period infectivity continues until the causative organism is no longer present in the discharges from nose and throat. The organism usually disappears from the nasopharynx within 24 hours after administration of specific treatment.
- All ages are susceptible; immunity is acquired by subclinical infection, clinical disease or vaccination. Infants derive passive immunity from the mother.
- Incubation period is 3 to 4 days, but may vary from 2 to 10 days.
- Transmitted by droplet infection.
- Treated with penicillin and chloramphenicol.
- Meningococcal vaccine is now available for immunization against the disease.

Meningococcal Meningitis	
Causative organism	: Neisseria meningitidis
Incubation period	: Average 3–4 days, may vary from 2–10 days
Mode of transmission	: Droplet transmission
Period of infectivity	: Until the causative organism is no longer present in the discharges from nose and throat

POLIOMYELITIS

- Primarily a viral infections disease of the human alimentary tract.
- May affect the brain, spinal cord and nerve resulting in paralysis.
- Faces and pharyngeal secretions of cases are the source of infection. The virus is found in the faces of cases for a few weeks and upto three months in young children. During the first five days, the virus is found in the secretions from the throat.
- Overcrowding and poor sanitation predisposes to infection.
- Most infection 7 to 10 days before and after the onset of symptoms.
- Transmitted by feco-oral route may also spread by droplet infection.
- Incubation period is 7 to 21 days.

Poliomyelitis	
Causative agent	: Virus, type I serotype
Incubation period	: 7–21 days
Mode of transmission	: Feco-oral route mostly, droplet infection is also possible
Period of infectivity	: 7–10 days before and after the onset of symptoms

- 90 percent of cases are asymptomatic, symptoms are fever, headache, diarrhea, vomiting and drowsiness. The warning sign are pain weakness and stiffness of the neck and back. There may be paralysis of the affected limb.

- Prevention by vaccination; oral polio vaccine (OPV) and injectable polio vaccine (IPV) are available, OPV is a sabin type of live attenuated vaccine when as IPV is a killed vaccine.

Polio vaccine should be stored at sub-zero temperature in a deep freezer to prevent inactivation.

- Pulse Polio Immunization (PPI) was started in December 1995. In PPI, oral polio vaccine is given to all children between 0 to 5 years of age on a single day irrespective of previous immunization. This will promote herd immunity.

HEPATITIS A

- Caused by Hepatitis A virus, an enterovirus.
- Clinically characterized by fever, malaise, nausea, vomiting and jaundice.
- Man is the only source of infection.
- Spread by feco-oral route; man's faces is the infective material.
- Incubation period: 15 to 50 days.

HEPATITIS B

- Formerly known as serum hepatitis, caused by Hepatitis B Virus (HBV)
- Cases and carriers are the source of infection; carrier state can persist for many years.
- Infection can lead to chronic liver disease.
- Blood and blood products are the infective material, body secretion such as saliva and semen are also infective.
- Transmitted by parenteral route through blood transfusion, inadequately autoclaved syringes and needles, ear piercing, tattooing and sexual contact. Can transmit from infected mother to a fetus in utero (vertical transmission). Incubation period is 60 to 80 days.
- Hepatitis B vaccine is available for prophylaxis. For immediate protection, Hepatitis B immunoglobulin should be given to those who are exposed to hepatitis B virus.

HEPATITIS C

- Parenterally transmitted hepatitis by Hepatitis C Virus (HCV).
- The incubation period is 6 to 7 weeks.

HEPATITIS E

- Caused by Hepatitis E Virus (HEV)
- Waterborne disease
- Incubation period is 2 to 9 weeks.

Hepatitis	Method of transmission	Incubation period
Hepatitis A	Feco-oral route	15–50 days
Hepatitis B	Parenteral, vertical	60–80 days
Hepatitis C	Parenteral	6–7 weeks
Hepatitis E	Waterborne	2–9 weeks

Types of Hepatitis	Causative agent
Hepatitis A	HAV
Hepatitis B	HBV
Hepatitis C	HCV
Hepatitis E	HEV

CHOLERA

- Acute infection disease caused by *Vibrio cholerae.*
- Characterized by repeated purging and vomiting leading to rapid dehydration, often resulting in death.
- Source of infection is a case or carrier.
- Stools and vomitus of the patient are infective. These contaminate water, food, flies and fomites.
- Cholera affects mainly low socioeconomic groups with poor personal and environmental hygiene.
- Transmitted by ingestion of contaminated water, food or drink.
- The immunity conferred by an attack lasts a few months only.
- Incubation period is few hours to five days (usually 1–2 days).

Cholera

Causative organism : *Vibrio cholerae*
Incubation period : Usually 1–2 days
Mode of transmission : Ingestion of contaminated water, food and drink or by stools and vomitus of patient

- Onset of symptoms is sudden with acute severe diarrhea (rice water stools) and vomiting. The loss of water and electrolytes lead to dehydration, acidosis and hypokalemia. Typical signs include sunken eyes, hollow cheeks, subnormal temperature, washer man's hands and feet, low BP, and suppression of urine. Dehydration eventually results in coma.
- Treatment is based on oral rehydration therapy.
- The oral rehydration solution contains:

Sodium chloride	3.5 gm
Sodium bicarbonate	2.5 gm
Potassium chloride	1.5 gm
Glucose (dextrose)	20.0 gm
Water	1 liter

- Treatment: Tetracycline is the antibiotic of choice. Septran has also been recommended.
- Disinfect stool, vomitus, clothes, feeding and cooking utensils and the room in which the patient is present.
- Parenteral vaccine (killed vaccine) in available which is given subcutaneously in two doses of 0.5 mL each at an interval of 4 to 6 weeks.

> Antibiotics should be avoided from one week before and one week after the administration of the oral live attenuated cholera vaccine.

FOOD POISONING

- Acute gastroenteritis caused by the ingestion of food or drink contaminated with either living bacteria or their toxin or chemical substances.
- **Types of food poisoning**
  1. **Non bacterial:** Caused by ingestion of chemical poisons such as arsenic.
  2. **Bacterial:** Caused by the ingestion of living bacteria, or their toxin. The bacterial food poisioning include *Salmonella* food poisoning, staphylococcal food poisoning and Botulism.
- ***Salmonella* food poisoning:** Caused by *Salmonella typhi* and *salmonella enteritidis*. Man gets infection through contaminated foods, e.g. milk and milk products, custard, eggs and egg products. Once ingested, the organism multiplies in the intestine and cause illness in about 12 to 24 hours. The prominent symptoms are nausea, vomiting, abdominal pain and diarrhea.
- **Staphylococcal food poisoning:** Man gets infection from eating food contaminated by staphylococci derived from another man (e.g. from boils, nose and throat discharges or pyogenic infection) or animals (e.g. milk and milk products). The organism is *Staphylococcus aureus* which produces a heat stable enterotoxin. The toxin acts on the intestine and produces nausea, vomiting, relating abdominal cramps, diarrhea and dehydration after an incubation period of 1 to 6 hours (usually 2–4 hours).
- **Botulism:** Caused by an enterotoxin which is a heat stable neurotoxin produced by *Clostridium botulinum* which occurs in soil, dust and intestinal tract of animals. Man gets the infection by eating foods which has been contaminated. Foods involved usually are improperly canned or bottled vegetables and fish.

> Cook and eat in the same day is the golden rule in the prevention of food poisoning.

TYPHOID FEVER (Enteric fever)

- Acute communicable disease caused by *Salmonella typhi.*
- Infection is marked by prolonged fever, toxic symptoms.
- Patients or carriers of typhoid fever are the source of infection.
- Faces and urine of the infected person are the infective materials. As long as the bacilli are present in faces and urine, a diseased person can infect another person.
- Poor sanitation and unsafe water are involved in transmission. Open air defecation, urination, low standards of food hygiene, health ignorance is responsible for spread of disease.
- Spread by feco-oral route.
- Incubation period: 7 to 28 days.

Typhoid Fever	
Causative organism	: *Salmonella typhi*
Incubation period	: 7–28 days
Mode of transmission	: Feco-oral
Period of infectivity	: As long as the bacilli are present in the faces and urine

- Chloramphenicol is the drug of choice in the treatment of typhoid fever.
- Control by proper disposal of faces and wine of infected person, disinfection of linen and fomites, safe water and sanitation.
- Anti-typhoid vaccine: Killed vaccine, given subcutaneously in two doses of 0.6 mL each for adults; given at an interval of 4 to 6 weeks. An oral typhoid vaccine is also available.

ASCARIASIS (Roundworm)

- Roundworm lives in the upper part of small intestine. The female worm lays eggs, passed out through faces and can contaminate soil or vegetable. The eggs take about 10 days to become infective. When these eggs are ingested, they reach the intestine and hatch into larvae. The larvae penetrate the intestine and migrate to liver and lungs and travel to trachea and pharynx to be swallowed by the lost. They reach intestine and become mature in about 6–10 weeks.
- The infestation is often symptomless, may produce malnutrition, abdominal pain and intestinal obstruction.
- Open field defection favors the spread of disease.
- Incubation period is about two months.
- Treatment is by mebendazole.

RABIES (Hydrophobia)

- Primarily a disease of warm blooded animals such as dogs, cats, jackals, wolfs, etc.

- Transmitted to man by the bite or lick of rabid animals.
- The causative agent is Lyssavirus Type I
- 95 percent of infection is due to dog bite.
- Saliva of the rabid animal is the infective material.
- Transmitted by the licks or bites and the viruses once entered the body, travel up the nerves and reaches the brain.
- Incubation period 1 to 3 months.

Rabies

Causative agent	: Lyssavirus Type I
Incubation period	: 1–3 month
Mode of transmission	: Bites or licks of rabid animal, 95% being dog bite

- The disease begins with headache, slight fever, malaise and perhaps twitching, pain and numbness at the site of bite. Soon the patient shows the classical symptoms of rabies viz. intolerance to noise and bright light, difficulty in swallowing, fear of water and intense spasms on being offered food or fluids. Death occurs due to respiratory paralysis.
- Anti Rabies vaccine available; given as 0.5 inoculation of 1 ml each subcutaneously or IM at 0, 3, 7, 14 and 30 days. A booster dose is given on day 90.
- An intradermal rabies vaccine (IDRV) is also available.

SEXUALLY TRANSMITTED DISEASES (STDS)

- Formerly known as venereal diseases.
- Transmitted predominantly by sexual contact and caused by a wide range of bacterial, viral protozoal, fungal agents and ecto parasites.

ACQUIRED IMMUNODEFICIENCY SYNDROME (AIDS)

Caused by Human Immunodeficiency Virus (HIV)

- AIDS breaks down the body's immune system exposing the individual to numerous lifethreatening infection, neurological disorders and malignancies.
- AIDS was first reported in the USA in 1981.
- In India, first case of AIDS was reported in 1986 from Tamil Nadu.
- HIV cases and carriers are the sources of infection.
- Blood and semen of infected person can spread the disease.
- Transmitted by sexual contact, blood transfusion, unsterilized injection equipments and peri natal transmission.
- Incubation period is six years or more.
- Anti-Retroviral Therapy (ART) consist of drugs viz. Azathioprine, Zidovudine, Lamivudine, etc.

Important sexually transmitted diseases

Pathogen	Disease or syndrome
Gonorrhea	*Neisseria gonorrhea*
Syphilis	*Treponema pallidum*
Chancroid (Soft sore)	*Haemophilus ducreyi*
Granuloma inguinale	*C. granulomatis*
Genital herpes	Herpes simplex virus
Acute and chronic hepatitis	Hepatitis B virus
Condyloma acuminata	Human papiloma virus (HPV)
AIDS	Human immunodeficiency virus

National AIDS control program was launched in India in 1987.

AIDS was first reported in USA in 1981. In India, first case of AIDS was reported in 1986 from Tamilnadu.

HOSPITAL ACQUIRED INFECTIONS

- Cross infection of one patient by another or by doctors, nurses and other hospital staff

WHO case definition for AIDS surveillance

For the purpose of AIDS surveillance an adult or adolescent (> 12 years of age) is considered to have AIDS if at least 2 of the following major signs are present in combination with at least 1 of the minor signs listed below:

Major signs

- Weight loss > 10% of body weight
- Chronic diarrhea for more than 1 month
- Prolonged fever for more than 1 month (intermittent or constant)

Minor signs

- Persistent cough for more than 1 month
- Generalized pruritic dermatitis
- Recurrent Herpes zoster
- Oropharyngeal candidiasis
- Chronic progressive or disseminated herpes simplex infection
- Generalized lymphadenopathy

The presence of either generalized Kaposi's Sarcoma or Cryptococcal meningitis is sufficient for the diagnosis of AIDS for surveillance purpose. For patients with tuberculosis persistent cough for more than 1 month should not be considered as minor sign.

- Sources may be hospital environment, patients and hospital staff
- Other common infections are skin infection, respiratory infection, urinary tract infections, wound infections, etc.

DEMOGRAPHY AND FAMILY WELFARE

DEMOGRAPHY

Demography is the scientific study of human population. India is the second populous country in the world, next to China.

According to 2001 census, the population of India is 1,027 million with an average annual growth rate of 1.93%.

Consequences of Population Growths

1. **Biological consequences:** Population growth affects the size and age composition of population. A high birth rate goes with a high death rate, infant mortality rate and a lower expectation of life.
2. **Economic consequences:** Population growth adversely affect the percapita income. Poverty leads to sickness and sickness leads to poverty.
3. **Social consequences:** Population explosion creates social problems like fewer job opportunities, inadequate schooling facilities, a high percentage of illiteracy, inadequate housing, etc.
4. **Health consequences:** Include higher mortality and morbidity rates, under nutrition, environmental hazards poor quality and quantity of health services, etc.

FAMILY PLANNING

WHO defines family planning as the practices that help individuals and couples to attain certain objectives:

- to avoid unwanted births
- to bring about wanted births
- to regulate the intervals between pregnancies
- to control the time at which births occur in relation to the ages of the parent
- to determine the number of children in the family.

Family Welfare

The term family welfare is broader than family planning which basically is related to quality of life. It includes education, nutrition, health, employment, women's welfare and rights, shelter, safe drinking water—all vital factors associated with the concept of welfare.

In 1977, the Government of India redesignated the "National Family Planning Program" as the "National Family Welfare Program".

Contraceptive Methods

Contraception aims to prevent pregnancy by preventing the union of ovum and sperm, by suppressing the ovulation or by interfering with the implantation of fertilized ovum in the uterus.

The various contraceptive methods may be broadly divided into spacing (non-terminal) and terminal (permanent) methods.

I. Spacing methods
- a. For men:
  1. Condom
  2. Withdrawal method
- b. For women:
  1. Intrauterine devices
     - i. Lippes loop
     - ii. Copper T
  2. Hormonal contraceptives
     - i. Oral pill
     - ii. Injectables (DMPA, NET-EN)
     - iii. Subdermal implants (Norplant)
  3. Diaphragm
  4. Foam tablets, jelly and cream
  5. Rhythm method (safe period)

II. Terminal methods
- a. For males: Vasectomy
- b. For females: Tubectomy

OCCUPATIONAL HEALTH

According to WHO, occupational health aims at:

1. The promotion and maintenance of the highest degree of physical, mental and social well-being of workers in all occupations.
2. The prevention among workers of departures from health caused by their working condition.
3. The protection of workers in their environment.

Health Promotion of Workers

- Nutrition
- Control of communicable diseases
- Environmental sanitation
- Mental health
- Health education
- Family planning.

Prevention of Occupational Diseases

a. **Medical measures:** Include preplacement examination, periodic examination, first aid and medical care, notification, safety of working environment, health education and maintenance of records.

b. **Engineering measures:** Include proper design of the factory building, maintenance of cleanliness, control of dust and fumes, providing protective devices to workers, etc.

c. **Legislation:** The most important factory laws in India are the Indian Factories Act, 1976 and the Employees State Insurance Act, 1975.

OCCUPATIONAL DISEASES

Occupational diseases may arise out of or in the course of employment. The important occupational diseases are:

Diseases due to physical agents:	
Heat	: Burns, heat cramps, heat exhaustion
Cold	: Frostbite, trench foot
Noise	: Occupational deafness
Pressure	: Air embolism, Caisson disease
Radiation	: Cancer, Leukemia
Dust diseases (Pneumoconiosis)	
Coal dust	: Anthracosis
Silica dust	: Silicosis
Asbestos dust	: Asbestosis
Cane fiber	: Bagassosis
Cotton dust	: Byssinosis
Chemical exposures	
Gases	: Carbon monoxide, etc.
Solvents	: e.g. benzene
Metals	: e.g. lead, arsenic
Organic	: e.g. insecticides
Biological factors	
Anthrax, Zoonoses	
Occupational cancer	
Occupational dermatitis	

HEALTH STATISTICS

Statistics: is the science of collection of numerical facts and data and the techniques of analyzing and drawing conclusion from such data.

Vital statistics are statistics relating to vital events of life namely, births, deaths, marriages and sickness that occur in a community.

Health statistics includes three measurements:

1. Measurements related to the state of health, i.e. sickness and death.
2. Measurements affecting health, i.e. nutrition, housing, social, economic and environmental factors.
3. Item of service, i.e. preventive, promotive and curative services.

Birth Rate

The number of live births during a year per 1,000 estimated mid-year population Birth rate =
No. of live births

$$\frac{\text{During the year}}{\text{Estimated mid-year population}} \times 1{,}000$$

Important Vital Statistical Rates and Indices
Birth rate
Death rate
Specific death rate
Infant mortality rate (IMR)
Neonatal mortality rate
Perinatal mortality rate
Under five mortality rate
Maternal mortality rate (MMR)
Expectation of life
General fertility rate

Specific Death Rate

The death rate due to specific diseases, in a specific groups or in a specific period of time.

Specific death rate = No. of death from

$$\frac{\text{Cholera during the year}}{\text{Mid-year population}} \times 1{,}000$$

Specific death rate =

$$\frac{\text{No. of deaths in 2001}}{\text{Mid-year population}} \times 1{,}000$$

Infant Mortality Rate (IMR)

Number of infant death under one year of age per 1,000 live births in one year.
IMR = No. of deaths under

$$\frac{\text{One year of age}}{\text{Total live births in the year}} \times 1{,}000$$

Neonatal Mortality Rate

Deaths occurring within four weeks or 28 days of birth per 1,000 live birth.

Neonatal mortality rate = No. of deaths under

$$\frac{\text{28 days of age}}{\text{Total live births}} \times 1{,}000$$

Perinatal Mortality Rate

Mortality of infants occurring during the period from 28th week of pregnancy to 7 days after birth per 1,000 total births.

Perinatal mortality rate = Late fatal deaths, i.e.

$$\frac{\text{Deaths under one week}}{\text{Total live + still birth}} \times 1{,}000$$

Under Five Mortality Rate

Annual number of deaths of children aged under five years, expressed as rate per 1,000 live births.

Under five mortality rate = No. of deaths of children less

$$\frac{\text{Than 5 years of age in a given year}}{\text{No. of live births in the same year}} \times 1{,}000$$

Maternal Mortality Rate (MMR)

Number of deaths from puerperal causes per 1,000 live births.

MMR = No. of deaths directly due to pregnancy or childbirth and occurs during pregnancy or within 42 days of the

$$\frac{\text{Delivery}}{\text{Total live births in the year}} \times 1{,}000$$

Expectation of life

The expectation of life is defined as the average number of years likely to be lived by a person who is subjected to the mortality risks of the whole population at any given time.

General Fertility Rate

Number of live births during a year per 1,000 women in the reproductive age group of 15 to 45 years.

General Fertility Rate =

$$\frac{\text{Number of live births}}{\text{No. of females in the}} \times 1{,}000$$

age group 15 to 45 years

HEALTH EDUCATION

Health Education is a process which effects changes in the health practices of people and in the knowledge and attitudes related to such changes.

Areas of Health Education

1. Human biology
2. Nutrition
3. Hygiene
4. Maternal and child health including family planning
5. Prevention of communicable diseases
6. Prevention of accidents
7. Use of health services
8. Mental health.

Principles of Health Education

1. Interest
2. Participation
3. Comprehension
4. Communication
5. Motivation
6. Reinforcement
7. Learning by doing
8. Good human relations.

Stages in Education

1. Awareness
2. Motivation
3. Action, adoption or acceptance.

Audio-visual Aids

No health education can be effective without Audio-visual aids. The different AV aids that can be used to impart health education can be:

1. **Auditory Aids**
   - Tape recorders
   - Microphones
   - Amplifiers
   - Earphones
2. **Visual Aids**
   - Black board
   - Flannel graph
   - Models
   - Specimens
   - Posters
   - Slides
   - Film strips
   - Epidiascope
   - Overhead projector

3. **Combined AV Aids**
   - Sound films
   - Slide tape combination
   - Television
   - LCD projector
   - Computers.

Methods of Group Teaching

1. One way or didactic methods
   - Group discussion
   - Panel discussion
   - Symposium
   - Workshop
   - Role playing
   - Demonstration
2. Methods of education to the general public
   - Posters
   - Health magazines
   - Press
   - Films
   - Radio and TV
   - Health exhibitions
   - Indigenous media.

HEALTH AND SOCIAL SERVICES IN INDIA

The health services in India are intended to promote and protect the health and welfare of people. The guidelines for organizing the health services in the country are taken from the following reports.

THE BHORE COMMITTEE

The Bhore Committee or the Health Survey and Development Committee was appointed in 1943 to survey the then existing health condition and health organization in the country and to make recommendations for the future development.

The recommendations of the Bhore Committee were:

- Integration of preventive and curative services at all administrative levels.
- Setting up of primary health units, secondary health units and district hospitals.

> Health Survey and Development Committee (The Bhore Committee) was appointed in 1943 to survey the existing health conditions and health organizations and to make recommendations for their development.

THE MUDALIAR COMMITTEE

The Mudaliar Committee or The Health Survey and Planning Committee was appointed in 1965 to look at the health needs and resources of the country in the period of five year plan.

The main recommendation of the Mudaliar Committee were:

1. To strengthen and expand the district hospitals.
2. The primary health center should not serve more than 40,000 population.
3. The output of public health nurses, lady health visitors and auxiliary nurses are to be increased.
4. Organize proper MCH services.

> The Health Survey and Planning Committee or The Mudaliar Committee was appointed in 1965 to evaluate the health needs and resources of the country in the context of five year plan.

THE CHADHA COMMITTEE

The Chadha Committee in 1963 suggested that the population to be covered by a subcenter of a PHC should not be more than 10,000 with an ultimate target of 50,000. Committee also recommended that each subcenter should be adequately staffed and the needed domiciliary health services should be provided.

> The Chadha Committee 1963 suggested that the subcenter under PHC should be adequately staffed and should cover a target population of 5,000.

THE MUKHERJI COMMITTEE

The Mukherji Committee in 1966 recommended additional staff at the PHC to take over the maintenance work of malaria and smallpox. The committee emphasized the need for building up strong administrative machinery from the center at the block level with adequate number of basic health workers and health supervisors.

> The Mukherji Committee in 1966 focussed on the basic health services and recommended that there should be adequate basic health workers and supervisors with good administrative control over them.

KARTAR SINGH COMMITTEE

The Kartar Singh Committee in 1972 looked into the need for the multipurpose workers for health and family planning. The broad recommendation of the committee were:

1. The multipurpose workers for the delivery of all health care services to the rural community and both feasible and desirable.

2. The present health workers should be replaced by Female Health Workers and Male Health Workers and one male and one female health workers should be there in one subcenter.
3. The subcenter should cover a population of 3000–3500.
4. The present day lady health visitors should be re-designated as Female Health Supervisor who should supervise the work of four female health workers.

> The Kartar Singh Committee in 1972 recommended the needs for male and female health workers in the health centers and there should be female health supervisors to supervise the work of female health workers.

SHRIVASTAV COMMITTEE

The Shrivastav Committee or the "Group on Medical Education and Support Manpower" was set up on 1974 and submitted their reports on 1975. The recommendations were:

1. Creation of bonds of para-professional and semi-professional health workers from within the community itself viz. school teachers, post- masters, etc.
2. Establishment of male and female multipurpose health workers.
3. Development of "Referral Services" complex between the primary health center, district hospital and medical colleges.
4. Establishment of a medical and health education commission for planning and implementing the reforms needed in health and medical education.

> The Shrivastav Committee or the "Group on Medical Education and Support Manpower" was set up in 1975 with the recommendation to create para-professionals from community itself, to establish a referral system and reforming the health and medical education.

NATIONAL HEALTH POLICY

The Ministry of Health and Family Welfare evolved a National Health Policy in 1983 in view of the national commitment to attain the goal of Health for all by the year 2000. The health strategies suggested include restructuring the health infrastructure development of health manpower, research and health development.

The National Health Policy laid down specific goals, to be achieved by 1985, 1990, 1995 and 2000 AD. A new National Health Policy-2002 was evolved to achieve goals by the year 2015.

FIVE YEAR PLANS

Plans	Period
First Five Year Plan	1951–56
Second Five Year Plan	1956–61
Third Five Year Plan	1961–66
Annual plans	1966–69
Fourth Five Year Plan	1969–74
Fifth Five Year Plan	1974–78
Annual Plans	1978–80
Sixth Five Year Plan	1980–85
Seventh Five Year Plan	1985–90
Annual Plans	1990–92
Eighth Five Year Plan	1992–97
Ninth Five Year Plan	1997–02
Tenth Five Year Plan	2002–07
Annual Plans	2002–03
Eleventh Plan	2007–12

INTERNATIONAL HEALTH AGENCIES

WORLD HEALTH ORGANIZATION (WHO)

The WHO is a specialized, non-political international health agency of the United Nations. Its headquarters is in Geneva, Switzerland. The constitution of WHO came into force on 7th April, 1948, which is celebrated every year as "World Health Day".

> World Health Day is celebrated on 7th April every year.

The WHO is the world's directing and coordinating authority on all international health work. It helps countries to strengthen and improve their own health services.

UNICEF (UNITED NATIONS INTERNATIONAL CHILDREN'S EMERGENCY FUND)

UNICEF is now called "UN Children's Fund"

UNICEF was established in 1946 with the headquarters in New York. UNICEF works in close collaboration with WHO, and other specialized agencies of United Nation to improve the health of mothers and children and to assist programs which would directly or indirectly benefit child health.

UNICEF was established in 1946, now called UN Children's Fund. The headquarters is in New York.

FAO (Food and Agricultural Organization)

FAO is a specialized agency of the United Nations to helps nations and raise their living standards and to better the condition of rural people by increasing the efficiency of farming, forestry and fisheries. It was established in 1945 with the headquarters at Rome.

FAO is a specialized agency of UN for improving farming, forestry and fisheries. FAO was established in 1945 and the headquarters is in Rome.

USAID (United States Agency for International Development)

Under USAID, India has been receiving assistance since 1952. The assistance include malaria control and eradication, national water supply and sanitation program; control of filariasis and assistance to medical colleges and allied institutions. It also supports agriculture and family planning programs.

THE RED CROSS

The red cross is a non-political, non-official, international, humanitarian organization quoted to the service of mankind in peace and war. It was founded by Henry Dunant in 1864.

The Indian Red Cross was established in 1920 with the triple objective of the improvement of health, prevention of disease and mitigation of suffering. The red cross promotes international friendliness understanding and cooperation.

International Red Cross Organization was founded by Henry Dunant in 1864. The Indian Red Cross was established in 1920 for the prevention of disease, promotion of health and mitigation of suffering.

UNDP (The United Nation Development Program)

UNDP was established in 1966 to help poorer nations develop their human and natural resources more fully. The UNDP projects cover agriculture, education, science, health, hospital administration, nursing services and health manpower development.

The United Nations Development Program (UNDP) was established in 1966 to help poorer nation develop their natural and human resources more fully.

THE WORLD BANK

The World Bank is a specialized agency of the United Nations. It functions to provide financial and technical assistance for the development of its poorer member countries. It supports projects resigned to raise living standards viz. agricultural, education, rural development, industry, energy and electric power.

OBJECTIVE QUESTIONS

1. **The causative organism of Dengue fever is**
   a. Enteric virus b. Arbovirus
   c. Variola virus d. Influenza virus
2. **Scurvy results from deficiency of**
   a. Vitamin C b. Vitamin B
   c. Vitamin D d. Vitamin A
3. **Poliomyelitis is transmitted through**
   a. Water b. Air
   c. Blood d. Vectors
4. **India's National Health Policy was approved in the Parliament in**
   a. 1961 b. 1980
   c. 1983 d. 1991
5. **Vaccines and toxoids produce**
   a. Natural immunity b. Active immunity
   c. Passive immunity d. Acquired immunity
6. **The measure of health status of children in a community is**
   a. Infant mortality rate b. Maternal mortality rate
   c. Crude birth rate d. Crude death rate
7. **Food constituents more required by pregnant woman**
   a. Calcium b. Iron
   c. Potassium d. Vitamin C
8. **A mechanical method of contraception**
   a. Vasectomy b. Mala-D
   c. Condom d. MTP
9. **Kartar Singh Committee is otherwise known as**
   a. Multipurpose workers committee
   b. Health survey and development committee
   c. Health survey and planning committee
   d. Committee on medical education

10. Drug which is not used in the treatment of leprosy

a. Streptomycin b. Rifampicin
c. Clofazimine d. INH

11. The desired quantity of 'free residual chlorine' in drinking water is

a. 1 mg/lit b. 0.5 mg/lit
c. 2 mg/lit d. 0.25 mg/lit

12. The vitamin which is involved in fat, protein and carbohydrate metabolism

a. Riboflavin b. Folic acid
c. Niacin d. Thiamine

13. The hormonal contraceptives are

a. Oral b. Injectable
c. Implant d. All of them

14. MCH service includes

a. Prenatal and postnatal care
b. Under fives care
c. Family planning service
d. All of them

15. The recommended maximum noise level for human beings

a. 85 dB b. 50 dB
c. 110 dB d. 160 dB

16. The best method of refuse disposal in a hospital is

a. Dumping b. Controlled tipping
c. Incineration d. Composting

17. MTP Act was passed in the year

a. 1983 b. 1977
c. 2000 d. 1972

18. The average amount of blood loss during normal delivery

a. 100 mL b. 300 mL
c. 500 mL d. 700 mL

19. The most frequent cause of maternal death during child birth is

a. Sepsis b. Toxemia
c. Asphyxia d. Hemorrhage

20. Which of the following is not an occupational disease?

a. Asbestosis b. Pneumoconiosis
c. Japanese encephalitis d. Silicosis

21. Carbohydrate is stores in the liver as

a. Glucose b. Sucrose
c. Glycogen d. Galactose

22. Causative organism of malaria is

a. Cryptococcus b. Leishmania
c. Plasmodium d. Klebsiella

23. Father of antiseptic surgery

a. Joseph Lister b. Louis Pasteur
c. William Harvey d. Ronald Ross

24. One gram of fat yields

a. 9 calories b. 6 calories
c. 8 calories d. 4 calories

25. Antisterility vitamin is

a. Vitamin A b. Vitamin E
c. Vitamin D d. Vitamin K

26. Koplik's spot is seen in

a. Chickenpox b. Measles
c. Mumps d. Variola

27. Immunization against DPT should be administered via

a. Oral route b. Intramuscular route
c. Subcutaneous route d. Intradermal route

28. World No Tobacco Day is observed on

a. 5th June b. 7th April
c. 10th August d. 31st May

29. World Heart Day is observed on

a. 21 September b. 28 September
c. 10 October d. 14 August

30. The ability of the body to recognize, destroy and eliminate antigenic material

a. Immunity b. Energy
c. Adaptation d. Resistance

31. Water soluble vitamin

a. Vitamin A b. Vitamin B complex
c. Vitamin D d. Vitamin K

32. Epidemiological triad comprises of

a. Agent, host and disease
b. Agent, host and organism
c. Agent, host and environment
d. Agent, host and infection

33. The best sources of calcium
a. Meat b. Vegetable
c. Fruits d. Milk

34. Separation of an infected person from noninfected persons
a. Incubation b. Isolation
c. Inoculation d. Immunization

35 The best indicator of infant nutrition
a. Height b. Weight
c. Vital signs d. Vital statistics

36. Permanent male sterilization
a. PPS b. Tubectomy
c. Vasectomy d. Mini lap

37. Care of the mother during delivery
a. Antenatal care b. Prenatal care
c. Postnatal care d. Intranatal care

38. Currently married couple, where woman is in the reproductive age
a. Potential couple b. High-risk couple
c. Eligible couple d. Able couple

39. Hydrophobia is a typical clinical feature of
a. Plague b. Rabies
c. Malaria d. Anthrax

40. Sexually transmitted diseases are also known as
a. Reproductive disorders b. Sexual disorders
c. Neurosis d. Venereal diseases

41. The test used to find out syphilis
a. Widal test b. ELISA test
c. VDRL test d. Shick test

42. Environmental barrier of communication is
a. Noise b. Deafness
c. Loss of concentration d. Loss of attention

43. The science of health and its preservation
a. Biology b. Nutrition
c. Sociology d. Hygiene

44. An outbreak of disease in a community in excess of normal expectation
a. Endemic b. Epidemic
c. Pandemic d. Sporadic

45. Scurvy is due to deficiency of
a. Vitamin D b. Vitamin K
c. Vitamin C d. Vitamin B complex

46. Supervised, community based Tuberculosis treatment
a. Chemotherapy b. MPO
c. DOTS d. Surveillance

47. World AIDS day
a. April 1st b. May 1st
c. December 1st d. July 1st

48. Oral polio vaccine is
a. Live attenuated vaccine b. Killed vaccine
c. Toxoid d. Combined vaccine

49. Total weight gain during pregnancy
a. 5 kg b. 10 kg
c. 15 kg d. 20 kg

50. Worm that is transmitted through meat
a. Hookworm b. Tapeworm
c. Roundworm d. Pinworm

51. Basic unit of society
a. Individual b. Panchayat
c. Family d. Block

52. The Panchayati Raj Institution at Block level
a. Grama Panchayat b. Zilla Parishad
c. Grama Sabha d. Panchayat Samiti

53. Horny or toad skin is due to the deficiency of
a. Proteins b. Essential fatty acid
c. Carbohydrates d. Essential minerals

54. Chemical substance used for purifying water
a. Lime b. Potassium permanganate
c. Bleaching powder d. Formaldehyde

55. A communicable disease that is eradicated from India
a. Chickenpox b. Rubella
c. Smallpox d. Rabies

56. Tuberculin test is commonly known as
a. Shick test b. Mantoux test
c. VDRL d. ELISA

57. The prime source of all water
a. Sea b. River
c. Rain d. Well

58. Committee on multipurpose worker
a. Mudaliar committee b. Kartar Singh committee
c. Bhore committee d. Shrivastav committee

59. Exchange of air between indoors and outdoors
a. Ventilation b. Air conditioning
c. Air change d. Wind

60. First step in the control of a communicable disease
a. Prevention b. Treatment
c. Notification d. Surveillance

61. Method used for diagnosing community health problem
a. Laboratory test b. Survey
c. Camp d. Health education

62. Total number of multipurpose workers in a subcenter
a. Two b. Four
c. Three d. Five

63. One subcentre is for a population of
a. 3,000 b. 5,000
c. 8,000 d. 10,000

64. The mosquito that transmit Malaria
a. Anopheles b. Culex
c. Aedes d. Mansonia

65. Most sensitive index of the health of a community
a. MMR b. IMR
c. Crude death rate d. Crude birth rate

66. The richest source of vitamin C
a. Milk b. Meat
c. Amla d. Liver

67. The daily requirement of folic acid for an adult is
a. 50 microgram b. 300 microgram
c. 200 microgram d. 100 microgram

68. Nucleus of health services in rural area
a. PHC b. Family
c. CHC d. Anganwadi

69. Backbone of public health nursing
a. Home visit b. Records
c. Health education d. Registers

70. Causative agent of diphtheria
a. Mycobacteria
b. Bordetella
c. Corynebacterium diphtheriae
d. Salmonella

71. Which is a didactic method of health teaching?
a. Symposium b. Workshop
c. Group discussion d. Lecture

72. ICN code of ethics for nurses was adopted in
a. 1948 b. 1973
c. 1978 d. 1958

73. Osteochondral beading is seen in deficiency of
a. Vitamin A b. Vitamin B_6
c. Vitamin C d. Vitamin D

74. Proponent of germ theory of disease
a. Louis Pasteur b. Robert Hook
c. Charles Darwin d. Robert Brown

75. Dose of vitamin A in vitamin A prophylaxis program
a. 1,00,000 IU b. 1,50,000 IU
c. 2,00,000 IU d. 2,50,000 IU

76. Panchayati Raj Institution at Rural level
a. Grama Sabha b. Grama Panchayat
c. Panchayat Samiti d. Zilla Parishad

77. Most sensitive index of the health and level of living of people
a. Crude death rate b. Birth rate
c. Infant mortality rate d. Maternal mortality rate

78. Cause of temporary hardness of water
a. Carbonates b. Sulphates
c. Chlorides d. Calcium

79. Characteristic smile in tetanus patients
a. Opisthotons b. Ataxia
c. Akinesia d. Risus sardonicus

80. Poor man's meat
a. Milk b. Cereals
c. Fish d. Pulses

81. Cracking or ulceration of lips and angles of mouth
a. Halitosis b. Glossitis
c. Stomatitis d. Cheilosis

82. A killed vaccine
a. BCG b. Measles
c. Typhoid d. Yellow fever

83. Anti-pellagra vitamin is
a. Niacin b. Thiamin
c. Pyridoxine d. Riboflavin

84. A live attenuated vaccine
a. Typhoid b. Cholera
c. Rabies d. Oral polio

85. Schick test is used to diagnose
a. Tuberculosis b. Diphtheria
c. Viral hepatitis d. Typhoid fever

86. Spore forming bacteria
a. *M. leprae* b. *V. cholerae*
c. *Cl. tetani* d. *Streptococcus*

87. The most effective room disinfectant is
a. Formalin and potassium permanganate
b. Bleaching powder
c. Ethylene oxide and carbon dioxide
d. Chlorhexidine

88. Which of the following is a protective food?
a. Fish b. Green leafy vegetables
c. Liver d. Egg

89. MiniLap operation is
a. Removal of a small piece of each fallopian tube and ligating each
b. The fallopian tubes are cut and ends are blocked
c. Removal of the fallopian tubes
d. Application of rings to occlude the fallopian tube

90. SARS is spread by
a. Virus b. Bacteria
c. Fungi d. Protozoa

91. An agent that has the power to kill micro-organisms
a. Bacteriocide b. Antiseptic
c. Bacteriostat d. Disinfectant

92. The incubation period of chickenpox is
a. 12–21 days b. 1–7 days
c. 5–10 days d. 3 weeks–1 month

93. Vector of malaria is
a. Female culex mosquito
b. Female anopheles mosquito
c. Male culex mosquito
d. Male anopheles mosquito

94. Megaloblastic anemia is due to the deficiency of
a. Iron b. Thiamine
c. Acetic acid d. Folic acid

95. Dr Salk discovered a vaccine for the prevention of
a. Measles b. Poliomyelitis
c. Smallpox d. Tetanus

96. The disease transferred through contact is called
a. Communicable disease b. Infectious disease
c. Epidemic disease d. Contagious disease

97. The following are examples of live vaccine except
a. Typhoid b. Oral polio
c. BCG d. Measles

98. A substance which suppress or neutralize bad odors is called
a. Deodorant b. Antiseptic
c. Disinfectant d. Antibiotic

99. Poliomyelitis is
a. Bacterial infection b. Viral infection
c. Fungal infection d. Spirochetal infection

100. Rabies is a fatal viral disease of
a. Cardiovascular system b. Muscular system
c. Central nervous system d. Skeletal system

101. A childhood psychiatric disorder characterized by abnormalities in communication and social interaction and by restricted repeated activities and interests
a. Phobia b. Obsession
c. Autism d. Illusion

102. Poisons alkaloid present in tobacco
a. Lead b. Nicotine
c. Alcohol d. Caffeine

103. Test used to detect typhoid
a. Widal test b. Millard's test
c. Kahn test d. Rorschach test

104. Local self government at District level
a. Zilla Parishad b. Grama Sabha
c. Municipality d. Panchayat Samiti

105. Under the ICDS program, there is an anganwadi worker for every
a. 3,000 population b. 1,000 population
c. 10,000 population d. 5,000 population

106. The very effective method of health teaching
a. Symposium b. Group discussion
c. Lecture d. Films and charts

107. Ovulation method of family planning is also known as
a. Calendar methods b. Billing methods
c. Symptothermal methods d. Spacing methods

108. The Government of India re-designated the "National Family Planning Program" as the "National Family Welfare Program" in the year

a. 1977 b. 1953
c. 1975 d. 1969

109. Which committee is known as the Health Survey and Planning Committee

a. Mudaliar Committee b. Kartar Singh Committee
c. Bhore Committee d. Shrivastav Committee

110. An international agency which assists in programs that benefit child health

a. UNO b. WHO
c. UNICEF d. Red Cross

111. Oral thrush is caused by

a. Bacteria b. Fungus
c. Virus d. Protozoa

112. The immunity acquired by suffering from a disease is

a. Natural immunity
b. Passive immunity
c. Active immunity
d Acquired natural immunity

113. Hospital acquired infection is termed as

a. Nosocomial infection b. Droplet infection
c. Auto infection d. Direct infection

114. Multipurpose workers for health and family planning was set up by

a. Bhore Committee
b. Mudaliar Committee
c. Kartar Singh Committee
d. Shrivastav Committee

115. National Filaria Control Program was

a. 1955 b. 1954
c. 1974 d. 1976

116. Occupational disease caused by coal dust is

a. Anthracosis b. Silicosis
c. Asbestosis d. Bagossosis

117. The population of a corporation is

a. 10,000 b. 1 lakh
c. 2 lakhs d. Above 2 lakhs

118. A safe, simple and reliable form of male contraception is

a. Use of condom b. Vasectomy
c. Coitus interrupts d. All the above

119. HIV can be transmitted to the child in the following way

a. Through fomites
b. Through droplet infection
c. Through being born to HIV infected mothers
d. Through food and water

120. The infant mortality rate of Kerala is

a. 70 b. 14
c. 60 d. 20

121. Sepsis means

a. Absence of infection
b. Presence of pathogenic organisms
c. Destroying of all organisms
d. Free from microorganisms

122. The bacillus of diphtheria is found in the

a. Throat b. Nasal passage
c. Upper respiratory tract d. All of these

123. The time interval between the entry of the disease agent into the body and the appearance of the first sign or symptom of the disease is

a. Incubation period b. Transmission
c. Infection d. Epidemic

124. Current net reproduction rate is

a. 1.4 b. 1.8
c. 1.2 d. 1

125. Malaria is a mosquito borne febrile disease caused by

a. Contamination b. Vector
c. Parasite d. Insects

126. The best and useful method of refuse disposal in rural area is

a. Dumping b. Composting
c. Incineration d. Controlled tipping

127. Growth means

a. Increase in size of the whole body
b. Increase in skill
c. Increase in health
d. Increase in abilities

128. Measles is caused by

a. Rotavirus b. Paramyxovirus
c. Astrovirus d. Variolavirus

129. Which one of the following is a noncommunicable disease?

a. Malaria b. Cholera
c. Hypertension d. Viral hepatitis

130. The National Malaria Eradication Program commenced from
a. 1963 b. 1956
c. 1958 d. 1953

131. Sources of vital statistics are
a. National sample surveys
b. Census
c. Report from different institutions
d. All of these

132. Live vaccine used for immunization is
a. BCG b. Cholera
c. Diphtheria d. Tetanus

133. The occurrence of a group of illness of similar nature in excess of natural expectation is
a. Endemic b. Epidemic
c. Pandemic d. None of these

134. World Health Day is on
a. August 10th b. May 12th
c. April 7th d. December 1st

135. The best time for insertion of IUD is
a. 40 days after delivery b. 6 weeks after abortion
c. Intermenstrual period d. All of these

136. Eye disease due to deficiency of vitamin A is
a. Pellagra b. Bitot's spot
c. Angular stomatitis d. Osteomalacia

137. Function of vitamin K is
a. helps in wound healing
b. helps in formation of healthy bones and teeth
c. helps for clotting of blood
d. helps in calcium absorption from the intestine

138. Pulse polio immunization is organized in India during the month
a. November to February b. May to September
c. March to May d. June to September

139. Which one of the following disease is transmitted through water?
a. Typhoid b. Tuberculosis
c. Measles d. Chickenpox

140. Limitation of freedom of movement of well person or domestic animal exposed to communicable disease for a period of time not longer than the longest incubation period of the disease is
a. Notification b. Isolation
c. Quarantine d. All of these

141. Birth should be registered with in
a. 45 days b. 21 days
c. 14 days d. 7 days

142. The cause of maternal mortality
a. Hemorrhage b. Anemia
c. Sepsis d. All of these

143. Which of the following destroys HIV?
a. Dettol b. Savlon
c. Sodium hypochlorite d. Lysol

144. Which of the following is a live vaccine?
a. TT b. DPT
c. BCG d. DT

145. Route of a administration of measles vaccine is
a. Intradermal b. Subcutaneous
c. Intramuscular d. Oral

146. Site of BCG vaccination is
a. Left thigh b. Right thigh
c. Left deltoid d. Right deltoid

147. The most precious and difficult resource to manage is
a. Man b. Money
c. Materials d. Machines

148. The best recommended Body Mass Index for adult is
a. 15–19 b. 20–25
c. 26–30 d. 31–35

149. Which of the following is a waterborne disease?
a. Filariasis b. Poliomyelitis
c. Dengue fever d. Influenza

150. The best method of disposal of hospital waste is
a. Dumping b. Burning
c. Composting d. Incineration

151. Which of the following disease is due to deficiency of calcium?
a. Kwashiorkor b. Marasmus
c. Rickets d. Beriberi

152. Pap Smear Examination is done to diagnose
a. Ca breast b. Ca cervix
c. Ca bladder d. Ca rectum

153. Immunization is a method of
a. Primary prevention b. Secondary prevention
c. Tertiary prevention d. Barrier prevention

154. The simplest method of prevent cross infection is

a. Disinfection b. Sterilization
c. Handwashing d. Fumigation

155. Which of the following is an antiretroviral agent?

a. Acyclovir b. Rifampicin
c. Nevirapine d. Cifran

156. Which of the following is a permanent method of contraception?

a. Oral pills b. Copper T
c. Condom d. Tubectomy

157. Anemia prophylaxis in pregnancy starts at the

a. First month b. Second month
c. Third month d. Fourth month

158. The most frequent side effect associated with the use of IUCD is

a. Ectopic pregnancy b. Expulsion of ICD
c. Rupture of uterus d. Excessive menstrual flow

159. After ovulation has occurred, the ovum remains viable for

a. 1 to 6 hours b. 12 to 24 hours
c. 24 to 36 hours d. 48 to 72 hours

160. Immunity transferred to fetus from the mother through placenta is

a. Active natural immunity
b. Active artificial immunity
c. Passive natural immunity
d. Passive artificial immunity

161. The most appropriate time to collect sputum specimen from a patient is

a. Before meals b. After meals
c. On awakening d. After activity

162. The most important complication of mumps in postpubertal males is

a. Hypopituitarism b. Sterility
c. Decrease in lifido d. Decrease in androgens

163. The nutrients essential to prevent nutritional anemia include proteins, iron, vitamin B12 and

a. Calcium b. Thiamine
c. Folic acid d. Iodine

164. The most important aspect of handwashing is

a. time b. soap
c. water d. friction

165. Peripheral most health care facility is

a. Primary health center b. Subcenter
c. Community health centerd. Taluk hospital

166. Dengue fever is caused by a

a. Bacteria b. Virus
c. Fungus d. Protozoa

167. Mode of transmission of Pertussis

a. Vector transmission b. Through contaminated water
c. Droplet infection d. Feco-oral

168. The following are the standard tuberculosis drug except

a. Chloromycin b. Streptomycin
c. INH d. PAS

169. Time required to measure the Mantoux test

a. 24–48 hours b. 48–72 hours
c. 10–12 hours d. 2–4 hours

170. Combination of Tripple Antigen

a. DPT b. BCG
c. TAB
c. ECG

171. Route of transmission of Hepatitis B

a. Oral b. Parenteral
c. Feco-oral d. Contaminated water

172. Site for Mantoux test

a. Outer and upper quadrant of gluteus maximus
b. Deltoid region
c. Thigh
d. Anterior left forearm

173. Media of transmission of bovine type of tubercle bacilli

a. Milk b. Water
c. Air d. Food

174. Cholera is caused by a kind of bacterium called

a. Tubercle bacillus b. Vibrio cholerae
c. Protozoa d. Entamoeba histolytica

175. Drinking of alcohol will severely effects the

a. Kidney b. Brain
c. Stomach d. Liver

176. A fungal infection

a. Malaria b. Athlets foot
c. Filariasis d. Typhus fever

177. The disease that spread through sexual contact

a. Leprosy b. AIDS
c. Itches d. Scabies

178. A disease caused by bacteria

a. Cold b. Typhoid
c. Typhus fever c. Chickenpox

179. Immunity get by the body after the first attack of disease

a. Natural immunity b. Passive immunity
c. Artificial immunity d. Acquired immunity

180. The cells that are responsible for the production of antibodies

a. Red blood cells b. Platelets
c. Plasma d. White blood cells

181. Number of times a healthy person can donate blood in an year

a. Six or seven b. Five or six
c. Three or four d. Two or three

182. The following are the contents of ORS except

a. Sodium chloride b. Sugar
c. Potassium chloride d. Calcium carbonate

183. The most common form of malnutrition are the following except

a. Beriberi
b. Protein energy malnutrition
c. Marasmus
d. Kwashiorkor

184. The first course of oral pills should be started on the .... day of menstrual cycle

a. 2nd b. 7th
c. 5th d. 10th

185. A permanent method of sterilization

a. MTP b. Diaphragm
c. Tubectomy d. D and C

186. Information given by the sufferer about his illness

a. Sign b. Symptom
c. Observation d. Diagnosis

187. Several persons in a town got the attack of leukemia. A possible reason may be

a. Exposed to radiation b. Drinking polluted water
c. Smoking d. Breathing impure air

188. The energy value is more in

a. Fats b. Starch
c. Protein d. Sugar

189. Amino acid molecules combine together to form

a. Nucleic acid b. Starch
c. Carbohydrate d. Proteins

190. Simple goiter is caused by the deficiency of

a. Sodium b. Iron
c. Iodine d. Calcium

191. Any waste which is generated during the diagnosis, treatment or research in the hospital is called

a. Biomedical waste b. Infected waste
c. Solid waste d. Pharmaceutical waste

192. Waste suspected of containing pathogens

a. Biomedical waste b. Infectious waste
c. Iodine d. Calcium

193. Sharp waste includes the following except

a. Needles b. Blades
c. Broken glasses d. Blood and body fluids

194. Complications of chikungunya include the following except

a. Encephalomyelitis b. Fulminant hepatitis
c. Erosive arthritis d. Carditis

195. CNS manifestation of chikungunya include

a. Photophobia b. Gastritis
c. Joint pain d. Myalgia

196. Incubation period of chikungunya

a. 2–3 days b. 2–3 weeeks
c. 10–15 days d. 10–20 days

197. Chikungunya is caused by

a. Arbovirus b. Aedes aegypti
c. Culex d. Anopheles

198. Inanimate objects that can transmit the disease

a. Droplet b. Dust
c. Fomites d. Reservoir

199. Drugs which cross the placental barrier

a. Bioactive drugs b. Teratogenic drugs
c. Genotoxic drugs d. None of these

200. A direct mode of transmission

a. Droplet infection b. Fomite borne infection
c. Vector borne infection d. Vehicle borne infection

201. Indirect mode of transmission includes the following except
a. Droplet infection b. Fomite borne infection
c. Vector borne infection d. Vehicle borne infection

202. First case of a common disease in a population
a. Index case b. Primary case
c. Secondary case d. Carrier

203. First case comes to the attention of the investigator
a. Index case b. Primary case
c. Secondary case d. Carrier

204. The natural habitat in which the infectious agent replicates
a. Agent b. Host
c. Source d. Reservoir

205. Person or animal or object from which the infectious agent is transmitted
a. Agent b. Host
c. Source d. Reservoir

206. Eradication of disease from a particular geographic region
a. Elimination b. Transmission
c. Surveillance d. Infestation

207. Physician induced infection
a. Opportunistic infection b. Nosocomial infection
c. Iatrogenic infection d. Indirect infection

208. Infection occurs when there is a defect in the defense of the host
a. Opportunistic infection b. Nosocomial infection
c. Iatrogenic infection d. Indirect infection

209. Infection occurring in a patient while in a hospital or health care agency
a. Opportunistic infection b. Nosocomial infection
c. Iatrogenic infection d. Indirect infection

210. Infection transmitted to man from vertebrate animals
a. Anthrapozoonosis b. Zooanthroponosis
c. Zoonosis d. Anthracosis

211. Infection transmitted to vertebrate animals from man
a. Anthrapozoonosis b. Zooanthroponosis
c. Zoonosis d. Anthracosis

212. Diseases imported into a country in which they do not occur otherwise
a. Endemic b. Exotic
c. Epidemic d. Pandemic

213. Epidemic affecting a large population
a. Endemic b. Exotic
c. Pandemic d. Outbreak

214. Cases widely separated and few and has no connection with each other
a. Endemic b. Exotic
c. Sporadic d. Pandemic

215. The extreme limit of noise tolerance is
a. 85 dB b. 100 dB
c. 120 dB d. 140 dB

216. Constant presence of a disease within a geographic area
a. Endemic b. Exotic
c. Pandemic d. Outbreak

217. Presence of offensive but not infectious matter in the atmosphere
a. Fomite b. Infection
c. Pollution d. Droplet

218. Illness due to specific infectious agent being transmitted directly or indirectly to man or animal
a. Infection b. Communicable disease
c. Endemic d. Epidemic

219. Man, animal or birds that permits lodgment to an infectious agent during natural condition
a. Agent b. Environment
c. Host d. Vector

220. Body's natural response to infection
a. Pyrexia b. Inflammation
c. Cachexia d. Weakness

221. Presence of infectious agent on a surface
a. Inflammation b. Fomite
c. Vector d. Contamination

222. Permanent male sterilization
a. Tubectomy b. Laparoscopy
c. NSV d. Vas deferens

223. In the normal 28 day menstrual cycle, ovulation usually occurs between
a. 10–18 days b. 15–25 days
c. 20–28 days d. 1–5 days

224. A natural family planning method
a. IUCD b. Condom
c. Tubectomy d. Cervical mucus method

225. Calendar method is otherwise known as
a. Abstinence b. Sympto-thermic method
c. Safe period method d. Withdrawal method

226. Withdrawal of penis from the vagina just before ejaculation
a. Abstinence b. Coitus interruptus
c. Mechanical method d. Rhythm method

227. The method of birth control in which sex urge is repressed
a. Abstinence b. Coitus interruptus
c. Mechanical method d. Rhythm method

228. MTP act permits abortion only up to
a. 20 weeks b. 24 weeks
c. 28 weeks d. 30 weeks

229. Legalization of abortion is made by
a. Family welfare program
b. UNFPA
c. MTP act
d. None of the above

230. Aspiration of uterine contents 6–14 days of a missed period
a. Abortion b. Hysterectomy
c. Hysterotomy d. Menstrual regulation

231. An injectable contraceptive
a. Mala-D b. NET-EN
c. Mala-L d. Cu-T

232. Male pill
a. Quinestrol b. Gossypol
c. Norethisterone d. NET-EN

233. The contraindication for IUD insertion
a. Pyrexia b. Irregular periods
c. Nullipara d. Multipara

234. III generation IUDs are
a. Copper impregnated b. Hormonal
c. Temporary d. Nylon

235. The cheap metal which is having strong anti- fertility effect
a. Iron b. Copper
c. Silver d. Gold

236. The tail of IUD are made of
a. Nylon b. Copper
c. Silicone d. Silastic

237. The most widely used barrier method
a. Copper-T b. Mala-D
c. Mala-N d. Condom

238. National Family Planning Program was renamed as National Family Welfare Program in the year
a. 1975 b. 1976
c. 1977 d. 1978

239. The indication of prevalence of contraceptive practices in the country
a. Eligible couple register b. NRR
c. Couple protection rate d. NPP

240. The basic document for family planning is
a. Eligible Couple register b. NRR
c. Couple protection rate d. NPP

241. Two child norm was introduced in the year
a. 1977 b. 1980
c. 1988 d. 1995

242. WHO was established in the year
a. 7th April 1948 b. 7th April 1946
c. 7th April 1956 d. 7th April 1950

243. Indian Red Cross Society was established in the year
a. 1910 b. 1915
c. 1920 d. 1922

244. RCH phase II was launched on
a. 2000 b. 2001
c. 2003 d. 2005

245. ESI Act was launched in the year
a. 1950 b. 1948
c. 1946 d. 1956

246. Community Development Program was launched in the year
a. 1950 b. 1952
c. 1954 d. 1962

247. Factory act was launched on
a. 1950 b. 1948
c. 1946 d. 1956

248. Chairman of ESI Corporation

a. Union minister for labor
b. State minister for labor
c. Union minister for health
d. State minister for health

249. Very effective method of communication

a. Seminar b. Symposium
c. Group discussion d. Lecture

250. Waste water from a community which does not contain human excreta

a. Sewage b. Contaminated water
c. Infected water d. Sullage

251. The first step in water purification

a. Sedimentation b. Filtration
c. Storage d. Chlorination

ANSWER KEY

1. b	2. a	3. a	4. c	5. d	6. a	7. b	8. c	9. a	10. c	11. b	12. a
13. d	14. d	15. a	16. c	17. d	18. c	19. d	20. c	21. c	22. c	23. a	24. a
25. b	26. b	27. b	28. d	29. b	30. a	31. b	32. c	33. d	34. b	35. b	36. c
37. d	38. c	39. b	40. d	41. c	42. a	43. d	44. b	45. c	46. c	47. c	48. a
49. b	50. b	51. c	52. d	53. b	54. c	55. c	56. b	57. b	58. b	59. a	60. d
61. b	62. a	63. b	64. a	65. b	66. c	67. d	68. a	69. a	70. c	71. d	72. b
73. d	74. a	75. c	76. b	77. c	78. a	79. d	80. d	81. d	82. c	83. a	84. d
85. b	86. c	87. a	88. b	89. b	90. a	91. a	92. a	93. b	94. d	95. b	96. d
97. a	98. a	99. b	100. c	101. c	102. b	103. a	104. d	105. b	106. d	107. c	108. a
109. a	110. c	111. b	112. d	113. a	114. c	115. a	116. a	117. d	118. a	119. c	120. b
121. b	122. d	123. a	124. d	125. c	126. b	127. a	128. b	129. c	130. c	131. d	132. a
133. b	134. c	135. d	136. b	137. c	138. a	139. a	140. c	141. b	142. d	143. c	144. c
145. b	146. c	147. a	148. b	149. b	150. d	151. c	152. b	153. a	154. c	155. c	156. d
157. d	158. d	159. b	160. c	161. c	162. b	163. c	164. d	165. a	166. b	167. c	168. a
169. b	170. a	171. b	172. d	173. a	174. b	175. d	176. b	177. b	178. b	179. d	180. d
181. c	182. d	183. a	184. c	185. c	186. b	187. a	188. a	189. d	190. c	191. a	192. b
193. d	194. d	195. a	196. a	197. b	198. c	199. b	200. a	201. a	202. b	203. a	204. d
205. c	206. a	207. c	208. a	209. b	210. a	211. b	212. b	213. c	214. c	215. d	216. a
217. c	218. b	219. c	220. b	221. d	222. c	223. a	224. d	225. c	226. b	227. a	228. a
229. c	230. d	231. b	232. b	233. c	234. b	235. b	236. a	237. d	238. c	239. c	240. a
241. b	242. a	243. c	244. d	245. b	246. b	247. b	248. c	249. c	250. d	251. c	

Chapter 6

Maternity Nursing

PUBERTY

A period during which the organs of reproduction mature and are prepare for their reproductive function.

Physical and Physiological Changes in Puberty

A. Physical Changes

In males

- Occur between 10 to 14 years of age; less dramatic in female.
- Heralded by deepening of the voice and growth of body hair on the face, axilla and genitalia.
- One year after onset, increased activity of the sweat glands and spermatogenesis occurs with periodic erections and emissions of mature sperm.
- Body growth spurt occurs.
- Ejaculation is the beginning of fertility and end of puberty.

In females

- Occurs between 9 and 13 years of age.
- Sudden enlargement of the breasts, growth of body hair on the axilla and genitalia, changes in size and vascularity of internal genital organs.
- Heralded by first menstrual flow called menarche, unlike the male's first ejaculation, many first menstrual cycles are anovulatory.

> Beginning of menstrual flow is called menarche. Many first menstrual cycles may be anovulatory.

B. Psychological Changes

- Age differs in maturation.
- Heterosexual interests: Girls earlier than boys, girls interested in older boys.
- Quarrels with parents.
- Desire for independence and desire for belonging for a peer group.

C. Menstrual Cycle

- Rhythmic reproductive cycle in females extending from the onset of a period of uterine bleeding to the onset of next period of bleeding; mean cycle length is 28 days, normal range is 20 to 45 days per cycle.
- During each cycle, about 20 follicles commence maturation, but usually only one reaches full maturity and rupture the contained ovum into the peritoneum (ovulation).
- The menstrual cycle is divided into three stages.

> The menstrual cycle has three stages viz. Menstruation, Follicular or Proliferative phase and Luteal or Secretory phase.

MENSTRUATION

It lasts 4 to 6 days, characterized by endometrial hemorrhage with the discharge through the vagina, estrogen and progesterone levels are low, the Follicle Stimulating Hormone (FSH) level is high and Luteinizing Hormone (LH) is low.

Follicular or Proliferative Phase

It lasts 8 to 10 days and ends in ovulation, endometrium repairs and proliferates in preparation for possible implantation and a single ovarian follicle approaches full maturation as the concentration of estrogen in the blood rises, estrogen exerts a negative feedback effect on FSH secretion and a positive feedback on LH secretion. LH induces ovulation.

Luteal or Secretory Phase

It beigns with ovulation and lasts for 9 to 13 days. LH promotes formation of corpus luteum from the ruptured follicle. If fertilization does not occur, the corpus luteum functions for 7 to 8 days after ovulation, and then involutes and becomes corpus albicans 7 to 12 days after ovulation. Progesterone and estrogen levels drop, the negative feedback effect of estrogen on FSH is released and the first stage begins again.

DEVELOPMENT OF THE EMBRYO

A. Formation of Gametes

- The ovum and spermatozoon each have one set of 23 chromosomes.

> The ovum and spermatozoon each have one set of 23 chromosomes and a special type of cell division called meiosis is occurring in them.

- The production of ova and spermatozoa requires a special type of cell division which occurs only in reproductive cells viz. meiosis in which the chromosome number is reduced from 2 sets (46 chromosomes) to one set (23 chromosomes).

B. Fertilization

- Spermatozoa are deposited in the vagina during sexual intercourse.
- Fertilization usually occurs in the ampulla of the fallopian tubes when the ovum is about one third of the way down the tube, usually this occurs about 24 hours after ovulation.
- The sperm must be in the genital tract 4 to 6 hours before they are able to fertilize an ovum, during this period 'capacitation' occurs and the ovum is penetrated by the sperm.
- Sperm enters the cytoplasm of the ovum a fertilization membrane is formed around the ovum to prevent entry of other sperms. Sperm tail is lost and male nucleus unites with the female nucleus and thus the chromosome number is restored in the resultant zygote (46 chromosomes).

> Fertilization usually occurs in the ampulla of the uterine tubes (fallopian tubes).

C. Cleavage

- In a short time after fertilization, the zygote undergoes rapid division to produce a mass of cells (morula) that descends in the uterine tube. As it descends, it also divides to form a hollow ball called blastocyst.

D. Implantation

- The blastocyst then implants into the uterine wall and differentiate into an inner cell mass and blastocele. Implantation occurs 7 to 8 days after fertilization, generally in the upper fundal portion.

E. Embryonic Period

- The zygote in the first two months is termed as embryo; after this period is called a fetus.
- About 12th day after fertilization a fetal membrane called amnion forms around the embryo. Amnion is fluid filled (amniotic fluid) and serves as a fetal shock absorber. A chorion also surrounds the embryo; this will eventually form the major part of the placenta. Finger like projections of the chorion called chorionic villi grow into the endometrium.

PLACENTA

Placenta is an organ of dual origin (maternal and embryonic portions) and helps for interchange of food and waste products between the mother and the fetus during pregnancy.

Placenta is formed from villous portion of chorion (chorionic frontosum) and the portion of the uterine endometrium (decidua basalis). Placenta functions as the fetal digestive tract and also fetal lungs, kidneys and as a major endocrine gland producing estrogen, progesterone, ACTH, growth hormone, gonadotropic hormones, human chorionic gonadotropin (HCG) and Human placental lactogen (HPL). It also serves as a protective barrier against harmful effects of some drugs and microorganism.

> Placenta is developed from chorionic frontosum and decidua basalis.

UMBILICAL CORD

It is inserted close to the central portion of the placenta and attached to the fetus. It has two arteries and one vein. Wharton's jelly, a protective covering, surrounds the entire cord.

FETAL CIRCULATION

Contains mixed blood.

- Ductus venosus is a connection between umbilical vein and inferior vena cava, bypassing the fetal liver.
- Ductus arteriosus is a connection between pulmonary artery and aorta during fetal life which bypasses the fetal lungs.
- Foramen ovale is an opening between the right and left atria during fetal life bypassing the fetal lungs.

PHYSICAL AND PHYSIOLOGICAL CHANGES IN THE MOTHER DURING PREGNANCY

Pregnancy is a normal physiological process that affects all body systems and results in both objective and subjective changes.

A. Endocrine Changes

- During pregnancy the placenta secretes HCG.
- The presence of HCG is an indicator of pregnancy; HCG reaches a peak in the third month and then drops.

- Estrogen and progesterone increases and continue to be secreted from the placenta during the last six months of pregnancy, progesterone inhibits uterine contraction.
- Thyroid activity is increased.
- Chorionic somatomammotrophin is increased, a diabetogenic hormone which decreases maternal use of glucose, leaving it available for fetal use.
- Serum estriol level increases, used as an indicator of fetal well-being.
- In the last month the uterine contents shift downward, so that the fetus is in contact with the cervix, this contact may induce oxytocin release from the posterior pituitary. Oxytocin stimulates uterine contractions, coupled with the drop in progesterone brings about labor, uterine contractions increase in intensity and frequency culminating in fetal expulsion or birth of the baby.

Serum estriol level during pregnancy may be used as an indicator of fetal well-being.

B. Reproductive Organ Changes

- Amenorrhea occurs, due to the inhibition of ovulation by the high level of circulating estrogen and progesterone.
- Breast changes such as fullness, tingling, soreness, darkening of the areola and nipples occur along with an increase in the hormone levels.
- Leukorrhea is increased as the hormone levels rise, and the increased activity is a protection from bacterial invasion.
- Softening of cervix—Goodell's sign.
- Softening of the lower uterine segment—Hegar's sign.
- Bluish discoloration of the vagina due to increased vascularity—Jacquimere's sign.
- Bluish discoloration of the cervix due to increased vascularity—Chadwick's sign.
- Uterus enlarges in size; in first trimester, uterus is in pelvic cavity, in second and third trimester it is in the abdominal cavity.

Pregnancy signs

Goodell's sign: Softening of cervix

Hegar's sign: Softening of the lower uterine segment

Jacquemier's sign: Bluish discoloration of the vagina due to increased vascularity

Chadwick's sign: Bluish discoloration of the cervix due to increased vascularity

Osiander's sign: Pulsations felt by the mother in the pelvic region due to increased vascularity.

C. Gastrointestinal System Changes

- Reduction in hydrochloric acid secretion interferes with gastric motility, causing nausea and vomiting (morning sickness) and pyrosis (heartburn).
- Elevated estrogen levels cause excessive salivation.
- Hyperemia and softening of the gums with accompanying hyperacidity of oral secretions results in gingivitis and gingival bleeds.
- Decreased emptying time of the gallbladder may precipitate development of gallstones.
- Food cravings may occur (pica).
- Hypoperistalsis leads to constipation.
- Pressure of enlarged uterus predispose to hemorrhoids in vulva and rectum.

D. Excretory

- Pressure of uterus on bladder in early and late pregnancy causes urinary frequency.
- Bladder tone is reduced due to the effect of hormones on the smooth muscles.
- Increased urinary output results in lowered specific gravity.
- Increased excretion of sugar caused by lowered renal threshold.
- Pressure of enlarging uterus causes dilatation of right ureter and kidney.

E. Circulatory System Changes

- Physiologic anemia occurs as a result of increased blood volume with no proportional increase in the RBC.
- Cardiac output increases 25–50% peaking at 7 to 8 months.
- Heart rate increases 10 beats/minute in the later half of pregnancy.
- Palpitation occurs in early months from sympathetic stimulation and in later months from increased thoracic pressure because of enlarged uterus.
- BP may drop slightly in second trimester.
- Supine Hypotension Syndrome: In supine position, weight of the enlarged uterus obstructs vena cava, which decreases blood return to the heart, decreased cardiac output ends up with hypotension, light headedness, faintness and palpitations.
- WBC, fibrinogen and other clotting factors increase.
- Varicose veins of the legs, vulva and perineal area may occur.
- Edema of the extremities common in the last six weeks of pregnancy because of stasis of blood.

Increased plasma volume with no proportional increase in RBC predispose to physiologic anemia during pregnancy.

Taking rest in the side lying position especially left lateral position release the weight of the gravid uterus on the inferior vena cava and improves blood return to the heart.

F. Respiratory System Changes

- Pressure of the enlarged uterus on the diaphragm and lungs may cause dyspnea around 36 to 38 weeks that subsides when lightening occurs.
- Oxygen consumption is increased by about 15 percent between the 16th and 40th weeks.
- Hyperventilation occurs to expel increased carbon dioxide transferred from the fetus.
- Nasal congestion occurs as a response to increased estrogen levels.

G. Integumentary System Changes

- Excretion of the waste through the skin causes diaphoresis.
- Skin changes: Darkening of the areola and the nipples, darkened patches on the face (chloasma), *linea nigra* on the abdomen, striae gravidarum present on the abdomen and legs due to skin stretching.

H. Skeletal System Changes

- Softening of all ligaments and joints especially symphysis pubis and sacroiliac joint, caused by increased hormonal action of estrogens and relaxin.
- Leg cramps may occur from the imbalance of calcium/ phosphorus ratio in the body and from the pressure of the gravid uterus on nerve supplying the lower extrimities.

I. Emotional Changes

- Acceptance of pregnancy, happens during first trimester.
- Acceptance of growing fetus as distinct from self occurs during second trimester.
- Preparation for birth usually occurs in third trimester.
- Ambivalence, mood swings, changes in sexual desire and anxiety about delivery occurs.

J. Confirmation of Pregnancy (Signs of Pregnancy)

1. **Presumptive signs: Mostly subjective, may be indicative of other illnesses**
   - Amenorrhea
   - Fatigue
   - Nausea and vomiting
   - Breast changes
   - Urinary frequency
   - Darkening or pigmentation on the face, breasts and stomach.
   - Quickening: First fetal movement felt by the mother.

Quickening usually occurs between 16–20 weeks of pregnancy.

2. **Probable signs:** Objective but still not definitive confirmations of pregnancy:
   - Uterine changes: Chadwick's sign, Hegar's sign, Goodell's sign, enlargement of the uterus and Jacquemier's sign
   - Fetal outline
   - Pregnancy tests: Presence of HCG in blood and urine of the mother
   - Ballottement
   - Braxton Hicks contractions.
3. **Positive signs:** Confirmatory signs of pregnancy
   - Fetal heart beats
   - Fetal outline and fetal movement as felt by examiner
   - USG
   - X-ray visualization of fetal skeleton

Expected Date of Confinement (EDD)
Naegele's rule—first day of the last menstrual period (LMP) + 9 months and 7 days.

K. Nutritional Needs During Pregnancy

- If nausea and vomiting: Limit fluids with meals, small frequent feeds, restricted fat, high carbohydrate feeds.

Solid foods and crackers are better tolerated than fluids if the patient has morning sickness.

- Constipation: Increase fluid, residue and fiber.
- Increased calories to meet increased metabolic needs (300 calories extra to the pre-pregnant state).
- Increased proteins to provide for growth demands (1.5 gm/ kg).
- Increased vitamins and minerals especially iron and folic acid supplementation.

A pregnant mother need 300 calories extra than the pre-pregnant state.

L. Medical Supervision During Pregnancy

- First medical check up: On missing periods
- History, physical examination and pelvic examination
- Height, weight, BP
- Blood and urine examination

Blood: Grouping, Rh typing, RBS, VDRL, HIV, HBsAg
Urine: Sugar, albumin

- Screening tests: AFP testing for neural tube defects
- Ultrasonography
- Immunization: Injection TT two doses at one month interval.

LABOR

Labor is a physiologic and mechanical process in which the baby, placenta and fetal membranes are propelled through the pelvis and expelled from the birth canal.

Bony Pelvis

- Comprises ilium, ischium, pubis, sacrum and coccyx.
- Joints are: Sacroiliac, sacrococcygeal and symphysis pubis.
- Divisions: False pelvis supports the enlarged uterus in abdominal cavity and true pelvis is the bony inner pelvis through which the baby must pass.
- Normal female pelvis (gynecoid pelvis) has an ample pubic arch, curved sacrum, curved sidewalls, blunt ischial spines and a movable coccyx.

CLINICAL FINDINGS PRIOR TO LABOR

1. **Physiologic**
    - Lightening: Fetus drops down into the true pelvis
    - Braxton Hick's contractions: Painless contractions in preparation for true labor, becomes more regular and frequent.
    - Increased vaginal secretions
    - Softening of the cervix and effacement (taking up of cervix)
    - Rupture of Membrane (ROM)
    - Bloody show—softening and effacement of the cervix causes mucus plug to be expelled, this is accompanied by small blood loss.
2. **Psychologic:** Mother shows signs of nesting (increased activity) caused by sudden rise in energy level.

CLINICAL FINDINGS OF TRUE LABOR

- Uterine contractions that increase in frequency, strength and duration and do not disappear when lying down or walking around.
- Effacement and progressive dilatation of the cervix.

Cervical effacement is recorded in percentage, i.e. 1/4th effaced (25%), 1/2 effaced (50%) and 3/4th effaced (75%).

Cervical dilatation is charted in centimeters (cm) and the maximum cervical dilatation is 10 cm.

MECHANISM OF LABOR

Rotation of vertex presentation through the true pelvis follows the following series of movements:

1. **Engagement, descent with flexion:** At onset of labor, head descends and chin flexes on the chest.
2. **Internal rotation:** As labor contractions and uterine forces move the fetus downward, the head internally rotates to pass through the ischial spines.
3. **Extension:** Occiput emerges under the symphysis pubis and the head is delivered by extension.
4. **External rotation of head:** Allows for internal rotation of the shoulders to an anteroposterior position.
5. **Expulsion:** The body is delivered by lateral flexion and the infant is born.

STAGES OF LABOR AND MATERNAL CHANGES

1. **First Stage:** From the onset of true labor pain to complete dilatation of the cervix; consists of latent phase, active phase and transition phase.
    a. ***Latent Phase:*** Mild, short contractions, cervix dilated upto 3 cm, mother excited and happy, some apprehension present.
    b. ***Active Phase:*** Moderate to strong contractions, five minutes apart, cervix 4 to 7 cm dilated, bloody show, membranes may rupture, breathing techniques help in relaxation, medications may be necessary for discomfort and mother has difficulty in following directions.
    c. ***Transition Phase:*** Strong contractions, 1 to 2 minutes apart, lasting 45 to 60 seconds with little gap in between, cervix 7 to 10 cm dilated, bloody show, mother becomes irritable, restless, agitated, highly emotional, belches, has leg tremors, perspires, pale, white ring around mouth (circumoral pallor), flushed face, feels need to have bowel movement because of pressure on the anus, unable to communicate or follow directions.

2. **Second Stage:** Beginning from full dilatation of the cervix and ending with birth of the infant, perineum bulges, mother pushing with contractions, grunting sounds present, behavior changes from great irritability to great involvement and leg cramps are common.
3. **Third Stage:** Following birth of the infant through expulsion of the placenta; placental separation starts 5 to 30 minutes, signs of placental separation are globular formation of uterus, lengthening of the umbilical cord and a sudden gush of fresh blood.
4. **Fourth Stage:** Following expulsion of placenta to 3–4 hours after delivery, fundus firm in the midline and at or slightly above the umbilicus, scant, bloody, vaginal discharge (Lochia Rubra), fatigue, thirst, chills, nausea, excitement and intermittent dozing.

OXYTOCICS

- Drugs that stimulate the uterus to contract.
- Used in the pregnant lady to initiate and accelerate labor, also capable of inducing contractions of the lacteal glands which aid in let down reflex for breast feeding, exert vasopressor and antidiuretic effect, used to control postpartum atony.
- Available as parenteral (IV, IM) and nasal preparations.
- For example, ergometrine, methylergometrine (methergine) and oxytocin (pitocin).
- **Major side effects**
  - Maternal: Hypertension, tachycardia, uterine tetany, water intoxication (antidiuretic effect), convulsions and coma due to water intoxication.
  - Fetal: Anoxia, asphyxia, premature ventricular contractions, bradycardia, hyperbilirubinemia.

MATERNAL ANALGESIA AND ANESTHESIA DURING LABOR

- Analgesia: Pethidine and morphine are used in active labor, may be given IM or IV; predisposes to respiratory distress in the fetus.
- Regional analgesia and anesthesia: Epidural, spinal and pudental blocks; local infiltration is most commonly used. Monitor mother for hypotension and urinary retention after epidural analgesia.

> Hypotension and urinary retention are the common side effects of epidural analgesia.

POSTPARTUM PERIOD

A. Puerperium

- Six week period following delivery in which the reproductive organs undergo physical and physiological changes (involution).
- Because of the many physiological and psychological stresses of the postpartum period, there is a trend to increase this period to three months following delivery and so called the fourth trimester of pregnancy.

B. Systemic changes during the puerperium

1. **Reproductive System**
   - Uterus: Intermittent contractions bring about involution, after pains may cause discomfort necessitating analgesics; occytocin release during breast feeding speeds up involution.
   - Lochia: Vaginal flow following delivery changes from lochia rubra to lochia serosa, then becomes lochia alba.
   - Vagina: Vagina returns to its pre-pregnant state through a healing of soft tissue.
   - Menstruation: Occurs about six weeks after delivery in non-nursing mothers and upto 24 weeks in fully nursing mothers.
   - Abdominal wall: Soft and flabby, but eventually regains tone.
   - Breasts
     - As placenta is delivered, there is activation of LH in the anterior pituitary, secretion of prolactin also stimulates milk production.
     - Posterior pituitary secretes oxytocin, which initiates the let down reflex with milk ejection as the baby suckles.
     - Breast engorgement occurs on the 2nd or 3rd day because of vasodilatation before lactation.
2. **Digestive System**
   - Added proteins and calories needed in the postnatal period (pregnancy + 200 kcal).
   - Increased amounts of fluids are needed.
   - Roughage and fluids along with exercise relieve constipation and abdominal distention.

> A mother during lactation requires 200 kcal extra to the pregnancy state, i.e. 500 kcal extra to the pre-pregnant state.

3. **Circulatory System**
   - Blood volume back to normal by 3rd week after delivery

- Blood fibrinogen levels increase during the first week
- WBC increases, may go as high as 30,000 cells/mm^3
- Hb and RBC drops on the 4th postpartum day.

4. **Excretory System**
   - Increased urinary output, second to fifth postpartum day.
   - Retention with overflow may occur since bladder tone is lost during pregnancy.
5. **Integumentary System**
   - Profuse diaphoresis occurs as wastes are being excreted.
6. **Vital Signs**
   - Temperature elevation upto 24 hours after delivery as a result of excretion and dehydration.
   - BP returns to baseline; drop suggests hemorrhage, elevation suggests PIH.
   - Pulse drops slightly due to decreased cardiac efforts.
   - Postpartal chills may be due to vasomotor changes.

THE NEWBORN

Adaptation to Extrauterine Life

A. Immediate needs at the time of delivery

- Aspiration of mucus to provide an open airway.
- Evaluation by use of APGAR score at 1 minute and 5 minutes following birth.
- Maintenance of body temperature.
- Constant observation of physical condition.
- Eye care and cord care.

B. Changes in the newborn during the first week of life

1. **Circulatory**
   - Tying of cord at birth brings changes in fetal circulation. Closure of the foramen ovale and ductus arteriosus and obliteration of the umbilical arteries produce an adult like circulation within one hour after birth.
   - Heart Rate regular, 120 to 160 beats/minute, but variable depending upon the infant's activity, soft heart murmur common for first month of life.
   - Clotting mechanisms poor because of low prothrombin concentration; injection vitamin K is necessary.
   - Liver immature, cannot destroy excessive RBC in the newborn, resulting in physiologic jaundice by about 3rd day.
   - Hb level high: 14 to 20 gm/100 mL of blood.
   - WBC count high: 6000 to 22000 cells/mm^3
2. **Respiratory:** Respirations diaphragmatic, irregular, abdominal, 30 to 50 per minute, quiet with periods of apnea.
3. **Excretory**
   - Kidneys immature, newborn should void during first 24 hours, albumin and urates (brick red staining on diaper) are common during first week because of dehydration.
   - Stools: First stool, black green and tenacious called meconium, by third day, becomes mixed with light yellow called transitional stool.
4. **Integumentary**
   - Lanugo: Fine, downy hair growth over the entire body.
   - Milia: Small, whitish, pinpoint spots over the nose caused by retained sebaceous secretions.
   - Mongolian spots: Blue-black discolorations on back, buttocks and sacral region that disappear by first year.
5. **Digestive**
   - Has a store of nutrients from intrauterine life.
   - Roots and sucks when anything is brought to the mouth.
   - Digests simple carbohydrates, fats and proteins readily.
   - Cardiac sphincter of stomach not well developed, therefore regurgitates if stomach is overfull.
   - Needs to be burped frequently to get rid of the air in the stomach.
6. **Endocrine**
   - Metabolic: All newborns normally lose 10 percent of their body weight by first week of life.

> All newborns normally lose 10 percent of their body weight by first week of life and regains birth weight by 10th day.

   - Hormonal: Enlarged breast in boys (gynecomastia) and girls is normal as a result of hormones transmitted to baby by the mother. Pseudomenstruation in girls also occurs due to hormonal effect.
7. **Neurological**
   - CNS and brain not well developed; infant needs constant supply of oxygen.
   - Breathing, sucking and crying are early neural activities necessary for infant's survival.
8. **Sleep**
   - Because sleep lowers body metabolism, it helps restore energy and assimilates nutrients for growth.

C. Nutrition

- Initial weight loss of 10 percent birth weight is normal and usually regained by 10th day of life.
- Nutritional needs are met by exclusive breast feeding.
- Breast feeding provides immunity, assists in involution of the uterus, less likely for allergic to mother's milk, and provides maternal antibodies through colostrum.
- Infant's suckling at the breast stimulates the maternal posterior pituitary to produce oxytocin which causes the let down of milk and also stimulates prolactin secretion.

> Breast feeding provides immunity, assists in involution of the uterus, less likely for allergic to mother's milk, and provides maternal antibodies through colostrum.

PREGNANCY-INDUCED HYPERTENSION (PIH), PRE-ECLAMPSIA AND ECLAMPSIA

1. **Pregnancy-induced Hypertension (PIH):** Sustained elevation of BP more than 140/90 mm of Hg in two occasions at least six hours apart, occurring after the 20th week of pregnancy.
2. **Pre-eclampsia:** Characterized by a triad of symptoms-edema, hypertension and proteinuria, occurs usually after the 20th week and disappears six weeks after delivery.
3. **Eclampsia:** Convulsions and/or coma associated with hypertension/proteinuria and edema.
4. **Blood parameters:** Rise in PCV, uric acid and BUN and decrease on CO_2 combining power indicates worsening of pre-eclampsia. Increase in urine albumin and/or decreased urinary output also indicates worsening of pre-eclampsia.
5. **Guidelines for prevention**
   - Sound nutrition counseling during pregnancy, labor and lactation.
   - Restriction of sodium is harmful during pregnancy; additional salt other than usual should be avoided.
   - Diuretics are usually contraindicated during pregnancy because they cause hypovolemia and deplete essential nutrients for mother and the fetus.

> Diuretics are usually contraindicated during pregnancy because they cause hypovolemia and deplete essential nutrients for mother and the fetus.

6. **Treatment of Pre-eclampsia**
   - High protein diet
   - Additional visits than routine
   - Frequent rest with foot elevated
   - Adhere to the therapeutic regimen.

> Alarming symptoms of pre-eclampsia include headache, disturbed sleep, diminished urinary output, epigastric pain and eye symptoms.

7. **Severe Pre-eclampsia or Eclampsia**
   - Hospitalization and complete bed rest.
   - Magnesium sulfate therapy.
   - Sedatives to ensure rest and sleep. Injection morphine is usually given.
   - Monitor intake and output.
   - Induce labor/LSCS if symptoms are under control.
   - Assess/monitor magnesium toxicity, reduced patellar reflexes, depressed respiration, urine output less than 30 mL/hour.
   - Monitor for HELLP syndrome (Hemolysis, Elevate Liver enzymes, Low Platelets) which is a complication of pIH.

> Reduced patellar reflexes, depressed respiration, urine output less than 30 mL/hour are the signs of magnesium toxicity.

BLEEDING DURING THE FIRST TRIMESTER

Abortion

Interruption of pregnancy in which there is complete/ partial expulsion of the products of conception.

Types

- **Threatened abortion:** Cervix closed, but bleeding, cramping and backache present.
- **Inevitable abortion:** Abortion has progressed to a state in which reversal is not possible, bleeding and cramping become more severe, cervix dilates and products of conception are expelled.
- **Complete abortion:** All products are expelled and cervix closed, bleeding minimal.
- **Incomplete abortion:** All the products of conception are not fully expelled.
- **Missed abortion:** Fetus dies in uterus, but not expelled, client must be monitored for disseminated intravascular coagulation (DIC).
- **Treatment**
  1. Complete bed rest.
  2. Assess vital signs.
  3. Blood—TC, grouping, Rh factor, cross matching.
  4. Alleviate fear and anxiety.
  5. Monitor for bleeding; assess BP and monitor for shock.
  6. Maintain fluid and electrolyte balance.

7. Dilatation and curettage or vaccum aspiration if products are not fully expelled.
8. Anti-D to Rh negative mother after abortion/ evacuation.

Ectopic Pregnancy

- Pregnancy in which implantation occurs outside the uterus.
- Most frequent site is fallopian tube, others being cervix, ovaries and abdomen.
- Early signs and symptoms are usually concealed.
- Spotting may occur after missed periods, sharp right or left lower abdominal pain radiating to shoulder, concealed bleeding from site of rupture leads to sudden shock.
- Diagnosis is confirmed by USG or culdocentesis.
- Surgical repair or removal of the ruptured tube is undertaken.

Vesicular Mole or Hydatidiform Mole

- An abnormal pregnancy in which there is a benign growth of the chorion.
- Spontaneous expulsion occurs between the 16th and 18th week of pregnancy.
- **Findings:** Uterus is unduly enlarged for period of gestation, fetal parts not palpable, symptoms of PIH develops, characteristic bleeding (white current in red current juice), sonographic findings (snow storm appearance), high HCG levels and expulsion of vesicles per vaginum.
- Chance for uterine perforation, hemorrhage and infection.

> "White current in red current juice" type of bleeding and "snow storm appearance" in USG are the characteristic features of vesicular mole.

- **Treatment:** If spontaneous evacuation does not occur, evacuation by curettage or hysterectomy may be done.
- Continued follow up of HCG is needed for one year to rule out choriocarcinoma.
- Family planning methods at least for one year.

> Choriocarcinoma is the dreaded complication of vesicular mole; so patients should be followed up with HCG values at least for one year.

Incompetent Cervix

- Cervix unable to hold the products of conception, cervical effacement and dilatation occurs in early mid trimester resulting in expulsion of products of conception.
- Cervical incompetency occurs due to congenital reasons or from forceful dilatation and curettage and difficult delivery.
- **Findings:** Painless contractions in mid trimester, delivery of dead or non-viable fetus.
- **Treatment:** Circlage procedures (Mc Donald and Shirodkar suture) during 14th to 16th week of gestation which is a suture placed beneath the cervical mucosa to close the cervix.
- Sutures are usually removed at 38 weeks or earlier if labor begins.

> Cervical encirclage procedures are done for incompetent cervix; the sutures put on cervix should be removed at 38 weeks of gestation or earlier if labor begins.

ANTEPARTUM HEMORRHAGE (APH)

- Bleeding from or into the genital tract after 28th week of pregnancy but before the birth of the baby.

> Bleeding from or into the genital tract after 28th week of pregnancy and before the birth of the baby is called Antepartum Hemorrhage (APH).

Placenta Previa

- Placenta is implanted partially or completely over the lower uterine segment.
- **Types of placenta previa**
  - Lateral: Major part of the placenta is in upper segment and only a small portion in the lower segment.
  - Marginal: Placental edge is reaching upto margin of internal os.
  - Incomplete central: Placenta covers internal os partially, but with the dilatation of the os, it is not covering the os at all.
  - Central: Placenta covers internal os fully even after full dilatation of the cervix.
- **Findings:** Painless bleeding in the later part of pregnancy is the only symptom.
- **Treatment:** Control of bleeding, replace blood loss, monitor FHR, prepare for delivery.

> Painless, causeless, bleeding that stops by its own is the characteristic bleeding pattern in placenta previa.

Abruptio Placenta

- Premature separation of a normally implanted placenta resulting in bleeding.
- **Types:** Concealed, revealed and mixed.
- **Findings**
  - Dark, blood may or may not be evident with partially detached placenta.

- Moderate to severe abdominal pain.
- Persistent uterine contraction.
- Normal to board like abdomen.
- Frequently associated with PIH.
- Predisposes mother to DIC and hypofibrinogenemia.

- **Treatment:** Replace blood loss, emergency LSCS if fetal distress, oxygen administration.

> Premature separation of a normally implanted placenta is termed as abruption-placenta.

POSTPARTUM HEMORRHAGE (PPH)

- Bleeding in excess of 500 mL within the first 24 hours following delivery.
- Usually associated with uterine atony, vaginal or cervical lacerations or retained placental fragments.
- **Findings**
  - Boggy uterus
  - Signs of hypotension
  - Signs of DIC (profuse, uncontrollable bleeding from uterus, oozing of blood from episiotomy, lacerations or IV site, fragmented RBC, decreased coagulation factors).
- **Treatment**
  - Massage uterine fundus to make it contracted.
  - Administer oxytocics.
  - Blood replacement.
  - Repair of vaginal and cervical lacerations.
  - Manual removal of retained placental fragments.
  - FFP or cryoprecipitate for DIC.

MULTIPLE PREGNANCY

- Defined as the occurrence or development of more than one fetus in the uterus simultaneously.
- **Types**
  - Twin pregnancy: two fetuses
  - Triplet : three fetuses
  - Quadruplets: four fetuses
  - Quintuplets: five fetuses
  - Sextuplets: six fetuses
- Commonest type is twin pregnancy.
- Increased incidence is seen in grand multipara (from 5th gravida onwards) and in those who have taken ovulation inducing drugs for fertility.
- **Findings:** Abdomen is unduly enlarged (barrel shaped), palpation of too many fetal parts, USG evidence of more than one fetuses, and unusual weight gain with exaggeration of minor ailments.
- **Complications:** Incresed association with abortion, anemia, pre-eclampsia, hydramnios, APH, preterm labor, malpresentations, PROM, PPH, asphyxia and fetal anomalies.
- Usually LSCS is undertaken for delivery.

POLYHYDRAMNIOS

- When liquor amni exceeds 2000 mL.
- AFI more than 20 cm.
- Congenital fetal malformations viz. anencephaly, open spina bifida, hydrops are associated with polyhydramnios.
- More commonly seen in multiple pregnancy, maternal diabetes, cardiac or renal diseases.
- **Findings:** Edema, varicosities, globular, markedly enlarged abdomen, fluid thrills over the uterus, fetal parts and FHR not get easily.
- Chance for pre-eclampsia, PROM, preterm labor, APH, PPH, cord prolapse and increased operative delivery.
- **Treatment:** Rest, salt restricted diet, vigilant monitoring, indomethacin (drug given to decrease amniotic fluid).

> Polyhydramnios is excessive amniotic fluid in the uterine cavity, i.e. amniotic fluid more than 2000 mL and AFI more than 20 cm.
> Normal amount of amniotic fluid at term is 1000 mL.

OLIGOHYDRAMNIOS

- When liquor amni is deficient, i.e. less than 100 mL.
- AFI less than 5 cm.
- Often associated with amnion nodosum, IUGR, renal agenesis.
- **Findings:** Abdomen full of fetus, less fetal movements, IUGR, AFI < 5 in USG.
- **Complications:** Chance for fetal part adhesions, fetal pulmonary hyperplasia, cord compression, PROM and prolonged labor.

> Oligohydramnios is reduced amount of liquor amni, i.e. amniotic fluid less than 100 mL and AFI < 5 cm.

VOMITING IN PREGNANCY

- Mild to moderate vomiting is normal in pregnancy called morning sickness which is attributed to the hormone HCG, usually disappears by the end of 3rd month.
- Excessive vomiting (hyperemesis gravidarum) if continues, endanger the life of mother and baby.

- Complications of hyperemesis include Wernicke's encephalopathy due to thiamine deficiency, stress ulcers and Korsakoff's psychosis.
- **Treatment:** Hospitalization and fluid replacement in severe cases, anti-emetic drugs, vitamin supplements, diet (bland, high carbohydrate, dry crackers are better tolerated).

> Excessive vomiting in pregnancy that affects the health of the mother is termed as hyperemesis gravidarum.

ABNORMALITIES OF PLACENTA AND CORD

- Battledore placenta-cord is attached to the margin of placenta.
- Velamentous placenta- abnormality in which the cord is attached to the membranes.
- Circumvallate placenta: Type of placental abnormality in which thin fibrous ring is present at the margin of the chorionic plate where fetal vessels appear to terminate.
- Placenta succenturiata: Type of placental abnormality in which one or more small lobes of placenta may be placed at varying distance from main placental margin.
- Short cord: When the length of the cord is less than eight inches or 20 cm.

HEART DISEASE IN PREGNANCY

- 90 percent rheumatic.
- Normal hemodynamics of pregnancy that adversely affect the lady with heart disease.
- Oxygen consumption increased 10 to 20 percent; related to the needs of the fetus.
- Plasma and blood volume increase and RBCs remain the same (physiologic anemia).
- **Classification**
  - Class I: No limitation of physical activity, no symptoms of cardiac insufficiency.
  - Class II: Slight limitation of physical activity, may experience fatigue, palpitation or dyspnea in last trimester.
  - Class III: Moderate to marked limitation of physical activity; bed rest indicated during most of pregnancy.
  - Class IV: Marked limitation of physical activity; pregnancy should be avoided; indication for medical termination of pregnancy.
- **Treatment**
  - Rest and avoid stress as far as possible.
  - Supervision by cardiologist throughout pregnancy.
  - Adequate calories, limited salt intake.
  - Digitalis, iron preparation and prophylactic antibiotics.
  - Labor in semi-fowler's or left lateral position.
  - Maternal and fetal monitoring.
  - Speed up second stage with vacuum/forceps to avoid pushing (vacuum is preferred since vacuum can be applied with the woman in sitting position).
  - Monitor for 48 hours postpartum.
  - Chance for congestive heart failure in the postpartum period since there is rapid return of blood after placental delivery. Signs of CHF include respiratory distress and tachycardia.

> Mother with heart disease should be monitored for 48 hours after delivery since rapid return of blood into the systemic circulation after placental delivery will predispose to congestive cardiac failure (CCF).

GESTATIONAL DIABETES

Normal physiology of pregnancy that affects pregnancy in woman with diabetes

- Vomiting during pregnancy, especially in first trimester, decrease carbohydrate intake resulting in acidosis.
- Increased activity of anterior pituitary decrease the tolerance for sugar.
- Elevated BMR and decrease in CO_2 combining power increase tendency towards education.
- Normal lowered renal threshold for glucose result in glucosuria.
- Muscular activity during labor depletes glycogen; therefore carbohydrate intake must be increased.
- During puerperium, hypoglycemia is common as involution and lactation occur.

Hazards of diabetes during pregnancy

- Often chance for repeated still births and fetal deaths.
- Fetal macrosomia (large babies weighing more than 4 kg).
- Neonatal deaths as a result of hypoxia, hypoglycemia, congenital anomalies and premature labor.
- PIH and hydramnios are common.
- Oral hypoglycemic contraindicated, insulin is used for treatment.
- Vigilant monitoring by obstetrician is needed throughout pregnancy and labor.
- LSCS is usually indicated owing to fetal macrosomia and unexplained fetal loss during the later weeks of pregnancy.

ANEMIA DURING PREGNANCY

- As per WHO, anemia during pregnancy is when Hb is less than 10 gm percent.
- Physiological anemia due to hemodilution and pathologic anemia can occur.
- Mild (Hb 8–10 gm%), moderate (Hb 7–8 gm%) and severe (Hb < 7 gm%).
- Dietary modification and iron therapy is indicated.
- Ferrous sulphate is the most common preparation used for oral iron supplementation.
- 1 iron tablet = 200 mg of ferrous sulphate which gives 60 mg of elemental iron.
- Iron dextran (imferon) is the common preparation for parenteral iron infusion/injection.
- 1 mL Imferon = 50 mg of elemental iron.
- Jectofer (Iron-Sorbitol-Citric acid complex) is also available for parenteral administrations.
- Blood transfusion is given if the labor is imminent.

> The type of iron preparation to be supplemented to correct anemia during pregnancy is determined by the Hb value and the period of gestation. If the labor is imminent and the Hb is low, blood transfusion is given.

INDUCTION OF LABOR

Elective induction: Initiation of labor contractions by:
- Pharmacologic means: Oxytocin, vaginal insertion of prostaglandins.
- Mechanical/surgical means: Artificial rupture of membranes (ARM).

May be done for medical or obstetrical reasons:
- Medical
- Obstetrical

Augmentation of labor: Assisting the client when the labor process is not progressing; normally done by pharmacologic and mechanical means.

> Induction and augmentation is not done if there is CPD, malpresentation of fetus, fetal distress, placenta previa or active vaginal herpes.

Bishop's Score: Gives an idea about whether cervix is favorable for induction; assessment parameters include cervical dilatation, length of cervix, consistency, position and station of fetal head; favorable score for induction is 6 to 13.

Factors	Score			
	0	1	2	3
Cervix				
Dilatation (cm)	closed	1–2	3–4	5+
Effacement (%)	0–30	40–50	60–70	80+
Consistency	firm	med	soft	–
Position	Post	mid	Ant	–
Head				
Station	–3	–2	–1,0	+1,+2
Favorable score 6–13 **Unfavorable score 0–5**				

PREMATURE RUPTURE OF MEMBRANES (PROM)

- Spontaneous rupture of membranes before the onset of labor.
- Chance for maternal infections if labor does not occur within 24 hours of ROM.
- Chance for prolapsed cord, fetal distress and ascending infections of the fetus.
- **Treatment:** Hospitalization and bed rest, amnioinfusion with isotonic saline is given in some cases.

> The ideal time for rupture of membrane is that when the cervix is fully dilated, i.e. 10 cm.

PRETERM OR PREMATURE LABOR

- Labor begins after 20th week, but before 37 completed weeks of gastation.
- Contributing factors include multiple abortions, abdominal surgery, incompetent cervix, multiple pregnancy and UTI.
- **Treatment:** Bed rest, sidelying position, tocolytic therapy (terbutaline or retodrine).
- Glucocorticoid therapy if the labor is imminent which reduces incidence of RDS in preterm infants.

> Administration of steroids will promote lung maturity in premature fetus; it should be given 24–48 hour before labor to get full benefit.

POSTTERM OR POST DATE LABOR

- Labor occurs 2 weeks beyond the EDD.
- **Fetal risks:** Excessive size may contribute to feto-pelvic disproportion, decreased placental function due to aging of the placenta, fetal asphyxia, skull bone calcification of fetal head prevent molding with resultant difficult labor.

- Treatment: If labor is not initiating by EDD, induction may be done.

DIFFICULT LABOR OR DYSTOCIA

Mechanical factors: Caused by contracted pelvis, obstruction in pelvis, malpresentation and position of fetus; treatment is cesarean delivery.

Functional: Caused by faulty uterine contractions, oxytocics can be given to augment labor considering the maternal and fetal condition.

PRECIPITATE LABOR

- Rapid labor and delivery of less than two hours duration.
- Chance for perineal lacerations and PPH.
- Hazards to the baby are anorexia and intracranial hemorrhage.

EPISIOTOMY

- Incision into the perineum to facilitate delivery and prevent lacerations and over stretching of the pelvic floor.
- Usually performed under local anesthesia and closed surgically.
- Postnatally assess mother for redness, edema, ecchymosis, discharge and approximation of wound (REEDA).

FAMILY PLANNING

CONTRACEPTIVE METHODS

Oral Contraceptives

- Used to prevent contraception, act by inhibiting ovulation causing a thickening of cervical mucus to inhibit sperm travel, also causes atrophic changes in the endometrium to prevent implantation.
- Available as progesterone only pills or estrogen progesterone combinations.
- Major side effects: Include thrombophlebitis, hypertension, libido changes, hyperglycemia, fluid retention, break through bleeding and breast tenderness.
- Contraindication for the use of oral contraceptives: Hypertension, thrombophlebitis, breast malignancy, cerebrovascular accident and breast feeding mothers.

> Major complications of oral contraceptives include thrombophlebitis, hypertension, libido changes, hyperglycemia, fluid retention, break through bleeding and breast tenderness.

> Contraindications for the use of oral contraceptives include hypertension, thrombophlebitis, breast malignancy, cerebrovascular accident and breast feeding mothers.

Intrauterine Devices

- Mechanical devices inserted into the isthmus of the uterus.
- Prevent pregnancy by increasing tubal motility, so that ovum gets to the uterus before lining is optimum for implantation.
- Not as effective as oral contraceptives because pregnancy may occur with device in place.
- May cause increased menstrual bleeding.

Diaphragms

- Mechanical device that fit over cervix and prevent sperm from entering cervical os.
- Used with spermicide for better results.
- Now, not in use.

Vaginal Sponge

- Plastic sponge impregnated with spermicide.
- Inserted into vagina before intercourse.
- Affords 48 hours of protection.

Condoms

- Rubber sheaths that cover the penis.
- Prevent semen from entering the cervical os.

> Vaginal creams, jellys, foam tablets are also available which are inserted into the vagina before intercourse.

Coitus Interruptus

Natural method of withdrawing the penis from the vagina before ejaculation; least effective method.

Rhythm Method or Safe Period Method

The plotting of basal body temperature to determine fertile period with abstinence from coitus during that time.

Surgical Sterilization (Permanent Methods of Family Planning)

- **Bilateral Vasectomy:** Small incision made into the scrotum and the vas deferens is ligated producing sterilization in the male by preventing ejaculation of the sperm; usually performed on an outpatient basis.
- **Bilateral Tubal Ligation:** Interruption in the continuity of the fallopian tubes by surgical transaction, electric cautery or compression with soft clamp preventing impregnation of ovum by the sperm; accomplished by laparotomy or laparoscopy; usually done on an outpatient basis.

MEDICAL TERMINATION OF PREGNANCY (MTP)

Abortion is induced for medical reasons by a registered medical practitioner.

a. **Menstrual extraction or menstrual regulation or mini suction:** Vacuum aspiration of uterine contents with a 50 mL syringe, done 5 to 7 weeks after last menstrual period.
b. **Vacuum aspiration:** Done in the first 12 weeks of pregnancy, the cervix is dilated and the products of conception are suctioned by a small hollow tube, the uterus is then curettaged to remove all fetal tissue.
c. **Dilatation and Curettage:** Performed during the first 12 weeks of pregnancy under local/general anesthesia, the cervix is dilated and uterus is curettaged.
d. **Saline injection:** Labor is induced when a pregnancy is 14–24 weeks in duration by injecting sterile hypertonic saline solution into the uterus by amniocentesis; labor usually begins within 20–36 hours after installation of saline and produce a macerated fetus. Not usually performed now a days.
e. **Prostaglandins:** Used during second trimester to trigger vasoconstriction and uterine contractions; interferes with endocrine function of placenta.
f. **Hysterotomy:** Performed after 16 weeks of pregnancy by surgically removing the fetus and placenta through an abdominal opening.

MTP act was passed in the year 1971.

MENOPAUSE

A period in woman's life when there is gradual cessation of ovarian function and menstrual cycles.

Physiologic Changes

- Ovaries lose their ability to respond to gonadotrophic hormone, vagina becomes dry and atrophied, hot flushes occur.
- Dramatic decrease in circulating estrogens and progesterone because the ovaries are atrophied.
- Increased FSH level in the blood, since production is no longer inhibited (negative feedback) by the ovaries, false positive pregnancy test may occur.

Therapeutic Management

- Support to release stress.
- Vaginal estrogen creams for vaginal dryness.
- Hormone replacement therapy: Small doses of estrogen and progesterone is now a days used to reduce menopausal discomforts.

OBJECTIVE QUESTIONS

1. **Most important muscle group supporting pelvic organs**
   a. Levator ani b. Pubococcygeal
   c. Iliococcygeal d. Ischiococcygeus
2. **Muscular partition which separates pelvic cavity from anatomical perineum**
   a. Pelvic muscle b. Pelvic diaphragm
   c. Peritoneum d. Fascia
3. **Transparent mucoprotein covering of ovum**
   a. Hyaluronidase b. Zona pellucida
   c. Corona radiata d. Chorionic leave
4. **Time required for maturation of spermatozoa**
   a. 16 days b. 31days
   c. 45 days d. 61 days
5. **Process of fusion of spermatozoa with mature ovum**
   a. Fecundation b. Fertilization
   c. Capacitation d. Fetation
6. **The part of uterine tube where fertilization occurs**
   a. Ampulla b. Infundibulum
   c. Cornua d. Fimbriae
7. **Fertilization span of oocyte**
   a. 12–24 hours b. 24–48 hours
   c. 48–72 hours d. > 72 hours
8. **Shape of human placenta**
   a. Oval b. Dome shaped
   c. Circular d. Discoid
9. **Average weight of placenta**
   a. 250 gms b. 500 gms
   c. 750 gms d. 1000 gms
10. **Color of amniotic fluid at term**
   a. Pale straw colored b. Golden yellow colored
   c. Greenish yellow colored d. Dark brown colored

11. **Color of amniotic fluid in Rh incompatibility**
a. Pale straw colored b. Golden yellow colored
c. Greenish yellow colored d. Dark brown colored

12. **Color of amniotic fluid in post maturity**
a. Pale straw colored b. Golden yellow colored
c. Greenish yellow colored d. Dark brown colored

13. **Color of amniotic fluid in IUD**
a. Pale straw colored b. Golden yellow colored
c. Greenish yellow colored d. Dark brown colored

14. **Average heart rate of newborn**
a. 100–120 bpm b. 120–140 bpm
c. 140–160 bpm d. >160 bpm

15. **Life span of fetal RBC**
a. 70 days b. 80 days
c. 100 days d. 120 days

16. **Surfactant is secreted by**
a. Alveolar epithelium b. Cuboidal epithelium
c. Squamous epithelium d. Keratinized epithelium

17. **Lecithin-Sphingomyelin ratio in amniotic fluid that indicates lung maturity**
a. 1:1 b. 1:2
c. 2:1 d. 2:2

18. **Endometrium in pregnancy is known as**
a. Decidua b. Decubitus
c. Trophoblast d. Gravid endometrium

19. **The non-pregnant uterus weighs**
a. 40 gm b. 60 gm
c. 80 gm d. 100 gm

20. **Painless, irregular contractions occurring in uterus in pregnancy**
a. Osiander's sign
b. Chadwick's sign
c. False pains
d. Braxton Hicks contractions

21. **Hypertrophic sebaceous glands around nipples during pregnancy**
a. Montgomery's tubercle b. Sebaceous cyst
c. Chloasma d. Linea nigra

22. **Pigmentation around neck, forehead and around eyes found during pregnancy**
a. Montgomery's tubercle b. Sebaceous cyst
c. Chloasma d. Linea nigra

23. **Brownish black pigmented area between xiphisternum and symphysis pubis in pregnancy**
a. Linea nigra b. Linea albicans
c. Striae gravidarum d. Striae albicans

24. **Pinkish linear marks found in abdominal wall, thighs and breasts during pregnancy**
a. Linea nigra b. Linea albicans
c. Striae gravidarum d. Striae albicans

25. **Postnatally, striae gravidarum becomes**
a. Linea nigra b. Linea albicans
c. Striae gravidarum d. Striae albicans

26. **Average total weight gain during pregnancy**
a. 8–10 kg b. 10–12 kg
c. 12–14 kg d. 15 kg

27. **Total iron requirement during pregnancy**
a. 500 gm b. 750 gm
c. 1000 gm d. 1500 gm

28. **The obstetrical conjugate measures**
a. 10 cm b. 11 cm
c. 12 cm d. 13 cm

29. **The strongest joint in the human body**
a. Sacroiliac joint b. Symphysis pubis
c. Sacrococcygeal joint d. Sacrospinous joint

30. **Fertilization takes place in fallopian tube in the**
a. Infundibulum b. Isthmus
c. Ampulla d. Fumbriae

31. **The ductus venosus connects the umbilical vein to the**
a. Superior vena cava b. Inferior vena cava
c. Aorta d. Pulmonary artery

32. **Drug of choice in controlling convulsions during eclamptic seizures**
a. Diazepam b. Phenobarbitone
c. Eptoin sodium d. Sodium valproate

33. **IUCDs are introduced postpartum at**
a. 4 weeks b. 6–8 weeks
c. 3 months d. 6 months

34. **Umbilical cord contains**
a. Two arteries and two veins
b. Two arteries and one vein
c. Two veins and one artery
d. One artery and one vein

35. Deep transverse arrest is a complication of
a. Occipito anterior position
b. Vertex presentation
c. Breech presentation
d. Occipito posterior position

36. A positive sign of pregnancy is
a. Hegar's sign
b. Osiander's sign
c. Fetal heart sounds
d. Morning sickness

37. Engaging diameter of vertex presentation
a. Suboccipito frontal
b. Suboccipito bregmatic
c. Submento bregmatic
d. Mento vertical

38. More common method of expelling placenta
a. Schultz method
b. Matthew Duncan method
c. Cord traction
d. Spontaneous expulsion

39. Objective method of accessing whether the cervix is favorable for induction of labor
a. APGAR score
b. Pinard's score
c. Downe's score
d. Bishop's score

40. Bluish discoloration of cervix during pregnancy
a. Jacquemier's sign
b. Hegar's sign
c. Chadwick's sign
d. Goodell's sign

41. The average amount of blood loss during a normal labor is
a. 500 mL
b. 800 mL
c. 1000 mL
d. 1500 mL

42. In prenatal development growth is most rapid in the
a. Implantation period
b. First trimester
c. Second trimester
d. Third trimester

43. The placenta does not produce
a. Chorionic gonadotrophin
b. Follicle stimulating hormone
c. Progesterone
d. Somatotropin

44. Physiologic anemia during pregnancy is a result of
a. Increased blood volume of the mother
b. Decreased dietary intake of iron
c. Decreased erythropoietin after first trimester
d. Increased detoxification of iron by the maternal liver

45. The pituitary hormone that stimulates the secretion of milk from the mammary glands
a. Oxytocin
b. Progesterone
c. Estrogen
d. Prolactin

46. The earliest clinical sign in respiratory distress syndrome in the newborn is
a. Sternal and subcostal retraction
b. Cyanosis
c. Rapid respirations
d. Grunting

47. Abruptio placenta is most likely to occur in a woman with
a. Cardiac disease
b. Hyperthyroidism
c. Pregnancy induced hypertension
d. CPD

48. The most effective position for a woman in labor when there is a prolapsed cord
a. Prone
b. Fowler's
c. Lithotomy
d. Trendelenburg

49. Signs and symptoms of placenta previa include
a. Sharp abdominal pain
b. Early rupture of membranes
c. Increased low back pain
d. Painless vaginal bleeding

50. In the female, evaluation of all the pelvic organs of reproduction is accomplished by
a. Cystoscopy
b. Hysterosalpingogram
c. Biopsy
d. Culdoscopy

51. During induction of labor, a woman should be observed carefully for signs of
a. Uterine tetany
b. Severe pain
c. Prolapse of the umbilical cord
d. Hypoglycemia

52. If the first day of last menstrual period was July 22, the estimated date of delivery would be
a. March 15
b. April 15
c. March 29
d. April 29

ANSWER KEY

1. a	2. b	3. b	4. d	5. b	6. a	7. a	8. d	9. b	10. a	11. b	12. c
13. d	14. b	15. b	16. a	17. c	18. a	19. b	20. d	21. a	22. c	23. a	24. c
25. d	26. b	27. c	28. b	29. a	30. c	31. b	32. a	33. b	34. b	35. d	36. c
37. b	38. a	39. d	40. c	41. a	42. d	43. b	44. a	45. d	46. a	47. c	48. d
49. d	50. b	51. a	52. d								

Chapter 7

Gynecologic Nursing

RELATED ANATOMY AND PHYSIOLOGY

The female pelvic organs are divided into two viz. external genitalia and internal genital organs.

EXTERNAL GENITALIA

External genitalia or vulva includes non-veneris, labia majora, labia minora, clitoris, vestibule and perineum.

Mons veneris is the pad of subcutaneous adipose tissue lying in front of the pubis. The vulva is bounded on each side by the elevation of skin and subcutaneous tissue which form the labia majora. Just within the labia majora, there are two thick folds of skin called labia minora. Clitoris in a small erectile body measuring about 2.5 cm situated in the most exterior part of the vulva. Clitoris is an analogue to the penis in the female. Vestibule is a triangular space pounded anteriorly by the clitoris, posteriorly by the fourchette and on either side by labia minora. There are four openings into the vestibule viz. urethral opening, vaginal orifice and openings of the Bartholin's ducts on either side.

INTERNAL GENITAL ORGANS

The internal genital organs in the females include vagina, uterus, fallopian tubes and the ovaries.

VAGINA

The vagina is a fibro musculomembranous sheath communicating the uterine cavity with the exterior at the vulva. It constitutes the excretory channel for the uterine secretion and menstrual blood. It is the organ of copulation and forms the birth canal of parturition. The canal is directed upwards and backwards forming an angle of 45° with the horizontal in erect posture.

The vagina has got an anterior, a posterior and two lateral walls. The length of the anterior wall is about seven cm and that of the posterior wall is about nine cm. vaginal fornices are at the top of the vagina due to the projection of the uterine cervix.

The layers of the vagina from within outwards are the muscles coat which is laid by stratified squamous epithelium submucous layer of loose vascular tissue, muscular layer, and fibroin coat derived from the endopelvic fascia.

The vaginal epithelium is under the control of sex hormones. At birth and upto 10 to 14 days, the epithelium is stratified squamous. Thereafter upto prepuberty and in postmenopause, the epithelium becomes thin, consisting of few layers only. From puberty till menopause, the vaginal epithelium is stratified squamous and devoid of any gland. The vaginal secretion is derived from the glands of the cervix, uterus, transudation of the vaginal epithelium and Bartholin's glands. The pH is acidic and ranges between 4 to 5.5 with an average of 4.5. There are a specialized type of gram-positive bacillus called Doderlein's bacilli in the vagina. Its function is to convert the glycogen present in the vaginal mucosa into lactic acid, so that the vaginal pH is maintained towards acidic side. This acid pH prevents growth of other pathogenic organisms.

The vagina is supplied by the cervico-vaginal branch of the uterine artery and the vaginal artery.

> The pH vaginal secretion is acidic and ranges between 4–5.5 with an average of 4.5.

> The function of Doderlein's bacilli is to convert the glycogen present in the vaginal mucosa into lactic acid, so that the vaginal pH is maintained towards acidic side. This acid pH prevents growth of other pathogenic organisms.

THE UTERUS

The uterus is a hollow pyriform muscular organ situated in the pelvis between the bladder in front and rectum behind. The uterus is normally anteverted and anteflexed. The uterus measures about 7.5 cm × 5 cm × 2.5 cm. The weight varies from 50 to 80 gm. The parts of the uterus are body or corpus, isthmus and cervix.

The uterus measures about 7.5 cm X 5 cm X 2.5 cm and the weight varies from 50–80 gm.

1. Body or Corpus

The body is further divided into fundus, the part which lies above the openings of the uterine tubes. The body proper is triangular and has the openings of the tubes and the isthmus. The superior-lateral angles of the body of the uterus project outwards from the junction of the fundus and the body and are called the cornua of the uterus. The uterine tube, round ligament and ligament of the ovary are attached to each cornua.

2. The isthmus is a constricted part measuring about 0.5 cm situated between the body and the cervix. It is limited above by the anatomical internal os and below by the histological internal os.

3. Cervix

The cervix is the lowermost part of the uterus. It extends from the histological internal os and ends at external os which opens into the vagina after perforating the anterior vaginal wall. It is about 2.5 cm in length and almost cylindrical in shape. It is divided into a supravaginal part, the part lying above the vagina and the vaginal part which lies within the vagina each measuring 1.25 cm.

Cavity of Uterus

The cavity of the uterine body is triangular on coronal section with the base above and the apex below. It measures about 3.5 cm. There is no cavity in the fundus. The cervical canal is fusiform and measures about 2.5 cm. The normal length of the uterine cavity including the cervical canal is usually 6 to 7 cm.

Layers of the Uterus

The body consists of three layers from outside inwards:

1. **Perimetrium:** Serous coat which covers the entire organ except on the lateral borders.
2. **Myometrium**: It consists of thick bundles of smooth muscle fibers held by connective tissue and are arranged in various directions; during pregnancy, three district layers can be identified —outer longitudinal, middle interlacing and the inner circular.
3. **Endometrium**: The mucous lining of the cavity is called endometrium. The endometrium is directly apposed to the muscle coat. The endometrium is changing during the menstrual cycle under hormonal action. The endometrium is changed to decidua during pregnancy.

The endometrium during pregnancy is called decidua.

The cervix is composed normally of fibrous connective tissue.

Secretion: The endometrial secretion is scanty and watery. The physical and chemical properties of the cervical secretion change with menstrual cycles and with pregnancy. The cervical glands secrete alkaline mucus with pH 7.8. Cervical mucus contributes significantly to the normal vaginal discharge. A part forms the mucus plug which functionally closes the cervical canal and has got bacteriolytic action.

The uterus is supplied with uterine artery—one on each side.

FALLOPIAN TUBES (UTERINE TUBES)

The uterine tubes are paired structures, measuring about 10 cm (4″) and are situated in the medial three-fourth of the upper free margin of the broad ligaments. Each tube has got two openings, one communicating with the lateral angle of the uterine cavity called uterine opening and measures 1 mm in diameter, the other is on the lateral end of the tube called pelvic opening or abdominal ostium and measures about 2 mm in diameter.

Parts of the Fallopian Tube

1. **Intramural or interstitial part** lying in the uterine wall and measures 1.25 cm in length and 1 mm in diameter.
2. **Isthmus** almost straight and measures about 2.5 cm in length and 2.5 mm in diameter.
3. **Ampulla**, tortuous part and measures about 5 cm in length.
4. **Infundibulum** measuring about 1.25 cm long with a maximum diameter of 6 mm.

The abdominal ostium is surrounded by a number of radiating fimbriae; one of these is longer than the rest and is attached to the outer pole of the ovary called ovarian fimbriae.

Layers of Fallopian Tube

1. **Serosa:** Consists of peritoneum on all sides except along the line of attachment of mesosalpinx.
2. **Muscular:** Arranged in two layers—outer longitudinal and inner circular.
3. Mucous membrane lined by columnar epithelium.

Functions: The important function of the tubes are transport of gamete and to facilitate fertilization and survival of zygote through its secretion.

Blood Supply

Arterial supply is from the uterine and ovarian artery.

OVARY

The ovaries are paired sex organ or gonads in female which are concerned with germ cell maturation, storage, release and steroidogenesis.

Each ovary is oval in shape and pinkish grey in color and the surface is scarred during reproductive period.

It measures about 3 cm × 2 cm × 1 cm. Each ovary presents two ends—tubal and uterine, two borders—mesovarium and free posterior and two surfaces—medial and lateral. The ovaries are intraperitoneal structures. The vary lies in the ovarian fossa on the lateral pelvic wall. The ovary is attached to the posterior layer of the broad ligament by the mesovarium.

Layers of Ovary

The ovary is covered by a single layer of cubical cell known as germinal epithelium. The substance of the gland consists of outer cortex and inner medulla.

The cortex consists of stromal cells which are thickened beneath the germinal epithelium to form tunica albuginea. During reproductive period, the cortex is studded with numerous follicular structures, called ovarian follicles which include primordial follicle, maturing follicle, Graafian follicle and corpus luteum.

Medulla consists of lose connective tissue, few unstriped muscles, blood vessels and nerves. There are small collection of cells called hilus cells which are homologous to the interstitial cells of the testes.

Ovary is supplied with ovarian artery, a branch of the abdominal aorta.

PELVIC FLOOR

Pelvic floor is a muscular partition which separates the pelvic cavity from the anatomical perineum. It consists of three sets of muscles on either side—pubococcygeus, Iliococcygeus and ischiococcygeus. These are collectively called levator ani. Its upper surface is concave and slopes downwards, backwards and medially and is covered by parietal layer of pelvic fascia. The inferior surface is convex an is covered by oval fascia. The muscle with the covering fascia is called the pelvic diaphragm.

Each levator ani arises from the back of the pubic rami, from the condensed fascia covering the obturator internus and from the inner surface of the ischial spine. These are two gaps in the middle, the anterior one is for the urethra and vagina and the posterior one is for the passage of the rectum.

Functions of Pelvic Floor

1. To support the pelvic organs.
2. To maintain intra-abdominal pressure.
3. Facilitates internal rotation of the presenting part when it presses on the pelvic floor.
4. Puborectalis plays an important role to the action of the external anal sphincter.
5. Ischiococcygeus helps to stabilize the sacroiliac and sacrococcygeal joints.
6. To steady the perineal body.

PERINEUM

The perineum is bounded above by the interior surface of the pelvic floor, below by the skin between the buttocks and thigh. Laterally, it is bounded by the ischiopubic rami, ischial tuberocities and sacrotuberous ligaments and posteriorly by the coccyx. The diamond shaped space of the bony pelvic outlet is divided into two triangular spaces with the common base formed by the free border of the urogenital diaphragm. The anterior triangle is called the urogenital triangle and the posterior one is called the anal triangle.

Musculofascial Structures in Perineum

1. **Fascia:** Two layers of superficial perineal fascia—superficial fatty layer and deeper layer called Colles fascia and the inferior and superior layer of urogenital diaphragm together called triangular ligament.
2. **Muscles:** Superficial and deep transverse perineal muscles, bulbocavernosus, levator ani, and external anal sphincter.

Importance of Perineum

1. It helps to support the levator ani which is placed above it.
2. By supporting the posterior vaginal wall, it indirectly supports the anterior vaginal wall, bladder and the uterus.
3. It is vulnerable to injury during childbirth.
4. Deliberate cutting of the structures during delivery is called episiotomy.

PELVIC PERITONEUM

The peritoneum covering the superior surface of the bladder reflects over the anterior surface of the uterus at the level of the internal os forming the uterovesical pouch. The peritoneum thereafter, is firmly attached to the anterior and posterior wall of the uterus and upper one third of the posterior vaginal wall where from it is reflects over the rectum. The pouch so formed is called rectouterine pouch or the pouch of Douglus.

BROAD LIGAMENT

The double fold of peritoneum which extends from the lateral border of the uterus to the lateral wall of the pelvis is called broad ligament.

Parts of the Broad Ligament:

1. Infundibulopelvic ligament

It includes the portion of the broad ligament which extends from the infundibulum of the fallopian tube to the lateral pelvic wall. It contains ovarian vessels and nerves and lymphatic from the ovary, fallopian tube and body of the uterus.

2. Mesovarium

The ovary is attached to the posterior layer of the broad ligament by a fold of peritoneum called mesovarium.

3. Mesosalpinx

The part of the broad ligament between the fallopian tube and the level of attachment of the ovary is the mesosalpinx.

4. Mesometrium

The part of the broad ligament below the mesosalpinx is called mesometrium.

Contents of Broad Ligament:

- Fallopian tubes.
- Uterine and ovarian arteries with their branches.
- Nerves and lymphatic from the uterus, fallopian tube and ovary.
- Proximal part of the round ligament which raises a peritoneal fold on the anterior leaf.
- Ovarian ligament which raises a peritoneal fold on the posterior leaf.
- Parametrium containing loose areolar tissue and fat.

NEUROENDOCRINOLOGY OF REPRODUCTION

HYPOTHALAMUS

Hypothalamus plays an important role in the neuro-endocrine regulation. The hypothalamus is connected with the anterior lobe of the pituitary through a special hypothalamopituitary system of vessels. It is directly connected with the posterior lobe of the pituitary by the supraoptic and paraventricular nuclei.

Secretions

The hypothalamus produces series of specific releasing and inhibiting hormones which have got effect on the specific pituitary hormones.

i. **Gonadotrophic releasing hormone (GnRH):** The GnRH is also names as luteinizing hormone releasing hormone (LHRH). GnRH is concerned with the release, synthesis and storage of both the gonadotrophins (FSH and LH) from the anterior pituitary.

ii. **Thyrotrophin releasing hormone (TRH):** The hormone TRH stimulates not only the release of thyrotrophin but also prolactin from the pituitary.

iii. **Hypothalamus** also recreates corticotrophin releasing hormone (CRH) and growth hormone releasing hormone (GHRH).

Feedback Mechanism

FSH and LH exert negative feedback effect on hypothalamic production of GnRH. Preovulatory sustained and high rise of estradiol results in increased GnRH secretion.

Among the specific releasing hormones from the hypothalamus, the important hormones are GnRH, TRH and CRH.

ANTERIOR PITUITARY

The anterior pituitary is a large, compact and highly vascular gland. The anterior pituitary produces gonadotrophins, thyrotrophin and corticotrophin.

The two gonadotrophic hormone secreted from the anterior pituitary are follicle stimulating hormone (FSH) and luteinizing hormone (LH). The FSH level tends to rise on following the onset of menstruation and attain its peak at the 12th day of the cycle (preovulatory) and gradually declines to attain the base level at about the 18th day.

LH causes ovulation, formation and maintenance of corpus luteum. LH levels remain almost static throughout the cycle except at least 24 hours prior to ovulation, which then attains its peak celled LH surge.

GnRH stimulates the release and synthesis of both LH and FSH from the anterior pituitary in a pulsatile manner.

TSH acts on the thyroid gland and regulates the production of thyroxin.

ACTH produced from anterior pituitary stimulates the production of corticosteroids in the adrenal cortex.

Pituitary also secretes somatotropin or growth hormone and melanocyte stimulating hormone (MSH) which is responsible for the pigmentary changes during puberty and in pregnancy.

POSTERIOR PITUITARY

Posterior pituitary produces vasopressin and oxytocin. Vasopressin or ADH is concerned with the maintenance of osmolarity of the plasma. Oxytocin acts on the myometrial contractile system, especially during labor and also causes contraction of the myoepithelial cells in the breast ductules during lactation.

OVARY

The functions of the ovary are ovulation and production of hormones (steroidogenesis). The principal hormones secreted from the ovaries are estrogens, progesterone, androgen and inhibin. Ovarian steroidogenesis is under the influence of LH and FSH.

During the follicular phase, under the influence of LH, androgens are aromatized to estrogens. After ovulation, the progesterone is synthesized under the influence of LH.

Estrogen exerts a negative feedback effect on the release of FSH by a direct action on pituitary decreasing the sensitivity of the gonadotrophins to GnRH. There is significant rise in the preovulatory period with the LH surge by its positive feedback action. The positive feedback effect of estradiol in the secretory phase is inhibited by progesterone.

> Ovarian hormones, estrogen and progesterone determine the cyclic pattern of FSH and LH release.

Production of androgen is primarily under the control of LH.

Inhibin is produced by the granulosa cells of the ovarian follicle. It has got a preferential negative feedback effect on FSH release.

Relaxin is secreted from the preovulatory follicle and corpus luteum. It probably facilitates follicular rupture during ovulation.

> FSH, in conjunction with LH, is involved in the maturation of oocyte and ovulation.

> LH stimulates meiosis, helps in ovulation and formation and maintenance of corpus luteum.

HYPOTHALAMIC PITUITARY OVARIAN AXIS

The hormones liberated from the hypothalamus, pituitary and ovary are dependent to one another. A well coordinated axis called hypothalamic pituitary ovarian axis which controls the secretion of hormones through feedback mechanism operating through this axis.

Feedback Loop

The long feedback loop refers to the feedback effects of the ovarian steroids on both the hypothalamus and pituitary. It is usually negative or inhibitory, but may be stimulatory or positive during preovulatory period.

The short feedback loop relates the secretion of GnRH by gonadotrophins by interplay between the neurotransmitters and the pituitary gonadotrophins. FSH and LH exert negative feedback effect on the hypothalamic production of GnRH.

Ultrashort feedback loop refers to autoregulation of the releasing hormones of the hypothalamus on its own synthesis.

> Estradiol exerts a negative feedback effect on the hypothalamo-pituitary axis. When the level is raised to more than 200 pg/mL and sustained for 24–48 hours, it has got positive feedback effects. The positive feedback effect cannot occur in the luteal phase because of progesterone.

> Progesterone has got negative feedback on the hypothalamo-pituitary axis, principally upon the mid-cycle gonadotrophin surge and is responsible for its short duration.

GYNECOLOGICAL DISEASES AND DISORDERS

PRECOCIOUS PUBERTY

* The girl exhibits secondary sex characteristics before the age 8 or menstruates before the age 10.

a. **Complete, central or true:** May be due to juvenile primary hypothyroidism, intracranial lesions, tumor or infection.
b. **Incomplete:** Includes premature thelarche, premature pubarche or premature menarche.
c. **Precocious pseudopuberty or peripheral:** May be due to granulosa cell tumor, theca cell tumor, leydig cell tumor, chorionic epithelioma, androblastoma, adrenal hyperplasia or tumor and estrogen or androgen intake.

> Premature thelarche is the isolated development of breast tissue before the age of 8. There are no other features of precocious puberty.

> Premature pubarche is isolated development of axillary and or pubic hair prior to the age of 8 without other signs of precocious puberty.

> Premature menarche is an isolated event of cyclic vaginal bleeding without any other sign of secondary sexual development.

Treatment

Depends on the cause

- The estrogen therapy or its inadvertent intake should be stopped.
- Cortisone therapy for adrenal hyperplasia.
- Surgery to remove adrenal or ovarian tumor.
- Neurosurgery for intractable tumors.
- For constitutional or idiopathic type, drugs used are medroxyprogesterone acetate, cyproterone acetate, GnRH analogues and Danazol are used.

DELAYED PUBERTY

Puberty is said to be delayed when the breast tissue and/or pubic hair have not appeared by 13 to 14 years or menarche appears as late as 16 years. The normal upper age limit of menarche is 15 years.

The delay may be constitutional secondary to chronic diseases endocrinal or systemic or due to true gonadal insufficiency, i.e. hypergonadotrophic hypogonadism (primary) or hypogonadotraphic hypogonadism (secondary).

Treatment is unsatisfactory. Assurance, improvement of general health and treatment of any illness may be helpful in non-endocrinal causes. In endocrine disorders, result may be unsatisfactory.

> Delayed puberty is when the breast tissue and or pubic hair leave not appeared by 13–14 years or menarche appears as late as 16 years.

PUBERTY MENORRHAGIA

- The initial periods may be heavy and or prolonged due to anovulatory cycles.
- Unopposed action of estrogen causes endometrial hyperplasia.
- Simple measures such as rest, reassurance, correction of anemia all will cure the condition in majority of cases.
- If simple measures fail, investigate for coagulation disorders and hypothyroidism.

Treatment

1. Treat any underlying pathological condition.
2. Hematinics and blood transfusion if Hb is less or any bleeding disorder present.
3. Progesterone preparation (e.g. nor-ethisterone, medroxy-progesterone acetate) are given 2 to 3 courses.
4. If all above fail uterine curettage may be needed.

> Common order of changes in puberty includes enlargement of the breast and beginning of growth spurt—Appearance of pubic hair—Axillary hair—Menstruation (menarche).

PELVIC INFECTIONS

Free anastomosis between the lymphatics and blood vessels causes the infection of one pelvic organ usually spreads to the other more frequently.

Defense of the Genital Tract

1. **Vulval defense**
   - Apposition of cleft by labia
   - Bartholin's glands
   - Fungicidal action of the apocrine glands
   - High resistance of the vulval and perineal skin to infection
2. **Vaginal defense**
   - Apposition of the anterior and posterior walls
   - Stratified epithelium devoid of glands
   - Presence of estrogen
   - Acidic vaginal PH due to the presence of Doderlein's bacilli
3. **Cervical defense**
   - Recemose type of glands
   - Mucus plug
   - Bactericidal effect of the mucus.
4. **Uterine defense**
   - Cyclic shedding of the endometrium
   - Closure of the uterine ostium of the fallopian tube with slightest inflammatory reaction in the endometrium
5. **Tubal defense**
   - Integrated mucus plicae and epithelial cilia
   - Peristalsis of the tube and the movement of the cilia towards the uterus
6. **Defense of the vagina**

PELVIC INFLAMMATORY DISEASE (PID)

- Disease of the upper genital tract.
- Due to ascending spread of microorganism from the cervicovaginal canal to the endometrium, fallopian tube and related pelvic structures.
- Includes endometritis, salpingitis, pelvic peritonitis and tubo-ovarian abscess.

> PID includes endometritis, salpingitis, pelvic peritonitis and tubo-ovarian abscess. The cervicitis is not included in the list.

	Newborn (0–10 days)	Up to puberty	Child bearing period	Postmenopause
Epithelium	Multi-layered	Thin	Multi-layered	Thin
Glycogen	++	-	++	-
Doderlein's bacillus	+	-	++	-
pH	Acidic (4–5)	Neutral or alkaline (6–8)	Acidic (4–5)	Neutral (6–7)

Vulnerable Groups

- Menstruating teenagers
- IUCD users
- Previous history of acute PID

Condom along with spermicidal chemicals containing Nonacynol-9 which is both bactericidal and viricidal offers protection against PID.

Progesterone content of oral pills produce thick mucus plug preventing ascend of bacteria.

Organisms Causing PID

1. The primary organism are sexually transmitted and limited approximately to *Neisseria gonorrhea, Chlamydia trachomatis* and *Mycoplasma hominis*.
2. The secondary organisms are aerobic organisms like non-herolytic *streptococcus*, *E coli*, group B *streptococcus* and *staphylococcus* anaerobic organism like bacterioids.

Mode of Infection

- Ascending infection from lower genital tract which is facilitated by the sexually transmitted vectors such as sperm and trichomonads.
- Reflux of menstrual blood along with gonococci into the fallopian tubes.
- Mycoplasma usually spreads across the parametrium to affect the fallopian tube.
- The secondary organism probably affect the tube through lymphatic.
- Organisms from the gut may affect the tube rarely.

Findings

- Bilateral dull lower abdominal and pelvic pain. The onset of pain is more rapid and acute in gonococcal infection (3 days) than in chlamydial infection (5–7 days).
- Fever, lassitude and headache.
- Irregular and excessive vaginal bleeding usually due to associated endometritis.
- Abnormal vaginal discharge which becomes purulent and or copious. Usually seen associated with lower genital tract infection.
- Nausea and vomiting.
- Dyspareunia.
- Pain and discomfort in the right hypochondrium due to concomittent perihepatitis associated with acute salpingitis.
- Tenderness on both the quadrants of lower abdomen.
- Enlarged, tender liver.
- Congested external urethral meatus or openings of Bartholin's ducts through which pus escapes while applying pressure.
- Bilateral tenderness on fornix palpation during bimanual examination.
- Thickening or mass felt through the fornices.

Investigations

- Culture and sensitivity of the pus or discharge collected from the urethra, Bartholin's gland, cervical canal, or pus from the fallopian tubes collected during laparoscopy/laparotomy.
- Blood TC elevated more than 10,000/cubic mm, elevated ESR more than 15 mm per hour.
- Serological test for syphilis.
- Laparoscopy.
- Sonography.
- Culdocentesis: aspiration of discharge/pus from the pouch of Douglas.
- Investigate partner also.

"Violin String" like adhesions of perihepatitis may be evident in chlamydial infection.

Complications

- Immediate: Pelvic peritonitis, generalized peritonitis, septicemia (leading to arthritis or myocarditis).
- Late: Infertility, chronic pelvic inflammation chronic pelvic pain and ill-health, increased chance of ectopic pregnancy.

Treatment

- **Antibiotics:** Penicillins, tetracycline, doxycycline, erythromycin, metronidazole.
- Laparotomy/laparoscopy.
- Treat partner also if sexually transmitted.

The only unequivocal proof of successful treatment after salpingitis is an intrauterine pregnancy.

PELVIC INFECTION FOLLOWING DELIVERY AND ABORTION

ABORTION

- The common organisms producing acute infection following delivery are anaerobic streptococcus, *Staphylococcus pyogenes*, nonhemolytic *streptococcus*, *E. coli* and *bacteroides*.

The normal defense of the reproductive organ is lost during childbirth and abortion.

An Infection is either localized to the cervix producing acute cervicitis or may affect the placental site producing endometritis. Infection can spread to the parametrium through the lymphatics or directly through the rest of the cervix. The infection can spread to tubes producing endosalpingitis. The ovary may also be affected producing a tubo-ovarian mass.

Findings

- Chief complaints include fever, lower abdominal pain, pelvic pain and offensive lochia following delivery or abortion.
- Patient restless and looks ill.
- Tenderness or rigidity in the lower abdomen.
- Vaginal examination is painful.
- Unilateral or bilateral tender indurated mass, bulging mass felt through the posterior fornix.

Complications

- Endotoxic shock
- Oliguria or anuria
- DIC
- Tubo-ovarian mass
- Peritonitis
- Parametritis
- Thrombophlebitis
- Pulmonary embolism.

Treatment

- Antibiotics.
- Symptomatic treatment.
- **Surgery:** Evacuation of the uterus, posterior colpotomy or laparotomy may be performed.

GENITAL TUBERCULOSIS

Genital tuberculosis is almost always secondary to primary infection elsewhere in the extragenital sites such as lungs, lymph nodes, urinary tract, bones and joints.

The fallopian tubes are the primary sites of pelvic tuberculosis from where secondary spread occurs to other genital organs.

Mode of spread: From any primary site, infection through blood stream and lymphatics.

Findings

- Menorrhagia, oligomenorrhea, amenorrhea.
- Infertility.
- Chronic pelvic pain.
- Pyrexia, anorexia, loss of weight, anorexia and anemia.
- The elongated and distended distal tube with the patent abdominal ostium gives the appearance of tobacco—pouch in genital TB.
- Irregular tender mass in the lower abdomen.
- WBC and ESR count elevated.
- Mantoux test is positive.
- Evaluation of diagnostic uterine curettage.
- Tobacco pouch appearance in hysterosalpingography (HSG).
- Diagnostic laparoscopy.

Treatment

- Anti-TB drugs: Three drug therapy for three months followed by two drug therapy further for a period of nine months. Three drug therapy is with INH, rifampicin and ethambutol and two drug therapy is continued using INH and rifampicin.
- Surgery: Indicated for tubercular pyosalpinx, ovarian abscess, pyometra, persistent menorrhagia or chronic pelvic pain. Total hysterectomy with salpingo-ophrectomy is done. In young women, one ovary may be preserved as far as possible.

SEXUALLY TRANSMITTED DISEASES

- Sexually Transmitted Diseases (STDs) include those diseases which are predominantly transmitted through sexual contact from an infected partner.
- Although transmission is mostly by sexual contact, other modes of transmission include placental (AIDS, Syphilis), by blood transfusion or infected needles (AIDS, hepatitis B or Syphilis) or by inoculation on to the infants mucosa when it passes through the birth canal (gonococcal, *Chlamydial* or herpes).

ACUTE GONORRHEA

- Causative organism is *Neisseria gonorrhea*—a gram-negative diplococcus.
- The incubation period is 3 to 7 days.
- Principal site of invasion is the columnar and transitional epithelium of the genitourinary tract.

Sexually transmitted diseases	
Gonorrhea	*Neisseria gonorrhoeae*
Non-gonococcus urethritis	*Chlamydia trachomatis* (D-K serotypes)
Syphilis	*Treponema pallidum*
Lymphogranuloma venereum	*Chlamydia trachomatis* (L serotypes)
Chancroid	*Haemophilus ducreyi*
Granuloma inguinale	*Donovania granulomatis*
Non-specific vaginitis	*Haemophilus vaginalis*
Mycoplasma infection	*Mycoplasma hominis*
AIDS	Human immunodeficiency Virus
Genital herpes	Herpes simplex virus (HSV 2)
Condyloma acuminata	Human papiloma virus (HPV)
Molluscum contagiosum	Pox virus
Viral hepatitis	Hepatitis B virus
C I N	HPV
Trichomonas vaginitis	*Trichomonas vaginalis*
Monilial vaginitis	*Candida albicans*
Scabies	Sarcoptes scabiei
Pediculosis pubis	*Crab louse (Phthirus pubis)*

> The squamous epithelium is resistant to gonococcal invasion, vaginitis in adult is not possible, but vulvo-vaginitis is possible in childhood.

- Gonococcal infection may ascend upto produce acute PID if not treated properly.
- Local symptoms of gonorrhea may be dysuria, frequency of micturition, excessive irritant vaginal discharge, swelling over labia due to involvement of Bartholin's gland.
- Speculum examination reveals congested ectocervix with increased mucopurulant cervical secretions escaping out through the external os.
- If untreated, signs and symptoms of PID develop.
- Spread of infection to liver capsule may produce perihepatitis.
- Diagnoses by culture and sensitivity of the secretion from urethra, Bartholin's glands and endocervix.
- Drugs used in acute gonorrhea are procaine penicillin, streptomycin, ampicillin, doxycycline, etc. Treat male partner simultaneously.

SYPHILIS

- Caused by *Treponema pallidum.*
- Acquired by direct contact with another person who has open primary or secondary syphilitic lesion.
- Incubation period ranges between 9 to 90 days.
- The primary lesion (chancre) may be single or multiple and is normally located in the labia. A small papule is formed which become an ulcer quickly.

> The ulcer in syphilis is painless without any surrounding inflammatory reaction.

- The primary chancre heals spontaneously in 1 to 8 weeks leaving behind a scar.
- Within 6 to 8 months from the onset of primary chancre, the secondary lesion may be present in the vulva as condyloma lata. These are coarse, flat-topped, moist and necrotic.

> The primary and secondary stage of syphilis can last upto two years and during the period, the woman is a source of infection.

- Serological test (VDRL) in done to diagnose syphilis.
- Treatment by benzathine penicillin or procaine penicillin.

HERPES GENITALIS

- The causative organism is herpes simplex virus (HSV) type 2.
- Usually transmitted sexually by an infected partner.
- Symptoms of the first attack usually appear less than seven days after sexual contact.
- Red inflammatory areas appear initially on the clitoris, labia and vestibule. Multiple vesicles appear which progress into multiple shallow ulcers and heal up spontaneously by crusting.

> Maternal transfer of herpes genitals to fetus occurs during vaginal delivery, if primary or recurrent attacks occur late in pregnancy.

- **Treatment:** No specific treatment available. Acyclovir is effective in acute cases.

ACQUIRED IMMUNODEFICIENCY SYNDROME (AIDS)

- The causative organism is human immunodeficiency virus (HIV) of strain HIV1 and HIV 2.
- Transmitted by sexual contact, transfusion of contaminated blood or blood products or by the use of contaminated needles.

> Vertical transmission to the neonates of the mothers infected with AIDS is about 25%.

- CD4 counts less than 200/cubic mm are taken as AIDS defining criteria.
- Following exposure to HIV infection, a patient develops antibodies against HIV in about 8 to 12 weeks.

> The development of antibodies against HIV marks the stage of sero conversion and in some cases manifest clinically as 'flu' like syndrome.

- After the initial exposure, the person remains asymptomatic for many years, the mean period being 7 to 10 years (known as window period).
- AIDS related complex (ARC): Refers to subjects having nonspecific clinical features of weight loss, fever, diarrhea, skin rash, herpes simplex, oral candidiasis without full blown pictures of AIDS.
- Common secondary infections are atypical TB, pneumonia (pneumocystis carinii pneumonia), systemic candidiasis and meningitis.
- Encephalitis, myelopathy and peripheral neuritis are neurological manifestations.

> Increased incidence of high grade lymphoma, Kaposi's sarcoma and non-Hodgkin's lymphoma is seen in AIDS.

- **Diagnostic tests:** ELISA and western blot tests.
- **Drug:** Anti-retro viral therapy (ART) using zidovudine, lamivudine, etc.

DISORDERS OF MENTSTRUAL CYCLES

DYSMENORRHEA

- Dysmenorrhea is painful menstruation
- Types: Primary or spasmodic and secondary or congestive.

Primary Dysmenorrhea

> Primary dysmenorrhea is one where there is no identifiable pelvic pathology.

> **Primary Dysmenorrhea**
> - Mostly confined to adolescents
> - Almost always confined to ovulatory cycles
> - The pain is usually caused following pregnancy and vaginal delivery
> - The pain is related to dysrhythric uterine contraction and uterine hypoxia.

Findings

- The pain begins a few hours before or just with the onset of menstruation.
- Severity of pain usually lasts for few hours, may extend to 24 hours but seldom persists beyond 48 hours.
- The pain is spasmodic and confined to lower abdomen; may radiate to back and medial aspect of thighs.
- Systemic discomforts such as nausea, vomiting, fatigue, diarrhea and headache may be associated.
- Vasomotor changes leads to pallor, cold sweats and occasional fainting. Rarely syncope and fainting occurs.

Pain in Dysmenorrhea

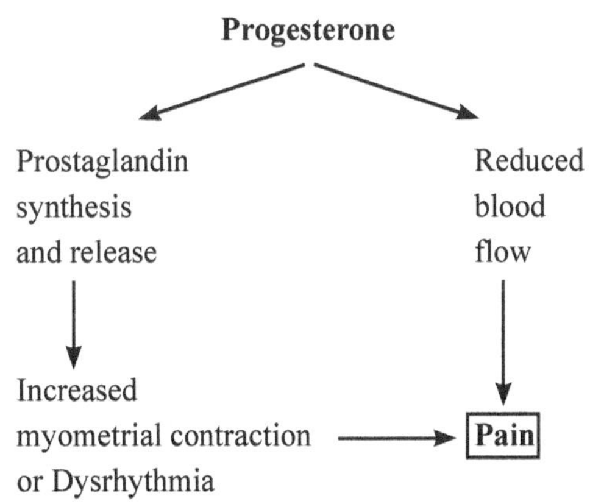

Treatment

- Improvement of general health.
- Psychotherapy.
- Analgesics and antipyretics.
- Prostaglandin synthetase inhibitors, e.g. mefenamic acid, naproxen, indomethacin.
- Oral contraceptives.
- In severe cases, dilatation of cervical canal, paracervical block, and presacral neurectomy, etc. may be performed.

Secondary Dysmenorrhea

- Menstruation associated pain occurring in the presence of pelvic pathology.

- Pain may be related to increasing tension in the pelvic tissue due to premenstrual pelvic congestion or increased vascularity in the pelvic organs.
- **Findings**: Dull pain, usually situated in the back without any radiation usually appears 3 to 5 days before the onset of menstruation and relieves with the start of bleeding.

Usually there is no systemic discomfort in secondary dysmenorrhea unlike in primary dysmenorrhea.

Treatment: Aims at the cause depending upon the age and parity of patient and severity of the symptoms.

MITTELSCHMERZ'S SYNDROME (OVULATORY PAIN)

- Pain appears in the mid-menstrual period.
- Pain is usually located in the hypogastrium or to one iliac fossa.
- Rarely lasts more than 12 hours.
- May be associated with high vaginal bleeding or excessive mucoid vaginal discharge.
- **Causes of pain:** Exact cause not known, thought to be due to
  1. Increased tension of the Graafian follicle just prior to rupture.
  2. Contraction of the tubes and uterus.
- **Treatment:** Reassurance, analgesics.
- In severe cases, make periods anovulatory with contraceptive pills.

PREMENSTRUAL SYNDROME (PMS)

- Change in mood or behavior or appearance of some abnormal vague symptoms are usual before menstruation.
- Often noticed in the second half of the menstrual cycle.
- Symptoms are spontaneously relieved following menstruation.

Criteria for diagnosing PMS
- Not related to any organic lesion
- Regularly occurs during the same phase of each menstrual cycle
- Symptom free period during rest of the cycle.

- Fluctuation in the level of estrogen and progesterone may be responsible for PMS.

Symptoms of PMS	
Related to water retention	Abdominal bloating
	Breast tenderness
	Swelling of the extremities
	Weight gain
Emotional instability or mood changes	Irritability
	Depression
	Insomnia
	Anxiety
	Dyspareunia
	Headache

Treatment

1. Assurance.
2. Salt restriction especially in the second half of cycle.
3. Diuretics in the second half of the cycle (frusemide).
4. Pyridoxine especially helpful in 'Pill' associated depression.
5. Tranquilizers and antidepressants in severe cases.
6. Hormones to suppress ovulation and to maintain a uniform hormonal milieu.
7. Oophorectomy in recurrent PMS and if the lady is approaching menopause.

PMS regularly occurs in the same phase of each menstrual cycle, the symptoms are not specific and there is usually no abnormal pelvic finding.

ABNORMAL MENSTRUAL BLEEDING

MENORRHAGIA

- Also called hypermenorrhea.
- Cyclic bleeding at normal intervals.
- Bleeding is either excessive in amount or duration or both.
- Causes may be organic (pelvic, systemic, blood dyscrasias) or endocrinal or functional.

Menorrhagia is seen in pelvic pathologic conditions like fibroid uterus, adenomyosis, tubo-ovarian mass, TB endometritis, retroverted uterus, IUCD, pelvic endometriosis and Granulosa cell tumor of the ovary.

- Treatment depends upon the cause.

EPIMENORRHEA (POLYMENORRHEA)

- Cyclic bleeding where the cycle is reduced to an arbitrary limit of 21 days or less.
- **Causes:**
  1. **Dysfunctional:** Seen during adolescence, preceding menopause and following delivery and abortion.
  2. Ovarian hyperemia as in PID or ovarian endometriosis.
- **Treatment:** Hormonal pills.

METRORRHAGIA

- Irregular, a cyclic bleeding from the uterus.
- Can be bleeding from any part of the genital tract.
- Treatment is based on the cause.

Menometrorrhagia is the term used when the bleeding is so irregular and excessive that the periods cannot be identified at all.

Causes of acyclic bleeding
- DUB: Usually during adolescence, following childbirth and abortion and preceding menopause
- Submucous fibroid
- Uterine polyps
- Carcinoma cervix and endometrial carcinoma.

Causes of contact bleeding
- Carcinoma cervix
- Mucous polyp of cervix
- Vascular erosion of the cervix specially during pregnancy, pill use or tubercular cervix
- Cervical endometriosis.

Causes of intermenstrual bleeding

Apart from the causes of contact bleeding, other causes are:
- Urethral caruncle
- Ovular bleeding
- Breakthrough bleeding in pill use
- IUCD inutero
- Decubitus ulcer.

OLIGOMENORRHEA

- Menstrual bleeding occurring more than 35 days apart and which remain constant at that frequency.
- Causes are usually related to endocrine or systemic disorders.
- Frequently seen during adolescence and preceding menopause.

HYPOMENORRHEA

- When the menstrual bleeding is unduly scanty and lasts for less than two days.
- Causes may be local (uterine synechiae or endometrial TB), endocrine (use of oral contraceptives, thyroid distinction and premenopausal period) or systemic (malnutrition).
- Treatment is directed towards the cause.

DYSFUNCTIONAL UTERINE BLEEDING (DUB)

- State of abnormal uterine bleeding without any clinically detectable organic pelvic pathology—tumor, inflammation or pregnancy.
- Classification
  1. **Primary:** DUB is due to the dysfunction present in the endometrium or in the hypothalamo-pituitary-ovarian axis.
  2. **Secondary:** DUB secondary to organic pathology outside the endometrium or hypothalamo-pituitary-ovarian axis.
  3. **Iatrogenic:** DUB is secondary to IUCD or steroidal contraceptives.
- The abnormal bleeding may be associated with or without ovulation and accordingly grouped into ovular bleeding and anovular bleeding.
- **Investigations**
  1. Pelvic examination
  2. Blood studies
  3. D and C
  4. Leparoscopy, Hysterosalpingography.
- **Treatment**
  1. General: Bed rest, assurance, diet and drugs to correct anemia, treat systemic or endocrine disorders.
  2. Conservative: Hormonal pills, prostaglandin synthetase inhibitors, antifibrinolytic drugs (tranexamic acid).
  3. Surgery: Uterine curettage, endometrial ablation/resection and hysterectomy.

Common causes of abnormal vaginal bleeding
- **Abnormal menstrual bleeding**

  Menorrhagia

  Epimenorrhea

  Metrorrhagia

  Oligomenorrhea

  Inappropriate (by age)
  - Precocious
  - Delayed menopause
  - Postmenopausal

Contd...

Contd...

- **Nonmenstrual bleeding**
  Foreign body
  Urethral caruncles
  Genital malignancy
  Postcoital
  Intermenstrual
  Abortion
  Breakthrough bleeding.

DISPLACEMENT OF THE UTERUS

- Uterus is not a fixed organ.
- It is anteverted and anteflexed.
- Minor variation in position in any direction occurs constantly with changes in posture, with straining, with full bladder or loaded rectum.

When the uterus rests continuously in a position beyond the limit of normal variation, it is known as displacement.

RETROVERSION

- When the long axes of the corpus and cervix are in line and the whole organ turns backwards in relation to the long axis of the birth canal.
- Retroflexion signifies bending backwards of the corpus on the cervix at the level of internal os.
- Retroversion and retroflexion usually occurs together and are called simply retroversion or retrodisplacement.
- **Degrees of retroversion**
  1. **First degree**: The fundus is vertical and pointing towards the sacral promontory.
  2. **Second degree**: The fundus lies in the sacral hollow but not below the internal os.
  3. **Third degree**: The fundus lies below the level of internal os.
- **Causes**
  1. **Developmental:** Lack of tone of uterine muscles due to developmental defects.
  2. **Acquired:** Due to puerperal causes, prolapse, tumors or pelvic adhesions.
- **Findings**
  - Chronic premenstrual pelvic pain
  - Backache
  - Dyspareunia
  - Infertility
  - Confirmed by bimanual examination and rectal examination.

In pregnancy, spontaneous correction of retroversion occurs by 12–14 weeks.

- **Prevention**
  - Empty bladder regularly after delivery or abortion.
  - Regular exercise to increase the tone of pelvic muscles.
  - Encourage lying in prone position for half to one hour once or twice daily in the postpartum period.
- **Treatment**
  - Pessary treatment used previously, now not in use.
  - Surgical correction.

GENITAL PROLAPSE

- Includes descent of the vaginal wall and or the uterus.

Supports of the Uterus

- The uterus is held in anteverted and anteflexed position by the three-tier support system viz. upper-tier, middle-tier and the inferior-tier.
- Upper-tier consisting of endopelvic fascia covering the uterus, round ligaments and broad ligaments. Comparatively weak.
- Middle-tier constituted by the cervicovaginal junction of pelvic cellular tissue, strongest support of the uterus.
- Inferior-tier comprising of the hollow vagina and the pelvic floor gives indirect support to the uterus.

The hammock like arrangement of condensed pelvic cellular tissue is the cardinal support of the uterus.

- **Causes**
  1. **Predisposing factors:** Repeated vaginal delivery, subinvolution, persistent full bladder in the puerperium, congenital weakness of supporting structures.
  2. **Aggravating factors:** Include postmenopausal atrophy, increased intra-abdominal pressure as in chronic cough or constipation, fibroid, malnutrition, cervical polyps, etc.

Types

Vaginal prolapse and uterine prolapse:

1. **Vaginal prolapse:** Anterior wall prolapse results in cystocele and urethrocele, posterior wall prolapse leads to relaxed perineum and rectocele and vault prolapse leads to enterocele.
2. **Uterine prolapse:** May be uterovaginal or congenital.

Degrees of Prolapse

1. **First degree:** The uterus descends down from its normal position (external os at the level of ischial spines) but the external os still remains inside the vagina.
2. **Second degree**: The external os protrudes outside the vaginal introitus but the uterine body still remains inside the vagina.
3. **Third degree (Procidentia or complete prolapse):** The uterine body descends to lie outside the introitus.

Morbid Changes

1. **Mucosal changes:** Vaginal mucosa becomes stretched and if exposed to air, becomes thickened and dry with surface keratinization.
2. Dependent part of the prolapsed mass lying outside the introitus becomes keratinized, leading to cracking, sloughing and ulcerations.
3. Chronic congestion of the vaginal part of the cervix, which lead to hyperplasia and hypertrophy of the fibro-musculo-glandular components.
4. Bladder shows incomplete emptying leading to cystitis.
5. Ureters are compressed and in chronic causes, it can lead to hydroureter.
6. Ascending infection from the bladder leads to pyelitis or pyelonephritis.
7. **Incarceration:** The entire prolapsed mass become edematous and congested.
8. Through the posterior vaginal wall, peritoneal infection may develop.

Signs and Symptoms

1. Feeling of something coming down per vaginum, difficulty in walking as the mass comes out of the introitus.
2. Backache or dragging pain in the pelvis.
3. Urinary symptoms (in cystocele) : Difficulty in passing urine, incomplete evacuation, cystitis, dysuria, stress incontinence, retention of urine.
4. Bowel symptom (in rectocele) difficulty in passing stool.
5. Excessive white or blood stained discharge per vaginun.

- **Treatment**
  1. **Preventive:** Effective arterial, antenatal and postnatal care.
  2. **Conservative:** Improve nutritional status, reassurance, pelvic floor exercises.
  3. Surgery vaginal hysterectomy with pelvic floor repair (PFR), fothergills operation, cervicopexy.

INFERTILITY

- Infertility is defined as a failure to conceive within one or more years of regular unprotected intercourse.
- Primary infertility denotes those patients who have never conceived.
- Secondary infertility indicates previous pregnancy but failure to conceive subsequently within one or more years of regular unprotected intercourse.

> Infertility is defined as a failure to conceive within one or more years of regular unprotected intercourse.

Causes of Infertility

1. **Male factors:** Defective spermatogenesis, destruction of the efferent duct system, failure to deposit sperm high in the vagina, errors in the seminal fluid, etc.
2. **Female factors:** Ovarian dysfunction, impaired tubal function, peritubal adhesions, endometriosis, fibroid uterus, inadequate secretory endometrium, congenital malformations of the uterus, uterine prolapse, acute retroversion of the uterus, anatomic defects of cervix, defect in composition of cervical mucus, chronic cervicitis, vaginal atresia, septate vagina, narrow introitus, vaginitis, etc.
3. **Combined factors:** Include the presence of factors both in the male and female partners causing infertility.

Investigations in Infertility

1. **In the males:** History, systemwise examinations, routine blood and urine examination, seminal fluid analysis, serum FSH, LH, testosterone and TSH, testicular biopsy, sex chromatin study and immunological studies.

Semen Analysis	Normal Study
Volume	2–6 mL
pH	Alkaline (7–9)
Liquefaction	Within half an hour
Count	60 million/mL
Motility	60% progressive forward motility
Morphology	60% normal form.

Semen Analysis	Abnormal Reports
Volume	< 1 mL or > 6 mL
Count	< 20 million/mL or > 350 million per mL.
Pus cells	Plenty (normal 1–2)

Semen Analysis	Other Findings
Acid phosphatase	25000–60000 IU/mL
Zinc	90–250 mg/mL
Fructose	150–600 mg/100 mL

Related Terminology

- **Aspermia:** Failure of formation or emission of semen
- **Oligospermia/Oligozoospermia:** Sperm count less than 20 million per mL.
- **Azoospermia:** No spermatozoa in the semen
- **Asthenospermia:** Reduction in the vitality of spermatozoa.
- **Necrospermia/Necrozoospermia:** The spermatozoa are dead or motionless.
- **Teratospermia/Teratozoospermia:** High number of malformed spermatozoa in the semen.

2. **In the females:** History, gynecologic examination, USG, laparoscopy, vaginal cytology, hormone studies (progesterone, LH, estradiol), endometrial biopsy, cervical mucus studies, ovarian biopsy, tubal insufflation studies, hysterosalpingography, etc.

Treatment of Male Infertility

- Psychological reassurance.
- Evaluate and treat coital problems.
- Avoid smoking/alcohol intake.
- Improvement of general health.
- Drugs: Gonadotrophins, GnRH analogues, testosterone.
- Steroids in case of antisperm antibodies.
- Microsurgery for obstruction of vas deferens.

Treatment of Female Infertility

- Psychological reassurance.
- Nutritional therapy.
- Weight reduction in obese patients.
- Drugs: Ovulogens, gonadotrophins.
- Treat hypothyroidism, diabetes, etc.
- Surgery in polycystic ovary, tuboplasty.
- Steroids in case of antisperm antibodies.
- Myomectomy in uterine fibroids.

ASSISTED REPRODUCTIVE TECHNOLOGY (ART)

Different Methods of ART

1. AIH—Artificial insemination by husband
2. AID—Artificial insemination by donor

Drugs used in induction of ovulation	
Stimulation of ovulation	Clomiphene citrate hMG FSH hCG GnRH
Reduction of increased level of androgen	Dexamethasone
Reduction of increased level of prolactin	Bromocriptine
Substitution therapy Hypothyroidism Diabetes mellitus	Thyroid extract Antidiabetic drugs

3. IUI—Intrauterine insemination
4. IVF—ET—In vitro fertilization and embryo Transfer
5. GIFT—Gamete intrafallopian transfer
6. ZIFT—Zygote intrafallopian transfer
7. MIST—Microinsemination sperm transfer.

Indications of IUI

Hostile cervical mucus
Cervical stenosis
Oligospermia
Immune factors (male and female)
Unexplained infertility

ZIFT was first described by Devroey in 1986. GIFT was first described by Asch in 1984.

Timing of IUI

- **Spontaneous cycles**
  Cervical mucus study and BBT chart, IUI twice on day 12 and 14
- **Clomiphene induced cycles**
  IUI is done on D5 and D7 after completion of CC
- **Urinary LH detection**
  IUI is done 24 hours after color change
- **hCG at 18 mm diameter of follicle**
  IUI done within next 2 days.

BENIGN LESIONS OF THE CERVIX

CERVICAL EROSION

- Condition where the squamous epithelium of the ectocervix is replaced by columnar epithelium which is continuous with the endocervix.

- May be congenital or acquired.
- **Acquired:** During pregnancy, continuous pill users, infection, etc.

Findings

1. Excessive mucoid vaginal discharge.
2. Contact bleeding especially during pregnancy and 'Pill use'.
3. Backache, pelvic pain and infertility in case of associated cervicitis.
4. Bright red area in the ectocervix during speculum examination.

Treatment

1. Cytological studies.
2. Stop contraceptive pills and advise barrier method.
3. Treatment is delayed at least 12 weeks postpartum if detected during pregnancy.
4. Thermal cauterization/cryosurgery/laser therapy, etc. in trouble some cases.

CERVICAL EVERSION (ECTROPION)

- Marked thickening of the cervical mucosa with underlying tissue edema in chronic cervicitis leads to eversion of endocervix.
- In eversion, the lips of the cervix curl upwards and outwards to expose the red looking endocervix, which may be confused with cervical erosion.

CERVICAL TEAR

- Varying degrees of cervical tear may occur during vaginal delivery.
- If there is no superimposed infection and the tear is small, the torn surfaces may appose leaving behind only a small notch.
- During operate procedures of dilation of the cervix, tear may also occur.
- Postmenopausal atrophy or chronic cervicitis predisposes to tear.

CERVICAL CYSTS

Nebothian Cyst: Formed due to blocking of the cervical gland mouth, usually as a result of healing of cervical erosion. The pent up secretion produces cysts of varying sizes. Treatment is directed towards chronic cervicitis.

Endometriotic Cysts: These are situated in the portio vaginalis part of the cervix. The cyst is small and reddish. The implantation of the endometrium occurs during delivery or surgery. The treatment is cauterization or excision.

ELONGATION OF THE CERVIX

- The normal length of the cervix is about 2.5 cm. The vaginal or supravaginal part may elongate.
- Vaginal part is always elongated congenitally.
- Elongation of the supravaginal part is commonly associated with the uterine prolapse.
- Patient may complain of something coming down, dyspareunia or infertility.
- **Treatment:** In congenital elongation, the excess length of the cervix is amputated. In supravaginal elongation, treat associated uterine prolapse.

BENIGN LESIONS OF THE UTERUS

FIBROID

- Commonest benign tumor of the uterus.
- Fibroid is an estrogen dependent tumor.
- Increased incidence is seen during pregnancy and during pill use.
- Growth potentiality is limited during child bearing period.
- Following menopause, there is cessation of growth.
- Types of fibroids:
  1. Interstitial or intramural
  2. Subperitoneal or subserous
  3. Submucous
  4. Pseudocervical
  5. Cervical.

Fate of submucous fibroid

- Surface necrosis
- Polypoid change
- Infection
- Degeneration including sarcomatous change.

- The fibroid consists of unstriped muscles and fibrous connective tissues of varying proportion. Originally, if consists of only muscle element, but later on fibrous tissues intermingle with the muscle bundles.

Secondary changes in fibroids

- Degenerations
- Atrophy
- Necrosis
- Infection
- Vascular changes
- Sarcomatous changes.

- Hyaline degeneration is the most common type of degeneration affecting all sizes of fibroids.
- Cystic degeneration usually occurs following menopause.
- Fatty degeneration is also found after menopause.
- Red degeneration occurs in large fibroid mainly during second half of pregnancy and puerperium.

Findings

1. The majority of fibroids remain symptomatic.
2. Patient may present with infertility.
3. Menorrhagia is the classic symptom of symptomatic fibroid.
4. Dysmenorrhea.
5. Sense of heaviness in the lower abdomen.
6. Myoma may be palpable during abdominal examination.
7. Pelvic examination reveals the swelling with enlarged uterus.

Life threatening complication of fibroids

- Persistent menorrhagia, metrorrhagia leading to severe anemia
- Severe intraperitoneal hemorrhage due to rupture of veins over subserous fibroid
- Severe infection leading to peritonitis or septicemia
- Sarcoma.

Treatment

1. **Symptomatic fibroids:** Drug therapy to reduce blood loss, to minimize the size and vascularity of the tumor. Drugs used are progestogens, androgens, danazol, GnRH analogues, etc.

   Surgery (Myomectomy, hysterectomy) may be done in unresponsive cases.

Hysterectomy is the operation of choice in symptomatic fibroid. The patients over the age of 40 years and in those desirous of further child are the classic indications.

2. **Asymptomatic fibroid:** Judicious observation may be followed if fibroid is less than the size of 12 weeks of pregnancy. If fibroid grows or if there is infertility, surgery may be performed.

BENIGN LESIONS OF THE OVARY

- The benign enlargement of the ovary is usually due to accumulation of fluid inside the functional unit of the ovary.
- The causes are:
  1. Follicular cysts.
  2. Corpus luteum cyst.
  3. Theca lutein and granulosae lutein cysts.
  4. Polycystic ovarian syndrome, endometrial cyst.

Follicular cysts, corpus luteum cyst, theca lutein and granulose lutein cyst and polycystic ovarian syndrome are all functional cysts of the ovary and are collectively called cystic ovary or ovarian cyst.

Features of functional cysts

1. Related to temporary hormonal disorders.
2. Rarely become complicated.
3. Usually not exceeding 5 cm.
4. Spontaneous regression occurs usually following correction of the functional disturbances.
5. Contain clear fluid inside unless hemorrhage occurs.
6. Living epithelium corresponds to the functional epithelium of the unit from which it arises.

FOLLICULAR CYST

- Commonest functional cyst
- Usually multiple and small
- The cause may be hyperestrinism
- Lined by typical granulose cells without lutein cells.
- Usually remain asymptomatic or may produce vague pain.
- Majority of cases are detected accidentally during bimanual examination, USG, laparoscopy or laparotomy.
- **Treatment:** In uncomplicated cases, it should be followed up and during that period combined pills may be given. If the size increases or if there is intracystic hemorrhage, laparotomy and removal is indicated.

Follicular cysts are the commonest functional cyst, usually asymptomatic, uncomplicated cases may be followed up with contraceptive pills, complicated ones may be surgically removed.

CORPUS LUTEUM CYST

- Usually occurs due to over activity of the corpus luteum.
- There is excessive bleeding inside the corpus luteum.
- Progesterone and estrogen secretion continues in the blood filled cyst, so the menstrual cycle is prolonged followed by heavy or continued bleeding.
- Acute intraperitoneal hemorrhage can occur if the intracystic bleeding is heavy.
- Laparotomy and enucleation of cyst is done if there are features of acute abdomen.

Follicular cyst and corpus luteum cysts are uncommon in women taking oral contraceptive pills. If the cyst persists after three months of pill therapy, it is more likely to be a neoplastic cyst.

LUTEIN CYST

- Usually bilateral and caused by excessive chorionic gonadotropin secreted in cases of gestational trophoblastic tumors.
- May also be formed with administration of gonadotropins or even clomiphene to induce ovulation.
- Can be lined by theca lutein cells (theca lutein cysts) or by granulose cells (granulosa lutein cysts).
- Spontaneous regression occurs following treatment with the gonadotropin level returning back to normal.

POLYCYSTIC OVARIAN SYNDROME (PCOS)

- Characterized by excessive androgen production by the ovaries/adrenals, which interferes with ripening of the ovarian follicles.
- First described in 1935 by Stein and Leventhal as a syndrome manifested by amenorrhea, hirsutism and obesity associated with enlarged polycystic ovaries.
- The ovaries are enlarged, thickened and pearly white and there is theca cell hypertrophy.
- **Findings**
  1. The patient complaints of increasing obesity, menstrual abnormalities in the form of oligomenorrhea or amenorrhea.
  2. Infertility.
  3. Hirsutism.
  4. Bilateral enlarged cystic ovaries on internal examination.
- Serum levels: LH level is elevated and/or the ratio LH:FSH is more than 3:1, reversible estradiol estrone ratio reduced SHBG, elevated androstenedione, marginally elevated serum testosterone and DHEA-5.
- Laparoscopy: Polycystic ovaries usually bilateral.

Serum values in PCOS

- Elevated LH level
- LH : FSH > 3 : 1
- Markedly elevated estrone level
- Reversible estradiol : estrone ratio
- Reduced SHBG
- Elevated androstenedione
- Marginally elevated serum testosterone and DHEA-5.

- **Treatment**
  1. **Patient in whom fertility is not confirmed:** Oral combined contraceptive and steroids. Steroids are not used in obese patients. Steroids are effective in minimizing excess adrenal androgen.
  2. **Patients wanting pregnancy:** Ovulation induction by clomiphene citrate with or without dexamethasone or bromocriptine.
  3. **Surgery:** Surgical removal is done in patients who are resistant to medical therapy.

ENDOMETRIAL CYST

- The Endometrium in the ectopic sites has got the potential to undergo changes under the action of ovarian hormones.
- If encysted, the endometrial cyst enlarges with cyclic bleeding. The serum gets absorbed in between the periods and the contact inside becomes chocolate cyst which is commonly located in the ovary.

OVARIAN TUMORS

- The ovary is composed of epithelial cells and derived from the coelomic epithelium, oocytes derived from the primitive germ cells and mesenchymal elements.
- Abnormal growth may occur from any of these elements and the classification is based on the structure from which the growth occurs.

CLASSIFICATION OF OVARIAN TUMOR

1. Epithelial tumor
   - Serous tumor
   - Mucinous cyst adenoma
   - Endometrioid tumors
   - Mesonephroid brenner tumor
   - Mixed epithelial tumors
   - Undifferentiated carcinoma
   - Unclassified epithelial tumors
2. Sex cord stromal tumors
   - Granulosa cell tumors
   - Thecoma
   - Fibroma
   - Androblastoma
   - Gynandroblastoma
   - Unclassified
3. Lipid cell tumor

4. Germ cell tumor
   - Dysgerminoma
   - Endometrial sinus tumor
   - Polyembryoma
   - Teratoma
   - Dermoid syst
5. Gonadoblastoma
6. Unclassified
7. Secondary metastasis.

> Mucinous cyst adenoma, serous cyst adenoma and dermoid cyst are the common varieties of ovarian tumor.

MUCINOUS CYST ADENOMA

- Arises from the totipotent surface epithelium of the ovary.
- Usually bilateral, chance of malignancy is about 5 to 10%.
- Largest benign ovarian tumor, if left uncared becomes a huge size.

SEROUS CYST ADENOMA

- Also arises from the totipotent surface epithelium of the ovary.
- Usually bilateral and has 30% chance of malignancy.
- Intracystic hemorrhage is more likely.

DERMOID CYST

- Arises from the germ cells arrested after the first meiotic division.
- Bilateral in about 15 to 20%, chance of malignancy is 1 to 25%.
- The content of the cyst is predominantly sebaceous material with hair, teeth and bones may also be found.

Findings of Tumors

- Predominantly manifest in the late child bearing period, dermoid cyst is more common during pregnancy.
- Most tumors are asymptomatic, accidently detected during routine abdominal palpation or by a gynecologist or during laparotomy.
- Patient may have heaviness in the lower abdomen.
- A gradually increasing mass in the lower abdomen.
- Dull aching pain in the lower abdomen.
- When huge tumor presses on the great veins, pitting edema of the legs may be present.

> Ascites and right side hydrothorax in association with fibroma of the ovary Brenner, thecoma and granulosa cell tumor are called Meig's syndrome.

Complication of Benign Ovarian Tumors

- Torsion of the pedicle
- Intracystic hemorrhage
- Infection
- Rupture
- Pseudomyxoma peritonei: Mucinous ascites usually secondary to mucinous of intra-abdominal origin.
- Malignancy.

> Torsion of ovaries pedicle is more common in dermoid cyst or serous cyst adenoma.

Treatment

Since complication can occur at any time and the nature of the tumor cannot be assessed clinically, the tumor should be surgically removed.

ENDOMETRIOSIS

The presence of functioning endometrium in sites other than uterine mucosa is called endometriosis.

> Ectopic endometrial tissue found in the myometrium is called endometriosis interna or adenomyosis.

Sites

Abdominal: Ovary, pouch of Douglas uterosacral ligament, broad ligament, rectovaginal septum, rectum and pelvic lymph nodes.

Extra-abdominal: Abdominal scar of hysterectomy, Cesarean section, tubectomy and myomectomy, umbilicus episiotomy scar, vagina and cervix.

Remote Sites

Pleura, lungs, deep tissues of arms and thighs.

> **Common sites of Endometriosis**
> Ovary
> Pouch of Douglas
> Uterosacral ligament
> Rectovaginal septum
> Abdominal scar following hysterectomy.

Causes

1. **Retrograde menstruation (Simpson's theory):** The retrograde flow of menstrual blood through the uterine tubes during menstruation leads to implantation of endometrial fragments in the peritoneal surface of pelvic organs.
2. **Celomic metaplasia:** Chronic irritation of the pelvic peritoneum by the menstrual blood may cause celomic metaplasia which results in endometriosis.
3. **Direct implantation:** The endometrial or decidual tissues start to grow in susceptible individuals when implanted in the new sites.
4. **Lymphatic theory:** Normal endometrium metastasis through the pelvic lymph nodes.
5. **Vascular theory:** Distant metastasis through blood occurs to lungs, pleura, arms, thighs, etc.
6. **Genetic and immunologic factors:** Increased incidence seen in first degree relatives.

> Small black dots called "Powder burns" are seen on the uterosacral ligaments and pouch of Douglas in pelvic endometriosis.

Finding

Symptoms are not related to the extent of the fexon, symptoms are mostly related to the site of lesion and its ability to respond to hormones.

Dysmenorrhea

Menorrhagia

Infertility

Dyspareunia

Pelvic pain

Abdominal pain

Bladder: Frequency of micturition, hematuria

Bowel: Painful defecation, diarrhea, rectal bleeding or malena.

Complications:

1. Endocrinopathy: Corpus luteum insufficiency, luteinized unruptured follicle, anovulation, elevated prolactin level, double LH peak (all leads to infertility).
2. Rupture of chocolate cyst.
3. Intestinal obstruction.
4. Urethral obstruction, hydroureter, hydronephrosis, pyelonephritis.

Treatment

1. **Preventive:** Avoid tubal patency test immediately after curettage or around the time of menstruation, avoid forceful pelvic examination during or shortly after menstruation, etc.
2. **Curative:** Hormonal pills, surgery.

> Conservative surgery in endometriosis includes any surgery for the removal of the uterus and preserving at least one ovary.

CERVICAL INTRAEPITHELIAL NEOPLASIA (CIN)

- Richard in 1966 put forward the concept of cervical intraepithelial neoplasia (CIN).
- CIN is a histopathological condition where part or whole thickness of cervical squamous epithelium is replaced by cells showing varying degrees of atypia.

Risk Factors of CIN

1. Early sexual intercourse
2. Early age of first pregnancy
3. Too many births/too frequent
4. Law socioeconomic status
5. Multiple sexual partners
6. Human papillomavirus (HPV) infection
7. Oral pill users
8. Smoking
9. Herpes simplex virus (HSV) infection.

Diagnosis

1. Cytologic screening by PAP smear
2. Colposcopy.

Treatment

1. **Preventive:** To delay sexual exposure, vulval hygiene, use of condom especially during the early sexual life.
2. **Treatment:** Treat local infection, electrocauterization, cryocauterization, carbon-dioxide laser through colposcopy, conization, total hysterectomy if the patient had completed the family.

Correlation of dysplasia and CIN (WHO)

Dysplasia	CIN	Limit of histology
Mild	CIN I	Basal one-third
Moderate	CIN II	Basal Half to two-third
Severe	CIN III	Whole thickness except one or two superficial layers
Carcinoma *in situ*	CIN III	Whole thickness

CARCINOMA CERVIX (CA CERVIX)

Cancer cervix is the most common cancer in women in most of the developing countries.

FIGO Staging of Carcinoma Cervix	
Preinvasive Carcinoma	
Stage O	Carcinoma *in situ* or intraepithelial carcinoma
Invasive Carcinoma	
Stage I a	Carcinoma strictly confined to the cervix
Stage I b	Depth of invasion more than 5 mm and horizontal spread more than 7 mm.
Stage II	The Carcinoma extends beyond the cervix but has not extended to the pelvic wall.
Stage II a	No obvious parametrial involvement
Stage II b	Obvious parametrial involvement
Stage III	The Carcinoma extends to the pelvic wall. The tumor involves the lower third of the vagina.
Stage III a	No extension to the pelvic wall but to the lower third of the vagina.
Stage III b	Extension on to the pelvic wall and/or hydronephrosis or non-functioning kidney.
Stage IV	The Carcinoma has extended beyond the true pelvic or has involved the bladder or rectum.
Stage IV a	Spread of growth to adjacent organs
Stage IV b	Spread to distant organs

The commonest variety is squamous cell carcinoma (90%) either well differentiated, moderately differentiated.

Mode of Spread

By direct implantation.

Staging

Staging of cervical cancer is based principally on clinical examination and investigation. In case of suspected pelvic inflammation, a course of antibiotic should be given.

Prognosis

- Depends upon the stage of the lesion.
- Endocervical tumors usually are diagnosed later, but grow fast.
- Well differentiated squamous cell carcinoma grows slowly and metastasizes lately.
- Well poorly differentiated squamous cell carcinoma is prognostically poor.
- Lymph node involvement reduces the survival rate by 50%.
- Associated pregnancy enhances the spread.

Findings

Menstrual abnormalities in the form of contact bleeding or bleeding on straining (during defecation), intermenstrual bleeding, excessive white discharge which may be offensive.

Red granular area on speculum examination which bleeds on touch cervix is freely mobile.

Rectal examination reveals the parametrium absolutely free.

Pelvic pain bladder and bowel symptoms, ureteric colic, cachexia anemia, edema of legs, etc. seen in advanced cases.

Complications

- Hydronephrosis
- Pyelonephritis
- Uremia
- Pyometra
- Vesicovaginal fistula
- Rectovaginal fistula
- Hemorrhage and shock
- Sepsis
- Anemia, cachexia
- Metastasis.

Treatment

1. **Preventive:** Identify high-risk cases and give education and screening with PAP smear.
2. **Curative:** Surgery, radiotherapy and combination therapy.

Stage	5 Year survival rate
I	85%
II	55%
III	30%
IV	10%

MALIGNANT OVARIAN TUMORS

20% of ovarian tumors are malignant.

Types

Can be primary or secondary primary can be epithelial or non-epithelial, secondary may be typical or atypical.

Primary	Secondary
Epithelial Non-epithelial	Atypical Typical

> The atypical ovarian malignancy is called Krukenberg tumor with signet ring appearance of cells.

Mode of Spread

1. Implantation
2. Lymphatics
3. Direct
4. Blood spread.

FIGO Staging of Ca Ovary

Stage I	Growth limited to the ovaries
Stage I a	Growth limited to one ovary; no ascites
Stage I b	Growth limited to both ovaries; no ascites
Stage II	Growth involving one or both ovaries with pelvic extension
Stage II a	Extension and/or metastases to the uterus and/or tubes
Stage II b	Extension to other pelvic tissues
Stage III	Tumor involving one/or both ovaries with peritoneal implants outside the pelvis and/or positive or retroperitoneal inguinal lymph nodes.
Stage III a	Tumor grossly limited to true pelvis with negative nodes.
Stage III b	Tumor of both ovaries with abdominal peritoneal surface implants of less than 2 cm; nodes are negative.

Clinical Features

1. Silent in early stage without any specific symptoms
2. Vague discomfort and feeling of abdominal distention
3. Dyspepsia, flatulence
4. Loss of appetite with a sense of bloating after meals
5. Dull aching pain and tenderness over one area
6. Loss of weight
7. Menstrual abnormalities
8. Cachexia, anemia
9. Respiratory distress—due to ascites or due to pleural effusion
10. Hepatomegaly and jaundice in case of liver metastasis.

Treatment

1. Early detection is difficult because of vague symptoms
2. Treatment options are surgery, chemotherapy, radiotherapy and combination therapy.

GENITAL FISTULA

- Abnormal communication between the urinary and genital tract either acquired or congenital with involuntary escape of urine into the vagina.

Types

1. Bladder
   - Vesicovaginal
   - Vesicouterine
   - Vesicourethrovaginal
   - Vesicocervical
2. Urethra
   - Urethrovaginal
3. Ureter
   - Ureterovaginal
   - Ureterouterine
   - Ureterocervical.

Vesicovaginal Fistula (VVF)

Communication between the bladder and vagina and the urine escapes into the vagina causing true incontinence.

Vesicovaginal fistula (VVF) is an abnormal communication between the bladder and the vagina and VVF is the commonest type of genito urinary fistula.

Causes

1. Obstetrical: Due to prolonged labor, traumatic as in case of instrumental delivery or destructive operation. It may also be produced by abdominal operation such as hysterectomy for rupture uterus or cesarean section specially a repeat one.
2. Gynecological: Surgeries like interior colporrhaphy, abdominal hysterectomy for benign or malignant lesions, traumatic (fall, fracture of pelvic bones), malignancy, ischemic necrosis due to radiation, chronic granulomatous infection such as vaginal TB, lympho granuloma venereum.

Types

Juxta cervical (close to the cervix)

Mid vaginal

Juxta urethral (close to the urethra).

Findings

1. History of difficult labor, surgeries, fall, etc.
2. Continuous escape of urine per vagina, patient has no urge to pass urine, pruritis vulvae.
3. Vulval inspection—Watery discharge with ammoniacal smell.
4. Excoriation of vaginal skin.
5. Bladder mucosa may be visibly prolapsed if the fistula is big.

Treatment of VVF

1. **Preventive:** Adequate antenatal care, anticipate obstructed labor and manage properly; take care to prevent bladder injury during pelvic surgery.
2. **Operative:** Assess the size, site and number of fistula, treat vulval and urinary infection if any, local repair of fistula, if fistula is big—skin or muscle grafting may be needed.

Rectovaginal Fistula (RVF)

Abnormal communication between the rectum and vagina with involuntary escape of flatus and or feces into the vagina.

Causes

1. **Congenital**
2. **Acquired:** Obstructed labor, instrumental delivery, trauma during gynecologic surgeries, fall, malignancy, radiation, TB vagina or lympho granuloma venereum, diverticulitis of the sigmoid colon, Crohn's disease involving the anal canal.

Findings

Involuntary escape of flatus and or feces into the vagina, if fistula is small there is incontinence of flatus and loose stool only but not of hard stool.

Rectovaginal examination reveals the size and site of the fistula.

Treatment

1. **Preventive:** Good intractable care, avoid injury to rectum during surgeries.
2. **Definitive:** Repair by flap method or by preliminary colostomy; local repair closure of colostomy method.

Rectovaginal fistula (RVF) is an abnormal communication between the rectum and the vagina with involuntary escape of flatus and or feces into the vagina. Complete perineal tear (CPT) is the commonest cause of RVF.

Complete Perineal Tear (CPT)

Tear of the perineal body involving the sphincter ani externus with or without involvement of the ano- rectal mucosa is called complete perineal tear or third degree perineal tear.

Tear is called old, when passed beyond an arbitrary period of three months following the injury.

Etiology

1. **Obstetrical:** Injury to perineum due to mis- management of second stage, over stretching of the perineum due to large baby, face delivery, outlet contraction with narrow public arch, forceps delivery without episiotomy, inelastic perineum as in perineal scar due to previous operations, extension of central episiotomy, etc.
2. **Gynecological:** Direct injury to perineum by all or physical abuse may lead to trauma on the perineum.

Findings

1. History of inadequate care during childbirth.
2. Inability to hold flatus or farces, soreness over perineal region, absence of perineum, vaginal and rectal mucosa is pinkish and rectal mucosa is reddish in color).
3. Absence of sphincteric grip evidenced when a finger is introduced into the rectum.

Treatment

1. **Preventive:** Proper conduct of the second stage of labor taking due care of the perineum, controlled delivery of the head, avoid delivery by early extension of head, deliver head only during contractions, perform timely episiotomy, take care during delivery of the shoulders.
2. **Operative:** Repair of the perineal tear with restoration of the perineal body (perineorrhaphy).

Important points to be remembered in the prevention of perineal tear.

- Delivery of the head by early extension is to be avoided.
- Controlled delivery of the flexed head in between uterine contractions.
- Timely and judicious mediolateral episiotomy specially in primigravida.
- Occipitoposterior, face, breech or forceps delivery.

INTERSEXUALITY

- Presence of both male and female external or internal genital organs in the same individual causing confusion in the diagnosis of true sex.
- Female intersex or female pseudohermaphrodite: An association of female gonads with male external genitalia.
- Male intersex or male pseudohermaphrodite: An association of male gonads with female external genitalia.
- True hermaphrodite: An individual possessing both ovaries and tests with ambiguity of genital organs.

FEMALE INTERSEX

Adrenal-genital syndrome (congenital adrenal hyperplasia)

- Autosomal recessive disorder.
- Due to inborn error of adrenal steroid metabolism.

- Lack of cortisol production resulting in excess of ACTH production from the pituitary.
- ACTH stimulates the adrenals to produce excess androgens with virilization of female off spring.
- Associated aldosterone deficiency may lead to excess salt depletion.
- Suspected anatomic defects at birth; an enlarged clitoris, presence of penile urethra or hypospadias, absence of tests in the scrotum, fusion of the labia minora.
- Hirsutism and amenorrhea may be the presenting feature around puberty in milder form.

Findings
Adrenogenital Syndrome
Positive bar body
Karyotype 46 XX
Serum 17-hydroxyprogesterone elevated beyond 8 ng/m
Sodium and chloride low, potassium raised
Urinary excretion of pregnanediol and 17-ketosteroids elevated.

Salt loosing syndrome (sodium and chloride less and potassium raises to a feature of congenital adrend hyperplastic or adrenogenital syndrome.

Masculinization due to increased androgen in maternal circulation.

- Drug induced androgenicity due to use of progesterone in early pregnancy complications.
- Danazol used in endometriosis may produce virilization in female offsprings.
- Androgen source may be adrenal tumor, androgen secreting tumor or crushings syndrome of the mother.
- Serum 17-hydroxyprogesterone is normal, history of androgenic drug intake present usually.

DISORDERS OF GONADAL DEVELOPMENT

- **Gonadal dysgenesis:** Patients with female habits in whom the gonads are imperfectly developed.
- Due to cytogenetic abnormality, the germ cells either fail to develop or fail to reach the gonads.
- Gonads are represented by white streaks without any germ cell.
- Turner's syndrome usually presents as primary amenorrhea with delayed secondary sex characters. Characterized by short stature, webbing of the neck, cubius valgus and poor development of secondary sexual characters, mental retardation often associated with coarctation of aorta. Vagina, uterus, fallopian tubes are present. Gonads are streaks without any follicle nor any potentiality to produce hormone.

Turner's syndrome
• Sex chromatin study negative
• Karyotype is 45 X0
• Serum Estriol very low
• Serum FSH and LH elevated.

Pure or True Gonadal Dysgenesis or Gonadal Agenesis

Usually present as primary amenorrhea with delayed development of secondary sex characters.

Average stature, the vagina, uterus and tubes are present, but infertile gonads are bilateral streaks without any potentiality to produce hormones. Uterus is responsive to exogenous estrogen.

Findings: Sex chromatic is doubtful, Karyotype is 46 XX or 46 XY.

Mixed Gonadal Dysgenesis

- Present with ambiguous, external genitalia at birth.
- Patients come around puberty for features of musculinization or primary amenorrhea.
- Features of partial musculinization of the external genitalia, the gonad of one side is testes and on the other side a 'steak'.
- The Karyotype is usually 45 X0/46 XY.

MALE INTERSEX

1. **Androgen insensitivity syndrome (testicular feminization)**
   - Inherited X-linked recessive gene
   - Underlying pathology is the ability of the end organs to respond to androgens.
   - Either there is lack of androgen cytosol receptor or the receptor is defective.
   - Rarely diagnosed prior to puberty; cases present with primary amenorrhea or infertility
   - Cases are female typically and psychologically female with adequate breast development, but there is absence of axillary and pubic hair. External genitalia looks normal. Vagina short and blind, testes are either present in the labia or inguinal canal or intra- abdominal, the gonads secrete MIF (Mullerian Inhibitory Factor).

Findings

- Sex chromatin negative karyotype is 46 XY.
- Serum testosterone is within average level for normal males.
- Serum estriol level high normal range for males.
- Diagnosis confirmed by gonadal biopsy.

KLINEFELTER'S SYNDROME

- Present with infertility, small penis and gynecomastia
- Sex chromatin positive
- Karyotype is XXY or XXXY
- Genitalia small and infertile
- Elevated serum gonadotropins.

TRUE HERMAPHRODITISM

- Both testicular and ovarian tissues are present in an individual in different combination.
- Bilateral Ovo-testis on both sided (commonest).
- Lateral: Ovary on one side and testis on other.
- Unilateral: Testis or ovary on one side and ovotestis on the other.
- Common presentation is ambiguity of external genitalia, the internal structures depend on the degree of differentiation of the associated gonads on that side.
- Sex chromatin is usually positive.
- Karyotype is usually 46 XX or 46 XY and rarely mosaic XX/YY.
- Confirmation of diagnosis by gonadal biopsy.

DIAGNOSIS OF INTERSEX

At Birth

- Ambiguity of sex detected at birth due to either congenital adrenal hyperplasia or to androgenic drugs administered to the mother in early pregnancy.

At Puberty

- Most cases presented at puberty are late manifestation of congenital adrenal hyperplasia, those of gonadal dysgenesis and rarely male intersexes. The child is usually reared up as girl and she is brought either for poor development or secondary sex characters or for primary amenorrhea with or without hirsutism.

MANAGEMENT OF INTERSEX

- Diagnose the correct nature of interest at birth or as early as possible.
- If diagnosis uncertain or the corrective surgery is deferred for the future, the baby is to be reared up as female.
- Adrenogenital syndrome: Suppress excess ACTH secretion by hydrocortisone, replace salt loss, once child is stable surgery to reduce enlarged clitoris should be done, surgery for labial fusion and vaginoplasty should be withheld until puberty.
- Gonadal dysgenesis: If Y chromatin present on karyotyping, remove gonads since there is chance of dysgerminoma or gonadoblastoma in such ovaries. Hormonal therapy help to develop secondary sex characters.
- Male intersex or androgen insensitive syndrome: Child should be reared up like a girl, testes which are azoospermic should be removed along with vaginoplasty, long-term estrogen replacement therapy after gonadectomy.

MENOPAUSE

- Permanent cessation of menstruation at the end of reproductive life due to ovarian follicular inactivity.
- Clinical diagnosis is confirmed following stoppage of menstruation for six consecutive months.
- Premenopause refers to the period prior to menopause.
- Postmenopause refers to the period after menopause.
- Perimenopause refers to the period around menopause.
- Climacteric is the physiologic period in woman's life during which there is regression of the ovarian function. This covers a wide period ranging 5 to 10 years on either side of menopause.
- Age at which menopause occurs is genetically predetermined, cigarette smoking and malnutrition may predispose to early menopause.
- The age of menopause ranges between 45 to 55 years, average being 50 years.

Endocrinology of Climacteric

- Few years prior menopause, along with depletion of the ovarian follicles, the follicles become resistant to pituitary gonadotropins.
- Folliculogenesis is impaired with diminished estradiol production. This decreases the negative feedback effect on hypothalamo-pituitary axis, resulting increases in follicle stimulating hormone, luteinizing hormone also increases subsequently.

- Disturbed folliculogenesis may result in anovulation, oligoovulation, premature corpus luteum and corpus luteal insufficiency.
- Sustained level of estrogens cause endometrial hyperplasia and clinical manifestation of menstrual abnormalities prior to menopause.
- When estradiol production drops down to the optimal level of 20 pg/mL, endometrial growth stops and there will be absence of menstruation.
- After menopause, the stroma cells of the ovary continue to produce androgens because of increase in luteinizing hormone.
- Adrenal glands also secrete androgen. Thus, cumulative effect is a decrease in estrogen- androgen ratio. This results increased facial hair growth and change in voice.

As the obese patient converts more androgens into estrone, they are less likely to develop symptoms of estrogen deficiency and osteoporosis, but more prone for endometrial hyperplasia and endometrial carcinoma.

The secretion of both luteinizing hormone and follicle stimulating hormone are increased due to absent negative feedback effect of estradiol or due to enhanced responsiveness of pituitary to GnRH. Ultimately due to physiologic aging, both follicle stimulating hormone and luteinizing hormone declines along with decline of estrogens.

Organ Changes Associated with Menopause

1. Ovaries shrink in size, become wrinkled and white, there is thinning of the cortex with increase in medullary components, stromal cells abundant with secretary activity.
2. **The uterus:** Becomes smaller and the ration between the body and the cervix reverts to the 1:1 ratio, endometrial becomes thin and atrophic, the cervical secretion becomes scanty.
3. **The vagina:** Becomes narrower due to gradual loss of elasticity, the vaginal epithelium becomes thin, rugae progressively flatten, there is no glycogen, Doderlein's bacilli are absent, pH becomes alkaline.
4. **The vulva:** Atrophic, labia flattened, pubic hair becomes thinner, introitus narrower.
5. **Breast:** Fat is absorbed and the glands atrophy, nipples decrease in size; eventually breast becomes flat and pendulous.
6. **Bladder and urethra:** Epithelium becomes thinner and more prone for damage and infection, dysuria present, frequency, urge or stress incontinence may be present.
7. **Loss of muscle tone:** Leads to pelvic relaxation, uterine descent, and anatomic changes in the urethra and neck of the bladder, pelvic cellular tissue becomes scanty, ligaments supporting the uterus and vagina lose their fore.

Menstruation Pattern Prior to Menopause

Any of the following patterns may be observed.

1. Sudden cessation of menstruation.
2. Gradual hypomenorrhea or infrequent cycles (oligomenorrhea).
3. Irregular with or without excessive bleeding.

> Genital malignancy should be excluded prior to diagnosing premenopausal pattern.

Menopausal Symptoms

Apart from cessation of menstruation, the following symptoms may be seen:

1. **Vasomotor:** Characteristic symptom is 'hot flush', may last for 1 to 2 minutes, frequently associated with profuse sweating, sleep may be disturbed due to night sweats. Associated palpitation and tachycardia may be there.

> Hot flushes are due to peripheral vascular instability; estrogen, progesterone and androgen are responsible.

2. **Genital and urinary:** Dyspareunia, features of atrophic vaginitis and endometritis, urinary urgency, dysuria, stress incontinence and recurrent UTI are seen.
3. **Psychological:** Increased frequency of anxiety, headache, insomnia, irritation and depression.
4. **Health hazards:** Osteoporosis and fracture, rise in lipid levels, triglycerides and cholesterol.

> After menopause, there is increased osteoclastic activity leading to bone resorption and fracture.

Low-density lipoprotein cholesterol increases compared to high-density lipoprotein, so chance of cardiovascular decrease is there.

Diagnosis of Menopause

1. Cessation of menstruation for consecutive six months during climacteric.
2. Appearance of menopausal symptoms, 'hot flush' and 'night sweats'.
3. Vaginal cytology shows features of low estrogen.
4. Serum estradiol < 20 pg/mL.
5. Serum FSH & LH > 100 mLu/mL.

Treatment

1. **Nonhormonal treatment:** Nutrition, diet with ample calcium, exercise, sedatives and tranquilizers to reduce psychological problems.
2. **Hormone replacement therapy (HRT):** Especially prescribed in gonadal agenesis, surgical or radiation menopause.

Contraindication to HRT

- History of breast cancer
- Presence of thrombophlebitis
- Recent history of endometrial cancer
- Active liver disease.

HRT preparations: Oral, subdermal implants transdermal patches and estrogen cream are available.

> Premature menopause is one when the menstruation stops at the age of 35 or earlier.
> Delayed menopause is one when menopause fails to occur even beyond 55 years.

OBJECTIVE QUESTIONS

1. **Starting of menstrual cycle is called**
   a. Ovulation b. Menstruation
   c. Menarche d. Menopause
2. **Pad of subcutaneous adipose connective tissue lying in front of the pubis in female**
   a. Labia majora b. Labia minora
   c. Mons pubis d. Clitoris
3. **The erectile structure in the female which is analogous to penis in male**
   a. Labia majora b. Labia minora
   c. Mons pubis d. Clitoris
4. **Vestibule contains openings except**
   a. Urethra b. Vagina
   c. Bartholin's glands d. Perineum
5. **Bacilli present in vaginal secretion**
   a. Doderlein's bacilli b. *Cl. tetani*
   c. *Cl. Welschii* d. *E. coli*
6. **Muscular layer of the uterus**
   a. Perimetrium b. Myometrium
   c. Endometrium d. Isthmus
7. **The part of the fallopian tube where fertilization takes place**
   a. Isthmus b. Interstitium
   c. Ampulla d. Infundibulam
8. **Gonads in the female**
   a. Testes b. Labia minora
   c. Ovaries d. Clitoris
9. **Skene's glands are homologous to**
   a. Testis b. Epididymis
   c. Prostate d. Penis
10. **Levator ani contains muscles except**
    a. Pubococcygeus b. Iliococcygeus
    c. Ischiococcygeus d. Symphysis pubis
11. **Pouch of Douglas is**
    a. Uterovesical pouch b. Rectouterine pouch
    c. Urethrovesical pouch d. Rectovesical pouch
12. **Fold of peritoneum attached to broad ligament**
    a. Mesovarium b. Ligament of ovary
    c. Ligamentum teres d. Mesometrium
13. **Average weight of uterus**
    a. 100 gms b. 50 gms
    c. 25 gms d. 10 gms
14. **Uterus is developed from the**
    a. Urogenital sinus b. Sinovaginal sinus
    c. Mullerian ducts d. Uterovaginal canal
15. **Cryptomenorrhea is**
    a. Early menarche
    b. Late menarche
    c. Pent up blood inside the vagina behind the hymen
    d. Narrow introitus
16. **Hematometra is**
    a. Collected blood in the uterine cavity
    b. Collected blood in the vagina
    c. Imperforate hymen
    d. Blood in the tubes
17. **Collected blood in the fallopian tubes**
    a. Pyometra b. Hematometra
    c. Hematocolpos d. Hematosalpinx
18. **Permanent cessation of menstruation**
    a. Menarche b. Menopause
    c. Menorrhagia d. Metrorrhagia
19. **Menopausal symptoms include the following except**
    a. Dry vagina b. Hot flushes
    c. Dysuria d. *S.estradiol* > 100 pg/mL
20. **Menopausal women are at risk for**
    a. Osteoporosis b. Hypotension
    c. High HDL d. Pregnancy

21. **The common complaint of a woman with IUCD is**
a. Vaginal bleeding b. Pelvic infection
c. Uterine perforation d. Abdominal pain

22. **Transparent mucoprotein covering of ovum**
a. Hyaluronidase b. Zona pellucida
c. Corona radiata d. Chorionic laeve

23. **Contraindications of HRT include all except**
a. Breast carcinoma b. Thrombophlebitis
c. Liver disease d. Gastritis

24. **GnRH is produced by**
a. Hypothalamus b. Anterior pituitary
c. Posterior pituitary d. Ovary

25. **Anterior pituitary produces all except**
a. FSH b. ADH
c. LH d. Prolactin

26. **TSH is produced from**
a. Posterior pituitary b. Anterior pituitary
c. Hypothalamus d. Uterus

27. **Oxytocin is produced from**
a. Posterior pituitary b. Anterior pituitary
c. Hypothalamus d. Uterus

28. **Menstrual function is significantly disturbed in**
a. Cardiovascular problems
b. GIT problems
c. Respiratory dysfunction
d. Thyroid dysfunction

29. **During menopause, the serum estradiol level falls below**
a. 110 pg/mL b. 100 pg/mL
c. 50 pg/mL d. 20 pg/mL

30. **The type of cell division occurring in the germ cell**
a. Mitosis b. Meiosis
c. Multiplication d. Mutation

31. **Ruptured Graphian follicle after ovulation is called**
a. Corpus albicans b. Granulosa cells
c. Corpus luteum d. Theca cells

32. **In menstrual cycle, FSH increases during the**
a. Follicular phase b. Menstruation
c. Secretory phase d. Postovulatory phase

33. **The life span of corpus luteum**
a. 30 days b. 280 days
c. 120 days d. 14 days

34. **Size of mature ovum**
a. 50 microns b. 70 microns
c. 100 microns d. 130 microns

35. **Absense of ferning in cervical mucus is a sign of**
a. Anovulation b. Ovulation
c. Infertility d. Fertilization

36. **Transvaginal aspiration of peritoneal fluid**
a. Culdocentesis b. Endometrial biopsy
c. Endoscopy d. Hysterography

37. **A viscid whitish discharge from the vagina**
a. Dysmenorrhea b. Leukorrhea
c. Menorrhagia d. Metrorrhagia

38. **Inflammation of vulva**
a. Vaginitis b. Cervicitis
c. Vulvitis d. Endometritis

39. **Inflammation of the Bartholin's glands**
a. Vaginitis b. Cervicitis
c. Bartholinitis d. Endometritis

40. **Use of stereoscopic binocular microscope to examine cervical epithelium, vagina and vulva**
a. Colposcopy b. Culdoscopy
c. Ultrasonography d. Hysteroscopy

41. **Soft tissue radiographic breast examination to detect breast lesions**
a. Culdoscopy b. Ultrasonography
c. Hysteroscopy d. Mammography

42. **Painful intercourse**
a. Dysmenorrhea b. Dyspareunia
c. Premenstrual syndrome d. Menorrhagia

43. **Emotional and physical disturbance that occur cyclically in female before menstruation**
a. Dysmenorrhea b. Premenstrual syndrome
c. Menorrhagia d. Metrorrhagia

44. **Most common benign tumor of female genital tract**
a. Fibroma b. Endometriosis
c. Adenoma d. Leiomyoma

45. **Surgical modification of the size or shape of the breast**
a. Mammogram b. Mammoplasty
c. Mammotomy d. Breast reduction

46. **Excessive growth of male breast**
a. Gynecomastia b. Mastodynia
c. Mammogram d. Mammoplasty

47. Surgically planned incision on the perineum and posterior vaginal wall during delivery

a. Perineorrhaphy b. Perineal tear
c. Vulval tear d. Episiotomy

48. Commonest obstetric operation performed

a. Perineorrhaphy b. Perineal tear
c. Vulval tear d. Episiotomy

49. The endometrium of pregnancy

a. Decidua b. Perimetrium
c. Corona radiata d. Chorionic frontosum

50. The part of fallopian tube lying in the uterine wall

a. Interstitium b. Isthmus
c. Ampulla d. Infundibulum

51. The part of the fallopian tube which lies nearer to the ovary

a. Interstitium b. Isthmus
c. Ampulla d. Infundibulum

52. Fingerlike projections in the fallopian tube

a. Interstitium b. Isthmus
c. Fimbriae d. Ampulla

53. Female gonads

a. Testes b. Ovaries
c. Fallopian tube d. Cervix

54. Ovary is attached to broad ligament by

a. Ovarian ligament b. Ligament of ovary
c. Mesovarium d. Posterior ligament

55. Pelvic floor consists of the following muscles except

a. Pubococcygeus b. Iliococcygeus
c. Ischiococcygeus d. Sacrococcygeal

56. Pelvic floor muscles are otherwise called

a. Perineal muscles
b. Levator animuscles
c. Puborectalis group
d. Anterior group of muscles

57. The muscle that controls the external and internal anal sphincter

a. Perineal muscles
b. Levator ani muscles
c. Puborectalis muscle
d. Anterior group of muscles

58. Deliberate cutting of perineum during delivery

a. Perineorrhaphy b. Episiotomy
c. Perineoplasty d. Herniorrhaphy

59. The peritoneal pouch between bladder and the uterus

a. Uterovesical pouch b. Retroperitoneal fold
c. Rectovaginal pouch d. Pouch of Douglas

60. The peritoneal pouch between the uterus and the rectum

a. Uterovesical pouch b. Retroperitoneal fold
c. Rectovaginal pouch d. Pouch of Douglas

61. The double fold of peritoneum extending from the uterus to the lateral wall of the pelvis

a. Round ligament b. Broad ligament
c. Uterosacral ligament d. Rectosacral ligament

62. GnRH is produced by

a. Hypothalamus b. Posterior pituitary
c. Anterior pituitary d. Ovaries

63. The other name for GnRH

a. FSH b. LH
c. LHRH d. TRH

64. The hormone concerned with the release of FSH and LH

a. TRH b. TSH
c. CRH d. GnRH

65. FSH and LH are produced by

a. Hypothalamus b. Posterior pituitary
c. Anterior pituitary d. Ovaries

66. The hormone responsible for the formation and maintenance of corpus luteum

a. FSH b. LH
c. LHRH d. TRH

67. LH surge occurs at

a. 24 hours before ovulation
b. 24 hours after ovulation
c. 48 hours before ovulation
d. 48 hours after ovulation

68. The production of corticosteroids in the adrenal cortex is stimulated by

a. FSH b. ACTH
c. LHRH d. TRH

69. **Hormone responsible for the pigmental changes during puberty and in pregnancy**
   a. TSH b. MSH
   c. GnRH d. LHRH

70. **Vasopressin is produced by**
   a. Hypothalamus b. Posterior pituitary
   c. Anterior pituitary d. Ovaries

71. **Oxytocin is produced by**
   a. Hypothalamus b. Posterior pituitary
   c. Anterior pituitary d. Ovaries

72. **Ovulation and steroidogenesis are the functions of**
   a. Hypothalamus b. Pituitary gland
   c. Ovaries d. Adrenals

73. **Contraction of myoepithelial cells during lactation is caused by**
   a. Vasopressin b. Prolactin
   c. Oxytocin d. FSH

74. **The hormone responsible for follicular rupture during ovulation**
   a. Estrogen b. Progesterone
   c. Relaxin d. Inhibin

75. **Isolated development of breast tissue before the age of 8 years**
   a. Premature puberty b. Premature pubarche
   c. Premature thelarche d. Premature menarche

76. **Development of secondary sexual characteristics before the age of 8 or menstruate before the age of 10 years**
   a. Precocious puberty b. Premature puberty
   c. Premature pubarche d. Premature menarche

77. **Delayed puberty is one when the menstruation occurs after the age of**
   a. 12 years b. 14 years
   c. 16 years d. 18 years

78. **Anovulatory cycles produce**
   a. Scanty menstrual bleeding
   b. Heavy and prolonged menstrual bleeding
   c. Delayed puberty
   d. Growth spurt

79. **Acidic vaginal pH is due to the presence of**
   a. Bartholin's glands b. Doderlein's bacilli
   c. *E. coli* d. Klebsiella

80. **The pH of vagina during child bearing period**
   a. 6–8 b. 6–7
   c. 4–5 d. 5–7

81. **PID includes all except**
   a. Endometritis b. Salpingitis
   c. Pelvic peritonitis d. Cervicitis

82. **Violin string like adhesions of perihepatitis is seen in**
   a. Chlamydial infection b. *E. coli* infection
   c. HIV d. HPV infection

83. **Proof of successful treatment after salpingitis**
   a. HSG b. USS
   c. Intrauterine pregnancy d. Ovulatory pain

84. **Primary site of pelvic tuberculosis may be**
   a. Uterus b. Ovaries
   c. Fallopian tubes d. Vagina

85. **Tobacco-pouch appearance of the tube is seen in**
   a. Pyosalpinx b. Salpingitis
   c. Genital TB d. Gonorrhea

86. **Gonorrhea is caused by**
   a. *Neisseria gonorrhoeae* b. *Chlamydia trachomatis*
   c. *Treponema pallidum* d. *Haemophilus ducreyi*

87. **Chancroid is caused by**
   a. *Neisseria gonorrhoeae* b. *Chlamydia trachomatis*
   c. *Treponema pallidum* d. *Haemophilus ducreyi*

88. **Nongonococcal urethritis is caused by**
   a. *Neisseria gonorrhoeae* b. *Chlamydia trachomatis*
   c. *Treponema pallidum* d. *Haemophilus ducreyi*

89. **Syphilis is caused by**
   a. *Neisseria gonorrhoeae* b. *Chlamydia trachomatis*
   c. *Treponema pallidum* d. *Haemophilus ducreyi*

90. **Monilial vaginitis caused by**
   a. *Neisseria gonorrhoeae* b. *Chlamydia trachomatis*
   c. *Treponema pallidum* d. *Candida albicans*

91. **The virus responsible for cervical intraepithelial neoplasm**
   a. Hepatitis B b. HIV
   c. HPV d. HCV

92. **Gonococcal vaginitis in adults usually does not occur due to the resistance offered by**
   a. Squamous epithelium b. Columnar epithelium
   c. Transitional epithelium d. Tubular cells

93. AIDS is caused by

a. Hepatitis B
b. Human immunodeficiency virus
c. HPV
d. HCV

94. Drug used in the treatment of gonorrhea

a. Procaine penicillin b. Nevirapine
c. Azithromycin d. Acyclovir

95. Painless ulcer without any surrounding inflammatory reaction is seen in

a. Chancroid b. AIDS
c. HPV infection d. Syphilis

96. Test done to diagnose syphilis

a. ELISA test b. Western blot test
c. VDRL d. HBsAg

97. Drug used in the treatment of syphilis

a. Procaine penicillin b. Nevirapine
c. Azithromycin d. Acyclovir

98. HSV type II produces

a. Syphilis b. Chancroid
c. Gonorrhea d. Herpis genitalis

99. Vertical transmission of AIDS occurs in

a. Man to woman b. Man to man
c. Mother to child d. Father to child

100. Drug used in the treatment of AIDS

a. Procaine penicillin b. Nevirapine
c. Azithromycin d. Acyclovir

101. Mittelschmerz's syndrome is

a. Premenstrual syndrome b. Ovulatory pain
c. Menorrhagia d. None of these

102. Cyclic bleeding at normal intervals either excessive in amount or duration

a. Menorrhagia b. Epimenorrhea
c. Metrorrhagia d. Polymenorrhea

103. Cyclical bleeding where the cycle is reduced to 21 days or less

a. Menorrhagia b. Epimenorrhea
c. Metrorrhagia d. Oligomenorrhea

104. Irregular acyclic bleeding from the uterus

a. Menorrhagia b. Epimenorrhea
c. Metrorrhagia d. Polymenorrhea

105. Epimenorrhea is otherwise called

a. Oligomenorrhea b. Polymenorrhea
c. Menorrhagia d. Metrorrhagia

106. Menstrual bleeding occuring more than 35 days

a. Oligomenorrhea b. Polymenorrhea
c. Menorrhagia d. Metrorrhagia

107. Unduely scanty menstrual bleeding lasting less than two days

a. Oligomenorrhea b. Hypomenorrhea
c. Menorrhagia d. Metrorrhagia

108. State of abnormal uterine bleeding without any clinically detectable pelvic organic athology

a. Menorrhagia
b. Metrorrhagia
c. Dysfunctional uterine bleeding
d. Epimenorrhea

109. Latrogenic dysfunctional uterine bleeding is due to

a. Salpingitis
b. HSG
c. IUCD insertion
d. Hypothalamic dysfunction

110. When the long axis of the uterus is in line with cervix and the whole organ is reflected backwards, it is called

a. Anteversion b. Anteflexion
c. Retroversion d. Retroflexion

111. Descend of vaginal wall and the uterus

a. Displacement b. Genital prolapse
c. Retroversion d. Anteversion

112. Third degree uterine prolapse is otherwise called

a. Procidentia b. Cystocele
c. Rectocele d. Urethrocele

113. Urinary symptoms are predominantly seen in

a. Procidentia b. Cystocele
c. Rectocele d. Vault prolapse

114. Bowel symptoms are predominantly seen in

a. Procidentia b. Cystocele
c. Rectocele d. Vault prolapse

115. Fothergill's operation is done for

a. Cervical tear b. Cervical cancer
c. Uterine infection d. Uterine prolapse

116. **Normal pH of semen**
a. 6–7 b. 5–6
c. 7–9 d. 8–10

117. **Normal sperm count**
a. 30 million/mL b. 20 million/mL
c. 60 million/mL d. 80 million/mL

118. **Failure of formation or emission of semen**
a. Aspermia b. Oligospermia
c. Azoospermia d. Asthenospermia

119. **No spermatozoa in the semen**
a. Aspermia b. Oligospermia
c. Azoospermia d. Asthenospermia

120. **Reduction in the vitality of the spermatozoa**
a. Aspermia b. Oligospermia
c. Azoospermia d. Asthenospermia

121. **Sperm count less than 20 million/mL**
a. Aspermia b. Oligospermia
c. Azoospermia d. Asthenospermia

122. **Dead or motionless spermatozoa is seen in**
a. Necrospermia b. Oligospermia
c. Azoospermia d. Asthenospermia

123. **High number of malformed spermatozoa in the semen**
a. Necrospermia b. Oligospermia
c. Teratospermia d. Asthenospermia

124. **Drug used for induction of ovulation**
a. Dexamethasone b. Thyroid extracts
c. Clomiphene citrate d. Bromocriptine

125. **Drug used to reduce the increased level of androgen**
a. Dexamethasone b. Thyroid extracts
c. Clomiphene citrate d. Bromocriptine

126. **Drug used to reduce the increased level of prolactin**
a. Dexamethasone b. Clomiphene citrate
c. hMG d. Bromocriptine

127. **hMG is used to**
a. Induce ovulation
b. Reduce the increased level of androgen
c. Reduce the increased level of prolactin
d. Improve thyroid function

128. **An assisted reproductive technique**
a. GIFT b. GERD
c. ECSL d. IUCD

129. **Condition where the squamous epithelium of the ectocervix is replaced by columnar epithelium**
a. Cervical tear b. Cervical erosion
c. Cervical polyp d. CIN

130. **Cervical erosion is precipitated by**
a. Polyps
b. Contraceptive pill use
c. IUCD
d. Assisted reproductive techniques

131. **Ectropion is**
a. Cervical erosion b. Cervical polyp
c. Cervical eversion d. Cervical tear

132. **D and C may predispose to**
a. Cervical erosion b. Cervical polyp
c. Cervical eversion d. Cervical tear

133. **Cyst formed due to blocking of cervical gland mouths**
a. Endometrial cyst b. Sebacious cyst
c. Bartholins' cyst d. Nabothian cyst

134. **Elongation of cervix may be associated with**
a. Cervical cysts b. Uterine prolapse
c. Cervical polyps d. Cervicitis

135. **Commonest benign tumor of the uterus**
a. Fibroid b. Endometritis
c. CIN d. Endometriosis

136. **Degeneration occurs to the fibroid during pregnancy**
a. Hyaline degeneration b. Cystic degeneration
c. Red degeneration d. Sarcomatous changes

137. **Commonest asymptomatic, functional cyst of the ovary**
a. Follicular cyst b. Theca lutein cyst
c. PCOD d. Granulosa lutein cyst

138. **Disease characterized by excessive androgen production in the ovary**
a. Ovarian cyst b. Polyps
c. PCOD d. Fibroids

139. **Hirsutism and obesity are seen in**
a. Follicular cyst b. Theca lutein cyst
c. Granulosa lutein cyst d. PCOD

140. **Ovarian cyst which contain sebaceous material, teeth, bone hair, etc.**
a. Mucinous cyst b. Serous cyst
c. Dermoid cyst d. Germ cell tumor

141. Presence of functioning endometrial tissue in sites other than the uterine mucosa

a. Endometritis b. Endometriosis
c. Endometrial cyst d. Ectropion

142. Powder burns in the uterosacral ligaments are seen in

a. Endometritis b. Ectropion
c. Endometrial cyst d. Endometriosis

143. Krukenberg tumor is

a. Atypical ovarian tumor b. Endometritis
c. Endometriosis d. PCOD

144. Signet ring appearance of cell is seen in

a. Krukenberg tumor b. Meig's syndrome
c. Gonadoblastoma d. Dysgerminoma

145. Abnormal communication between bladder and the vagina

a. VVF b. RVF
c. UVF d. VCF

146. Commonest type of genitourinary fistula

a. VVF b. RVF
c. UVF d. VCF

147. Abnormal communication between rectum and the vagina

a. VVF b. RVF
c. UVF d. VCF

148. Cervical tear is the commonest cause of

a. VVF b. VCF
c. RVF d. UVF

149. Surgery performed for perineal tear

a. Perineotomy b. Perineorrhaphy
c. Fistulectomy d. None of these

150. Salt loosing syndrome is a feature of

a. Congenital adrenal hyperplasia
b. Intersex
c. Gonadal dysgenesis
d. Testicular feminization

151. 45 XO karyotype is seen in

a. Turner's syndrome
b. Congenital adrenal hyperplasia
c. Cushing's syndrome
d. Gonadal dysgenesis

152. XXY or XXXY karyotype is seen in

a. Gonadal dysgenesis
b. Klinefelter's syndrome
c. Congenital adrenal hyperplasia
d. Cushing's syndrome

153. Permanent cessation of menstruation

a. Menarche b. Menorrhagia
c. Metrorrhagia d. Menopause

154. Menstruation stops when the estradiol production is less than

a. 40 pg/mL b. 50 pg/mL
c. 20 pg/mL d. 10 pg/mL

155. The following symptoms are seen after menopause except

a. Hot flushes b. Tachycardia
c. Atrophic vaginitis d. Bradycardia

156. Women after menopause are prone for

a. Dysmenorrhea b. Osteoporosis
c. Hypotension d. Breast cancer

157. Contraindication for HRT include the following except

a. History of breast cancer
b. Thrombophlebitis
c. Cardiovascular disease
d. Gastritis

158. Induction of abortion is permitted up to

a. 10 weeks of pregnancy b. 12 weeks of pregnancy
c. 18 weeks of pregnancy d. 22 weeks of pregnancy

159. Commonest site of tubal pregnancy

a. Infundibulum b. Ampulla
c. Isthmus d. Interstitial

160. Signs of ectopic pregnancy includes the following except

a. Amenorrhea b. Abdominal pain
c. Abdominal distension d. Vaginal bleeding

161. Average menstrual blood loss is

a. 80 mL b. 30 mL
c. 20 mL d. 50 mL

162. Causative organism of genital warts

a. HPV b. Poxvirus
c. Staphylococcus d. Streptococcus

163. Gene thought to be responsible for breast cancer
a. BRCA gene
b. CRP
c. ANA
d. Carcino embryonic antigen

164. Organ homologous to male scrotum
a. Labia minora b. Clitoris
c. Labia majora d. Mons pubis

165. The male sex hormone is called
a. Vasopressin b. Gonadotropic hormone
c. FSH d. Testosterone

166. Urinary bladder is line with
a. Simple epithelium
b. Stratified epithelium
c. Transitional epithelium
d. Pseudostratified epithelium

167. MCH service includes
a. Prenatal and postnatal care
b. Under fives care
c. Family planning service
d. All of them

168. A packet of oral pill (Mala-N) contains
a. 28 pills b. 30 pills
c. 31 pills d. 42 pills

169. Hormone having anti-inflammatory effect
a. Estrogen b. Progesterone
c. Corticosteroids d. Gonadotropins

170. The position used to treat shock and decreased blood pressure
a. Lithotomy position
b. Genupectoral position
c. Dorsal recumbent position
d. Trendelenburg position

171. Minilap operation is
a. Removal of a small piece of each fallopian tube and ligating each
b. The fallopian tubes are cut and ends are blocked
c. Removal of the fallopian tubes
d. Application of rings to occlude the fallopian tube

172. Copper carrying contraceptive devices acts by
a. Preventing ovulation
b. Prevent spermatozoa coming in contact with ovum
c. Destruction of spermatozoa
d. Making cervical mucus thick to prevent penetration of spermatozoa

173. How many chromosomes are found in a cell of human being?
a. 23 b. 28
c. 46 d. 48

174. A cartilaginous joint between the pubic bone is
a. Symphysis pubis b. Sacroiliac joint
c. Synovial joint d. Coccyx

175. In addition the OS is closed in case of
a. Complete abortion b. Inevitable abortion
c. Septic abortion d. Threatened abortion

176. Which of the following destroys HIV?
a. Dettol b. Savlon
c. Sodium hypochlorite d. Lysol

177. Abnormal opening between rectum and vagina
a. Rectovaginal fistula b. Urethrovaginal fistula
c. Vesicovaginal fistula d. Genital prolapse

178. The most frequent side effect associated with the use of IUCD is
a. Ectopic pregnancy b. Expulsion of IUCD
c. Rupture of uterus d. Excessive menstrual flow

179. Abnormal opening between bladder and vagina
a. Rectovaginal fistula b. Urethrovaginal fistula
c. Vesicovaginal fistula d. Genital prolapse

ANSWER KEY

1. c	2. c	3. d	4. d	5. a	6. b	7. c	8. c	9. c	10. d	11. b	12. a
13. b	14. c	15. c	16. a	17. d	18. b	19. d	20. a	21. a	22. b	23. d	24. a
25. b	26. b	27. a	28. d	29. d	30. b	31. c	32. a	33. d	34. d	35. a	36. a
37. b	38. c	39. c	40. a	41. d	42. b	43. b	44. a	45. b	46. a	47. d	48. d
49. a	50. a	51. d	52. c	53. b	54. c	55. d	56. b	57. c	58. b	59. a	60. d
61. b	62. a	63. c	64. d	65. c	66. b	67. a	68. b	69. b	70. b	71. b	72. c
73. c	74. c	75. c	76. a	77. c	78. b	79. b	80. c	81. d	82. a	83. c	84. c
85. c	86. a	87. d	88. b	89. c	90. d	91. c	92. a	93. b	94. a	95. d	96. c
97. a	98. d	99. c	100. b	101. b	102. a	103. b	104. c	105. b	106. a	107. b	108. c
109. c	110. c	111. b	112. a	113. b	114. c	115. d	116. c	117. c	118. a	119. c	120. d
121. b	122. a	123. c	124. c	125. a	126. d	127. a	128. a	129. b	130. b	131. c	132. d
133. d	134. b	135. a	136. c	137. a	138. c	139. d	140. c	141. b	142. d	143. a	144. a
145. a	146. a	147. b	148. c	149. b	150. a	151. a	152. b	153. d	154. c	155. d	156. b
157. d	158. b	159. b	160. c	161. d	162. a	163. a	164. c	165. d	166. c	167. d	168. a
169. c	170. d	171. b	172. d	173. c	174. a	175. d	176. c	177. a	178. d	179. c	

Chapter 8

Nutrition

Nutrition is the science of food and its relationship to health. It is concerned primarily with the role of nutrients in body growth, development and maintenance.

Dietetics is the practical application of the principles of nutrition, and includes the planning of meals for the well and the sick.

FUNCTIONS OF FOOD

1. Supply of energy
2. Body building and repair
3. Maintenance and regulation of tissue formation.

CONSTITUENTS OF FOOD

- Carbohydrates
- Proteins
- Fats
- Vitamins
- Minerals
- Water.

Proteins, fats and carbohydrates are called "proximate principles" or energy yielding foods. Together with water, they form the bulk food.

Composition of human body	
Constituents	**Percentage**
Water	63
Protein	17
Fat	12
Minerals	7
Carbohydrates	1

CLASSIFICATION OF FOODS

1. **Classification by origin:**
   i. Foods of animal origin
   ii. Foods of plant origin.
2. **Classification by chemical composition:**
   i. Proteins
   ii. Fats
   iii. Carbohydrates
   iv. Vitamins
   v. Minerals.
3. **Classification by predominant function:**
   i. Body building foods, e.g. milk, meat, poultry, fish, eggs, pulses, groundnuts, etc.
   ii. Energy-giving foods, e.g. cereals, sugars, roots and tubers, fats and oils.
   iii. Protective foods, e.g. vegetables, milk, fruits.
4. **Classification by nutritive value:**
   i. Cereals and millets
   ii. Pulses (legumes)
   iii. Vegetables
   iv. Nuts and oilseeds
   v. Fruits
   vi. Animal foods
   vii. Fats and oils
   viii. Sugar and jiggery
   ix. Condiments and spices
   x. Miscellaneous foods.

NUTRIENTS

Nutrients are organic and inorganic complexes contained in food. Each nutrient has specific function in the body. Most natural foods contain more than one nutrient. They may be divided into:

1. **Macronutrients:** These are proteins, fats and carbohydrates, which are often called "proximate principles" because they form the main bulk of food. In the Indian menu, they contribute to the total energy intake in the following proportion:

Constituents	Percentage
Protein	7–15%
Fat	10–30%
Carbohydrates	65–80%

2. **Micronutrients:** These are vitamins and minerals. They are called micronutrients because they are required in small amounts which may vary from a fraction of a milligram to several grams.

PROTEINS

Proteins ate compounds of carbon, hydrogen, oxygen, nitrogen and sulfur. They are made up of simpler substances called amino acids. There are around 22 amino acids needed in the human body; out of which eight are called essential. These are called essential because the body cannot synthesize them in sufficient quantity and therefore they must be obtained from the food we eat.

FUNCTIONS OF PROTEINS

1. For growth and development.
2. For repair of body tissues and their maintenance.
3. For synthesis of antibodies, enzymes and hormones.

Proteins are also a source of energy.

1 gm protein yields 4 calories.

SOURCES OF PROTEINS

1. **Animal sources:** Milk, egg, meat, fish, etc.
2. **Plant sources:** Pulses, cereals, nuts, etc.

Protein content of some foods

Food	Protein (g per 100 g of food)
Animal foods	
Milk	3.2–4.3
Meat	18.0–26.0
Egg	13.0
Fish	15.0–23.0
Plant foods	
Cereals	6.0–13.0
Pulses	21.0–28.0
Vegetables	1–4
Fruits	1–3
Nuts	4.5–29.0
Soybean	43.2
Others	
Oils and fats	Nil
Sugar and jaggery	Nil

Pulses are called poor man's meat.

Soybean is unique among the pulses because it contains over 40% protein.

PROTEIN REQUIREMENTS

Indian Council of Medical Research (ICMR) recommends 1gm/kg body weight for an Indian adult.

EFFECTS OF PROTEIN DEFICIENCY

The effects of protein deficiency are:

1. **During pregnancy:** Still birth, low birth weight, anemia.
2. **Infancy and early childhood:** Marasmus, kwashiorkor, mental retardation, stuned growth and development.
3. **Adults:** Loss of weight, under weight, poor musculature, anemia, increased susceptibility to infection, frequent loose stools, general lethargy, incapacity to sustained work, delay in wound healing, cirrhosis of liver, edema, ascites, etc.

FATS

Fats are composed of carbon, hydrogen and oxygen. They are composed of smaller units called fatty acids. Some fats are liquid at room temperature (e.g. groundnut oil, gingeli oil). Some fats such as ghee and butter are solid at room temperature.

CLASSIFICATION OF FATS

Fats are classified into saturated and unsaturated fats. Animal fats are saturated fats and vegetable oils and fats are unsaturated fats.

Recommended protein allowances	
Group	**Protein allowance gm/kg/day**
Man (60 kg)	1.00
Woman (50 kg)	1.00
Infants	
0–3 months	2.50
3–6 months	1.80
6–9 months	1.65
9–12 months	1.50
Children	
1–3 years	1.83
4–6 years	1.52
7–9 years	1.48
Adolescent—Male	
10–12 years	1.46
13–15 years	1.40
16–18 years	1.31
Adolescent—Female	
10–12 years	1.45
13–15 years	1.33
16–18 years	1.21

Cardiovascular disease is attributed to excessive consumption of saturated fats.

Functions of Fats

1. Dietary fat is a concentrated source of energy.
2. Fats are acrriers of fats soluble vitamins viz. vitamin A, D, E and K.
3. Dietary fats supplies essential fatty acids.

Linoleic acid, one of the essential fatty acids (EFA) prevents skin scaling.

4. The fat layer under the skin helps to maintain body temperature.
5. Fats provide support for many organs in the body such as heart, kidney, intestine, etc.

Sources

1. **Animal sources:** Ghee, butter, fat of meat, fish oils.
2. **Vegetable sources:** Vegetable oils viz. groundnut, gingelly, mustard, cotton seed, sunflower and coconut oil.

1 g of fat give 9 calories

Fat Requirements

Dietary fats provides 30 to 40 % of total energy intake. WHO expert committee now recommends only 20 to 30% of total dietary energy to be provided by fats.

- Excessive intake of fat predisposes to coronary artery disease.
- Deficiency of essential fatty acids causes dry and rough skin or toad skin (Phrenoderma).

CARBOHYDRATES

Carbohydrates are composed of carbon, hydrogen and oxygen. They are the cheapest source of energy.

In balanced diets, carbohydrates provide not more than 50 to 60% of total calories.

Carbohydrates, when taken in excess, are converted to body fat.

Sources of Carbohydrates

1. **Starches:** Cereals (rice, wheat), roots and tubers (potatoes).
2. **Sugars**
   a. Monosaccharides: Glucose, fructose and galactose.
   b. Disaccharides: Sucrose, lactose and maltose.
3. **Cellulose:** Vegetables, fruits and cereals.

Cellulose acts as a roughage and prevents constipation.

Daily energy requirements		
Age group	**Weight in kg**	**Energy kcal**
Birth–6 months	3–7	600
6 months–1 year	7–9	800
1–3 years	9–13	1200
4–6 years	15–17	1500
7–9 years	18–21	1800
10–12 years	23–28	2100
Reference man	60 kg	2700
Reference woman	50 kg	2000

VITAMINS

Vitamins are complex chemical substances. They are required by the body in very small amounts. They do not yield energy like fats or carbohydrates. They are vital for the very survival of man because they take part as catalysts in various body processes. They protect the body against ill health, infection and disease.

Around 13 vitamins are needed for the well-being of the body. Since the body cannot manufacture vitamins in sufficient quantity, they must be supplied through the diet.

Classification of Vitamins

1. **Fat soluble vitamins:** Vitamin A or retinol, vitamin D, E and K.
2. **Water soluble vitamins:** Vitamin B_1 or thiamine, vitamin B_2 or riboflavin, nicotinic acid, pyridoxine or vitamin B_6, pantothenic acid, folic acid, vitamin B_{12} and ascorbic acid or vitamin C.

VITAMIN A

Vitamin A is a fat soluble vitamin, the chemical name being retinol.

Functions

1. It is needed for the normal vision and health of the eyes.
2. It is needed for the health of the epithelial tissue (e.g. skin, mucous membrane) of the body.
3. It is connected with growth, especially skeletal growth.
4. It is anti-infective. It protects the body against microbial infection.

Sources

1. **Animal sources:** Foods of animal origin such as butter, ghee, egg, milk, liver and fish are good sources of vitamin A.
2. **Plant sources:** The cheapest source of vitamin A is green leafy vegetables, such as spinach, amaranth, coriander and drum stick leaves. Vegetables such as carrots, pumpkin and ripe fruits, e.g. mangoes, papaya, tomatoes, etc. are also rich sources.

A daily intake of 100 gm of leafy vegetables provide the daily requirement of vitamin A.

In vegetables and fruits, vitamin A occurs in a precursor form called carotene. The greener the leafy vegetable, the higher the carotene content. The carotene is converted to vitamin A in the small intestine and stored in the liver.

3. **Fish liver oils:** The richest natural sources of vitamin A are the fish liver oils.

1 teaspoonful of shark liver oil supplies about 6000 IU of vitamin A.

4. **Synthetic:** Vitamin A is available in the synthetic form as capsules (soft gels) and syrups.

Daily Requirement

The recommended daily intake of vitamin A is 750 μg for adults.

Under vitamin A prophylaxis program, children below 6 years are given every 6 months an oral dose of 2,00,000 IU of vitamin A to prevent/control the nutritional blindness.

Vitamin A Deficiency

1. **Night blindness:** Inability to see in dim light is the earliest symptom of vitamin A deficiency.
2. **Xerophthalmia:** Early clinical sign of vitamin A deficiency in which the conjunctiva becomes dry. Conjunctiva also appears muddy and wrinkled.
3. **Bitot's spots:** Brownish, triangular, raised foamy patches seen on the conjunctiva.
4. **Keratomalacia:** The cornea becomes soft and loses its transparency. If not treated early it leads to complete collapse or destruction of the eye ball, resulting in blindness.

Night blindness, Xerophthalmia, Bitot's spots and Keratomalacia are the clinical signs of vitamin A deficiency. Nutritional blindness is blindness due to vitamin A deficiency.

Dietary sources of vitamin A

Sources	IU of vitamin A per 100 gm
Milk, whole	180
Fish	100
Egg	2200
Ghee	2500
Spinach	5500
Amaranth	2500–11000
Cabbage	2000
Carrots	2000–4300
Mangoes, ripe	4800
Papaya, ripe	2020
Cod liver oil	6000
Shark liver oil	9000–60000

VITAMIN D

Vitamin D exists in vitamin D_2 or ergocalciferol and vitain D_3 or cholecalciferol.

Functions

1. Vitamin D is required for the formation of healthy bones and teeth. It has a direct action on the mineralization of the bones.
2. It promotes the intestinal absorption and utilization of calcium and phosphorus.

> Vitamin D is required for the formation of healthy bones and teeth.

Sources

Sunlight: The provitamin 7-dehydrocholesterol present in the skin is converted to vitamin D_3 by the action of the ultraviolet rays of the sunlight. The synthesis if vitamin D_3 depends upon the amount of melanin present in the skin and the exposure to the sun.

> The heavier the melanin in the skin, the lesser will be the synthesis of vitamin D_3.

Dietary Sources of Vitamin D

Item	μg per 100 g
Egg	1.5
Butter	0.5–1.5
Liver	30–40
Milk	0.1

Daily Requirement

Adults need 2.5 μg (100 IU) of vitamin D per day. Normal adults usually obtain enough amounts by exposure to sunlight.

Hypervitaminosis can occur if vitamin D is taken in excessive amounts as it is stored in the body. Symptoms of hypervitaminosis D include nausea, vomiting, loss of appetite, excessive urination, etc. In case of extreme toxicity, soft tissues like kidneys, lungs and heart can be calcified leading to death.

Vitamin D Deficiency

Deficiency leads to rickets in children and osteomalacia in adults. In both these conditions the bones contains less calcium.

> Vitamin D deficiency leads to rickets in children and osteomalacia in adults.

VITAMIN E

The role of vitamin E in human body is not clear. Animal studies have shown that deficiency of vitamin E is associated with habitual abortion, testicular and myocardial degeneration.

> Vitamin E or tocopherol is known as anti-sterility vitamin.

The richest sources of vitamin E are vegetable oils. For example, oils of sunflower seeds, cotton seeds and safflower seeds. Vitamin E is available in small quantities in meat, fruits and vegetables.

VITAMIN K

Vitamin K is synthesized to some extent by intestinal bacteria. It is necessary for proper clotting of blood.

> Vitamin K is synthesized by intestinal bacteria. So malabsorption can lead to vitamin K deficiency.

The vitamin K requirement of man is met by a combination of dietary intake and microbial synthesis in the gut. The normal daily requirement is about 0.03 mg/kg of body weight for the adult.

> Newborn infant tend to be deficient in vitamin K due to minimal stores of prothrombin at birth and lack of an established intestinal flora.

Since newborn infants are having deficiency of vitamin K, all infants should receive a single intra-muscular dose of vitamin K preparation (0.5 mg of vitamin K).

VITAMIN B_1 OR THIAMINE

Vitamin B_1 is a water soluble vitamin, otherwise known as thiamine.

Functions

1. Thiamine plays an important part in carbohydrate metabolism.
2. Thiamine is also essential for the proper functioning of the nervous system.

Sources

Thiamine is widely distributed in small amounts in all natural foods. The richest sources are un milled cereals, pulses and nuts, especially groundnut.

Thiamine is readily lost from cereals during the process of washing and cooking. The milling of rice results in considerable loss of thiamine. Parboiled and home pounded rice are better sources. Thiamine in fruits and vegetables is partly lost during prolonged storage.

Thiamine in Food Stuffs

Deficiency: Thiamine deficiency leads to beriberi and Wernicke's encephalopathy.

> Moderate deficiency of thiamine manifests itself in the form of loss of ankle and knee jerks and calf tenderness.

Food stuff	mg/100 gm
Wheat, whole	0.54
Rice, home pounded	0.21
Milled rice	0.06
Gingelly seeds	1.01
Groundnut	0.90
Liver	0.36
Hen's egg	0.13
Milk, whole	0.05

VITAMIN B_2 OR RIBOFLAVIN

Riboflavin is involved in the protein, fat and carbohydrate metabolism.

Sources: Good sources of riboflavin are milk and milk products, eggs, liver and green leafy vegetable. Wheat, millets and pulses are fair sources, but rice is a poor source.

> Riboflavin is synthesized by the bacteria in the large intestine which is an additional source.

Daily requirement: 0.6 mg per 1000 calories intake.

Deficiency of riboflavin leads to angular stomatitis, cheilosis, soreness of the tongue, redness and burning sensation in the eyes and dermatitis.

> Riboflavin is essential for protein, fat and carbohydrate metabolism. The signs of riboflavin deficiency include angular stomatitis, cheilosis, soreness of the tongue, redness and burning sensation in the eyes and dermatitis.

NIACIN

Niacin or nicotinic acid is required by the body for the utilization of carbohydrate and for tissue respiration.

Sources: Whole grain cereals, pulses, nuts, meat, liver and chicken.

The daily requirement: 6.6 mg per 1000 calories intake.

Deficiency of niacin leads to pellagra which is characterized by soreness of the tongue, pigmented scaly skin and diarrhea. Severe deficiency leads to mental disturbances.

> Niacin is required for the utilization of carbohydrate and tissue respiration. Deficiency of niacin leads to pellagra characterized by soreness of the tongue.

VITAMIN B_6 OR PYRIDOXINE

Pyridoxine plays an important role in the metabolism of amino acids, fats and carbohydrate.

Sources: Liver, meat, fish, whole cereals and legumes.

Deficiency: Pyridoxine deficiency leads to skin lesions, cheilosis, glossitis and convulsions in children.

Adults require 2 mg per day of pyridoxine.

FOLIC ACID

Folic acid is essential for the synthesis of DNA.

Sources: Green leaves, liver, pulses, nuts and whole grain.

Deficiency: Deficiency leads to anemia.

Requirement: For healthy adults, the daily requirement is 100 microgram, during pregnancy, the requirement increases to 400 microgram.

VITAMIN B_{12}

Necessary for the synthesis of DNA, carbohydrate, fat and protein metabolism.

Sources: Liver, egg, fish and milk.

> Foods of vegetable origin do not contain vitamin B_{12}. So, B_{12} deficiency is seen in strict vegetarians who do not even take milk.

Deficiency: Deficiency of vitamin B_{12} leads to pernicious anemia characterized by marked decrease in the number of RBC. Vitamin B_{12} deficiency also affects the nervous system including spinal cord.

Requirement: For adults, the daily requirement is 1 microgram.

> For proper utilization of vitamin B_{12}, an intrinsic factor secreted by the parietal cells of gastric mucosa is essential. So patients after gastrectomy usually suffer from pernicious anemia.

VITAMIN C OR ASCORBIC ACID

Vitamin C is a water soluble vitamin. It gets destroyed by high temperature, oxidation, drying or storage.

> Vitamin C is the most unstable of all the vitamins.

Functions

1. Needed for the formation of collagen, the protein substance that binds the cells together.
2. Helps in blood clotting.
3. Increases the absorption of iron.
4. Increases the general resistance of the body to fight infection.

Sources: All fresh fruits, green leafy vegetables. Amla is the richest source; citrous fruits and guava are also rich sources. Meat and milk contain very small amounts.

> Amla is the richest source of Vitamin C; citrous fruits and guava are also rich sources.

Deficiency: Deficiency leads to scurvy, a bleeding disorder.

Requirement: Adults need 40 mg of vitamin C per day.

> Vitamin C deficiency leads to scurvy, a disease characterized by bleeding phenomena.

MINERALS

- The body contains about 24 minerals; all of which should be supplied from the diet.
- They are classified into major elements and trace elements.
- **Major minerals:** Iron, calcium, phosphorous, sodium, etc.
- **Trace elements:** Fluorine, iodine, cobalt, zinc.

Functions

1. Calcium, phosphorous and magnesium are needed for bones and teeth.
2. Some minerals form part of body fluids and maintain osmotic pressure.
3. Iron is needed for blood formation.

> 99% of body calcium is found in the bones. Calcium is needed by the body for the formation and maintenance of bones and teeth, for blood coagulation and for regulation of neuromuscular activity. Iron is required for the formation of hemoglobin and also for oxygen transport. Iron deficiency leads to anemia.

REVIEW QUESTIONS

1. **Science of food**
   a. Dietetics b. Nutrition
   c. Food hygiene d. Diet therapy
2. **An energy yielding food**
   a. Fish b. Liver
   c. Meat d. Rice
3. **Proteins are**
   a. Energy yielding foods b. Body building foods
   c. Protective foods d. Fatty foods
4. **Water constitutes**
   a. 35% of body weight b. 40% of body weight
   c. 63% of body weight d. 90% of body weight
5. **All of the following are macronutrients except**
   a. Carbohydrates b. Proteins
   c. Fats d. Vitamins
6. **Proteins are made up of**
   a. Fatty acids b. Amino acids
   c. Glycerol d. Glucose
7. **Fatty acids that the body cannot synthesis by its own**
   a. Essential fatty acids b. Trans fatty acids
   c. Keto acids d. Ketone bodies
8. **The repair of body tissues and their maintenance requires**
   a. Carbohydrates b. Fats
   c. Proteins d. Minerals
9. **1 gm of protein yields**
   a. 2 kcals b. 4 kcals
   c. 6 kcals d. 9 kcals
10. **Richest source of protein**
    a. Oils b. Nuts
    c. Egg d. Soybean
11. **Poor man's meat**
    a. Carbohydrates b. Proteins
    c. Fats d. Minerals
12. **Protein requirement of adult per day**
    a. 0.5 gm/day b. 0.1 gm/day
    c. 1 gm/day d. 1.5 gm/day
13. **Fatty acids are smaller units of**
    a. Carbohydrates b. Minerals
    c. Proteins d. Fats
14. **A source of fat which is liquid at room temperature**
    a. Groundnut oil b. Ghee
    c. Butter d. Vanaspati

15. Cardiovascular disease is attributed to excessive consumption of

a. Coconut oil b. Proteins
c. Saturated fats d. Gingelly oil

16. Fats are carriers of the following vitamins

a. Vitamin C b. Vitamin A
c. Vitamin B_1 d. Vitamin B_2

17. One gram of fat provides

a. 4 kcals b. 6 kcals
c. 7 kcals d. 9 kcals

18. Deficiency of EFA predisposes to

a. Scleroderma b. Phrenoderma
c. CAD d. PEM

19. 'Toad skin' is due to the deficiency of

a. EFA b. Carbohydrates
c. Vitamins d. Minerals

20. Carbohydrates, when taken in excess, are converted to

a. Glucose b. Proteins
c. Body fat d. Starches

21. A fat soluble vitamin

a. Vitamin D b. Vitamin C
c. Vitamin B_{12} d. Vitamin B_2

22. The following are fat soluble vitamins except

a. Vitamin A b. Vitamin D
c. Vitamin E d. Vitamin C

23. Vitamin needed for the health of the epithelial tissues

a. Vitamin E b. Vitamin D
c. Vitamin A d. Vitamin C

24. A water soluble vitamin

a. Vitamin A b. Vitamin C
c. Vitamin D d. Vitamin E

25. Precursor of vitamin A

a. Nicotinic acid b. Cholecalciferol
c. 7-dehydrocholesterol d. Carotene

26. Richest source of vitamin A

a. Butter b. Fish liver oil
c. Ghee d. Liver

27. The dose of vitamin A given in vitamin A prophylaxis program

a. 100000 IU b. 200000 IU
c. 250000 IU d. 300000 IU

28. Nutritional blindness is caused by

a. Cataract
b. Retrolental fibroplasias
c. Deficiency of vitamin A
d. Glaucoma

29. Deficiency of vitamin A produces all of the following except

a. Night blindness b. Xerophthalmia
c. Bitot's spots d. Pellagra

30. Brownish, triangular, raised, foamy patches seen on the conjunctiva due to vitamin A deficiency

a. Keratomalacia b. Xerophthalmia
c. Scleroderma d. Bitot's spots

31. Keratomalacia is

a. Toad skin
b. Phrenoderma
c. Loss of transparency of lens due to deficiency of vitamin A
d. Inability to see in dim light

32. Vitamin needed for healthy bones and teeth

a. Vitamin A b. Vitamin C
c. Vitamin D d. Vitamin E

33. Deficiency of vitamin D leads to

a. Keratomalacia b. Rickets
c. Pellagra d. Sterility

34. Osteomalacia is due to the deficiency of

a. Vitamin A b. Vitamin E
c. Vitamin C d. Vitamin D

35. Tocopherol is

a. Vitamin A b. Vitamin C
c. Vitamin E d. Vitamin B_2

36. Anti-sterility vitamin

a. Vitamin A b. Vitamin D
c. Vitamin C d. Vitamin E

37. Rich source of vitamin E

a. Sunflower oil b. Meat
c. Vegetables d. Fruits

38. Vitamin needed for blood clotting

a. Vitamin A b. Vitamin B
c. Vitamin E d. Vitamin K

39. Malabsorption syndrome can lead to the deficiency of

a. Vitamin A b. Vitamin E
c. Vitamin K d. Vitamin C

40. As a routine, all newborns are given an intra-muscular dose of vitamin

a. A b. B
c. C d. K

41. Thiamine is

a. Vitamin B_1 b. Vitamin B_2
c. Vitamin B_6 d. Vitamin B_{12}

42. The B-vitamin lost during milling of rice

a. Vitamin B_{12} b. Vitamin B_6
c. Vitamin B_2 d. Vitamin B_1

43. Thiamine deficiency leads to

a. Rickets b. Beriberi
c. Pellagra d. Xerophthalmia

44. Niacin deficiency causes

a. Pellagra b. Rickets
c. Beriberi d. Bitot's spots

45. Pyridoxine is

a. Vitamin B_1 b. Vitamin B_2
c. Vitamin B_6 d. Vitamin B_{12}

46. Pernicious anemia is due to the deficiency of

a. Vitamin A b. Vitamin D
c. Vitamin B_1 d. Vitamin B_{12}

47. Ascorbic acid is the other name for

a. Vitamin A b. Vitamin C
c. Vitamin D d. Vitamin E

48. Deficiency of vitamin C leads to

a. Night blindness b. Scleroderma
c. Rickets d. Scurvy

49. Mineral needed for the development of bones and teeth

a. Iron b. Magnesium
c. Iodine d. Calcium

50. Mineral needed for the formation of hemoglobin

a. Iron b. Iodine
c. Calcium d. Magnesium

ANSWERS

1. b	2. d	3. b	4. c	5. d	6. b	7. a	8. c	9. b	10. d	11. b	12. c
13. d	14. b	15. c	16. b	17. d	18. b	19. a	20. a	21. a	22. d	23. c	24. b
25. d	26. b	27. b	28. c	29. d	30. d	31. c	32. c	33. b	34. d	35. c	36. d
37. a	38. d	39. c	40. d	41. a	42. d	43. b	44. a	45. c	46. d	47. b	48. d
49. d	50. a										

Chapter 9

Objective Questions on Nursing Research

1. **The variable which is known from the beginning and does not change is called the**
   a. Confounding variable
   b. Extraneous variable
   c. Dependent variable
   d. Independent variable

2. **Random sampling or probability sampling includes all the following techniques, except**
   a. Purposive sampling
   b. Cluster sampling
   c. Simple random sampling
   d. Stratified random sampling

3. **The degrees of freedom in a table with 3 rows and 2 columns**
   a. 1
   b. 2
   c. 3
   d. 4

4. **The phenomenon of those who obtain extreme scores at pretest tending to obtain less extreme scores at post-test, at both the high and low ends of the measure is**
   a. Internal validity
   b. Statistical validity
   c. Statistical regression
   d. Statistical power

5. **The concept of statistical power in the social and behavioral sciences was first introduced by**
   a. Kolmogrov
   b. Carl Pearson
   c. Spearman
   d. Jacob Cohen

6. **Gender, age-class, religion, type of disease, and blood group are measured as**
   a. Ratio
   b. Nominal
   c. Ordinal
   d. Interval

7. **Which scale of measurement has an absolute zero?**
   a. Nominal
   b. Ordinal
   c. Ratio
   d. Interval

8. **The degrees of freedom for a 2 × 2 contingency table for Chi-squire distribution is**
   a. 0.05
   b. 1
   c. 2
   d. 4

9. **The probability that a given effect will be detected using a sample of a specified size, with the probability level of the statistical test being set at a predetermined level is**
   a. Internal validity
   b. Power of a statistical test
   c. Reliability of a study
   d. External validity

10. **The variable which is influenced by the intervention of the researcher is called**
    a. Dependent
    b. Independent
    c. Extraneous
    d. Discrete

11. **Type I errors occur**
    a. Accepting the null hypothesis when it should have been rejected.
    b. When the null hypothesis is rejected but it should have been retained.
    c. When the obtained p-value is higher than 0.05.
    d. Considering the alternate hypothesis as false when it actually it was true.

12. **The statistical approach which helps the investigator to decide whether the outcome of the study is a result of factors planned within design of the study or determined by chance**
    a. Normal distribution
    b. Standard deviation
    c. Descriptive statistics
    d. Inferential statistics

13. **The degree of flatness or peakedness of a graph of a frequency distribution is termed as**
    a. Standard deviation
    b. Mode
    c. Skewness
    d. Kurtosis

14. **The standards of critiquing qualitative research include, except**
    a. Methodological congruence
    b. Heuristic relevance
    c. Chance for committing Type-I error
    d. Analytical and interpretative preciseness

15. **History as a threat to the internal validity of a particular study refers to**
 a. Groups that are formed not on randomization basis.
 b. An event that takes place between pretest and post-test.
 c. Natural change during the period between baseline and post-test.
 d. The phenomenon of differential attrition during the course of treatment.

16. **A form of graphical presentation of data**
 a. Line diagram b. Histogram
 c. Pie diagram d. Bar diagram

17. **In a negatively skewed distribution, the mean generally falls to**
 a. The right of the median and the median usually lies to the right of the mode.
 b. The middle of median and mode.
 c. The left of the median and the median usually lies to the left of the mode.
 d. The center of the distribution.

18. **All the following are measures of central tendency, except**
 a. Mode b. Mean
 c. Median d. Variance

19. **Which statement about normal distribution is false**
 a. 50% of the observations fall within one standard deviation sigma of the mean
 b. 68% of the observations fall within one standard deviations sigma of the mean
 c. 95% of observation fall within two standard deviations
 d. 99.7% of observations fall within three standard deviations of the mean

20. **The parameters of power analysis are the following, except**
 a. The size of the effect hypothesized or to be detected
 b. The alpha or probability level of the significance test
 c. The size of the sample being studied
 d. Reliability of the rating scale

21. **The measure of central tendency which is influenced by extreme scores and skewed distributions**
 a. Mean b. Median
 c. Mode d. Range

22. **A measure used to standardize the central tendency away from the mean across different samples**
 a. mode b. Range
 c. Skewness d. Z-score

23. **The qualitative method which focuses on description and interpretation of cultural behavior**
 a. Ethnography b. Phenomenology
 c. Grounded theory d. Symbolic interactionism

24. **The probability of making a Type II error in any statistical test**
 a. Alpha b. Beta
 c. Delta d. Theta

25. **A measure of central tendency calculated by numbers arranging in numerical order is**
 a. Mode b. Median
 c. Range d. Standard deviation

26. **The term triangulation was coined by**
 a. Heidegger b. Denzin (1989)
 c. Leininger (1985) d. Glaser and Strauss (1967)

27. **Probability values fall on scale between**
 a. – 3 to + 3 b. – 1 to +1
 c. 0.05 to 0.01 d. 0 and 1.

28. **A characteristic feature of qualitative research**
 a. Inductive process
 b. Deductive process
 c. Control over the context
 d. Fixed research design

29. **The area of inquiry in grounded theory approach is**
 a. Social structural processes within social setting
 b. Holistic view of culture
 c. Lived experiences
 d. Behavior observed over time in natural context

30. **In qualitative research, a guiding principle in deciding sample size is**
 a. Number of variables b. Effect size
 c. Sub-group analysis d. Data saturation

31. **The research design in which the area inquiry is the manner by which people make sense of social interactions**
 a. Ethnography b. Grounded theory
 c. Phenomenology d. Symbolic interactionism

32. Characteristics of qualitative research design are

a. Flexible and elastic design
b. Use of mixed methodologies
c. Ongoing analysis to formulate subsequent strategies
d. All of the above

33. A pharmacology trial concluded that 'a new antipsychotic reduced negative symptoms when in reality it did not'; is an example of

a. Type I error b. Type II error
c. Type III error d. Type IV error

34. The proportion of observations fall above the median is

a. 68% b. 50%
c. 75% d. 95%

35. A qualitative research design

a. Cohort design b. Emergent design
c. Correlative design d. Experimental design

36. Phenomenological study involves all the following features, except

a. Manipulation b. Intuition
c. Analysis d. Description

37. The term refers to the use of multiple referents to draw conclusions about what constitutes the truth

a. Item analysis b. Factor analysis
c. Triangulation d. Error measurement

38. The tendency in qualitative research to derive a complex array of data from a variety of sources, using variety of methods is termed as

a. Conformability b. Triangulation
c. Bricolage d. Cross-tabulation

39. The correlation coefficient provides all of the following types of information, except

a. The strength of the relationship between the variables.
b. Whether or not there is a relationship between the variables.
c. The direction of the relationship between the variables.
d. The cause of the relationship between the variables.

40. Kappa coefficient of reliability is related to

a. Continuous variables
b. Ratio scale of measurement
c. Nominal scale of measurement
d. Interval scale of measurement

41. The indices used to measure variation or dispersion among scores are the following, except

a. Mean b. Range
c. Variance d. Standard deviation

42. Standard error is calculated by

a. Dividing number of nominated outcome by number of possible outcome
b. Dividing standard deviation by the square root of the sample size
c. Adding all the numbers and then dividing by the numbers of observations
d. Arranging the numbers in numerical order, and then taking the middle one

43. Effect size is used to calculate

a. Sample size b. Reliability
c. Predictive validity d. Internal consistency

44. For a two-group comparison study, a standardized measure of effect size is

a. Square of the Pearson correlation coefficient.
b. Chi-square value
c. Eta-squared value
d. The difference between the two means, divided by the average of the standard deviations.

45. The sum of the values of a variable for a set of observations, divided by the number of the observations in the set refers to

a. Mean b. Median
c. Variance d. Standard deviation

46. A measure of dispersion of a set of observations in which it is calculated by the difference between the highest and lowest values produced is called

a. Mode b. Range
c. Standard deviation d. Variance

47. When explaining the direction of the linear association between two numerical paired variables, a positive correlation is stated when

a. One variable increases and the other variable decreases or vice versa
b. Dependent variable increases and independent variable decreases
c. Correlation coefficient is stated close to 0
d. Both variables increase and decrease at the same time

48. Another name for a bar graph is

a. Line graph b. Polygon
c. Histogram d. Normal curve

49. The F-statistic is calculated in

a. Chi-squire test b. ANOVA
c. T-test d. Correlation analysis

50. A non-parametric "Analysis of Variance"

a. Mann-Whitney U-test b. Wilcoxon Rank test
c. Friedman's test d. Kruskal-Wallis test

51. The degrees of freedom for the chi-square test is

a. (R + 1) (C – 1) b. (R – 1) (C – 1)
c. (R × C) – 1 d. (R – 1) (C + 1)

52. A statistic which describes the interval of scores bounded by the 25th and 75th percentile ranks

a. Confidence interval b. Standard deviation
c. Variance d. Inter-quartile range

53. The Median value is the

a. 25th percentile b. 50th percentile
c. 75th percentile d. 95th percentile

54. Large standard deviations suggest

a. The scores not normally distributed.
b. There is very little deference among scores.
c. Scores are probably widely scattered.
d. Mean, median and mode are the same.

55. A type of graphical presentation data used to explain correlation between dependent and independent variable

a. Frequency curve b. Histogram
c. Frequency polygon d. Scatter plot

56. Components required for estimating power (1-beta) of a study are the following, except

a. The population effect size
b. Sample size
c. Level of significance (alpha)
d. Standard deviation

57. Power analysis builds on the concepts of

a. Effect size b. Reliability
c. Validity d. Internal consistency

58. Chi-square test is used to test

a. Difference in means of two independent variables
b. Difference in proportions
c. Relationship between two bivariate variables
d. Difference in means of three or more set of variables

59. Which of the following is not a multivariate statistical approach

a. Analysis of variance
b. Analysis of covariance (ANCOVA)
c. Multiple regression
d. Factor Analysis

60. The formula given below is computational formula for+

$$\sqrt{\frac{\Sigma(x-x)^2}{(n-1)}}$$

x = each score
x = mean
n = the number of values
$\sum$ = sum

a. Mean b. Variance
c. Standard deviation d. t-statistic

61. The reliability of a measuring tool has the following aspects, except

a. Equivalence b. Stability
c. Internal consistency d. Efficiency

62. Studies that produce basic estimates of the rates of disorder in a general population and its subgroups is

a. Descriptive epidemiology
b. Qualitative epidemiology
c. Analytic epidemiology
d. Experimental epidemiology

63. A table that shows how often different scores appear in a set of scores is called

a. Normal curve b. Polygon
c. Distribution d. Histogram

64. The stability index of a measuring tool is derived through procedures that evaluate

a. Test-retest reliability b. Inter-rater reliability
c. Internal consistency d. Cronbach's alpha

65. The number of new cases that occur within a specific population within a defined time interval is

a. Point prevalence b. Incidence
c. Lifetime prevalence d. Period prevalence

66. Correlation coefficient ranges from

a. – 3 to + 3 b. – 1 to + 1
c. 0.01 to 0.05 d. 0 to 1

67. Deductive Reasoning is applied in

a. Qualitative research b. Applied research
c. Quantitative research d. Action research

68. The following is not a criterion for Fisher's exact test

a. When proportions derived from independent groups are compared
b. When there are cells with a value of 0
c. Sample size is small (less than 30)
d. When testing difference between three or more group means

69. The degree of consistency with which an instrument measures the attribute it is supposed to measure

a. Objectivity b. Validity
c. Reliability d. Sensitivity

70. The extent to which the same results are obtained on repeated administrations of the instrument

a. Validity b. Internal consistency
c. Sensitivity d. Stability

71. The Spearman's-Brown formula is used to estimate

a. Validity b. Test-retest reliability
c. Internal consistency d. Equivalence

72. The statistic used to explain the chances of being exposed to a risk among those with the diagnosis divided by exposure to the risk among those without the diagnosis is

a. Kappa b. Phi coefficient
c. Chi-square d. Odds ratio

73. In biomedical research survival analysis is typically used to evaluate

a. Lifetime prevalence b. Incidence of a disease
c. Point prevalence d. Life expectancy

74. The square of the standard deviation is the

a. Variance b. Standard deviation
c. Standard error d. Z-score

75. When doing power analysis in an ANOVA context, the estimate of effect size is

a. Correlation coefficient b. Eta-squared
c. Standard error d. Chi-squire value

76. 95% confidence interval refers to

a. Considering 1 out of 100 chances are taken as wrong.
b. Considering 95 out of 100 chances are taken as wrong.
c. Considering 1 out of 20 chances are taken to be wrong.
d. Considering 5 out of 20 chances are taken as wrong.

77. The Z-score for 97.5th percentile in a distribution

a. – 1.96 b. 0.05
c. + 1.96 d. + 2.5

78. The phi coefficient is used for correlations between

a. Two dichotomous variables
b. Two continuous variables
c. Two set of means
d. Two rating scales

79. A systematic method for continuous monitoring of diseases in a population, in order to be able to detect changes in disease patterns and then to control them is

a. Surveillance b. Conditional probability
c. Screening d. Prevalence

80. Kruskal-Wallis test is used to

a. Test the difference among the means of 3+ related groups
b. Test the difference between two independent group means
c. Test the difference in ranks of scores of 3+ independent groups
d. Test the difference among the means of 3+ independent groups

81. The most appropriate inferential analysis to test the difference among the means of 3+ related group's to sets of scores

a. Friedman test
b. Repeated-measures ANOVA
c. Wilcoxon signed-rank test
d. Paired T-test

82. Which of the following is not a type of validity index of a research instrument

a. Homogenous validity b. Construct validity
c. Content validity d. Concurrent validity

83. The degree to which an instrument measures what it is supposed to be measure

a. Sensitivity b. Validity
c. Internal consistency d. Equivalence

84. A hypothesis which a researcher tries to disprove is

a. Alternate hypothesis b. Research hypothesis
c. Null hypothesis d. Positive hypothesis

85. A contingency table (2×2) is used to calculate

a. Chi-squire statistic b. t-statistic
c. Correlation coefficient d. Variance

86. A qualitative research design in which lived experiences of individuals is examined in their "life-world".

a. Grounded theory b. Ethnography
c. Ethnology d. Phenomenology

87. Using power analysis, the value of estimated effect size (gamma) for large effects in two group test of mean difference is

a. 0.5 b. 0.8
c. 1.0 d. 0-2

88. Analysis of variance (ANOVA) test is used to

a. Test the difference between two related group means
b. Test the difference between two independent group means
c. Test the difference among the means of 3+ independent groups
d. Test the difference in ranks of scores of 3+ independent groups

89. The adequacy of an instrument in differentiating between the performance or behavior on some future criterion is termed as

a. Construct validity b. Predictive validity
c. Concurrent validity d. Content validity

90. In epidemiology research, if the relative risk is greater than 1.0, the group with the suspected risk factor

a. Have a higher incidence rate of the disorder
b. Have a lower incidence rate of the disorder
c. Is having no relationship with the risk factor
d. No conclusive predictions can be done

91. Which of the following is not a method of quantitative research

a. Correlational research
b. Grounded theory research
c. Quasi-experimental research
d. Experimental research

92. The term 'grounded theory' was developed by

a. Denzin b. Heidegger
c. Glaser and Strauss d. Husserl

93. The most common type of composite scale

a. Likert scale b. Questionnaire
c. Visual analog scale d. Checklists

94. Which is not a characteristic of normal distribution

a. Symmetric b. Bell-shaped
c. Negative skewness d. Mean = median = mode

95. Skewness is a measure

a. Which decides whether the distribution may have high or low variance
b. Of the asymmetry of the probability distribution
c. Of central tendency
d. None of the above

96. A tentative explanation/statement of a declaration of the expected outcome of a research study based on observations

a. Hypothesis b. Relationships
c. Analysis d. Variables

97. Multi-trait-multi-matrix (MTMM) is a procedure developed to establish

a. Content validity b. Internal consistency
c. Inter-rater reliability d. Construct validity

98. Which of the following is not a procedure for establishing construct validity of an instrument

a. MTMM b. Known-group technique
c. Factor analysis d. Cronbach's alpha

99. The term "action research" was coined by

a. Jacob Cohen b. Kurt Lewin
c. Glaser and Strauss d. Karl Pearson

100. The formula given below is used to calculate

$$\Sigma\frac{(O-E)^2}{E}$$

O = Observed frequency,
E = Expected frequency

a. Correlation coefficient b. t-test statistic
c. Chi-squire statistic d. Standard deviation

101. In a naturalistic observation, the phenomenon in which the behavior of the subjects being observed changes because they are being watched

a. Representative sampling
b. Observer bias
c. Observer effect
d. Participant observation

102. In the scientific investigation, the first step is:

a. Testing hypothesis b. Reporting your results
c. Drawing conclusion d. Perceiving a question

103. The listed observations 1, 2, 3, 4, 100 suggest the distribution

a. Is negatively skewed
b. Is positively skewed
c. Has zero skewness
d. Is left-skewed

104. The entire group of people or animals in which the researcher is interested

a. Controls
b. Sample
c. Experiment group
d. Population

105. A careful appraisal of the strengths and weaknesses of the study is

a. Evidence-based practice
b. Research critique
c. Research proposal
d. Action Research

ANSWER KEY

1. d	2. a	3. b	4. c	5. d	6. c	7. d	8. b	9. b	10. a	11. b	12. d
13. d	14. c	15. b	16. b	17. c	18. d	19. a	20. d	21. a	22. d	23. a	24. b
25. b	26. b	27. d	28. a	29. a	30. d	31. d	32. d	33. a	34. b	35. b	36. a
37. c	38. c	39. d	40. c	41. a	42. b	43. a	44. d	45. a	46. b	47. d	48. c
49. b	50. d	51. b	52. d	53. b	54. c	55. d	56. d	57. a	58. b	59. a	60. c
61. d	62. a	63. c	64. a	65. b	66. b	67. c	68. d	69. c	70. d	71. c	72. d
73. d	74. a	75. b	76. c	77. c	78. a	79. a	80. c	81. b	82. a	83. b	84. c
85. a	86. d	87. b	88. c	89. b	90. a	91. b	92. c	93. a	94. c	95. b	96. a
97. d	98. d	99. b	100. c	101. c	102. d	103. b	104. d	105. b			

Appendices

Normal Values

Blood Test Reference Range Chart	
Test	**Reference Range (conventional units)**
17-Hydroxyprogesterone (men)	0.06–3.0 mg/L
17-Hydroxyprogesterone (women) Follicular phase	0.2–1.0 mg/L
25-hydroxyvitamin D (25 (OH) D)	8–80 ng/mL
Acidity (pH)	7.35–7.45
Alcohol	0 mg/dL (more than 0.1 mg/dL normally indicates intoxication) (ethanol)
Ammonia	15–50 µg of nitrogen/dL
Amylase	53–123 units/L
Ascorbic acid	0.4–1.5 mg/dL
Bilirubin	Direct: up to 0.4 mg/dL Total: up to 1.0 mg/dL
Blood volume	8.5–9.1% of total body weight
Calcium	8.5–10.5 mg/dL
Carbon dioxide pressure	35–45 mm Hg
CD4 cell count	500–1500 cells/µL
Chloride	98–106 mEq/L
Complete blood cell count (CBC)	Tests include: Hemoglobin, hematocrit, mean corpuscular hemoglobin, mean corpuscular hemoglobin concentration, mean corpuscular volume, platelet count, white blood cell count
Copper	Total: 70–150 µg/dL
Creatine kinase (CK or CPK)	Male: 38–174 units/L; Female: 96–140 units/L
Creatinine	0.6–1.2 mg/dL
Erythrocyte sedimentation rate (ESR)	Male: 1–13 mm/h; Female: 1–20 mm/h
Glucose (fasting)	70–110 mg/dL

Contd...

Contd...

Hematocrit	Male: 45–62%; Female: 37–48%
Hemoglobin	Male: 13–18 g/dL; Female: 12–16 g/dL
Iron	60–160 µg/dL (normally higher in males)
Lactate (lactic acid)	Venous: 4.5–19.8 mg/dL; Arterial: 4.5–14.4 mg/dL
Lactic dehydrogenase	50–150 units/L
Lead	40 µg/dL or less (normally much lower in children)
Lipase	10–150 units/L
Zinc	70–102 µmol/L
Lipids:	
Cholesterol	Less than 225 mg/dL (for age 40–49 years; increases with age)
Triglycerides	10–29 years 53–104 mg/dL
	30–39 years 55–115 mg/dL
	40–49 years 66–139 mg/dL
	50–59 years 75–163 mg/dL
	60–69 years 78–158 mg/dL
	> 70 years 83–141 mg/dL
Liver function tests	Tests include bilirubin (total), phosphatase (alkaline), protein (total and albumin), transaminases (alanine and aspartate), prothrombin (PTT)
Magnesium	1.5–2.0 mEq/L
Mean corpuscular hemoglobin (MCH)	27–32 pg/cell
Mean corpuscular hemoglobin concentration (MCHC)	32–36% hemoglobin/cell
Mean corpuscular volume (MCV)	76–100 cu µm
Osmolality	280–296 mOsm/kg water
Oxygen pressure	83–100 mm Hg
Oxygen saturation (arterial)	96–100%
Phosphorus	3.0–4.5 mg/dL (inorganic)
Platelet Count	150,000–350,000/mL
Potassium	3.5–5.0 mEq/L
Prostate-specific antigen (PSA)	0–4 ng/mL (likely higher with age)
Proteins:	
Total	6.0–8.4 g/dL
Albumin	3.5–5.0 g/dL
Globulin	2.3–3.5 g/dL

Contd...

Contd...

Prothrombin (PTT)	25–41 sec
Pyruvic Acid	0.3–0.9 mg/dL
Red blood cell count (RBC)	4.2–6.9 million/µL/cu mm
Sodium	135–145 mEq/L
Thyroid-stimulating hormone (TSH)	0.5–6.0 µ units/mL
Transaminase:	
Alanine (ALT)	1–21 units/L
Aspartate (AST)	7–27 units/L
Blood urea nitrogen (BUN)	7–18 mg/dL
BUN/creatinine ratio	5–35
Uric acid	Male: 2.1 to 8.5 mg/dL (likely higher with age)
	Female: 2.0 to 7.0 mg/dL (likely higher with age)
Vitamin A	30–65 µg/dL
WBC (leukocyte count and white blood cell count)	4.3–10.8 × $10^3/mm^3$
White blood cell count (WBC)	4,300–10,800 cells/µL/cu mm

ABBREVIATIONS

k = kilo
d = deci
c = centi
m = milli
µ = micro
< = less than
> = greater or more than
m = meter
L = liter
dL = deciliter
g = gram
mg = milligram
mg/dL = milligram per deciliter
ng = nanogram
cells/µcl = cells per microliter
g/dL = grams per deciliter
pg/cell = picograms per cell
mol = mole
mmol = millimole
Osm = osmoles
mOsm = milliosmoles
Eq = Equivalents
mEq = milliequivalent
IU = International unit

Approximate Equivalents Chart		
1 teaspoonful	=	5 mL
1 tablespoonful	=	15 mL
1/4 grain	=	15 mg
1/2 grain	=	30 mg
1 grain	=	60 mg
1.5 grains	=	100 mg
5 grains	=	300 mg
10 grains	=	600 mg

Previous Solved Question Papers Staff Nurse (Kerala Public Service Commission)

STAFF NURSE (Insurance Medical Service)

{Exam held on 17-01-2004}

1. **Which of the following is a common symptom of active tuberculosis?**
   a. Marked weight loss b. Dyspnea on exertion
   c. Mental status changes d. Constipation
2. **The most common symptoms of hypoglycemia are**
   a. Nervousness and diaphoresis
   b. Anorexia and incoherent speech
   c. Kussumaul's respiration and confusion
   d. Bradycardia and blurred vision
3. **Antisterility vitamin**
   a. Vitamin K b. Vitamin D
   c. Vitamin C d. Vitamin E
4. **Progesterone is secreted by**
   a. Corpus luteum b. Corpus albicans
   c. Pituitary gland d. Graafian cells
5. **Cessation of menstrual cycle is called**
   a. Ovulation b. Puberty
   c. Menopause d. Implantation
6. **Hormones are produced by**
   a. Exocrine glands b. Endocrine glands
   c. Holocrine glands d. Apocrine glands
7. **Islets of Langerhans are present in**
   a. Brain b. Stomach
   c. Ovary d. Pancreas
8. **The male sex hormone is called**
   a. Vasopressin b. Gonadotropic hormone
   c. FSH d. Testosterone
9. **Number of spinal nerves in man are**
   a. 11 pairs b. 12 pairs
   c. 31 pairs d. 33 pairs
10. **The function of choroid plexus is**
    a. To produce lymph
    b. To produce blood
    c. To produce cerebrospinal fluid
    d. To produce endolymph
11. **The cerebellum is concerned with**
    a. Coordination of muscular movements
    b. Perception
    c. Memory
    d. Vision
12. **The commonest cause of CVA is**
    a. Cerebral hemorrhage b. Cerebral thrombosis
    c. Cerebral embolism d. Cerebral spasm
13. **The pH of fresh urine is about**
    a. 7.1 b. 5.0
    c. 8.4 d. 9.9
14. **Rh factor can produce**
    a. AIDS b. Erythroblastosis fetalis
    c. Turner's syndrome d. Sickle cell anemia
15. **Pulse pressure is**
    a. Diastolic pressure
    b. Systolic pressure
    c. Differences between diastolic and systolic pressure
    d. Pressure in pulmonary veins
16. **Edema is due to**
    a. Increased permeability of capillary walls
    b. Reduced return of lymph
    c. Increased capillary pressure
    d. All of these

17. Removal of gallbladder in man could lead to

a. Impairment of fat digestion
b. Impairment of digestion of protein
c. Jaundice
d. Increased acidity in intestine

18. Loss of appetite, gastrointestinal disorders and muscular weakness are deficiency symptoms of

a. Vitamin A b. Vitamin B
c. Vitamin C d. Vitamin D

19. Largest gland in human body is

a. Liver b. Thyroid
c. Pituitary d. Pancreas

20. The blood vessel in which the oxygen content is highest in the fetus is

a. Aorta b. Umbilical vein
c. Pulmonary artery d. Inferior vena cava

21. India's National Health Policy was approved in the parliament in

a. 1961 b. 1980
c. 1983 d. 1991

22. The measure of health status of children in a community is

a. Infant mortality rate b. Maternal mortality rate
c. Crude birth rate d. Crude death rate

23. Which of the following food constituents are more required by pregnant woman?

a. Iron b. Calcium
c. Potassium d. Vitamin C

24. An antenatal mother is ordered to have a diet that contains 90 grams of protein each day. How many calories will the protein contribute to her daily weight?

a. 180 calories b. 360 calories
c. 540 calories d. 810 calories

25. The antidote of magnesium sulphate is

a. Calcium gluconate b. Diazepam
c. Calcium chloride d. Nalorphine hydrochloride

26. The approximate volume of blood at birth is

a. 60 mL/kg body weight b. 85 mL/kg body weight
c. 110 mL/kg body weight d. 125 mL/kg body weight

27. Which of the following signs and symptoms indicate salycilate toxicity?

a. Chest pain b. Pink colored urine
c. Slow pulse rate d. Ringing in ears

28. Urinary bladder is lined with

a. Simple epithelium
b. Stratified epithelium
c. Transitional epithelium
d. Pseudostratified epithelium

29. Sprain is due to pulling of

a. Muscles b. Tendons
c. Ligaments d. Nerves

30. Rickets is due to deficiency of

a. Vitamin D b. Vitamin A
c. Vitamin B d. Vitamin C

31. Which of the following is a mechanical method of contraception?

a. Vasectomy b. Mala-D
c. Condom d. MTP

32. Kartar Singh Committee is otherwise known as

a. Multipurpose workers committee
b. Health survey and development committee
c. Health survey and planning committee
d. Committee on medical education

33. Which of the following drugs has not been used in the treatment of leprosy?

a. Streptomycin b. Rifampicin
c. Clofaximin d. INH

34. Which of the following is a potassium sparing diuretic?

a. Fursemide b. Aldactone
c. Mannitol d. Dimox

35. The position most suited for an unconscious patient is

a. Fowlers position b. Prone position
c. Supine position d. Semiprone position

36. Temperature of water for preparing hot water bag is

a. 60–65°C b. 65–70°C
c. 70–75°C d. 90–100°C

37. 39°C is equal to

a. 100.2°F b. 102.2°F
c. 101.2°F d. 103.2°F

38. Sand bags are used to prevent

a. Foot drop
b. Wrist drop
c. Internal rotation of thigh
d. All of them

39. Hemoptysis is

a. Blood in urine b. Blood in vomitus
c. Blood in sputum d. Blood in feces

40. For continuous oxygen administration for longer period, the nasal catheter should be changed

a. Every 6 hours b. Every 12 hours
c. Every 24 hours d. Every 48 hours

41. The causative organism of dengue fever is

a. Enteri virus b. Arbovirus
c. Variola virus d. Influenza virus

42. The desired quantity of 'free residual chlorine' in drinking water is

a. 1 mg/L b. 0.5 mg/L
c. 2 mg/L d. 0.25 mg/L

43. The vitamin which is involved in fat, protein and carbohydrate metabolism

a. Riboflavin b. Folic acid
c. Niacin d. Thiamine

44. The hormonal contraceptives are

a. Oral b. Injectable
c. Implant d. All of them

45. Poliomyelitis is transmitted through

a. Water b. Air
c. Blood d. Vectors

46. MCH service includes

a. Prenatal and postnatal care
b. Under fives care
c. Family planning service
d. All of them

47. The recommended maximum noise level for human beings

a. 85 dB b. 50 dB
c. 110 dB d. 160 dB

48. The best method of refuse disposal in a hospital is

a. Dumping b. Controlled tipping
c. Incineration d. Composting

49. MTP Act was passed in the year

a. 1983 b. 1977
c. 2000 d. 1972

50. The maximum amount of blood loss during delivery that is considered to be within normal limit is approximately

a. 100 mL b. 300 mL
c. 500 mL d. 700 mL

51. The most frequent cause of maternal death during child birth is

a. Sepsis b. Toxemia
c. Asphyxia d. Hemorrhage

52. Mrs. Mary's LMP (Last Menstrual Period) was on July 13th 2003. Her expected date of delivery is

a. March 6th 2004 b. March 20th 2004
c. April 6th 2004 d. April 20th 2004

53. The unit of measure commonly used to describe effacement of cervix is

a. Decimal b. Percentage
c. Centimeter d. Finger breadth

54. Mrs. Leela has placenta previa. The most likely symptom she will present is

a. Painless bleeding
b. A board like abdomen
c. Intermittent pain with spotting
d. A dull pain in the lower abdomen

55. Which of the following combination of blood types is most likely to produce hemolytic disease of the new born?

a. Negative mother and positive father
b. Positive mother and negative father
c. Negative mother and negative father
d. Positive mother and positive father

56. The vein which will most likely be used to give exchange transfusion in the

a. Jugular vein b. Femoral vein
c. Temporal vein d. Umbilical vein

57. Which of the following is not an occupational disease?

a. Asbestosis b. Pneumoconiosis
c. Japanese encephalitis d. Sillicosis

58. Carbohydrate is stored in the liver as

a. Glucose b. Sucrose
c. Glycogen d. Galactose

59. Which of the following signs and symptoms indicate salycilate toxicity?

a. Chest pain
b. Pink colored urine
c. Slow pulse rate
d. Ringing in ears

60. Which of the following symptoms might indicate that a client is developing tetany following subtotal thyroidectomy?

a. Backache
b. Hoarseness
c. Dyspnea
d. Tingling in the fingers

61. The master gland of the body is

a. Liver
b. Pituitary
c. Thyroid
d. Adrenal

62. Causative organism of malaria is

a. Cryptococcosis
b. Leishmania
c. Plasmodium
d. Klebsiella

63. Sepsis means

a. Absence of infection
b. Presence of pathogenic organisms
c. Destruction of pathogenic organisms
d. Infection in the blood

64. Father of antiseptic surgery

a. Joseph Lister
b. Louis Pasteur
c. William Harvey
d. Ronald Ross

65. Vaccines and toxoids produce

a. Natural immunity
b. Active immunity
c. Passive immunity
d. Acquired immunity

66. One gram of fat yields

a. 9 calories
b. 6 calories
c. 8 calories
d. 4 calories

67. Antisterility vitamin is

a. Vitamin A
b. Vitamin E
c. Vitamin D
d. Vitamin K

68. Where is the vomiting center located?

a. Cerebellum
b. Cerebrum
c. Medulla oblongata
d. Diencephalon

69. The most common complication that can occur after renal biopsy is

a. Infection
b. Tenderness
c. Renal failure
d. Hemorrhage

70. Which of the following is a side effect of morphine?

a. Increased blood pressure
b. Decreased respiratory rate
c. Reduced mucus secretion
d. Visual disturbance

71. Koplik's spot is seen in

a. Chickenpox
b. Measles
c. Mumps
d. Variola

72. Which of the following vitamin deficiency results in scurvy?

a. Vitamin C
b. Vitamin B
c. Vitamin D
d. Vitamin A

73. An example of a congenital cyanotic heart disease is

a. Rheumatic heart disease
b. Ventricular septal defect
c. Aortic stenosis
d. Tetralogy of Fallot

74. Approximate time for introduction of solid food in the diet of a child is

a. 1–3 months
b. 5–6 months
c. 6–8 months
d. 10–12 months

75. Expected time of closure of antierior fontannel is

a. 4–6 weeks
b. 6–8 months
c. 9–12 months
d. 16–18 months

76. Wilm's tumor is a condition affecting

a. Kidney
b. Bone
c. Blood
d. Brain stem

77. Which of the following is the reason for chest pain associated with myocardial infarction?

a. Decreased oxygen in heart muscle
b. Left ventricular overload
c. Circulatory collapse
d. Electrolyte imbalance

78. Which of the following would be a priority assessment for a client receiving blood transfusion?

a. Urine output
b. Skin turgor
c. Anaphylactic reaction
d. Level of consciousness

79. Which of the following symptoms must be reported to the doctor by a patient receiving warfarin?

a. Hematuria
b. Constipation
c. Dyspnea
d. Pruritus

80. In a patient receiving paritoneal dialysis, which of the following signs indicate peritonitis?

a. Swelling in the legs
b. Redness at the catheter insertion site
c. Poor drainage of the dialysate fluid
d. Cloudy dialysate fluid

81. Non-invasive method of oxygen saturation monitoring can be done by

a. Arterial blood gas studies
b. Capillary blood gas studies
c. Venoclysis
d. Pulse oxymetry

82. Drug of choice for respiratory depression in a new born whose mother received morphine during labor

a. Naloxone b. Digoxin
c. Lidocaine d. Adrenaline

83. Immunization against DPT should be administered via

a. Oral route b. Intramuscular route
c. Subcutaneous route d. Intradermal route

84. Which of the following is a typical sign of tracheo-esophageal fistula?

a. Continuous drooling
b. Diaphragmatic breathing
c. Slow response to stimuli
d. Passage of frothy meconium

85. Best method of oxygen administration in a 2-month-old baby is via

a. Oxyhood b. Oxygen mask
c. Nasal canula d. Nasal prongs

86. Absence of ganglion cells in colon is a feature of

a. Ulcerative colitis
b. Hirschsprung's disease
c. Anorectal malformation
d. Reye's syndrome

87. A 4-year-old child is having a weight of 7.8 kg. To which grade of protein energy malnutrition does this child belong.

a. Grade I b. Grade II
c. Grade III d. Grade IV

88. Gastric lavage is contraindicated after ingestion of which of the following

a. Aspirin
b. Organophosphorous compound
c. Corrosive alkali
d. Odolum

89. In an underwater seal drainage system cessation of fluid fluctuation in the drainage tubes generally means that

a. Lung has fully expanded
b. Lung has collapsed
c. Mediastinal space has decreased
d. Chest tube is in the pleural space

90. Which of the following is a complication associated with the presence of tracheostomy tube?

a. Pneumothorax
b. Decreased cardiac output
c. Respiratory distress syndrome
d. Damage to laryngeal nerve

91. What is the compression-ventilation ratio for two rescuer CPR?

a. 4 : 2 b. 5 : 1
c. 5 : 2 d. 15 : 2

92. Which of the following would be the best indication that fluid replacement for the client in hypovolemic shock is adequate?

a. Skin feels warm
b. Systolic BP above 100 mm Hg
c. Diastolic BP above 90 mm Hg
d. Urine output greater than 30 mL/h

93. Which of the following is the best technique to determine whether a nasogastric tube is positioned in the stomach?

a. Irrigating with normal saline
b. Aspirating with syringe for gastric contents
c. Placing free end of tube in water
d. Instilling air and auscultating over epigastric area

94. Patients with upper abdominal surgery are advised to use an incentive spirometer during the postoperative period in order to

a. Stimulate circulation
b. Prepare for ambulation
c. Strengthen abdominal muscles
d. Increase respiratory effectiveness

95. Which of the following test result is useful to assess the liver function?

a. Glucose tolerance test b. Creatine clearance test
c. Serum transaminase d. Serum electrolytes

96. World No Tobacco Day is observed on

a. 5th June b. 31st May
c. 10th August d. 7th April

97. Which of the following manifestations indicate that a client with cirrhosis is developing hepatic encephalopathy?

a. Change in vital signs
b. Altered level of consciousness
c. Change in respiratory status
d. Decreased urine output

98. A normal local tissue response to radiation is

a. Atrophy of the skin
b. Scattered pustule formation
c. Redness of surface tissue
d. Sloughing of two layers of skin

99. Automatic rhythmic contractility is characteristic of

a. Cardiac tissue
b. Nervous tissue
c. Connective tissue
d. Muscular tissue

100. World Heart Day is observed on

a. 21 September
b. 28 September
c. 10 October
d. 14 August

ANSWERS

1. a	2. a	3. d	4. a	5. c	6. b	7. d	8. d	9. c	10. c	11. a	12. b
13. a	14. b	15. c	16. a	17. a	18. b	19. a	20. b	21. c	22. a	23. a	24. b
25. a	26. a	27. d	28. c	29. c	30. a	31. c	32. a	33. a	34. b	35. d	36. b
37. b	38. a	39. c	40. c	41. b	42. b	43. a	44. d	45. a	46. d	47. a	48. c
49. d	50. c	51. d	52. d	53. b	54. a	55. a	56. d	57. c	58. c	59. d	60. d
61. b	62. c	63. b	64. a	65. b	66. a	67. b	68. c	69. d	70. b	71. b	72. a
73. d	74. b	75. d	76. a	77. a	78. c	79. a	80. d	81. d	82. a	83. b	84. a
85. a	86. b	87. b	88. c	89. b	90. c	91. b	92. b	93. b	94. d	95. c	96. b
97. b	98. c	99. a	100. b								

JUNIOR PUBLIC HEALTH NURSE – GRADE II
Municipal Common Service

(Exam held on 08-07-2006)

1. **The ability of the body to recognize, destroy and eliminate antigenic material is called**
   a. Energy b. Immunity
   c. Adaptation d. Resistance

2. **Inflammation of mouth is called**
   a. Glossitis b. Stomatitis
   c. Cystitis d. Gingivitis

3. **Painful urination**
   a. Dysuria b. Anuria
   c. Pyuria d. Hematuria

4. **Exercises that a patient does for himself**
   a. Passive exercises b. Isotonic exercise
   c. Isometric exercises d. Active exercises

5. **One gram of fat supplies**
   a. 9 calories b. 4 calories
   c. 6 calories d. 12 calories

6. **Water soluble vitamin is**
   a. Vitamin A b. Vitamin B complex
   c. Vitamin D d. Vitamin K

7. **Epidemiological triad comprises of**
   a. Agent, host and disease
   b. Agent, host and organism
   c. Agent, host and environment
   d. Agent, host and infection

8. **The best sources of calcium**
   a. Meat b. Vegetable
   c. Fruits d. Milk

9. **Separation of an infected person from non-infected persons**
   a. Incubation b. Isolation
   c. Inoculation d. Immunization

10. **Condition in which the placenta situated in the lower uterine segment**
    a. Vasa previa b. Placenta accreta
    c. Placenta previa d. Abruptio placenta

11. **Normal hemoglobin level**
    a. 4–8 g% b. 1–5 g%
    b. 15–25 g% d. 10–14 g%

12. **The best indicator of infant nutrition**
    a. Height b. Weight
    c. Vital signs d. Vital statistics

13. **Permanent male sterilization**
    a. PPS b. Vasectomy
    c. Tubectomy d. Mini lap

14. **Care of the mother during delivery**
    a. Antenatal care b. Prenatal care
    c. postnatal care d. Intranatal care

15. **Currently married couple, where woman is in the reproductive age**
    a. Potential couple b. High risk couple
    c. Eligible couple d. Able couple

16. **The diameter of the fetal skull that stretches the vulva during normal delivery**
    a. Biparietal diameter
    b. Bitemporal diameter
    c. Occipito bregmatic diameter
    d. Suboccipito frontal

17. **Dryness of the eye due to vitamin A deficiency**
    a. Bitot's spot b. Night blindness
    c. Xerophthalmia d. Keratomalacia

18. **Hydrophobia is a typical clinical feature of**
    a. Plague b. Rabies
    c. Malaria d. Anthrax

19. **Sexually transmitted diseases are also known as**
    a. Reproductive disorders b. Sexual disorders
    c. Neurosis d. Venereal diseases

20. **Diagnostic procedure done in heart disease**
    a. EEG b. USG
    c. EMG d. ECG

21. **Reagent used for urine sugar test**
   a. Acetic acid b. Benedict's solution
   c. Gentian violet d. Methylene blue

22. **One ounce is**
   a. 5 mL b. 15 mL
   c. 30 mL d. 50 mL

23. **The hormone that is detected during urine pregnancy test.**
   a. HPL b. hCG
   c. Estrogen d. Progesterone

24. **Loss of appetite is**
   a. Asphyxia b. Anorexia
   c. Nausea d. Dysphagia

25. **Change in the shape of fetal head when it passes through the birth canal**
   a. Moulding b. Casting
   c. Shaping d. Spalding

26. **Loss of three or more consecutive pregnancies**
   a. Threatened abortion b. Missed abortion
   c. Spontaneous abortion d. Habitual abortion

27. **Universal donors are persons having**
   a. Blood group A b. Blood group B
   c. Blood group O d. Blood group AB

28. **The test used to find out syphillis**
   a. Widal test b. ELISA test
   c. VDRL test d. Shick test

29. **Environmental barrier of communication is**
   a. Noise b. Deafness
   c. Loss of concentration d. Loss of attention

30. **Temperature of water used for bed bath**
   a. 37°–42°F b. 96°–99°F
   c. 120°–130°F d. 110°–115°F

31. **The placenta that is adhered to myometrium and difficult to remove**
   a. Placenta succenturiate b. Placenta previa
   c. Placenta accrete d. Placenta circumvallate

32. **Artificial rupture of fetal membranes**
   a. Amniocentesis b. Stripping
   c. Amniotomy d. Fetoscopy

33. **Birth injury due to damage of brachial plexus**
   a. Facial palsy b. Erb's palsy
   c. Cephal hematoma d. Subdural hematoma

34. **Hot and dry vagina during labor is a feature of**
   a. Prolonged labor b. Normal labor
   c. Obstructed labor d. Precipitate labor

35. **The science of health and its preservation**
   a. Biology b. Nutrition
   c. Sociology d. Hygiene

36. **An outbreak of disease in a community in excess of normal expectation**
   a. Endemic b. Epidemic
   c. Pandemic d. Sporadic

37. **Scurvy is due to deficiency of**
   a. Vitamin D b. Vitamin K
   c. Vitamin C d. Vitamin B complex

38. **Device used to raise the head or foot end of bed**
   a. Bed cradle b. Bed block
   c. Sand bag d. Foot rest

39. **The position used for vaginal examination is**
   a. Fowler's b. Dorsal recumbent
   c. Prone d. Sim's lateral

40. **Abortion is the termination of pregnancy before**
   a. 12 weeks b. 28 weeks
   c. 37 weeks d. 42 weeks

41. **A packet of oral pill (Mala-N) contains**
   a. 28 pills b. 30 pills
   c. 31pills d. 42 pills

42. **Nurse's day celebrated on**
   a. April 7th b. May 12th
   c. August 15th d. December 15th

43. **Weaning starts at**
   a. 6th month b. 9th month
   c. 12th month d. 15th month

44. **Feeling with hand to note the size of internal organs**
   a. Auscultation b. Percussion
   c. Palpation d. Vibration

45. **Drug used to control bleeding during third stage of labor**
   a. Drotin b. Methergin
   c. Prostaglandin d. Epidosyn

46. **Blood vessels present in the umbilical cord**
   a. 2 arteries and 1 vein b. 2 veins and 1 artery
   c. 1 vein and 1 artery d. 2 veins and 2 arteries

47. Nature's tooth brush
a. Coal b. Neem stick
c. Drum stick d. Food

48. The simplest method for removing stains is
a. Bicarbonates b. Bleaching powder
c. Cold water d. Ammonia

49. Normal volume of amniotic fluid at term
a. 500 mL b. 1000 mL
c. 2000 mL d. 3000 mL

50. Infection in a hospital, with a disease other than for which the patient was admitted
a. Cross infection b. Reinfection
c. Immediate infection d. Postinfection

51. Temperature, pulse, respiration and BP are called
a. Vital statistics b. Vital functions
c. Vital signs d. Vital symptoms

52. Tachycardia is
a. Elevated BP b. Rapid pulse
c. Elevated temperature d. Rapid respiration

53. A breech with extended leg
a. Complete breech b. Frank breech
c. Footling breech d. Kneeling breech

54. Positive sign of pregnancy
a. Fetal movement b. Amenorrhea
c. Morning sickness d. Uterine growth

55. Supervised, community based tuberculosis treatment
a. Chemotherapy b. MPO
c. DOTS d. Surveillance

56. World AIDS day
a. April 1st b. May 1st
c. December 1st d. July 1st

57. Oral polio vaccine is
a. Live attenuated vaccine b. Killed vaccine
c. Toxoid d. Combined vaccine

58. Total weight gain during pregnancy
a. 5 kg b. 10 kg
c. 15 kg d. 20 kg

59. Solution used for cleaning enema
a. Soap and water b. Plane water
c. Warm water d. Rice water

60. The strength of Dettol solution used to disinfect clinical thermometer
a. 1:20 b. 1:40
c. 1:60 d. 1:100

61. Person who is practical, active and easily mixes with others
a. Introvert b. Ambivalent
c. Extrovert d. Dependent

62. Worm that is transmitted through meat
a. Hook worm b. Tape worm
c. Round worm d. Pin worm

63. Vomiting during pregnancy that seriously affects the woman
a. Morning sickness b. Hyperemesis gravidarum
c. Night sickness d. HELLP syndrome

64. MTP Act was passed in
a. 1971 b. 1986
c. 1961 d. 1976

65. Basic unit of society
a. Individual b. Panchayat
c. Family d. Block

66. Hypertensive disorder of pregnancy
a. Vesicular mole b. Supine hypotension
c. Eclampsia d. Placenta previa

67. False perception is called
a. Hallucination b. Illusion
c. Delusion d. Imperception

68. The Panchayat Raj Institution at block level
a. Grama Panchayat b. Zilla Parishad
c. Grama Sabha d. Panchayat Samiti

69. Horny or toad skin is due to the deficiency of
a. Proteins b. Essential fatty acid
c. Carbohydrates d. Essential minerals

70. Chemical substance used for purifying water
a. Lime b. Potassium permanganate
c. Bleaching powder d. Formaldehyde

71. A communicable disease that is eradicated from India
a. Chickenpox b. Rubella
c. Smallpox d. Rabies

72. **Tuberculin test is commonly known as**

a. Shick test b. Mantoux test
c. VDRL d. ELISA

73. **Abbreviation of 'OD' denotes**

a. Once a day b. At bed time
c. Whenever necessary d. After meals

74. **The prime source of all water**

a. Sea b. River
c. Rain d. Well

75. **A 'Saucer' shaped depression at or just below umbilicus indicates**

a. Breech presentation
b. Occipito posterior position
c. Transverse lie
d. Occipito anterior position

76. **Committee on multipurpose worker**

a. Mudhaliar Committee b. Kartar Singh Committee
c. Bhore Committee d. Srivastav Committee

77. **During labor, the descent of fetal head is checked in relation to**

a. Ischial tuberosity b. Symphasis pubis
c. Ischial spines d. Cervix

78. **The body of fetus is delivered by**

a. Extension b. Lateral extension
c. Flexion d. Lateral flexion

79. **Exchange of air between indoors and outdoors**

a. Ventilation b. Air conditioning
c. Air change d. Wind

80. **First step in the control of a communicable disease**

a. Prevention b. Treatment
c. Notification d. Surveillance

81. **Third stage of labor is**

a. Cervical dilatation b. Birth of baby
c. Cervical effacement d. Delivery of placenta

82. **Method used for diagnosing community health problem**

a. Laboratory test b. Survey
c. Camp d. Health education

83. **Total number of multipurpose workers in a sub centre**

a. Two b. Four
c. Five d. Ten

84. **Antibiotics are the drugs used to treat**

a. Infection b. Inflammation
c. Pain d. Itching

85. **One sub-center is for a population of**

a. 3,000 b. 5,000
c. 8,000 d. 10,000

86. **The mosquito that transmit malaria**

a. Anopheles b. Culex
c. Aedes d. Mansonia

87. **Insulin is usually administered**

a. Intramuscularly b. Subcutaneously
c. Intradermally d. Orally

88. **Normal body temperature**

a. 99.60°F b. 97.6°F
c. 98.6°F d. 99°F

89. **Most sensitive index of the health of a community**

a. MMR b. IMR
c. Crude death rate d. Crude birth rate

90. **The richest source of vitamin C**

a. Milk b. Meat
c. Amla d. Liver

91. **The daily requirement of folic acid for an adult is**

a. 50 microgram b. 300 microgram
c. 200 microgram d. 100 microgram

92. **Nucleus of health services in rural area**

a. PHC b. Family
c. CHC d. Anganwadi

93. **First 6 weeks after delivery is called**

a. Antepartum period b. Puerperium
c. Recovery period d. Motherhood period

94. **Umbilical cord behind the unruptured membrane during PV examination**

a. Short cord b. Cord prolapse
c. Long cord d. Cord presentation

95. **LMP is on 12th June 2003, then EDC is on**

a. 12th March 2004 b. 18th June 2004
c. 19th March 2004 d. 21st March 2004

96. **Back bone of public health nursing**

a. Home visit b. Records
c. Health education d. Registers

97. The return of uterus to prepregnant state after delivery
a. Regression b. Inversion
c. Involution d. Eversion

98. BCG vaccine give protection against
a. Typhoid b. Tuberculosis
c. Leprosy d. Whooping cough

99. Relationship of fetal head and limbs to trunk
a. Lie b. Presentation
c. Attitude d. Position

100. Freedom from disease producing organisms
a. Clean b. Hygiene
c. Sepsis d. Asepsis

ANSWERS

1. b	2. b	3. a	4. d	5. a	6. b	7. c	8. d	9. b	10. c	11. d	12. b
13. b	14. d	15. c	16. a	17. c	18. b	19. d	20. d	21. b	22. c	23. b	24. b
25. a	26. d	27. c	28. c	29. a	30. d	31. c	32. c	33. b	34. c	35. d	36. b
37. c	38. b	39. d	40. b	41. a	42. b	43. a	44. c	45. b	46. a	47. b	48. b
49. b	50. a	51. c	52. b	53. b	54. a	55. c	56. c	57. a	58. b	59. a	60. b
61. c	62. b	63. b	64. a	65. c	66. c	67. b	68. d	69. b	70. c	71. c	72. b
73. a	74. c	75. b	76. b	77. c	78. d	79. a	80. a	81. d	82. b	83. a	84. a
85. b	86. a	87. b	88. c	89. b	90. c	91. d	92. a	93. b	94. d	95. c	96. a
97. c	98. b	99. c	100. d								

STAFF NURSE (HEALTH DEPARTMENT)

{Exam held on 16-09-2006}

1. **In adult during ear irrigation to straighten the ear canal hold the pinna**
   a. Upward b. Downward and backward
   c. Straight backward d. Upward and backward
2. **The following is an iron chelating agent**
   a. Chlorpheniramine b. Deferoxamine
   c. Sulfonamide d. EDTA
3. **Electrolyte imbalance potentiate digitalis toxicity**
   a. Hyperkalemia b. Hyponatremia
   c. Hypokalemia d. Hypernatemia
4. **Psychosexual disorder in which sexual behavior is directed to animals**
   a. Fetishism b. Bestiality
   c. Frotteurism d. Transvestism
5. **Hormone that helps to confirm pregnancy**
   a. Human chorinonic gonadotropin
   b. Human placental lactogen
   c. Estriol
   d. Progesterone
6. **Which of the following is a mydriatic?**
   a. Atropine b. Adrenaline
   c. Novocaine d. Silver nitrate
7. **Blood clots floating in the circulating blood**
   a. Emboli b. Thrombus
   c. Plaque d. Aneurysm
8. **Baby doubles birth weight by**
   a. 3 months b. 6 months
   c. 12 months d. 18 months
9. **The drug used for aversion therapy in alcoholics.**
   a. Dantrolene b. Bentropine
   c. Bromocriptine d. Disulfiram
10. **Drug of choice for diabetes insipidus**
    a. Oxypocin b. Vasopressin
    c. Lasix d. Calcium glucomate
11. **Couvelaire uterus occurs in**
    a. Placenta previa b. Placental abruption
    c. DIC d. Hydatidiform mole
12. **Pernicious anemia is due to deficiency of**
    a. Vitamin B b. Intrinsic factor
    c. Gastrin d. Pancreatic enzyme
13. **Cholecystectomy is a**
    a. Restorative surgery b. Corrective surgery
    c. Curative surgery d. Palliative surgery
14. **Best and cheapest investment in the health of children**
    a. Nutrition b. Immunization
    c. Breastfeeding d. Growth cards
15. **Sudden voluntary repetitive meaningless movement of voluntary muscles**
    a. Chorea b. Tetany
    c. Tremor d. Tic
16. **.......................... is an obstetric emergency**
    a. Cord presentation
    b. Involution of uterus
    c. Occipitoposterior position
    d. Inversion of uterus
17. **The apical pulse is located at ....in the midclavicular line**
    a. 2nd intercostal space b. 3rd intercostal space
    c. 5th intercostal space d. 7th intercostal space
18. **The condition in which the patient is conscious but is non-responsive to the environment**
    a. Delirium b. Stupor
    c. Coma d. Confusion
19. **Regional enteritis is also called**
    a. Ulcerative colitis
    b. Conn's disease
    c. Irritable bowel syndrome
    d. Crohn's disease

20. Among eligible couple the age of woman
a. 18–45 years b. 15–44 years
c. 15–50 years d. 18–50 years

21. The congenital deformity in which foot is dorsiflexed and the toes are higher than heel
a. Talipes calcaneus b. Talipes aquines
c. Talipes valgus d. Talipes varus

22. The best time to collect sputum specimen
a. Before brushing teeth in the morning
b. After an antiseptic mouth wash
c. After nebulization
d. After steam inhalation

23. Test used to check the patency of ureter
a. Barlow test b. Plethysmography
c. Buret test d. Sulkowitch test

24. The Employees State Insurance Act was in
a. 1975 b. 1976
c. 1948 d. 1952

25. The term schizophrenia was coined by
a. Bleuler b. Pinel
c. Emil Kraeplin d. Philippe Pinel

26. Spalding sign in X-ray indicates
a. IUGR b. Preterm pregnancy
c. Intrauterine death d. Post-term pregnancy

27. Causative agent of diphtheria
a. Coryne bacteria b. Bordetella
c. Klebs-Loeffler bacillus d. Salmonella

28. Unintentional filling of gaps of memory with untrue of fanciful ideas
a. Confabulation b. Paramnesias
c. Dejavu d. Hyperamnesia

29. Which is a didactic method of health teaching?
a. Symposium b. Workshop
c. Group discussion d. Lecture

30. Dilation of spermatic vein
a. Hydrocele b. Varicocele
c. Spermatocele d. Torsion of testicle

31. Terminology used to refer normal eye
a. Emmetropia b. Ametropia
c. Hyperopia d. Metropia

32. ICN code of ethics for nurses was adopted in
a. 1948 b. 1973
c. 1978 d. 1958

33. Osteochondral beading is seen in deficiency of
a. Vitamin A b. Vitamin B_6
c. Vitamin C d. Vitamin D

34. Proponent of germ theory of disease
a. Louis Pasteur b. Robert Hook
c. Charles Darwin d. Robert Brown

35. Inability of the eyes to move together in coordinated manner
a. Diplopa b. Stye
c. Nystagmus d. Strabismus

36. The chemical agent used for testing albumin in urine
a. Iodine b. Sulphur powder
c. Sodium nitroprusside d. Acetic acid

37. Anterior fontanelle is also called
a. Bregma b. Lambda
c. Vertex d. Glabella

38. An ototoxic drug
a. Aspirin b. Digoxin
c. Chlorpromazole d. Dapson

39. Frequent cyanotic spells occurs in
a. VSD b. Coarctation of aorta
c. PDA d. Tetralogy of Fallot

40. The temperature of water for tepid sponge
a. 65°–85°F b. 85°–100°F
c. 100°–105°F d. 105°–110°F

41. Surgical Management of Chronic sinusitis
a. Caldwell luc operation b. Shirodkar operation
c. Mc Donald operation d. Hypophysectomy

42. During labor the station of fetal head is assessed in relation to
a. Ischial spine b. Ischial tuberosity
c. Sacral pomontory d. Pelvic brim

43. Drugs that inhibit the cough reflex
a. Antihistamines b. Antiasthamatics
c. Antitussives d. Expectorants

44. Macewen's sign in a manifestation of
a. Hydrocephalus b. Meningomyelocele
c. Cerebral palsy d. Meningitis

45. **How much of 15% solution is required to give 100 mg of the drug?**
   a. 0.5 mL b. 0.7 mL
   c. 0.1 mL d. 1.5 mL

46. **Water seal drainage is not indicated in**
   a. Thoractotomy b. Lobectomy
   c. Pneumonectomy d. Wedge resection

47. **The relationship of different parts of fetus to one another**
   a. Lie b. Presentation
   c. Attitude d. Denominator

48. **Urethral meatus is on the penile dorsal surface in**
   a. Paraphimosis b. Epispadias
   c. Phimosis d. Hypospadias

49. **Huge tumor like overgrowth of scar tissues**
   a. Chancroid b. Cellulitis
   c. Eczema d. Keloids

50. **Pus in the pleural cavity**
   a. Pleural effusion b. Empyema
   c. Emphysema d. Pyorrhea

51. **For administering 3000 mL of fluid for 24 hours, the flow rate is**
   a. 31 drops/min b. 15 drops/min
   c. 45 drops/min d. 52 drops/min

52. **Birth injury due to damage of starnocleido mastoid muscle**
   a. Chignon b. Facial palsy
   c. Torticollis d. Klumpkee's palsy

53. **Which of the following is a complication of blood transfusion?**
   a. Citrate toxicity b. Calcium overload
   c. Magnesium toxicity d. Hypotension

54. **Dose of vitamin A in vitamin A prophylaxis programme**
   a. 1,00,000 IU b. 1,50,000 IU
   c. 2,00,000 IU d. 2,50,000 IU

55. **Central separation of placenta**
   a. Controlled cord traction
   b. Schultze method
   c. Mathews Duncan method
   d. Expectant management

56. **Preinduction assessment score**
   a. Bishop's score b. Apgar score
   c. Latch score d. Ones

57. **The risk of vasa previa is more in**
   a. Bipartite placenta
   b. Battle door placenta
   c. Circumvallate placenta
   d. Velamentous insertion of cord

58. **Panchayat Raj Institution at block level**
   a. Grama Sabha b. Grama Panchayat
   c. Panchayat Samiti d. Zilla Parishad

59. **Which of the following is a complication of hyperemesis gravidarum?**
   a. Eclampsia
   b. Miscarriage
   c. Wernick's encephalopathy
   d. Vesicular mole

60. **The second heart sound is due to closure of**
   a. Aortic valve b. Mitral valve
   c. Tricuspid valve d. Foramen ovale

61. **Endometrium of pregnant uterus**
   a. Trophoblast b. Blastocyst
   c. Decidua d. Mesoderm

62. **Most sensitive index of the health and level of living of people**
   a. Crude death rate b. Birth rate
   c. Infant mortality rate d. Maternal mortality rate

63. **Hormone having anti-inflammatory effect**
   a. Estrogen b. Progesterone
   c. Corticosteroids d. Gonadotropins

64. **A patient who is fond of his daughter finds the nurse of the same age and height as his daughter. This is**
   a. Identification b. Projection
   c. Transference d. Reaction formation

65. **Destruction of all the pathogenic organisms is called**
   a. Sterilization b. Disinfection
   c. Disinfestation d. Cleaning

66. **The hormone that help in milk ejection reflex**
   a. Prolactin b. Oxytocin
   c. Estrogen d. Progesterone

67. **Umbilical cord contains**
   a. 2 artery and 1 vein b. 2 vein and 1 artery
   c. 1 artery and 1 vein d. 2 artery and 2 vein

68. **Proponent of theory of learning by conditioning**
   a. Sigmund Freud b. Pavlov
   c. Pinel d. Kraeplin

69. Characteristic smile in tetanus patients
a. Opisthotonus b. Ataxia
c. Akinesia d. Risus sadonicus

70. Cause of temporary hardness of water
a. Carbonates b. Sulphates
c. Chlorides d. Calcium

71. 104°F is.......................... °C
a. 40 b. 45
c. 50 d. 70

72. The liver enzyme that helps in bilirubin metabolism
a. Urobilinogen b. Pancreatic lipase
c. Glucoranyl transferase d. Trypsin

73. The fetal blood flow through placenta
a. 200–400 mL/mt b. 400–500 mL/mt
c. 500–600 mL/mt d. 600–800 mL/mt

74. Full volume but rapidly collapsing pulse
a. Bounding pulse b. Bigeminal pulse
c. Water hammer pulse d. Dicrotic pulse

75. Sign of hypocalcemia
a. Cullen's sign b. Homan's sign
c. Goodell's sign d. Trousseau's sign

76. The recommended level of free residual chlorine in drinking water
a. 25 mg/L b. 0.5 mg/L
c. 0.1 mg/L d. 1.5 mg/L

77. Respiration is controlled by
a. Cerebrum b. Cerebellum
c. Medulla oblongata d. Hypothalamus

78. Presence of alfa fetoprotein in amniotic fluid indicates
a. Hydrocephalus
b. Tetralogy of Fallot
c. Tracheoesophageal fistula
d. Spina bifida

79. Reflex elicited by stroking the sole of the foot with a sharp instrument
a. Patellar reflex b. Achilles reflex
c. Triceps reflex d. Plantar reflex

80. Benign tumor of outer layers of skin
a. Squamous cell carcinoma
b. Papilloma
c. Melanoma
d. Lipoma

81. Poor man's meat
a. Milk b. Cereals
c. Fish d. Pulses

82. Cracking or ulceration of lips and angles of mouth
a. Halitosis b. Glossitis
c. Stomatitis d. Cheilosis

83. Inflection of soft tissues around and under the nail
a. Felon b. Carbuncle
c. Cellulitis d. Paronychia

84. The creamy substance that cover the umbilical cord
a. Vernix caseosa b. Wharton's jelly
c. Smegma d. Milia

85. Misperception of external stimuli
a. Hallucination b. Depersonalization
c. Delusion d. Illusion

86. Projectile vomiting is seen in
a. Intussusception b. Duodenal atresia
c. Pyloric stenosis d. Megacolon

87. The formula of calculating EDC
a. Haase's rule b. Young's rule
c. Clark's rule d. Naegele's rule

88. Antibiotic used as chemotherapeutic agent
a. Augmentin b. Vincristine
c. Actionomycin d. Streptomycin

89. A killed vaccine
a. BCG b. Measles
c. Typhoid d. Yellow fever

90. Pregnancy mask
a. Linea nigra b. Butterfly rashes
c. Chloasma d. Erythema

91. The position used to treat shock and decreased blood pressure
a. Lithotomy position
b. Genupectoral position
c. Dorsal recumbent position
d. Trendelenberg position

92. Human chorionic gonadotropin is produced by
a. Cytotrophoblast b. Decidua
c. Mesoderm d. Syncytiotrophoblast

93. Ribbon like stool is seen in
a. Intussusception b. Hirshsprung's disease
c. Ulcerative colitis d. Diverticulitis

94. **Therapeutic serum level of lithium**
 a. 4 mEq/L–6 mEq/L b. 0.6 mEq/L–8 mEq/L
 c. 0.8 mEq/L–2 mEq/L d. 1.2 mEq/L–4 mEq/L

95. **The amount of potassium chloride in oral rehydration mixture**
 a. 3.5 g b. 2.5 g
 c. 0.5 g d. 1.5 g

96. **Increased pulsation of lateral vaginal fornices during pregnancy**
 a. Jacqumere's sign b. Chadwick's sign
 c. Goodell's sign d. Osiander's sign

97. **Which of the following is a fundamental symptom of Schizophrenia?**
 a. Ambivalence b. Delusion
 c. Hallucination d. Mannerism

98. **Absence of recognizable 'QRS' complex in ECG indicate**
 a. Atrial fibrillation b. Ventricular fibrillation
 c. Sinus arrhythmias d. Paroxysmal ventricular tachycardia

99. **The drug of choice for eclampsia**
 a. Magnesium sulfate b. Calcium gluconate
 c. Adrenergic blockers d. Diazepam

100. **Puerperium is the period**
 a. 6 weeks after delivery
 b. 28 days after delivery
 c. 6 months after delivery
 d. 28 weeks after delivery

ANSWERS

1. d	2. b	3. a	4. b	5. a	6. a	7. a	8. b	9. d	10. b	11. b	12. b
13. c	14. c	15. a	16. d	17. c	18. b	19. d	20. b	21. a	22. a	23. b	24. a
25. c	26. c	27. a	28. a	29. d	30. b	31. a	32. b	33. d	34. a	35. d	36. d
37. a	38. a	39. d	40. b	41. a	42. a	43. c	44. a	45. b	46. c	47. c	48. b
49. d	50. b	51. a	52. c	53. d	54. c	55. b	56. a	57. d	58. c	59. c	60. a
61. c	62. c	63. c	64. a	65. b	66. a	67. a	68. b	69. d	70. a	71. a	72. c
73. b	74. c	75. d	76. b	77. c	78. d	79. d	80. c	81. d	82. d	83. d	84. b
85. d	86. c	87. d	88. c	89. c	90. c	91. d	92. a	93. b	94. c	95. d	96. d
97. a	98. b	99. a	100. a								

STAFF NURSE (STATE FARMING CORPORATION)

{Exam held on 12-03-2006}

1. **APGAR score for color done at 5 minutes after birth is recorded as 2. It indicates**
   a. Pallor
   b. Body pink, extremities blue
   c. Cyanosed
   d. Pink

2. **Sudden jarring causes sudden extension and abduction of extremities and funning of fingers in a newborn is called**
   a. Moro reflex b. Startle reflex
   c. Tonic neck reflex d. Rooting reflex

3. **Persistence of foramen ovale leads to**
   a. VSD b. ASD
   c. PDA d. TOF

4. **Diabetes insipidus is due to deficiency of**
   a. Insulin b. Antidiuretic hormone
   c. Glucocorticolid d. Thyroxine

5. **Pawlik's maneuvre is used**
   a. To give fundal pressure
   b. To locate fetal pressure
   c. To assess the size and mobility of the fetal head
   d. To diagnose the lie and presentation of fetus

6. **The part of the fetus that lies at the pelvic brim is called**
   a. Lie b. Denominator
   c. Presentation d. Attitude

7. **For giving soap and water enema the height of the enema from the anus is**
   a. 10 inches b. 8 inches
   c. 25 inches d. 18 inches

8. **PRN means.**
   a. If necessary in emergency
   b. Every hourly
   c. When required
   d. Each night

9. **Which of the following is a natural family planning method?**
   a. Abstinence b. CU-T
   c. Condom d. Tubectomy

10. **Which of the following is true for cephalhematoma?**
    a. Swelling appears immediately after birth
    b. Pitting on pressure
    c. Scalp is movable
    d. It does not cross a suture

11. **Adenoma is a tumor originating from the**
    a. Glands b. Fibrous tissue
    c. Mucous membrane d. Muscles

12. **In face presentation, the attitude of the head is**
    a. Extension b. Complete extension
    c. Flexion d. Deflexion

13. **Deep transverse arrest is a complication in**
    a. Brow presentation
    b. Occipitoanterior position
    c. Occipitoposterior position
    d. Breech presentation

14. **Antipellagra vitamin is**
    a. Niacin b. Thiamin
    c. Pyridoxine d. Riboflavin

15. **Ophthalmia neonatorum is caused by**
    a. *Candida albicans* b. *E. coli*
    c. *Staphylococcus* d. *Gonococci*

16. **False belief is called**
    a. Hallucination b. Illusion
    c. Delusion d. Perseveration

17. **Polyhydramnios is usually associated with**
    a. Esophageal atresia b. ASD
    c. Congenital megacolon d. Down syndrome

18. In the mechanism of normal labor, flexion is followed by
a. Extension of the head
b. Internal rotation of the head
c. Descent
d. Internal rotation of shoulders

19. Dystocia is
a. Prolonged labor
b. Ineffective uterine contractions
c. Difficult labor
d. Involuntary expulsion

20. The personality type in which a person think that other people will harm him
a. Cyclothymic b. Schizoid
c. Hysterical d. Paranoid

21. The outermost layer of meninges is
a. Pia mater b. White matter
c. Dura mater d. Arachnoid

22. Hypothyroidism occurring in adults
a. Myxedema b. Cretinism
c. Simple goiter d. Toxic goiter

23. Anopheles mosquitoes transmit
a. Filaria b. Encephalitis
c. Malaria d. Yellow fever

24. Which of the following is a live attenuated vaccine?
a. Typhoid b. Cholera
c. Rabies d. Oral polio

25. Repeated small movements of a habitual kind
a. Mannerism b. Tics
c. Compulsion d. Overactivity

26. Wilms tumor is affecting the
a. Liver b. Kidney
c. Bone d. Skin

27. Developmental task during the toddler period is
a. Trust vs mistrust
b. Autonomy vs shame and doubt
c. Initiative vs guilt
d. Industry vs role confusion

28. The endometrium during pregnancy is called
a. Corpus luteum b. Trophoblast
c. Corpus albicans d. Decidua

29. Circumvallate placenta means
a. Presence of an opaque ring on the placenta
b. Cord is attached at the edge of the placenta
c. Cord is inserted into the membrane
d. Presence of an extralobo of placenta

30. Blood group A contain
a. Alpha agglutinins
b. Beta agglutinins
c. No agglutinins
d. Both alpha and beta agglutinins

31. Menghini needle is used for
a. Thoracentesis b. Renal biopsy
c. Liver biopsy d. Lumbar punture

32. Which of the following chemical is used to test urine for albumin?
a. Ammonium sulfate b. Sodium nitroprusside
c. Acetic acid d. Liquor ammonia

33. Antitussives are drugs which
a. Inhibit cough reflex
b. Causes contraction of tissues
c. Arrest discharges
d. Dilates blood vessels

34. One teaspoon is approximately
a. 50 drops b. 75 drops
c. 100 drops d. 120 drops

35. A small division on a tuberculin syringe is equivalent to
a. 0.1 mL b. 0.01 mL
c. 1.0 mL d. 0.5 mL

36. Pyorrhea is
a. Foul smelling breath
b. Bleeding gums
c. Pus in the sockets of teeth
d. Brown crusts on the teeth

37. Pressure exerted by plasma protein is called
a. Hydrostatic pressure b. Filtration pressure
c. Systolic blood pressure d. Oncotic pressure

38. Antidiuretic hormone is secreted by
a. Adrenal cortex
b. Anterior pituitary
c. Posterior lobe of pituitary
d. Adrenal medulla

39. The fifth cranial nerve is names as

a. Trigeminal b. Trochlear
c. Facial d. Abducens

40. Dysarthria is

a. Difficulty in swallowing
b. Difficulty in speaking
c. Difficulty in joint movement
d. Abnormal involuntary movements

41. Right ventricular enlargement due to pulmonary problem is called

a. Cardiac tamponade b. Cor pulmonale
c. Cardiomyopathy d. Emphysema

42. The difference between systolic and diastolic blood pressure is called

a. Pulse deficit
b. Pulse pressure
c. Mean arterial pressure
d. Peripheral vascular resistance

43. T-tube drainage is used after

a. Lobectomy b. Billroth I
c. Cholecystectomy d. Ileostomy

44. The specific intervention included in secondary prevention is

a. Early diagonsis b. Health promotion
c. Disability limitation d. Rehabilitation

45. Destruction of all microorganisms including their spores is called

a. Disinfection b. Sterilization
c. Antisepsis d. Asepsis

46. Schick test is used to diagnose

a. Tuberculosis b. Diphtheria
c. Viral hepatitis d. Typhoid fever

47. Which of the following vaccination should be taken for a 10-year-old child as per the national immunization schedule?

a. Tetanus toxoid b. TAB
c. DT d. Hepatitis B

48. One packet of oral rehydration mixture contain

a. 2.5 g of sodium chloride
b. 1.5 g of sodium chloride
c. 3.5 g of sodium chloride
d. 1.0 g of sodium chloride

49. Coining of new words is

a. Word salad b. Aphasia
c. Circumstantiality d. Neologism

50. Inflammation of payers patches is associated with

a. Typhoid fever b. Hepatitis
c. AIDS d. Cholera

51. Ramsteds operation is done for

a. Hiatus hernia b. Pyloric stenosis
c. Congenital megacolon d. Repair of cleft lip

52. Trismus is

a. Inability to swallow
b. Inability to open the jaw
c. Spasm of facial muscles
d. Paralysis muscles

53. Flag sign is positive in

a. Marasmus b. Beriberi
c. Kwashiorkor d. Scurvy

54. A baby with diaphragmatic hernia is nursed with

a. Foot end elevated b. Prone
c. Supine d. Head slightly elevated

55. The most common cause of apnea in a preterm baby is

a. Pulmonary surfactant deficiency
b. Pneumonia
c. Aspiration
d. Hypoglycemia

56. Spore forming bacteria

a. *M. Leprae* b. *V. Cholerae*
c. *Cl. Tetani* d. *Streptococcus*

57. The umbilical cord contain

a. One artery and one vein
b. Two arteries and two veins
c. Two veins and one artery
d. Two arteries and one vein

58. Coronal suture separates

a. Frontal bones from parietal bones
b. Occipital bones from parietal bones
c. The two frontal bones
d. The two parietal bones

59. **Brauns splint is used for**
   a. Fracture of the arms
   b. Fracture of pelvis
   c. Fracture of the lower limbs
   d. Fracture of collar bone

60. **The strength of Dettol solution used for disinfecting thermometers**
   a. 1:10 b. 1:20
   c. 1:30 d. 1:40

61. **A harsh, vibrating, shrill sound produced during respiration seen in laryngitis is**
   a. Rale b. Wheeze
   c. Stertorous d. Stridor

62. **Glycerine enema is an example of**
   a. Astringent enema b. Purgative enema
   c. Emolient enema d. Retention enema

63. **Human albumin is an example of**
   a. Crystalloid b. Amino acid solution
   c. Colloid solution d. Fat emulsion

64. **Pancuronium bromide is**
   a. Vasoconstrictor b. Analgesic
   c. Anticoagulant d. Muscle relaxant

65. **Signs of meningeal irritation include all the following except**
   a. Neck rigidity b. Brudzinski sign
   c. Babinski sign d. Kernig sign

66. **Which of the following is an antifungal agent?**
   a. Amphoteracine B b. Adenocine arabinocide
   c. Adriamycin d. Amantidine

67. **Submucosal resection is the surgical correction of**
   a. Cleft palate b. Deviated nasal septum
   c. Aneurysm d. Glaucoma

68. **The volume of air inhaled with normal respiration is called**
   a. Vital capacity b. Tidal volume
   c. Inspiratory capacity d. Lung capacity

69. **Endoxan is**
   a. Adriamycin b. Methotrexate
   c. Cyclophosphamide d. Mustargen

70. **Stimulation of alpha adrenergic receptors produce**
   a. Vasodilation
   b. Increased heart rate
   c. Increased myocardial contractility
   d. Vasoconstriction

71. **Which of the following is an acyanotic cardiac defect?**
   a. Transposition of great vessels
   b. Tetralogy of Fallot
   c. Pulmonary atresia
   d. Ventricular septal defect

72. **The most effective room disinfectant is**
   a. Formalin and potassium permanganate
   b. Bleaching powder
   c. Ethylene oxide and carbon dioxide
   d. Chlorhexidine

73. **Which of the following is a protective food?**
   a. Fish b. Green leafy vegetables
   c. Liver d. Egg

74. **Minilap operation is**
   a. Removal of a small piece of each fallopian tube and ligating each
   b. The fallopian tubes are cut and ends are blocked
   c. Removal of the fallopian tubes
   d. Application of rings to occlude the fallopian tube

75. **Rice water stool is characteristic of**
   a. Cholera b. Typhoid fever
   c. Dysentery d. Polimyelitis

76. **Presistent irrational fear of an object**
   a. Obsession b. Phobia
   c. Compulsion d. Delusion

77. **Filling the gap of memory with fabrication is**
   a. Amnesia b. Dejavu
   c. Hyperamnesia d. Paramnesia

78. **Children with TOF assumes**
   a. Squatting b. Fowlers
   c. Sitting d. Legs down

79. **The birth weight of a baby will be doubled by**
   a. 3 months b. 6 months
   c. 9 months d. 1 year

80. **Bitots spots is due to deficiency of**
   a. Vitamin B_{12} b. Vitamin A
   c. Niacin d. Pyridoxin

81. **Deficiency of clotting factor IX leads to**
   a. Hemophilia b. Thrombocytopenea
   c. Christmas disease d. Thalassemia

82. **Which of the following food contain first class protein?**
   a. Dhal b. Green leafy vegetable
   c. Soybeans d. Cereals

83. The biparietal diameter of the fetal skull is

a. 9.5 cm b. 8.2 cm
c. 10 cm d. 11.5 cm

84. Which of the following is a probable sign of pregnancy?

a. Quickening
b. Palpable fetal parts
c. Palpable fetal movements
d. Blueing of vagina

85. Which of the following is a definite indication of cesarean section?

a. Breech presentation
b. Diabetes mellitus
c. Moderate preeclampsia
d. Cephalo pelvic disproportion

86. Copper carrying contraceptive devices acts by

a. Preventing ovulation
b. Prevent spermatozoa coming in contact with ovum
c. Destruction of spermatozoa
d. Making cervical mucus thick to prevent penetration of spermatozoa

87. 37°C is equal to

a. 98.6°F b. 98.4°F
c. 98.8°F d. 98°F

88. One gram of protein yields

a. 4 calories b. 8 calories
c. 5 calories d. 9 calories

89. How much drug is contained in 100 mL of 1:1000 solution?

a. 1.0 g b. 10 g
c. 0.01 g d. 0.1 g

90. The enzyme which helps in digestion of fat is

a. Ptyalin b. Lactase
c. Lipase d. Pepsin

91. The most common side effect of streptomycin is

a. Nephrotoxicity b. Hepatotoxicity
c. Optic neuritis d. 8th nerve damage

92. Which of the following parameter should be monitored in patients after heart valve replacement?

a. Prothrombin time b. Clotting time
c. Bleeding time d. Platelet count

93. Patients after gastrectomy can develop

a. Hemolytic anemia
b. Pernicious anemia
c. Iron deficiency anemia
d. Folic acid deficiency anemia

94. *Helicobactor pylori* is associated with

a. Ulcerative colitis b. Typhoid fever
c. Peptic ulcer d. Crohn's disease

95. Outbreak of disease in the community in excess of normal expectation is

a. Pandemic b. Sporadic
c. Endemic d. Epidemic

96. Kopliks spots are characteristics of

a. German measles b. Measles
c. Oral cancer d. Purpura

97. SARS is spread by

a. Virus b. Bacteria
c. Fungi d. Protozoa

98. Waxy flexibility is a clinical feature of

a. Somnambulism b. Hypochondriasis
c. Mania d. Schizophrenia

99. Disturbance in the content of thinking is called

a. Obsession b. Compulsion
c. Flight of ideas d. Elation

100. Which of the following is a neuroleptic?

a. Lithium carbonate b. Phenelzine
c. Lorazepam d. Chloropromazine

ANSWERS

1. d	2. a	3. b	4. b	5. c	6. c	7. d	8. c	9. a	10. d	11. a	12. a
13. c	14. a	15. d	16. c	17. a	18. b	19. c	20. d	21. c	22. a	23. c	24. d
25. b	26. b	27. b	28. d	29. a	30. a	31. c	32. c	33. a	34. b	35. b	36. c
37. d	38. c	39. a	40. b	41. b	42. b	43. c	44. a	45. b	46. b	47. a	48. c
49. d	50. a	51. b	52. b	53. c	54. d	55. a	56. c	57. d	58. a	59. c	60. d
61. d	62. c	63. c	64. d	65. c	66. a	67. b	68. b	69. c	70. a	71. d	72. a
73. b	74. b	75. a	76. b	77. d	78. a	79. b	80. b	81. c	82. c	83. a	84. d
85. d	86. d	87. a	88. a	89. d	90. c	91. d	92. a	93. b	94. c	95. d	96. b
97. a	98. d	99. c	100. d								

STAFF NURSE GRADE II (Health Department)

{Exam held on 18-10-2007}

1. ....is the inflammation of the tongue.
   a. Gingivitis b. Gastritis
   c. Glossitis d. Parotitis

2. Heat regulating center is
   a. Thalamus b. Hypothalamus
   c. Basal nuclei d. Central cortex

3. Position used for giving enema
   a. Left lateral b. Right lateral
   c. Dorsal recumbent d. Lithotomy

4. Strength of normal saline is
   a. 1% b. 10%
   c. 19% d. 0.9%

5. An agent that has the power to kill microorganisms
   a. Bacteriocide b. Antiseptic
   c. Bacteriostat d. Disinfectant

6. 1 gram of fat give ....calories of heat
   a. 10 b. 4
   c. 2 d. 9

7. Strength of savlon for disinfecting thermometer is
   a. 1:30 b. 1:20
   c. 1:40 d. 1:10

8. Reaction of normal urine is
   a. Acidic b. Slight acidic
   c. Neutral d. Alkaline

9. Loss of appetite is termed as
   a. dyspepsia b. dysphagia
   c. anorexia d. nausea

10. Amount of solution administered for evacuant enema for adults
    a. 250–500 mL b. 500–1000 mL
    c. 1000–1500 mL d. 1500–2000 mL

11. The temperature of the water used for tepid sponging is
    a. 65°–85°F b. 85°–100°F
    c. 100°–105°F d. 105°–110°F

12. One pint is equal to
    a. 250 mL b. 500 mL
    c. 750 mL d. 1000 mL

13. Size of needle for intramuscular injection
    a. 18–20 gauge b. 21–23 gauge
    c. 24–25 gauge d. 26–27 gauge

14. Rate of oxygen administration through nasal catheter
    a. 0.5–1 liter b. 1.0–2 liter
    c. 2–4 liter d. 4–6 liter

15. Instrument used to examine the rectum
    a. Autoscope b. Proctoscope
    c. Endoscope d. Ophthalmoscope

16. Florence nightingale was born on
    a. January 12 b. April 12
    c. May 5 d. May 12

17. Drugs used to induce vomiting is
    a. Emetic b. Antiemetic
    c. Pyretics d. Antipyretics

18. Acetic acid is used for testing urine for
    a. Sugar b. Acetate
    c. Albumin d. Bile salts

19. Enema given to destroy or expel the worms form the intestine
    a. Astringent enema b. Anthelmintic enema
    c. Purgative enema d. Carminative enema

20. The important person in the hospital
    a. Doctor b. Nurse
    c. Patient d. Technician

21. Examination with the help of stethoscope is called
    a. Percussion b. Palpation
    c. Auscultation d. Inspection

22. When pulse rate is less than 60 beats per minute, it is called
    a. Bradycardia b. Bradypnea
    c. Tachycardia d. Tachypnea

23. Lock Jaw develops in

a. Typhoid b. Tetanus
c. Meningitis d. Diphtheria

24. The process of incising the ear drum to promote drainage is called

a. Trephening b. Mobilization
c. Myringotomy d. Fenestration

25. The most common complication during the first 24 hours following an amputation

a. Infection b. Flexion contraction
c. Hemorrhage d. Sloughing of the sutures

26. The doctor ordered for a patient 1,00,000 units of penicillin. At hand there is a vial containing 2,00,000 units diluted in 10 mL. How many mL will be given to the patient?

a. 5 mL b. 0.75 mL
c. 1.25 mL d. 2.5 mL

27. Profuse menstrual flow during regular period is called

a. Metrorrhagia b. Menorrhagia
c. Amenorrhea d. Polymenorrhea

28. The most serious complication of frature is

a. Infection b. Fat embolism
c. Hemorrhage d. Air embolism

29. Buck's extension is a method of

a. Skin traction b. Skin grafting
c. Skeletal traction d. Born grafting

30. The incubation period of chickenpox is

a. 12–21 days b. 1–7 days
c. 5–10 days d. 3 weeks–1 month

31. Shick test is used for the determination of person's susceptibility to

a. Scarlet fever b. Tuberculosis
c. Diphtheria d. Typhoid fever

32. Which of those effected is expected following the administration of a mydriatic medication?

a. Dilatation of the pupils
b. Improved power of accommodation
c. Inflammation of the nasolacrimal duct
d. Increased drainage of the aqueous humor.

33. Common type of fracture in children

a. Simple fracture b. Colli's fracture
c. Greenstick fracture d. Complicated fracture

34. The most important point in nursing care of a patient after tracheostomy is

a. Administration of antibiotics
b. Maintenance of intake output
c. Oxygen administration
d. Suctioning

35. Quickening takes place between

a. 10th and 16th weeks b. 16th and 20th weeks
c. 20th to 24th weeks d. After 24th weeks

36. The diuretic phase begins in burns within

a. 48–72 hours b. 12–24 hours
c. 36–48 hours d. 24–36 hours

37. The main side effect of streptomycin is

a. Hepatotoxicity b. Blood dyscrasias
c. Ototoxicity d. Visual disturbance

38. Vector of malaria is

a. Female culex mosquito
b. Female anopheles mosquito
c. Male culex mosquito
d. Male anopheles mosquito

39. Megaloblastic anemia is due to the deficiency of

a. Iron b. Thiamine
c. Acetic acid d. Folic acid

40. The normal serum bilirubin is

a. 0.1–1 mg/dL b. 2–4 mg/dL
c. 1.5–3.5 mg/dL d. 10–12 mg/dL

41. The symptom of enlarged prostrate include

a. Pyuria b. Difficulty in micturition
c. Ototoxicity d. Visual disturbance

42. A degenerative disease of the brain associated with liver failure

a. Uremia b. Diabetic coma
c. Septicemia d. Hepatic coma

43. Severe pain occur in the right quadrant of the abdomen radiating the back and to the right shoulder

a. Renal Colic b. Internal Colic
c. Biliary Colic d. Abdominal Colic

44. To lower the acidity of gastric secretion give

a. Gelusil b. Belladona
c. Aspirin d. Carminative mixture

45. **Diabetes mellitus is usually recognized by**
a. Albuminuria b. Lack of appetite
c. Glycosuria d. Urea in the urine

46. **Tuberculosis of the spine is also called**
a. Osteomalacia b. Charcot's disease
c. Erving's disease d. Pott's disease

47. **Nitroglycerine is given sublingually to relieve pain by vasodilatation of**
a. Pulmonary artery b. Coronary artery
c. Aortic artery d. Carotid artery

48. **The cause of ascites in cirrhosis of the liver is**
a. General fluid imbalance
b. Portal obstruction
c. Kidney trouble
d. All of these

49. **Dr Salk discovered a vaccine for the prevention of**
a. Measles b. Poliomyelitis
c. Smallpox d. Tetanus

50. **Pneumothorax is the condition in which there is**
a. Water in the visceral space
b. Air in the visceral space
c. Water in the pleural space
d. Air in the pleural space

51. **The cause of anemia in renal failure is**
a. Erythropoietin deficiency
b. Repeated hemodialysis
c. Excessive use of diuretics
d. Restriction of protein in the diet

52. **Group 'O' patients can receive blood belonging to group**
a. O b. B
c. A d. AB

53. **Xerophthalmia is due to deficiency of**
a. Vitamin K b. Vitamin C
c. Vitamin A d. Vitamin D

54. **Best therapeutic measure for empyema is**
a. Chest drainage b. Postural drainage
c. Breathing exercise d. Fowler's position

55. **Allergen causes**
a. Bronchitis b. Asthma
c. Bronchiectasis d. Pneumonia

56. **Serum cholesterol level will be low in case of**
a. Hypothyroidism b. Hyperthyroidism
c. Cretinism d. Diabetes

57. **Normal bleeding time is**
a. 1–3 minutes b. 6–10 minutes
c. 3–6 minutes d. 10–12 minutes

58. **Excessive salivation and drooling is seen in**
a. Esophageal atresia
b. Diaphragmatic hernia
c. Omphalocele
d. Trachea esophageal fistula

59. **Koplik's spot is seen in**
a. Chickenpox b. Measles
c. Mumps d. Smallpox

60. **The bilirubin encephalopathy due to high concentration of indirect bilirubin on brain and basal ganglia in the neonatal period is**
a. Status epileptics b. Kerning's sign
c. Kernicterus d. Jaundice

61. **Diabetes insipidus is caused by**
a. Growth hormone b. Insulin metabolism
c. Antidiuretic hormone d. Carbohydrate metabolism

62. **A congenital hemolytic disease caused by Rh incompatibility is**
a. Sickle cell anemia b. Erythroblastosis fetalis
c. Megaloblastic anemia d. Jaundice

63. **On an average, the normal infant triples their birth weight when they reach the age approximately**
a. 6 months b. 12 months
c. 18 months d. 24 months

64. **A nurse is assisting with the care of a child receiving oxygen by cannula. In what way it may differ from the way it is normally administering an adult.**
a. The oxygen need to be humidified before administering to a child.
b. The cannula for a child has only one nasal prong whereas an adult cannula has two nasal prongs.
c. The amount of oxygen administered to a child should be less than the amount administered to an adult.
d. The technique used for this therapy is same for an adult and child.

65. The commonest type of jaundice in new born
a. Hemolytic b. Physiological
c. Obstructive d. Hepatogenic

66. The most common cause of heart disease in adolescence or young adult is
a. Rheumatic fever b. Congenital heart disease
c. Anemia d. Melanization

67. Manifestation of anger in children
a. Thump sucking b. Temper tandrum
c. Nightmare d. Regression

68. Kwashiorkor is developed due to lack of
a. Protein b. Calories
c. Fat d. Protein and calories

69. Accidents are the largest single cause of mortality and disability between the age of
a. 1–4 years b. 5–7 years
c. 9–10 years d. 10 years onwards

70. One of the following drug is not an anticonvulsant.
a. Diazepam b. Phenobarbitone
c. Carbamazepine d. Penicillin

71. Increased concentration of oxygen in capillaries causing vasoconstriction and dilated vision of eyes is seen in
a. Conjunctivitis b. Cataract
c. Strabismus d. Retrolental fibroplasia

72. Liver enzymes which converts lipid soluble bilirubin
a. Low density lipoprotein
b. Acetylcholine
c. Glucoronyl transferase
d. High density lipoprotein

73. Expected weight of a child at 1 year whose birth weight was 3.5 kg would be
a. 7.5 kg b. 12.5 kg
c. 11.5 kg d. 10.5 kg

74. The disease transfered through contact is called
a. Communicable disease b. Infectious disease
c. Epidemic disease d. Contagious disease

75. The following are examples of live vaccine except
a. Typhoid b. Oral polio
c. BCG d. Measles

76. A substance which suppress or nutralize bad odors is called
a. Deodorant b. Antiseptic
c. Disinfectant d. Antibiotic

77. Poliomyelitis is
a. Bacterial infection b. Viral infection
c. Fungal infection d. Spirochetal infection

78. Rabies is a fatal viral disease of
a. Cardiovascular system b. Muscular system
c. Central nervous system d. Skeletal system

79. A childhood psychiatric disorder characterized by abnormalities in communication and social interaction and by restricted repeated activities and interests
a. Phobia b. Obsession
c. Autism d. Illusion

80. Misperception of external stimuli is called
a. Phobia b. Hallucination
c. Addiction d. Illusion

81. A syndrome in which the central features are over activity, mood change and self-important ideas
a. Mania b. Schizophrenia
c. Depression d. Hallucination

82. Voltage of current applied for ECT is
a. 35–75 volts b. 75–100 volts
c. 75–120 volts d. 100–150 volts

83. An artificially induced stage in which the person is relaxed and unusually suggestible
a. Phobia b. Play therapy
c. Epilepsy d. Hypnosis

84. Senile dementia occurs during
a. Childhood b. Teenage
c. Adult d. Old age

85. The ability to enter into the life of another person to accurately perceive his or her current feeling and to communicate this feeling to the patient is
a. Sympathy b. Empathy
c. Self-disclosure d. Role playing

86. Weight of uterus is
a. 30 g b. 60 g
c. 90 g d. 120 g

87. **The volume of amniotic fluid at term**
a. 500 mL b. 750 mL
c. 1000 mL d. 1250 mL

88. **Tobacco is not only in cigarettes, but is chewed by many people. Which is the poisons alkaloid that is present in tobacco?**
a. Lead b. Nicotine
c. Alcohol d. Caffeine

89. **After blood circulation stops, how long does the brain function**
a. 3 minutes b. 5 minutes
c. 8 minutes d. 10 minutes

90. **At what age does our brain stop further growth**
a. After 5 years b. After 10 years
c. After 15 years d. After 20 years

91. **How many bones are present in the entire framework of the human skeleton?**
a. 106 b. 206
c. 306 d. 406

92. **How many chromosomes are found in a cell of human being?**
a. 23 b. 28
c. 46 d. 48

93. **Which part of the heart is responsible for circulating blood through the lungs?**
a. Left ventricle b. Right ventricle
c. Left atrium d. Right atrium

94. **When the lens of the eyes become cloudy and opaque, the condition is known as**
a. Glaucoma b. Long sightedness
c. Cataract d. Short sightedness

95. **Which refers to the treatment of mental disease with the help of electric shock?**
a. Electroconvulsive therapy
b. Electroencephalography
c. Electrocardiography
d. Electric wave

96. **Which term is applied for the sensation of noise as roaring or ringing in the ears?**
a. Tinnitus b. Tetanus
c. Murmur d. Peristalsis

97. **Paralysis of the lower half of the torso and of both legs**
a. Quadriplegia
b. Hemiplegia
c. Paraplegia
d. Paralysis of lower extremity

98. **Which test is used to detect typhoid?**
a. Widal test b. Millard's test
c. Kahn test d. Rorschach test

99. **Obstruction of the artery or vein by a clot of blood?**
a. Thrombosis b. Embolism
c. Thrombophlebitis d. Phlebitis

100. **What should be the duration of full term pregnancy?**
a. 250 days b. 280 days
c. 300 days d. 310 days

ANSWERS

1. c	2. b	3. a	4. d	5. a	6. d	7. b	8. b	9. c	10. b	11. b	12. b
13. b	14. c	15. b	16. d	17. a	18. c	19. b	20. c	21. c	22. a	23. b	24. c
25. c	26. a	27. b	28. b	29. a	30. a	31. c	32. a	33. c	34. d	35. b	36. a
37. c	38. b	39. d	40. a	41. b	42. d	43. c	44. a	45. c	46. d	47. b	48. b
49. b	50. d	51. a	52. a	53. c	54. a	55. b	56. b	57. c	58. a	59. b	60. c
61. c	62. b	63. b	64. c	65. b	66. a	67. b	68. a	69. a	70. d	71. d	72. c
73. d	74. d	75. a	76. a	77. b	78. c	79. c	80. d	81. a	82. c	83. d	84. d
85. b	86. b	87. c	88. b	89. a	90. c	91. b	92. c	93. b	94. c	95. a	96. a
97. c	98. a	99. a	100. b								

STAFF NURSE (Plantation Corporation)

{Exam held on 08-11-2008}

1. **A cartilaginous joint between the pubic bone is**
   a. The symphysis pubis b. The sacro iliac joint
   c. The synovial joint d. The coccyx

2. **Largest cranial nerve is**
   a. Vagus b. Trigeminal
   c. Sciatic d. Optic

3. **Painful micturition is called**
   a. Anuria b. Dysuria
   c. Enuresis d. Oliguria

4. **Temperature regulating center in human body is**
   a. Hypothalamus b. Medulla oblongata
   c. Cerebellum d. Cerebrum

5. **The position of the patient while giving enema is**
   a. Lithotomy b. Dorsal recumbent
   c. Sidelying d. Left lateral position

6. **The temperature used for autoclaving or sterilization by steam under pressure is**
   a. 110°C b. 160°C
   c. 98.6°C d. 121°C

7. **The body of the uterus is known as**
   a. Fundus b. Cornua
   c. Infundibulum d. Corpus

8. **Normal pH of fetal blood is**
   a. 7.25 to 7.3 b. 7.35 to 7.45
   c. 7.2 d. 7

9. **The type of pelvis more suitable for child bearing**
   a. An oval brim b. A round brim
   c. A heart shaped brim d. A kidney shaped brim

10. **Fertilization of the ovum normally takes place in the**
    a. Corpus luteum
    b. Ampullary part of fallopian tube
    c. Fimbriated end of the fallopian tube
    d. Interstitial part of the fallopian tube

11. **In addition the OS is closed in case of**
    a. Complete abortion b. Inevitable abortion
    c. Septic abortion d. Threatened abortion

12. **When the umblical cord is attached to the very edge of the placenta is called**
    a. Placenta circumvallatta b. Velamentous insertion
    c. Battledore insertion d. Placenta accreta

13. **Placenta is developed from**
    a. Decidua b. Trophoblasticlayer
    c. Fallopian tube d. Amnion

14. **There is no mechanism of**
    a. Breech presentation
    b. Face presentation
    c. Shoulder presentation
    d. Occipito posterior presentation

15. **Expected time of closure of anterior fontannel is**
    a. 4–6 weeks b. 6–8 weeks
    c. 9–12 weeks d. 16–18 months

16. **The leader of health of the primary health center is**
    a. Patient b. Medical officer
    c. Health assistant d. Health inspector

17. **Colostrum is formed at**
    a. 16 weeks b. 20 weeks
    c. 24 weeks d. 10 weeks

18. **Local self government at district level**
    a. Zilla parishad b. Grama sabha
    c. Municipality d. Panchayat samiti

19. **Under the ICDS program, there is an anganwadi worker for every**
    a. 3000 population b. 1000 population
    c. 10,000 population d. 5000 population

20. **The very effective method of health teaching**
    a. Symposium b. Group discussion
    c. Lecture d. Films and charts

21. **Ovulation method of family planning is also known as**
    a. Calendar methods
    b. Billing methods
    c. Sympto thermal methods
    d. Spacing methods

22. **The Government of India redesignated the "National Family Planning Program" as the "National Family Welfare Program" in the year**
    a. 1977 b. 1953
    c. 1975 d. 1969

23. **Instrument used for high rupture of membranes in polyhydramnios**
    a. Kochers forceps b. Amniohook
    c. Drew smythe catheter d. Wrigley's forceps

24. **Temporary hardness is due to the presence of**
    a. Sulfate of calcium and magnesium
    b. Carbonates of calcium and magnesium
    c. Bicarbonates of calcium and magnesium
    d. Nitrates of calcium and magnesium

25. **The most sensitive measure of growth is**
    a. Weight b. Height
    c. Length d. Mid arm circumference

26. **Understand the situation and feelings of others**
    a. Empathy b. Sympathy
    c. Affection d. Emotion

27. **Which committee is known as the Health Survey and Planning Committee?**
    a. Mudaliar Committee b. Kartar Singh Committee
    c. Bhore Committee d. Shrivastav Committee

28. **Which one of the following is an international agency which assist in programs that benefit child health most?**
    a. UNO b. WHO
    c. UNICEF d. Red cross

29. **Formation of urea is a function of**
    a. Liver b. Kidney
    c. Spleen d. Gallbladder

30. **Oral thrush is caused by**
    a. Bacteria b. Fungus
    c. Virus d. Protozoa

31. **The immunity acquired by suffering from a disease is**
    a. Natural immunity
    b. Passive immunity
    c. Active immunity
    d. Acquired natural immunity

32. **Scrub typhus is caused by**
    a. Rickettsiae b. Varicella virus
    c. Leptospirosis d. *Haemophilus influenzae*

33. **Hospital acquired infection is termed as**
    a. Nosocomial infection b. Droplet infection
    c. Auto infection d. Direct infection

34. **The longest diameter of the fetal skull is**
    a. Biparietal b. Bitemporal
    c. Occipitofrontal d. Mentovertical

35. **The ovarian hormone responsible for the first half of the menstrual cycle is**
    a. Estrogen
    b. Progesterone
    c. Prolactin
    d. Human chorinic gonadotrophin

36. **Multipurpose workers for health and family planning was set up by**
    a. Bhore Committee
    b. Mudaliar Committee
    c. Kartar Singh Committee
    d. Shrivastav Committee

37. **National Filaria Control Program was initiated in**
    a. 1955 b. 1954
    c. 1974 d. 1976

38. **Montgometry Tubercles around the nipple of breast appear at**
    a. 6 weeks b. 4 weeks
    c. 8 weeks d. 10 weeks

39. **Vaginal examination is carried out in promigravida to determine the pelvic size and shape at**
    a. 34–36 weeks b. 38 weeks
    c. 40 weeks d. 30–32 weeks

40. **Occupational disease caused by coal dust is**
    a. Anthracosis b. Silicosis
    c. Asbestosis d. Bagossosis

41. **The population of a corporation is**
   a. 10000 b. 1 lakh
   c. 2 lakhs d. Above 2 lakhs

42. **A safe, simple and reliable form of male contraception is**
   a. Use of condom b. Vasectomy
   c. Coitus interrupts d. All of the above

43. **Vaccine and toxoids produce**
   a. Natural immunity b. Active immunity
   c. Passive immunity d. Racial immunity

44. **HIV can be transmitted to the child in the following way**
   a. Through fomites
   b. Through droplet infection
   c. Through being born to HIV infected mothers
   d. Through food and water

45. **The infant mortality rate of Kerala is**
   a. 70 b. 14
   c. 60 d. 20

46. **Sepsis means**
   a. Absence of infection
   b. Presence of pathogenic organisms
   c. Destroying of all organisms
   d. Free from microorganisms

47. **The bacillus of diphtheria is found in the**
   a. Throat b. Nasal passage
   c. Upper respiratory tract d. All of these

48. **The most common symptom of perception is**
   a. Delusion b. Hallucination
   c. Passivity d. Dementia

49. **The most common cause of early abortion is**
   a. Abnormalities of embryo
   b. Severe systemic infections of the mother
   c. Psychic and physical trauma
   d. Diabetes

50. **Pregnant women should be advised**
   a. To avoid contact with infectious disease
   b. To refrain from taking drugs and to stop smoking
   c. To take foods rich in body builders
   d. All of these

51. **Quickening is the movement of the fetus in utero where the first recognized the mother usually between**
   a. 16th to 20th week b. 20th to 24th week
   c. 8th to 10th week d. None of these

52. **The presence of excessive amounts of gases in the intestine leading to the distention of the abdomen is**
   a. Constipation b. Fecal impaction
   c. Flatulence d. None of these

53. **Instillation of drug means**
   a. Introducting solid forms of drugs into the body orifices
   b. Putting a drug in liquid form into a body cavity
   c. Administration of drugs in the form of powder into a body cavity
   d. Putting in a solid drug into the body tissues

54. **A substance that dilate the pupil of the eye is**
   a. Myotics b. Mydriatics
   c. Narcotics d. None of these

55. **A bath which is taken in a sitting position is**
   a. Bed bath b. Partial bath
   c. Sitz bath d. Tepid sponge

56. **The patient can breath only in a upright position is**
   a. Hyperpnea b. Orthopnea
   c. Apnea d. Bradypnea

57. **Presence of blood in the sputum is called as**
   a. Hemetemesis b. Hemoptysis
   c. Melena d. None of these

58. **Pus formation in the sockets of teeth is**
   a. Pyuria b. Pyorrhea
   c. Cheilosis d. Gingivitis

59. **Enzyme produced by the pancreas which helps in the digestion of carbohydrate is**
   a. Lipids b. Trypsin
   c. Amylase d. None of these

60. **Which is not a social problem?**
   a. Prostitution b. Alcoholism
   c. Drug addiction d. Dementia

61. **A tendency to blame others for his mistakes or failure is**
   a. Projection b. Rationalization
   c. Compensation d. Regression

62. **A reflection of one's personality is**
a. Trait b. Behavior
c. Intelligent d. Habit

63. **The time interval between the entry of the disease agent into the body and the appearance of the first sign or symptom of the disease is**
a. Incubation period b. Transmission
c. Infection d. Epidemic

64. **Current net reproduction rate is**
a. 1.4 b. 1.8
c. 1.2 d. 1

65. **Progesterone is secreted by**
a. Corpus luteum b. Corpus albicans
c. Graffian follicles d. Pituitary gland

66. **The normal body temperature of a person is**
a. 98.6°F b. 99.6°F
c. 97.4°F d. 97.6°F

67. **Malaria is a mosquito borne febrile disease caused by**
a. Contamination b. Vector
c. Parasite d. Insects

68. **The normal pulse rate for infants**
a. 110–120/min b. 120–130/min
c. 120–140/min d. 140–160/min

69. **A baby below 6 months needs**
a. 80 calories/kg body weight/day
b. 120 calories/kg body weight/day
c. 100 calories/kg body weight/day
d. 150 calories /kg body weight/ day

70. **The cheapest source of vitamin D is**
a. Milk b. Fish liver oil
c. Butter and cheese d. Sunlight

71. **The lifespan of RBC is**
a. 125 days b. 140 days
c. 120 days d. 150 days

72. **The most likely symptom will present in placenta previa is**
a. A board like abdomen
b. Painless bleeding
c. Intermittent pain with spotting
d. A dull pain in the lower abdomen

73. **The maximum amount of blood loss during delivery that is considered to be within normal limit is approximately**
a. 300 mL b. 100 mL
c. 500 mL d. 700 mL

74. **Apgar score of a healthy baby is**
a. 5 b. 10
c. 7 d. 4

75. **Neonate is one who is**
a. Less than 1 year b. Less than 42 days old
c. Less than 1 month old d. Less than 7 days old

76. **The best and useful method of refuse disposal in rural area is**
a. Dumping b. Composting
c. Incineration d. Controlled tipping

77. **Growth means**
a. Increase in size of the whole body
b. Increase in skill
b. Increase in health
d. Increase in abilities

78. **Measles is caused by**
a. Rotavirus b. Paramyxovirus
c. Astrovirus d. Variolavirus

79. **Which one of the following is a non-communicable disease?**
a. Malaria b. Cholera
c. Hypertension d. Viral hepatitis

80. **The National Malaria Eradication program commenced from**
a. 1963 b. 1956
c. 1958 d. 1953

81. **Sources of vital statistics are**
a. National sample surveys
b. Census
c. Report from different institutions
d. All of these

82. **Live vaccine used for immunization is**
a. BCG b. Cholera
c. Diphtheria d. Tetanus

83. The occurrence of a group of illness of similar nature in excess of natural expectation is

a. Endemic b. Epidemic
c. Pandemic d. None of these

84. World Health Day is on

a. August 10th b. May 12th
c. April 7th d. December 1st

85. The best time for insertion of IUD is

a. 40 days after delivery b. 6 weeks after abortion
c. Intermenstrual period d. All of these

86. Eye disease due to deficiency of vitamin A is

a. Pellagra b. Bitot's spot
c. Angular stomatitis d. Osteomalacia

87. Function of vitamin K is

a. Helps in wound healing
b. Helps in formation of healthy bones and teeth
c. Helps for clotting of blood
d. Helps in calcium absorption from the intestine

88. Pulse polio immunization is organized in India during the month

a. November to February b. May to September
c. March to May d. June to September

89. Which one of the following disease is transmitted through water?

a. Typhoid b. Tuberculosis
c. Measles d. Chickenpox

90. Limitation of freedom of movement of well person or domestic animal exposed to communicable disease for a period of time not longer than the longest incubation period of the disease is

a. Notification b. Isolation
c. Quarantine d. All of these

91. The largest gland in the body is

a. Pituitary gland b. Spleen
c. Pancreas d. Liver

92. The hormone produced by the posterior lobe of pituitary gland is

a. Growth hormone b. Vasopressin
c. Cortisone d. Adrenalin

93. Premature baby means

a. Baby born at 38 weeks
b. Baby born at 28–37 weeks
c. Baby born at 40 weeks
d. Baby born after 40 weeks

94. In a malnourished child, the arm circumference is

a. 16 cm b. 15 cm
c. 14 cm d. below 13 cm

95. Birth should be registered within

a. 45 days b. 21 days
c. 14 days d. 7 days

96. The cause of maternal mortality

a. Hemorrhage b. Anemia
c. Sepsis d. All of these

97. The longest vein in the body is

a. Femoral vein b. Cephalic vein
c. Long saphenous vein d. Umbilical vein

98. Universal recipient blood group is

a. A b. B
c. AB d. O

99. A group of biologically related individuals living together is known as

a. Society b. Family
c. Clean d. Community

100. Knee joint is an example for

a. Gliding joint b. Saddle joint
c. Hinge joint d. Synovial joint

ANSWERS

1. a	2. b	3. b	4. a	5. d	6. d	7. d	8. b	9. b	10. b	11. d	12. c
13. b	14. c	15. d	16. b	17. a	18. a	19. b	20. b	21. c	22. a	23. c	24. c
25. a	26. a	27. a	28. c	29. b	30. b	31. d	32. a	33. a	34. d	35. a	36. c
37. a	38. c	39. a	40. a	41. d	42. b	43. b	44. c	45. b	46. b	47. d	48. b
49. a	50. d	51. a	52. c	53. b	54. b	55. c	56. b	57. b	58. b	59. c	60. d
61. a	62. b	63. a	64. d	65. a	66. a	67. c	68. c	69. a	70. d	71. c	72. b
73. c	74. b	75. c	76. b	77. a	78. b	79. c	80. c	81. d	82. a	83. b	84. c
85. d	86. b	87. c	88. a	89. a	90. c	91. d	92. b	93. b	94. d	95. c	96. d
97. c	98. c	99. b	100. c								

STAFF NURSE(48/2008)

{Exam held on 19-06-2009}

1. **Which of the following destroys HIV?**
   a. Dettol b. Savlon
   c. Sodium hypochlorite d. Lysol
2. **Which of the following is a live vaccine?**
   a. TT b. DPT
   c. BCG d. DT
3. **Recommended population coverage of an Anganwadi is**
   a. 1000 b. 3000
   c. 5000 d. 10000
4. **Route of a administration of measles vaccine is**
   a. Intradermal b. Subcutaneous
   c. Intramuscular d. Oral
5. **Site of BCG vaccination is**
   a. Left thigh b. Right thigh
   c. Left deltoid d. Right deltoid
6. **The most precious and difficult resource to manage is**
   a. Man b. Money
   c. Materials d. Machines
7. **The best recommended body mass index for adult is**
   a. 15–19 b. 20–25
   c. 26–30 d. 31–35
8. **Nurse—Patient relationship is**
   a. Human to human relation
   b. Superior subordinate relation
   c. Subordinate superior relation
   d. Employer employee relation
9. **Which of the following is a waterborne disease?**
   a. Filariasis b. Poliomyelitis
   c. Dengue fever d. Influenza
10. **The best method of disposal of hospital waste is**
    a. Dumping b. Burning
    c. Composting d. Incineration
11. **Which of the following disease is due to deficiency of calcium?**
    a. Kwarshiorkor b. Marasmus
    c. Rickets d. Beriberi
12. **Temperature regulating center of the body is**
    a. Medulla oblongata b. Thalamus
    c. Hypothalamus d. Pituitary gland
13. **The best position to give enema is**
    a. Left lateral b. Right lateral
    c. Prone d. Supine
14. **Bleeding between menstrual period is called**
    a. Menorrhagia b. Metrorrhagia
    c. Amenorrhea d. Dysmenorrhea
15. **Which of the following is a zoonosis?**
    a. Chikungunya b. Malaria
    c. Rabies d. AIDS
16. **Outbreak of a diseases in the community in excess of normal expectation is**
    a. Endemic b. Pandemic
    c. Epidemic d. Sporadic
17. **Pap smear examination is done to diagnose**
    a. Ca breast b. Ca cervix
    c. Ca bladder d. Ca rectum
18. **Total score of Glasgow coma scale is**
    a. 5 b. 10
    c. 15 d. 20
19. **The most preferred intramuscular injection site for children is**
    a. Deltoid b. Ventrogluteal
    c. Dorsogluteal d. Vastus lateralis
20. **One ounce is**
    a. 10 g b. 20 g
    c. 30 g d. 40 g

21. **Drugs that cause expulsion of gas from the intestinal tract is**
    a. Astringents b. Cathartics
    c. Carminatives d. Emetics

22. **Administration of a medicine just below the skin is called**
    a. Intramuscular b. Intradermal
    c. Intravenous d. Subcutaneous

23. **The difference between oral and rectal temperature is**
    a. 1°F b. 2°F
    c. 3°F d. 4°F

24. **An agent that inhibit the growth of bacteria is**
    a. Bacteriostat b. Bactericide
    c. Carrier d. Vaccine

25. **Immunization is a method of**
    a. Primary prevention b. Secondary prevention
    c. Tertiary prevention d. Barrier prevention

26. **The position recommended for a patient with epistaxis is**
    a. Supine
    b. Prone
    c. Sitting with head turning forward
    d. Sitting with head turning backward

27. **Which of the following is an independent nursing function?**
    a. Administration of oral medicine
    b. Administration of injection
    c. Giving blood transfusion
    d. Health education

28. **Priority attention required for an unconscious patient is**
    a. Nutrition b. Elimination
    c. Airway patency d. Exercise

29. **Which of the following is related to vision testing?**
    a. Tuning fork b. Snellen's chart
    c. Litmus paper d. Acetic acid

30. **Head circumference and chest circumference of child becomes equal at the age of**
    a. 1 year b. 2 years
    c. 3 years d. 4 years

31. **The simplest method of prevent cross infection is**
    a. Disinfection b. Sterilization
    c. Handwashing d. Fumigation

32. **Neonates are prone to**
    a. Hypoglycemia b. Hyperglycemia
    c. Hypocalcemia d. Hypercalcemia

33. **Which of the following is a sign of toxemia in pregnancy?**
    a. Low blood pressure b. High blood pressure
    c. Low blood sugar d. High blood sugar

34. **Intrauterine contraceptive device are introduced postpartum at**
    a. 6 weeks b. 12 weeks
    c. 6 months d. 12 months

35. **Which of the following is an antiretroviral agent?**
    a. Acyclovir b. Rifampicin
    c. Nevirapine d. Cifran

36. **Which of the following is a barrier method of contraception?**
    a. Oral pills b. Copper T
    c. Condom d. Tubectomy

37. **Anemia prophylaxis in pregnancy starts at the**
    a. First month b. Second month
    c. Third month d. Fourth month

38. **The fundal height is at the level of xiphisternum at**
    a. 28 weeks b. 32 weeks
    c. 36 weeks d. 40 weeks

39. **While receiving blood transfusion, the patient develops chills and headache. The nurse's first action is to**
    a. Lightly cover the patient
    b. Slow the blood flow
    c. Notify the physician
    d. Stop the transfusion immediately

40. **The basic emotional task for the toddler is**
    a. Trust b. Industry
    c. Independence d. Identification

41. **A nursing diagnosis represents the**
    a. Proposed plan of care
    b. Client's health problems
    c. Assessment of client data
    d. Actual nursing intervention

42. **Mentally healthy individuals can be defined as those who**
   a. Have insight into their own problems
   b. Do not exhibit pathological symptoms
   c. Are able to meet their own basic needs
   d. Are free from both physical and emotional problems.

43. **Which of the following side effect should be monitored in a patient on rifampicin?**
   a. Skin rashes b. Headache
   c. Jaundice d. Giddiness

44. **The ability to tolerate frustration is an example of one of the functions of the**
   a. ID b. Ego
   c. Superego d. Unconscious

45. **A person seeing a design on the wallpapers perceives it as an animal. This is an example of**
   a. Illusion b. Delusion
   c. Hallucination d. Idea of reference

46. **Fertilization usually occurs in the**
   a. Ovary b. Fallopian tube
   c. Uterus d. Vagina

47. **Which of the following vitamin prevents neural tube defects in fetus?**
   a. Vitamin. A b. Vitamin C
   c. Vitamin E d. Folic acid

48. **The most frequent side effect associated with the use of IUCD is**
   a. Ectopic pregnancy b. Expulsion of IUCD
   c. Rupture of uterus d. Excessive menstrual flow

49. **After ovulation has occurred, the ovum remains viable for**
   a. 1 to 6 hours b. 12 to 18 hours
   c. 24 to 36 hours d. 48 to 72 hours

50. **The first fetal movement felt by the mother is known as**
   a. Lightening b. Quickening
   c. Engagement d. Ballottement

51. **The safest position for a woman in labor with prolapse cord is**
   a. Supine b. Fowler's
   c. Lithotomy d. Trendelenburg

52. **If the first day of a woman's last menstrual period was July 22, the estimate date of child birth would be**
   a. April 15 b. April 29
   c. May 5 d. May 14

53. **Physiologic anemia during pregnancy is a result of**
   a. Decreased dietary intake of iron.
   b. Increased plasma volume of the mother.
   c. Decreased erythropoiesis in the pregnancy.
   d. Increased demands of the fetus.

54. **A patient in active labor spontaneously ruptures membranes. The nurse should first**
   a. Monitor the fetal heart rate.
   b. Call the doctor.
   c. Check vital signs.
   d. Monitor contractions.

55. **Early ambulation in the postpartum period is encouraged to**
   a. Promote respiration
   b. Increase tone of bladder
   c. Increase tone of abdominal muscles
   d. Increase peripheral vasomotor activity

56. **Immunity transferred to fetus from the mother through placenta is**
   a. Active natural immunity
   b. Active articifical immunity
   c. Passive natural immunity
   d. Passive artificial immunity

57. **The most appropriate time to collect sputum specimen from a patient is**
   a. Before meals b. After meals
   c. On awakening d. After activity

58. **Scheduled dose of digoxin is withheld and notify physician when the adult patient's pulse rate drop below**
   a. 50/min b. 60/min
   c. 70/min d. 80/min

59. **The primary task to be accomplished between 12 to 15 months of age is to learn to**
   a. Walk erect b. Climb stairs
   c. Use a spoon d. Say simple words

60. **To instill eardrops to a small child, pull the pinna**
a. Forward b. Up and back
c. Straight back d. Down and back

61. **The most important complication of mumps in postpubertal males is**
a. Hypopituitarism b. Sterility
c. Decrease in lifido d. Decrease in androgens

62. **The most important nursing action in the first 48 hours of hospitalization of a patient with full thickness burns over 30% of the body is directed towards preventing**
a. Pneumonia b. Shock
c. Contractures d. Hypertension

63. **An infection caused by canadia albicans often occuring in infants and defilitated individuals is**
a. Dysentery b. Hepatitis
c. Thrush d. Typhoid fever

64. **Which of the following is an isotonic solution?**
a. 5% dextrose b. Normal saline
c. 10% dextrose d. 5% dextrose saline

65. **A 5% dextrose saline 1000 mL is ordered for a patient to run in 8 hours. A drip set with a drop factor of 15 per mL is used. What is the flow rate to be set?**
a. 11 drops/min b. 21 drops/min
c. 31 drops/min d. 41 drops/min

66. **Which of the following drug is to be infused fast?**
a. Aminophylline b. Mannitol
c. Dopamine d. Potassium chloride

67. **A common finding in most children with cardiac anomalies is**
a. Mental retardation
b. Cyanosis
c. Family history of cardiac anomalies
d. Delayed physical growth

68. **The nutrients essential to prevent nutritional anemia include proteins, iron, vitamin B_{12} and**
a. Calcium b. Thiamine
c. Folic acid d. Iodine

69. **The action of ranitidine is**
a. Increase gastric motility
b. Neutralize gastric acidity
c. Increase histamine release
d. Inhibit gastric acid secretion

70. **The percentage of fluid in the infant's body is**
a. 20% b. 40%
c. 60% d. 80%

71. **The most important electrolyte of intracellular fluid is**
a. Sodium b. Potassium
c. Chloride d. Calcium

72. **Normal pH for arterial blood is**
a. 7.0 b. 7.30
c. 7.42 d. 7.50

73. **Position to be given to a patient recovering from general anesthesia is**
a. Supine position b. Side lying position
c. Fowler's position d. Trendelenburg position

74. **A patient has an IV infusion. If the IV infusion infiltrates, the nurse should first**
a. Elevate the IV site b. Discontinue the infusion
c. Flush the tube d. Apply warm, moist soaks

75. **Infection with Group A β-hemolytic streptococci is associated with**
a. Hepatitis b. Rheumatoid arthritis
c. Rheumatic fever d. Meningitis

76. **The position in which a patient with dyspnea should be placed is**
a. Sims b. Orthopneic
c. Supine d. Prone

77. **Airborne precautions for a patient with pulmonary tuberculosis has to be taken until**
a. Tuberculin test is negative
b. The patient no longer has the disease
c. No tubercle bacilli in the sputum
d. Patient's temperature has returned to normal

78. **When suctioning a patient with tracheostomy the nurse must remember to**
a. Use new sterile catheter with each suction
b. Insert catheter until cough reflex is stimulated
c. Initiate suction as the cathter is being withdrawn
d. Remove inner cannula before inserting suction catheter

79. **When a Ryle's tube is being inserted, the best position to be given to the patient is**
a. Supine position b. Side lying position
c. High fowler's position d. Trendelenburg position

80. Nasogastric tube feeding is to be given slowly to reduce the hazard of

a. Distention b. Flatulence
c. Indigestion d. Regurgitation

81. Which of the following is a blood borne infection?

a. Hepatitis B b. Chikungunya
c. Weil's disease d. Plague

82. Before doing paracentesis for a patient with ascites, instruct the patient to

a. Eat foods low in fat b. Remain NPO for 24 hours
c. Empty the bladder d. Assume supine position

83. The diet should be followed by a patient with colostomy is

a. Rich in protein
b. Low in fiber
c. High in carbohydrate
d. As close to normal as possible

84. Which of the following vitamin is administered with Isoniazid (INH)?

a. Vitamin B_1 b. Vitamin B_2
c. Vitamin B_6 d. Vitamin B_{12}

85. The hormone controlling the use of glucose by the cell is

a. Thyroxin b. Steroids
c. Insulin d. Growth hormone

86. The most important aspect of hand washing is

a. Time b. Soap
c. Water d. Friction

87. Which of the following is an indication of hypoglycemic reaction?

a. Pallor, perspiration, tremors
b. Excessive thirst, dry hot slain
c. Fruity odor of breath, acetonuria
d. Anorexia, glycosuria, tachycardia

88. Which of the following would predispose a patient to the occurrence of diabetic ketoacidosis?

a. Taking too much insulin
b. Doing too much exercise
c. Running a fever with infection
d. Eating less calories

89. The temperature of water for a tepid sponge bath should be approximately

a. 92° to 94°F b. 95° to 97°F
c. 98° to 100°F d. 101° to 103°F

90. Hemiplegia means

a. Paralysis of both lower extremities
b. Paralysis of one side of the body
c. Paralysis of upper and lower extremities
d. Paresis of one side of the body

91. The first aid treatment for a patient who had been bitten by a dog involves

a. Administering antirabies vaccine
b. Applying a wound dressing
c. Cleaning the wound with soap and water
d. Applying tourniquet proximal to the wound

92. A person's body temperature of 98.6°F is converted to

a. 36.5°C b. 37.0°C
c. 37.7°C d. 38.2°C

93. When a person is unconscious, the person is unable to

a. Hear voice b. Control elimination
c. Move spontaneously d. React to painful stimuli

94. The position of an unconscious patient should be changed at least every

a. 2 hours b. 4 hours
c. 6 hours d. 8 hours

95. Infection from urinary catheters can be best prevented by

a. Encouraging adequate fluid intake
b. Changing position frequently
c. Cleansing around the meatus periodically
d. Irrigating the catheter daily

96. Gonorrhea is highly infectious and

a. Is easily cured
b. Occurs very rarely
c. Is limited to external genitalia
d. Can produce sterility

97. Birth weight doubles at the age of

a. 2 months b. 3 months
c. 6 months d. 9 months

98. Peripheral most health care facility is

a. Primary health center
b. Subcenter
c. Community health center
d. Taluk hospital

99. Dengue fever is caused by a

a. Bacteria
b. Virus
c. Fungus
d. Protozoa

100. A patient is to have an enema. The rectal tube should be inserted

a. 2 inches
b. 4 inches
c. 6 inches
d. 8 inches

ANSWERS

1. c	2. c	3. a	4. b	5. c	6. a	7. b	8. a	9. b	10. d	11. c	12. c
13. a	14. b	15. c	16. c	17. b	18. c	19. d	20. c	21. c	22. b	23. a	24. a
25. a	26. c	27. d	28. c	29. b	30. b	31. c	32. a	33. b	34. a	35. a	36. c
37. d	38. c	39. d	40. c	41. b	42. a	43. c	44. b	45. a	46. b	47. d	48. d
49. b	50. b	51. d	52. b	53. b	54. a	55. d	56. c	57. c	58. b	59. a	60. d
61. b	62. b	63. c	64. b	65. c	66. b	67. d	68. a	69. d	70. c	71. b	72. c
73. a	74. b	75. c	76. b	77. c	78. a	79. c	80. d	81. a	82. c	83. a	84. d
85. c	86. a	87. a	88. d	89. c	90. b	91. c	92. b	93. b	94. a	95. a	96. d
97. c	98. a	99. b	100. b								

QUALIFYING EXAMINATION FOR KNMC REGISTRATION

{Exam held in November 2009}

1. **Which of the following is a complication of prolonged bed rest?**
   a. Jaundice b. Diarrhea
   c. Kidney stone d. Fever
2. **The best time for administration of diuretics is**
   a. 9 am b. 1 pm
   c. 4 pm d. 6 pm
3. **Dumping syndrome is a postoperative complication of**
   a. Cholecystectomy b. Gastrostomy
   c. Appendicectomy d. Gastrectomy
4. **Condition in which the endometrial cells seeded outside the uterine cavity is**
   a. Endometritis b. Fibroid
   c. Procidentia d. Endometriosis
5. **Inner force that moves the individual to a certain action**
   a. Motive b. Attitude
   c. Behavior d. Mind
6. **Inborn allround mental efficiency of an individual is called**
   a. Emotion b. Intelligence
   c. Behavior d. Drives
7. **Difficulty in getting off to sleep or in maintaining sleep is called**
   a. Amnesia b. Insomnia
   c. Narcolepsy d. Hypersomnia
8. **A group of drug to treat extrapyramidal side effect is**
   a. Antipsychotic drugs b. Antiparkinsonism drugs
   c. Antidepressant drugs d. Anticonvulsants
9. **The strongest joint in the human body**
   a. Sacroiliac joint b. Symphysis pubis
   c. Sacrococcygeal joint d. Sacrospinous joint
10. **Genital anomalies in which the urethral opening is below its normal location on the glans of the penis is termed**
    a. Epispadias b. Hypospadias
    c. Chordee d. Phimosis
11. **An elevated ASO titer is seen in which of the following conditions**
    a. Nephrotic syndrome b. Rheumatic fever
    c. Gastric ulcer d. Ulcerative colitis
12. **The common complaint of a woman with IUD is**
    a. Vaginal bleeding b. Pelvic infection
    c. Uterine perforation d. Abdominal pain
13. **A basic document for organizing family planning work is**
    a. Family record b. Eligible couple register
    c. MCH record d. Birth and death register
14. **Expected weight of a child at one year whose birth weight was 3 kg is**
    a. 7 kg b. 9 kg
    c. 10.5 kg d. 12 kg
15. **Children with Tetralogy of Fallot assumes**
    a. Squatting b. Fowler's
    c. Sitting d. Legs down
16. **Do not suction the patient more than 10–15 seconds at a time after tracheostomy because there is the danger of**
    a. Anoxia b. Hypoxia
    c. Anorexia d. Ataxia
17. **A hereditary form of arthritis with an excess of uric acid in the blood occurs in**
    a. Syringomyelia b. Still's disease
    c. Gout d. Spondylitis
18. **The client with gastric lavage or prolonged vomiting must be assessed for**
    a. Acidosis
    b. Alkalosis
    c. Loss of oxygen from the blood
    d. Loss of osmotic pressure of the blood
19. **For a patient with pulmonary edema, the oxygen flow rate should be at**
    a. 2 L b. 6 L
    c. 8 L d. 10 L

20. Accidental removal of a parathyroid gland during thyroidectomy would cause

a. Myxedema
b. Tetany
c. Hypovolemic shock
d. Adrenocortical stimulation

21. Dysphasia is a defect that cause difficulty in

a. Walk b. Speech
c. Swallowing d. Vision

22. Goiter, hyperthyroidism and exophthalmos are characteristic symptoms of

a. Grave's disease b. Thyroiditis
c. MNG d. Thyroid adenoma

23. Repair of tympanic membrane is

a. Tympanoplasty b. Myringoplasty
c. Myringotomy d. Septoplasty

24. CSF is secreted by

a. Cerebral aqueduct b. Arachnoid granulations
c. Choroid plexus d. Falx cerebri

25. Area where the optic nerve leaves the eye is called

a. Macula lutea b. Choroid
c. Ciliary body d. Optic disc

26. The two outstanding characteristic symptoms of diabetes mellitus are

a. Hypoglycemia and glycosuria
b. Hyperglycemia and glycosuria
c. Hypoglycemia and hypokalemia
d. Hyperglycemia and hypokalemia

27. A defense mechanism where the individual transfer unacceptable thoughts or feeling to another object is

a. Rationalization b. Sublimation
c. Displacement d. Substitution

28. The ductus connects the umbilical vein to the

a. Superior vena cava b. Inferior vena cava
c. Aorta d. Pulmonary artery

29. The drug of choice in controlling convulsions in eclamptic seizures

a. Diazepam b. Phenobarbitone
c. Eptoin sodium d. Sodium valproate

30. Which of the following development milestone is expected from a 2-year-old child

a. Uses a spoon to eat
b. Uses a cup to drink
c. Uses a knife for cutting food
d. Pour milk into a cup

31. A complication that can occur due to unwise administration of oxygen to a newborn

a. Retrolental fibroplasia
b. Pneumothorax
c. Tachycardia
d. Hyaline membrane disease

32. The only safe and effective drug against filarial infection

a. Chloroquine
b. Rifampicin
c. Diethyl Carbamazepine Citrate
d. Pyrazinamide

33. An epidemic which spreads from country to country or over the whole world is called

a. Sporadic b. Pandemic
c. Endemic d. Epidemic

34. Koplik's spots are characteristic of

a. Measles b. Oral cancer
c. Purpura d. Mumps

35. Worm that is transmitted through meat is

a. Hookworm b. Tapeworm
c. Round worm d. Pinworm

36. An instrument used to measure intraocular pressure

a. Gonioscope b. Tonometer
c. Bifocal lens d. Ophthalmoscope

37. A serious possible complication of mastoidectomy

a. Meningitis b. Otitis
c. Sinusitis d. Keratitis

38. The nurse should position a client recovering from general anesthesia in a

a. Supine position b. Sidelying position
c. High Fowler's position d. Trendelenburg position

39. Postoperatively, if a patient's colostomy stoma is viable, its color will be

a. Gray b. Brick red
c. Pale pink d. Dark purple

40. Subdural hematoma is a blood collection between

a. Skull and dura mater
b. Dura and pia mater
c. Arachnoid and pia mater
d. Dura and subarachnoid mater

41. Obstruction due to twisting of intestine is

a. Volvulus b. Intussusception
c. Diverticulum d. Megacolon

42. Trendelenburg's test is simple non-invasive diagnostic tool to assess

a. Varicose veins b. TAO
c. Raynaud's disease d. Thrombophlebitis

43. Postoperative cardiac arrhythmia is caused by

a. Hypotension b. Hypovolemia
c. Hypoventilation d. Hypoxia

44. An important mineralocorticoid by adrenal cortex

a. Cortisone b. Corticosterone
c. Aldosterone d. Androgen

45. False perception are called

a. Illusions b. Hallucinations
c. Hyperesthesia d. Paresthesia

46. Persistent irrational fear of an object is

a. Obsession b. Phobia
c. Compulsion d. Delusion

47. IUCDs are introduced postpartum at

a. 4 weeks b. 6–8 weeks
c. 3 months d. 6 months

48. Umbilical cord contains

a. 2 arteries and 2 veins b. 2 arteries and 1 vein
c. 2 veins and 1 artery d. 1 artery and 1 vein

49. Following surgery a child has an intravenous infusion running at 20 mL per hour. The infusion set delivers 60 drops per mL. The nurse regulates the drops per minute at

a. 12 drops per minute b. 5 drops per minute
c. 10 drops per minute d. 20 drops per minute

50. When an infant's cheek is stroked, he turns his head in the direction of the stroked cheek. This reflex which is present at birth is known as

a. Rooting reflex b. Moro reflex
c. Tonic neck reflex d. Sucking reflex

51. Temporary hardness of water is due to the presence of

a. Bicarbonates of calcium and magnesium
b. Nitrates of calcium and magnesium
c. Chlorides of calcium and magnesium
d. All the above

52. How much salt must be added to 1 liter of water to make a solution of normal saline (0.9%).

a. 19 g b. 0.9 g
c. 9 g d. 90 g

53. Vincristine is a drug administered for the treatment of

a. Heart disease b. Bleeding
c. Leukemia d. Asthma

54. A high malignant sarcoma that arises in the bone marrow

a. Morton's neuroma b. Ewing's tumor
c. Osteosarcoma d. Osteochondritis

55. In influenza, there are opaque coating on the anterior part of the vocal cords and laryngeal inlet named

a. Chronic laryngitis b. Edema of the larynx
c. Chorditis fibrinosa d. Laryngeal stridor

56. The immediate complication in a patient who has sustained a fracture of femur is

a. Electrolyte imbalance b. Fat embolism
c. Fluid volume deficit d. Disuse syndrome

57. In Cushing's syndrome, there will be

a. Dehydration and menorrhagia
b. Buffalo hump and hypertension
c. Pitting edema and frequent cold
d. Migraine headache and dysmenorrhea

58. The surgical management of cholelithiasis is

a. Colectomy b. Gastrectomy
c. Nephrectomy d. Cholecystectomy

59. Bell's palsy is due to the compression of

a. Olfactory nerve b. Facial nerve
c. Optic nerve d. Occulomotor nerve

60. X-ray visualization of trachea bronchial tree after introducing contrast medium is

a. Bronchoscopy b. Fluoroscopy
c. Tomography d. Bronchography

61. Normal level of serum bicarbonate is

a. 15 mEq/L b. 27 mEq/L
c. 40 mEq/L d. 20 mEq/L

62. An abnormal curvature of the spine, where the spine is found twisted

a. Kyphosis b. IVDP
c. Lordosis d. Scoliosis

63. The tendency of an organism to behave in the same way as it has behaved before

a. Motive b. Drive
c. Behavior d. Habit

64. A positive sign of pregnancy is

a. Hegar's sign b. Osiander's sign
c. Fetal heart sounds d. Morning sickness

65. Engaging diameter of vertex presentation

a. Suboccipitofrontal b. Suboccipitobragmatic
c. Submentobregmatic d. Mentovertical

66. Protrusion of intestinal contents into the chest through the defect in the diaphragm is termed as

a. Indirect hernia
b. Inguinal hernia
c. Omphalocele
d. Congenital diaphragmatic hernia

67. Which of the following is a cause for physiological jaundice?

a. Immaturity of the liver b. Bile duct obstruction
c. ABO incompatibility d. Rh incompatibility

68. An eye disease characterized by increased intraocular pressure

a. Cataract b. Strabismus
c. Trachoma d. Glaucoma

69. The arthritis affecting the spine and sacroiliac joints before puberty

a. Still's disease b. Atrophic arthritis
c. Spondylitis d. Rheumatoid arthritis

70. In the immediate postoperative period following thyroidectomy, the first priority is to

a. Maintain a patent airway
b. Assess for hemorrhage
c. Monitor for hypocalcemia
d. Prevent strain on the suture line

71. The most reliable investigation in coronary artery disease is

a. Dardiac catheterization
b. Electrocardiography
c. Coronary angiography
d. Computerized tomography

72. Slow shuffling gait is characteristic of

a. Myasthenia gravis b. Guillain-Barre syndrome
c. Parkinson's disease d. Tic disorder

73. Normal central venous pressure is

a. 60–120 mm of H_2O b. 4–10 mm of H_2O
c. 15–20 mm of H_2O d. 50–100 mm of H_2O

74. Wound dehiscence is

a. Delayed wound healing
b. Separation of wound edges
c. Wound sepsis
d. Protrusion of visceral organs through wound

75. Cardiogenic shock results from

a. Myocardial insufficiency
b. Decreased blood volume
c. Vasodilatation
d. Suppressed sympathetic system

76. The process of destroying microorganisms including spores is

a. Disinfection b. Sterilization
c. Infection control d. Isolation

77. Accepted ways of behaving in a society are called

a. Customs b. Norms
c. Folkways d. Culture

78. Bluish discoloration of cervix during pregnancy

a. Jacquemier's sign b. Hegar's sign
c. Chadwick's sign d. Goodell's sign

79. The average amount of blood loss during a normal labor is

a. 500 mL b. 800 mL
c. 1000 mL d. 1500 mL

80. During phototherapy, baby's eyes are covered to prevent

a. Bronze baby syndrome b. Dehydration
c. Retinal damage d. Conjunctivitis

81. Common type of fracture in children is

a. Simple fracture b. Colli's fracture
c. Greenstick fracture d. Complicated fracture

82. Soon after tonsillectomy, the position provided for the patient is

a. Sim's b. Dorsal
c. Prone d. Trendelenburg

83. Rice water stool is found in case of

a. Amebic dysentery b. Food poisoning
c. Bacillary dysentery d. Cholera

84. Tarry stool is evidence of

a. Gastric hemorrhage b. Hemorrhoids
c. Anal fissure d. Intestinal obstruction

85. Systemic lupus erythematosis is a disease of

a. Joint b. Bone
c. Connective tissue d. None of the above

86. Muscle present at the back of the thigh which helps for the flexion of the knees

a. Quadriceps femoris b. Sartorius
c. Gastrocnemius d. Hamstring

87. Physiologic anemia during pregnancy is a result of

a. Increased blood volume of the mother
b. Decreased dietary intake of iron
c. Decreased erythropoiesis after first trimester
d. Increased detoxification of iron by the maternal liver

88. Abruptio placentae is most likely to occur in a woman with

a. Cardiac disease
b. Hyperthyroidism
c. Pregnancy induced hypertension
d. CPD

89. While doing ear irrigation in an adult, the ear lobe is

a. Lifted upward and forward
b. Lifted upward and backward
c. Pulled downward and forward
d. Pulled downward and backward

90. The surgical procedure for otosclerosis is known as

a. Mastectomy b. Mastoidectomy
c. Otoplasty d. Stapedectomy

91. Pacemaker perform the function of

a. SA node b. AV node
c. Bundle of His d. Purkinje fibers

92. Oral hypoglycemic agents may be used for clients with

a. Ketosis
b. Obesity
c. Type I diabetes
d. Minimal insulin production

93. Signs and symptoms of placenta previa include

a. Sharp abdominal pain
b. Early rupture of membranes
c. Increased low back pain
d. Painless vaginal bleeding

94. In the female evaluation of all the pelvic organs of reproduction is accomplished by

a. Cystoscopy b. Hysterosalpingogram
c. Biopsy d. Culdoscopy

95. Acromegaly is produced by an over production of

a. Testosterone b. Growth hormone
c. Thyroid hormone d. ACTH

96. The frequently used drug for angina pectoris is

a. Lasix b. Anticoagulants
c. Nitroglycerin d. Analgesics

97. During induction of labor a woman should be observed carefully for signs of

a. Uterine tetany
b. Severe pain
c. Prolapse of umbilical cord
d. Hypoglycemia

98. The term used for generalized edema is

a. Anasarca b. Pitting edema
c. Periorbital edema d. Septicemia

99. Morphine is a

a. Tranquilizer b. Analgesic
c. Narcotic analgesic d. Sedative

ANSWER KEY

1. c	2. a	3. d	4. d	5. a	6. b	7. b	8. b	9. a	10. b	11. b	12. a
13. b	14. b	15. a	16. b	17. c	18. b	19. a	20. b	21. b	22. a	23. a	24. c
25. d	26. b	27. c	28. b	29. a	30. b	31. a	32. c	33. b	34. a	35. b	36. b
37. a	38. b	39. c	40. d	41. a	42. a	43. a	44. c	45. a	46. b	47. b	48. b
49. d	50. a	51. a	52. c	53. c	54. b	55. c	56. b	57. b	58. d	59. b	60. d
61. b	62. d	63. d	64. c	65. b	66. d	67. a	68. d	69. a	70. a	71. c	72. c
73. b	74. b	75. a	76. b	77. b	78. c	79. a	80. c	81. c	82. a	83. d	84. a
85. c	86. d	87. a	88. c	89. b	90. d	91. a	92. d	93. d	94. b	95. b	96. c
97. a	98. a	99. c									

QUALIFYING EXAMINATION FOR KNMC REGISTRATION

{Exam held in April 2010}

1. **Florence Nightingale was born on**
   a. 12th May b. 10th May
   c. 15th June d. 12th June
2. **Branch of medicine dealing with the problems of the ageing and diseases of the elderly**
   a. Geriatrics b. Pediatrics
   c. Gerontological nursing d. Gerontology
3. **Backflow of partly digested food into the mouth from the stomach is**
   a. Vomiting b. Nausea
   c. Regurgitation d. Dyspepsia
4. **World Health Day is celebrated on**
   a. April 7 b. October 10
   c. November 14 d. January 30
5. **Lack of oxygen in the blood stream is**
   a. Anoxemia b. Anoxia
   c. Asphyxia d. Hypoxia
6. **The most preferred site for IM injection for the children**
   a. Ventrogluteal site b. Vastuslateralis site
   c. Mid-feltoid site d. Dorsogluteal site
7. **Acetone in urine is tested by**
   a. Smith's test b. Hey's test
   c. Rothera's Test d. Benedict's test
8. **Sudden severe attack of shivering in which the body temperature rises rapidly**
   a. Stadium b. Fastigium
   c. Crisis d. Rigor
9. **Abnormal condition of the vertebral column characterized by increased convexity in the thoracic spine**
   a. Kyphosis b. Scoliosis
   c. Lordosis d. Sretorius
10. **Substances used to counteract the effect of poison**
    a. Antidotes b. Antiseptics
    c. Antibiotics d. Antifungal
11. **One ounce is equal to**
    a. 60 mL b. 30 mL
    c. 15 mL d. 45 mL
12. **Hospital acquired infection is known as**
    a. Droplet infection b. Opportunistic infection
    c. Nosocomial infection d. Contamination
13. **Application of the drug to the skin by friction is called**
    a. Instillation b. Insertion
    c. Insufflation d. Inunction
14. **Bland diet is used for patients with**
    a. Diabetes mellitus
    b. Gastrointestinal disturbances
    c. Hypertension
    d. Cardiac disorders
15. **The term stomatitis is**
    a. Inflammation of the stomach
    b. Inflammation of the mouth
    c. Inflammation of the lungs
    d. Inflammation of the gums
16. **The term dyspepsia is**
    a. Difficulty in swallowing
    b. Indigestion
    c. Loss of appetite
    d. Breathing difficulty
17. **Antitussives are drugs that are used to treat**
    a. Diarrhea
    b. Relieve itching
    c. Inhibit cough reflex
    d. Prevent the progress of inflammation
18. **An increase in the depth of respiration is**
    a. Orthopnea b. Hyperpnea
    c. Apnea d. Dyspnea
19. **Bluish discoloration of the skin and mucous membrane is**
    a. Cyanosis b. Anoxia
    c. Anoxemia d. Hypoxia

20. The serious side effect of streptomycin is

a. Peripheral neuritis b. Ototoxicity
c. Hepatotoxicity d. Respiratory depression

21. Ketone bodies appear in the blood and urine when fats are oxidized in great amounts. This condition is associated with

a. Starvation
b. Alcoholism
c. Positive nitrogen balance
d. Bone healing

22. Disinfection means

a. Destroying all pathogenic microorganisms
b. Destroying all microorganisms
c. Inhibiting growth of microorganisms
d. Killing only bacteria

23. Payer's patches are situated in

a. Large intestine b. Small intestine
c. Stomach d. Esophagus

24. Acetabulum is the part of

a. Scapula b. Femur
c. Tibia d. Hip bone

25. Which of the following is a retrovirus

a. Rotavirus b. HIV
c. Herpes simplex virus d. Measles

26. Mitral valve is situated

a. In the pulmonary vein
b. Between left atria and left ventricle
c. Between right atria and right ventricle
d. In the aorta

27. Renin is a hormone secreted by

a. Liver b. Kidney
c. Adrenals d. Pancreas

28. The muscular layer of uterus is termed as

a. Endometrium b. Perimetrium
c. Myocardium d. Myometrium

29. In the absence of pathology, the client's respiratory center is stimulated by

a. Oxygen b. Lactic acid
c. Calcium ions d. Carbon dioxide

30. Normal pH of arterial blood is

a. 7.0 b. 7.3
c. 7.42 d. 7.5

31. A client with fractured rib may develop

a. Scoliosis b. Pneumothoraxes
c. Obstruction of lungs d. Diaphragmatic hernia

32. The extreme limit of noise tolerance is

a. 85 decibels b. 140 decibels
c. 100 decibels d. 120 decibels

33. The placenta does not produce

a. Chorionic gonadotrophin
b. Follicle stimulating hormone
c. Progesterone
d. Somatotropin

34. The nurse realize that pain associated with coronary occlusion is caused primarily by

a. Arterial spasm
b. Ischemia of heart muscle
c. Blocking of coronary artery
d. Irritation of nerve endings in cardiac plexus

35. Before administering morphine to a client, the nurse should assess the client's

a. Blood pressure b. Respiratory rate
c. Pulse d. Temperature

36. X-ray visualization of trachea bronchial tree after introducing contrast medium is

a. Bronchoscopy b. Tomography
c. Bronchography d. Fluoroscopy

37. Inability to recognize familiar objects is called

a. Ataxia b. Apraxia
c. Amnesia d. Agnosia

38. Which of the following is not a sign of thromboembolism?

a. Redness b. Swelling
c. Coolness d. Edema

39. After a bronchoscopy, with biopsy, which of the following sign should be reported immediately?

a. Green sputum b. Laryngeal stridor
c. Hemoptysis d. Dry cough

40. A common nursing diagnosis for a client with hypothyroidism and complaints of fatigue, muscular weakness and muscle cramp would be

a. Activity intolerance b. Anxiety
c. Hopelessness d. Ineffective family coping

41. Abnormal production of erythrocytes are termed as

a. Leukocytosis b. Anemia
c. Polycythemia d. Thrombocytopenia

42. **The normal value of potassium in the blood is**
   a. 3.5–5.4 mEq/L b. 3–4 mEq/L
   c. 5.6–7 mEq/L d. 10–12 mEq/L

43. **Sterilizing articles by means of steam under pressure is known as**
   a. Boiling b. Autoclaving
   c. Pasteurization d. Incineration

44. **The causative organism of typhoid fever is**
   a. *Clostridium welchii* b. *Salmonella typhi*
   c. *Escherichia coli* d. *Treponema pallidum*

45. **Oxygenated blood from the lungs to left atrium is carried by**
   a. Coronary arteries b. Pulmonary arteries
   c. Pulmonary veins d. Inferior venacava

46. **Thyroid stimulating hormone is secreted by**
   a. Adrenal gland b. Pituitary gland
   c. Thyroid gland d. Parathyroid

47. **Active immunity is developed by the administration of the following**
   a. Antitetanus serum b. Tetanus toxoids
   c. Antibiotics d. Vitamin supplements

48. **Respiratory center is situated in the**
   a. Cerebellum b. Cerebrum
   c. Medulla oblongata d. Ventricles

49. **The following are cranial nerves except**
   a. Trigeminal nerve b. Olfactory nerve
   c. Sciatic nerve d. Glossopharyngeal nerve

50. **The largest gland in the body is**
   a. Thyroid b. Adrenal
   c. Liver d. Pituitary

51. **A client with iron deficiency anemia takes iron supplements. The nurse emphasize to the client that the drug will have increased absorption if taken with**
   a. Milk b. Orange juice
   c. Food d. Beta carotene

52. **A fatty meal is given in cholecystogram**
   a. To know the size of the gallbladder
   b. To know the function of the gallbladder
   c. To know the liver function
   d. To know the contractibility of the gallbladder

53. **Calculation of pediatric dosage of medicine is by using**
   a. Young's rule b. Clark's rule
   c. Fried's rule d. All of the above

54. **The supply of oxygen must be equipped with a regulator**
   a. To know the amount of gas
   b. To prevent the bursting of the cylinder
   c. To prevent fire
   d. To control flow of gas

55. **Moving a part of the body to note the flexibility**
   a. Percussion b. Palpation
   c. Auscultation d. Manipulation

56. **Windows may be cut in plaster cast**
   a. To relieve excessive pressure
   b. To treat surgical wound
   c. To inspect the area of discomfort
   d. All of the above

57. **Cover the mouth piece of the inhaler**
   a. To prevent burns of the lips
   b. To prevent heat loss
   c. To prevent spilling of fluid
   d. None of the above

58. **National rural health mission (NRHM) was launched on**
   a. 2002 b. 2003
   c. 2005 d. 2006

59. **The vector of dengue fever**
   a. *Aedes aegypti* b. *Culex*
   c. *Anopheles* d. *Brugia malayi*

60. **Mental Health Act was passed in India in**
   a. 1912 b. 1947
   c. 1987 d. 1995

61. **Polio vaccine is stored at**
   a. 0°C b. 2°C
   c. -10°C d. -20°C

62. **When performing cardiac compression of adult client, the nurse should exert downward vertical pressure on the lower sternum**
   a. 1.3–2 cm b. 2–2.5 cm
   c. 2.5–4 cm d. 4–5 cm

63. What is the normal respiratory rate of a new born?
a. 16–20 breaths per minute
b. 20–30 breaths per minute
c. 30–60 breaths per minute
d. 40–80 breaths per minute

64. Expand BFHI
a. Baby first hospital induction
b. Breastfeeding hospitals in India
c. Baby-friendly hospital initiative
d. Breastfeeding, hide infection

65. The system of transporting and storing vaccine at the recommended temperature
a. Cold chain b. Deep freezer
c. Day carrier d. Vaccine carrier

66. A sanitary well should be located not less than the meters from likely source of contamination
a. 50 meters b. 15 meters
c. 10 meters d. 5 meters

67. The common complaint of a woman with an IUD is
a. Vaginal bleeding b. Pelvic infection
c. Uterine perforation d. Abdominal pain

68. Children with Tetralogy of Fallot assumes
a. Squatting b. Fowler's
c. Sitting d. Legs down

69. Koplik's spots are characteristic of
a. Measles b. Oral cancer
c. Purpura d. Mumps

70. Which of the following is the cause for physiologic jaundice?
a. Immaturity of liver b. Bile duct obstruction
c. ABO incompatibility d. Rh incompatibility

71. The most reliable investigation in coronary artery disease is
a. Cardiac catheterization
b. Electrocardiography
c. Coronary angiography
d. Computerized tomography

72. Normal central venous pressure is
a. 60–120 mm of H_2O b. 4–10 mm of H_2O
c. 15–20 mm of H_2O d. 50–100 mm of H_2O

73. The average amount of blood loss during a normal labor is
a. 500 mL b. 800 mL
c. 1000 mL d. 1500 mL

74. The two outstanding characteristic symptoms of diabetes mellitus are
a. Hypoglycemia and glycosuria
b. Hyperglycemia and glycosuria
c. Hypoglycemia and hypokalemia
d. Hyperglycemia and hypokalemia

75. Painful micturition is called
a. Dysuria b. Anuria
c. Glycosuria d. Oliguria

76. A person who harbors pathogenic organisms of a disease in his body without showing signs and symptoms of the disease
a. Fomites b. Rodents
c. Carrier d. Pathogen

77. Antibodies are produced by
a. Eosinophils b. Plasma cells
c. Erythrocytes d. Lymphocytes

78. Human Papilloma virus is important in its possible role in the development of
a. Cervical cancer b. Skin cancer
c. Lung cancer d. Oral cancer

79. Most specific feature of digoxin toxicity
a. Increased urinary output b. Tachycardia
c. Nausea and vomiting d. Hyperkalemia

80. The administration of a medicine just below the skin is called
a. Intradermal b. Subcutaneous
c. Intramuscular d. Intrathecal

81. The main indication of hemodialysis for a patient who has CRF is
a. Ascites b. Acidosis
c. Hypertension d. Hyperkalemia

82. The most important observation for a burns victim after 48 hours of fluid therapy
a. Peripheral perfusion b. Weight
c. Urinary output d. Dehydration

83. A defense mechanism, in which blaming others for one's own mistake

a. Regression b. Sublimation
c. Projection d. Substitution

84. The patient with liver cirrhosis and hepatic coma should be assessed for

a. Icterus b. Urticaria
c. Uremic frost d. Hemangioma

85. Pacemaker perform the function of

a. AV node b. SA node
c. Bundle of His d. Purkinje fibers

86. Acromegaly is produced by an overproduction of

a. Testosterone b. Growth hormone
c. Thyroid hormone d. ACTH

87. The best time for administration of diuretics is

a. 9 am b. 1 pm
c. 4 pm d. 6 pm

88. Condition in which endometrial cells seeded outside the uterine cavity is

a. Endometritis b. Fibroid
c. Procidentia d. Endometriosis

89. The temperature for the sponge bath

a. 110°–115°F b. 100°–110°F
c. 90°–100°F d. 120°–125°F

90. Difficulty in getting off to sleep or in maintaining sleep is called

a. Amnesia b. Narcolepsy
c. Insomnia d. Hypersomnia

91. Complication of prolonged bed rest include

a. Fever b. Pain
c. Renal stone d. Jaundice

92. Voiding during normal sleeping hours is termed as

a. Dysuria b. Nocturia
c. Anuria d. Oliguria

93. Blood concentration of calcium is regulated by

a. Thyroxine b. Parathormone
c. Prolactin d. Glucocorticoids

94. Pulmonary edema may be a complication of

a. Heart block b. Congestive heart disease
c. Coronary artery disease d. CVA

95. Application of drug in liquid form into a body cavity

a. Inunction b. Instillation
c. Insertion d. Implantation

96. Primary effect of cold application

a. Vasodilation b. Violation
c. Ventilation d. Vasoconstriction

97. Pulse pressure is

a. Difference between diastolic and systolic
b. Diastolic pressure
c. Aortic pressure
d. Systolic pressure

98. Suitable position for lumbar puncture

a. Lateral position of spine
b. Knee flexed position
c. Any desired position
d. Full flexion of spine

99. Which part of the nursing process includes the statement of the client's actual or potential problems?

a. Assessment b. Implementation
c. Nursing diagnosis d. Planning

100. The best method of sterilizing gloves

a. Boiling b. Drying
c. Soaking d. Steam under pressure

ANSWER KEY

1. a	2. a	3. c	4. a	5. a	6. b	7. c	8. d	9. a	10. a	11. b	12. c
13. d	14. b	15. b	16. b	17. c	18. b	19. a	20. b	21. a	22. a	23. b	24. d
25. b	26. b	27. b	28. d	29. d	30. c	31. b	32. b	33. b	34. b	35. b	36. c
37. d	38. c	39. b	40. a	41. c	42. a	43. b	44. b	45. c	46. b	47. b	48. c
49. c	50. c	51. b	52. d	53. d	54. d	55. d	56. d	57. a	58. c	59. a	60. c
61. d	62. d	63. c	64. c	65. a	66. b	67. a	68. a	69. a	70. a	71. c	72. b
73. a	74. b	75. a	76. c	77. d	78. a	79. d	80. b	81. d	82. c	83. c	84. a
85. b	86. b	87. a	88. d	89. a	90. c	91. c	92. b	93. b	94. b	95. b	96. d
97. a	98. d	99. c	100. d								

QUALIFYING EXAMINATION FOR KNMC REGISTRATION

{Exam held in August 2010}

1. **World Health Day is celebrated on**
   a. April 7 b. May 12
   c. November 15 d. January 30
2. **The best method of sterilizing gloves is**
   a. Steam under pressure b. Boiling
   c. Fumigation d. Sterilization by hot air
3. **Which of the following bed is very useful to prevent bed sore**
   a. Fracture bed b. Blanket bed
   c. Occupied bed d. Water bed
4. **Tapping an area to elicit sound is termed as**
   a. Percussion b. Palpation
   c. Observation d. Auscultation
5. **Increased pulsation in the lateral vaginal fornices is**
   a. Hegar's sign b. Jacquemier's sign
   c. Osiander's sign d. Chadwick's sign
6. **The amount of amniotic fluid at term is**
   a. 500 mL b. 800 mL
   c. 1000 mL d. 700 mL
7. **The presentation which does not have mechanism is**
   a. Shoulder b. Face
   c. Breech d. Vertex
8. **Cheapest source of vitamin A**
   a. Milk b. Green leafy vegetables
   c. Fish liver oil d. Citrus fruits
9. **Average daily reduction of fundal height during postnatal period**
   a. 2.5 cm b. 5 cm
   c. 1 cm d. 1.5 cm
10. **Multipurpose worker scheme was introduced in**
    a. 1975 b. 1980
    c. 1977 d. 1972
11. **Metastasis of neoplasm**
    a. Spread to adjacent tissues
    b. Recurrence after removal
    c. Spread to distant areas through blood or lymph
    d. Suppressed growth of neoplasm
12. **Protamine sulfate is**
    a. An anticoagulant b. Heparin antagonist
    c. Vasodilator d. An antiarrhythmic
13. **Varicocele is**
    a. Dilatation of spermatic vein
    b. Esophageal varices
    c. Dilated anorectal veins
    d. Dilated umbilical veins
14. **A group of persons who work together to promote better health in the community**
    a. Multi-purpose health workers
    b. Dais
    c. Health team
    d. Community health nurse
15. **The basic unit of the system of Panchayati Raj**
    a. Grama Panchayat b. Grama Sabha
    c. Nyaya Panchayat d. Panchayat Samiti
16. **The headquarters of UNICEF**
    a. Geneva b. Rome
    c. New York d. New Delhi
17. **In the postoperative period coughing is encouraged as it**
    a. Keeps airway patent
    b. Prevents atelectasis
    c. Facilitates re-expansion of the lung
    d. All of the above
18. **Hematocrit measures**
    a. Volume of red blood cells per 100 mL of blood
    b. Measures hemoglobin content of erythrocytes
    c. Measures concentration of red blood cells in cubic mm of blood
    d. None of the above
19. **Exophthalmos is a characteristic sign of**
    a. Hyperthyroidism
    b. Hypothyroidism
    c. Increased intracranial pressure
    d. Hyperpituitarism

20. Deep transverse arrest occur in

a. Occipitoanterior position
b. Occipitoposterior position
c. Breech presentation
d. Transverse lie

21. During labor +1 station indicates that the presenting part is

a. On the perineum
b. Slightly below ischial spines
c. High in the false pelvis
d. Slightly above ischial spines

22. Rectal temperature is higher than the oral temperature:

a. 0.5°F b. 0.5°C
c. 1°C d. 1°F

23. Which of the following procedures relieve the congestion of the pelvic organs?

a. Sitz bath b. Hot bath
c. Cold bath d. Catheterization

24. Painful micturition is known as

a. Enuresis b. Anuria
c. Pyuria d. Dysuria

25. Anorexia means

a. Indigestion b. Feeling of fullness
c. Loss of appetite d. Back flow of food

26. The condition in which the fetal blood vessels lie in front of the presenting part is

a. Vasa previa b. Cord prolapse
c. Placenta previa d. Hydramnios

27. The condition that is contraindicated for administration of injection ergometrine is

a. Cardiac disease b. Renal disease
c. Respiratory disease d. Liver disease

28. The usual prevalence of a given disease in a particular area

a. Endemic b. Epidemic
c. Sporadic d. Pandemic

29. Backbone of public health nursing

a. Bag technique b. Recording
c. Home visiting d. Community survey

30. Recommended maximum noise level

a. 140 decibels b. 90 decibels
c. 85 decibels d. 120 decibels

31. Aplastic anemia is due to

a. Iron deficiency
b. Absence of intrinsic factor
c. Bone marrow depression
d. Abnormal RBCs

32. H1N1 infection spreads through

a. GIT b. Percutaneous
c. GUT d. Respiratory tract

33. Rhinoplasty is

a. Reconstruction of nose
b. Face lifting
c. Fat removal
d. Reconstruction of ear drum

34. The Indian Red Cross society was established

a. 1973 b. 1920
c. 1925 d. 1948

35. The most popular method of health teaching

a. Lecture b. Group discussion
c. Panel discussion d. Symposium

36. The scientific study of human population

a. Vital statistics b. Demography
c. Statistics d. Census

37. Vitamin B_6 is given with INH because it

a. Enhances tuberculostatic effect of INH
b. Improves immunologic response of the patient
c. Replaces vitamin as INH interferes with natural vitamin synthesis
d. None of the above

38. Symptoms of morphine overdose include

a. Slow pulse, slow respirations, sedation
b. Slow respirations, dilated pupils, restlessness
c. Profuse sweating, pin point pupils, deep sleep
d. Slow respirations, constricted pupils, deep sleep

39. A patient is to receive 200 mL of IV fluid in 12 hours. The drop factor is 10 drops per mL. The nurse should regulate the flow so the number of drops per minute is approximately

a. 27–29 b. 30–32
c. 40–42 d. 48–50

40. Important side effects of $MGSO_4$ (Magnesium sulfate)

a. Hemorrhage b. Hypertension
c. Hyporeflexia d. Headache

41. Premature separation of normally situated placenta is called

a. Placenta circumvallata b. Placenta previa
c. Abruptio placentae d. Placenta accreta

42. In the active phase of labor cervical dilatation in a primigravida should be at the rate of

a. 1 cm per hour b. 1.5 cm per hour
c. 2 cm per hour d. 2.5 cm per hour

43. One tea spoon is equal to

a. 5 mL b. 1 mL
c. 0.5 mL d. 10 mL

44. Inflammation of the mucous membrane of the mouth is termed as

a. Gastritis b. Glossitis
c. Stomatitis d. Gingivitis

45. Which of the following drug will soften, soothe and protect mucous membrane

a. Emollient b. Caustics
c. Demulcents d. Astringent

46. The forceps that is used to deliver fetal head at or above the pelvic brim

a. Keilland's b. Simpsons
c. Wrigley's d. Kelly's

47. The neonatal complication that can develop in a GDM mother

a. Hypoglycemia b. Hyperglycemia
c. Anemia d. Albuminuria

48. Treatment of PPH is

a. Change position b. Give perineal care
c. Empty the uterus d. IV Fluids

49. Visualization of pelvic structures through an incision in the pouch of Douglas is known as

a. Cystoscopy b. Salpingoscopy
c. Culdoscopy d. Colonoscopy

50. The principal screening test used for carcinoma of cervix is

a. Culture b. Pap smear
c. Cytology d. Cervical biopsy

51. The causative organism for syphilis is

a. *Treponema pallidum* b. *Chlamydia trachomatis*
c. *Trichomonas* d. *E. coli*

52. Socratic method of group teaching

a. Workshop b. Lecture
c. Seminar d. Symposium

53. Incubation period of polio myelitis

a. 7–21 days b. 15–50 days
c. 7–14 days d. 4–6 days

54. Act prescribes maximum of 48 working hours per week for employees

a. ESI act b. Indian Factories Act
c. Indian Lunacy Act d. Labor Act

55. Sudden blockage of one of the branches of coronary arteries causes:

a. Angina pectoris b. Myocardial infarction
c. Vincent's Angina d. TIA

56. Surgical fusion of a joint is

a. Arthroplasty b. Arthrodesis
c. Arthrotomy d. Dysarthria

57. Following are causes of conductive hearing loss except

a. Otitis media b. Otosclerosis
c. Ear wax d. Meniere's disease

58. According to Central Birth and Death Registration Act, the time limit for registration of birth:

a. 7 days b. 11 days
c. 14 days d. 19 days

59. The best and cheapest investment in the health of children:

a. Weaning b. Family planning
c. Immunization d. Feeding

60. The population of a corporation is

a. < 2 lakhs b. > 2 lakhs
c. 5000–10000 d. 1 lakh

61. The term bradycardia means

a. Grossly irregular heart beat
b. A heart rate over 90 per minute
c. A heart rate less than 60 per minute
d. A heart beat that has regular skipped beats

62. During blood transfusion, a patient develops chills and headache. The nurse should

a. Cover the patient with blanket
b. Inform the physician immediately
c. Slow the blood flow to keep the vein open
d. Stop the transfusion immediately

63. Expectoration of blood stained sputum is termed

a. Hematuria b. Hematoma
c. Hemoptysis d. Hemetemesis

64. The increased caloric need in pregnancy is

a. 300 b. 550
c. 800 d. 400

65. Increased pulsation felt in lateral fornices of vagina in pregnancy is termed as

a. Chadwick's sign b. Osiander's sign
c. Goodell's sign d. Hegar's sign

66. Physiological changes in pregnancy include the following except

a. Increase in intravascular volume
b. Increase in cardiac output
c. Increase in peripheral vascular resistance
d. Increase in stroke volume

67. Commonly used vasodilator is

a. Nitroglycerine b. Nitrazepam
c. Digoxin d. Furosemide

68. Caldwell Luc surgery is surgical treatment for

a. Chronic mastoiditis
b. Ascites
c. Chronic frontal sinusitis
d. Chronic maxillary sinusitis

69. Inflammation of cornea is

a. Blepharitis b. Uveitis
c. Keratitis d. Stye

70. The last census in India was taken

a. 1981 b. 1881
c. 2001 d. 2005

71. Daily requirement of iron during pregnancy

a. 40 m b. 40 g
c. 400 g d. 50 g

72. The leader of health team at primary health center

a. Medical officer b. Lady health visitor
c. Dais d. Block extension educator

73. One of the most common complication of chronic asthma is

a. Atelectasis b. Emphysema
c. Pneumothorax d. Pulmonary fibrosis

74. The nurse should position a patient recovering from general anesthesia in

a. Supine position b. Trendelenburg position
c. High fowler's position d. Side lying position

75. During the immediate postoperative period the nurse should give the highest priority to

a. Observing for hemorrhage
b. Checking vital signs every 15 minutes
c. Recording the intake and output chart
d. Maintaining a patent airway

76. Macrosomia is a common complication in

a. Preeclampsia
b. Polyhydramnios
c. Gestational diabetes mellitus
d. Multiple pregnancy

77. Massaging of uterus to make it hard is important in

a. Traumatic PPH b. Atonic PPH
c. Inversion of uterus d. Subinvolution

78. The following are the classic features of ectopic pregnancy except

a. Amenorrhea b. Irregular vaginal bleeding
c. Vomiting d. Abdominal pain

79. All are means of immobilization of fractured bone except

a. Reduction b. Traction
c. Splinting d. Plaster cast

80. Trendelenburg test is non-invasive simple diagnostic test to assess

a. Varicose veins b. Thrombophlebitis
c. Embolism d. Raynaud's disease

81. Paroxysmal nocturnal dyspnea is a sign of

a. Right ventricular failure b. Myocardial infarction
c. Left ventricular failure d. Arrhythmia

82. An example of subdermal implants method of family planning

a. Oestradiol b. Norplant
c. Depo provera d. Copper T

83. Revised National Tuberculosis Control Program (RNTCP) was established in

a. 1990 b. 1994
c. 1992 d. 2000

84. A communicable disease eradicated from India
a. Chickenpox b. Rubella
c. Smallpox d. Rabies

85. Method used for diagnosing community health problem
a. Laboratory test b. Survey
c. Camp d. Health education

86. Most sensitive index of the health of the community
a. Maternal mortality rate b. Crude death rate
c. Infant mortality rate d. Crude birth rate

87. When suctioning a patient with tracheostomy, the nurse must
a. Initiate suction as the catheter is being withdrawn
b. Use new sterile catheter with each insertion
c. Insert catheter until the cough reflex is stimulated.
d. Remove the inner cannula before inserting the suction catheter

88. After thoracentesis, the nurse should observe the patient for
a. Periods of confusion
b. Expectoration of blood
c. Increased breath sounds
d. Decreased respiratory rate

89. The type of hepatitis most frequently transmitted by transfusion is
a. Hepatitis A b. Hepatitis B
c. Hepatitis C d. Hepatitis D

90. The total score in APGAR rating system is
a. 5 b. 8
c. 10 d. 14

91. Which of the following is not a component of Bishop's score
a. Cervical length b. Position of head
c. Cervical dilatation d. Station of the head

92. The state reporting the lowest neonatal mortality in India is
a. Delhi b. Maharashtra
c. Kerala d. Gujarat

93. State of increased pressure within the anterior chamber of the eye is
a. Trachoma b. Sarcoma
c. Chondroma d. Glaucoma

94. Inherited sex linked bleeding disorder is
a. Hemophilia b. Thalassemia
c. Sickle cell disease d. Purpura

95. After radical mastectomy arm on affected side should be observed for
a. Cyanosis b. Erythema
c. Ischemia d. Lymphedema

96. Neomycin sulfate is administered to a patient before colon surgery to
a. Destroy intestinal bacteria
b. Increase the production of vitamin K
c. Decrease incidence of any secondary infection
d. Decrease the possibility of postoperative urinary tract infection

97. Hemorrhoids generally result from
a. Hypertension b. Constipation
c. Eating spicy foods d. Poor bowel control

98. Immediately following a thyroidectomy, patient should be monitored for
a. Decreased blood pressure
b. Urinary retention
c. Signs of restlessness
d. Signs of respiratory obstruction

99. A skin graft that is taken from another portion of a patient's own body is known as
a. An allograft b. A kenograft
c. An autograft d. A homograft

100. HIV transmission from mother to newborn is most common during
a. First trimester b. Second trimester
c. Third trimester d. Delivery

ANSWER KEY

1. a	2. a	3. d	4. a	5. c	6. b	7. a	8. b	9. c	10. a	11. c	12. b
13. a	14. c	15. b	16. c	17. d	18. a	19. a	20. b	21. b	22. b,d	23. a	24. d
25. c	26. a	27. a	28. a	29. c	30. c	31. c	32. d	33. a	34. b	35. a	36. b
37. c	38. d	39. a	40. c	41. c	42. b	43. a	44. c	45. c	46. a	47. a	48. c
49. c	50. b	51. a	52. c	53. a	54. b	55. b	56. b	57. d	58. c	59. c	60. b
61. c	62. d	63. c	64. a	65. b	66. c	67. a	68. d	69. c	70. c	71. a	72. a
73. b	74. d	75. d	76. c	77. b	78. c	79. a	80. a	81. c	82. b	83. c	84. c
85. b	86. c	87. a	88. d	89. b	90. c	91. b	92. c	93. d	94. a	95. d	96. a
97. b	98. d	99. c	100. d								

SENIOR LECTURER IN NURSING-KERALA PSC

(Exam held on 2-09-2010)

1. **Concept of Public Health was born in**
   a. Mesopotamia b. Rome
   c. Greek d. China
2. **A newborn exhibits respiratory distress, distension of neck veins, low BP and diminished breath sounds, most likely diagnosis is**
   a. Pulmonary air leak syndrome
   b. Hyaline membrane disease
   c. Primary atelectasis
   d. Transient tachypnea
3. **Bone age is less than chronological age in all, except**
   a. Chondrodystrophies b. Hypothyroidism
   c. Hypopituitarism d. Malnutrition
4. **The syndrome of recurrent infections, partial albinism, photophobia and nystagmus are seen in**
   a. Bodian-Shwachman syndrome
   b. Chronic granulomatous disease
   c. DiGeorge syndrome
   d. Chediak-Higashi syndrome
5. **The intrauteric ridge forming the base of trigonal structure is also called**
   a. Bell' muscle b. Mercier's bar
   c. Rice's bar d. White line of Toldt
6. **Myiasis refers to**
   a. Foreign body in nose b. Maggots in nose
   c. Fungal infection d. Tuberculosis
7. **Chondroma is the most common in**
   a. Cricoid b. Thyroid
   c. Asytenoid d. Epiglottis
8. **Keshan's disease is due to deficiency of**
   a. Zinc b. Copper
   c. Selenium d. Manganese
9. **Grommet is used in**
   a. Glue ear b. ASOM
   c. Cholesteatoma d. CSOM
10. **The pioneers of the immunization are**
    a. Chinese b. Egyptians
    c. Indians d. Romans
11. **Non-sedative antihistamine drug is**
    a. Diphenhydramine b. Promethazine
    c. Astemizole d. Chlorpheniramine
12. **The most reliable landmark in otoscopy is**
    a. Handle of malleus
    b. Umbo
    c. Cone of light
    d. Lateral process of malleus
13. **Opioid analgesic inhibit the release of**
    a. ADH b. LH
    c. Prolactin d. Somatotropin
14. **A patient has been admitted in the hospital with gastroenteritis. During assessment, the nurse is expected to find:**
    a. Hypoactive bowel sounds
    b. Hyperactive bowel sounds
    c. Rigid and broad like abdomen
    d. Rebound tenderness
15. **The most frequent complication arising from hyperviscosity of polycythemia is**
    a. Thrombosis b. Cardiomyopathy
    c. Pulmonary fibrosis d. Leukemia
16. **The nurse while taking care of a patient with cervical level spinal cord injury should give priority to the following nursing diagnosis**
    a. Risk for hypertension
    b. Ineffective airway clearance
    c. Ineffective thermoregulation
    d. Impaired physical mobility
17. **When variables are not measurable, which of the following is to be represented?**
    a. Nominal b. Ordinal
    c. Interval d. Ratio

18. **Best method of variability is**
    a. Mean b. Median
    c. Range d. Standard deviation
19. **Mortality experience is taken into consideration, when finding**
    a. General fertility rate b. Total fertility rate
    c. Net reproduction rate d. Gross reproduction rate
20. **In which one pair, indicating a vicious circle of cardiac deterioration, is set-up in cardiogenic shock?**
    a. Ventricular force-cardiac output
    b. Venous return-right atrial pressure
    c. Arteria wall-peripheral resistance
    d. Arterial pressure-coronary blood flow
21. **The correct value of refractory index of air**
    a. 1.001 b. 1.000
    c. 0.009 d. 1.010
22. **In response to hypoglycemia, the hormone cause hepatic glycogenolysis and gluconeogenesis**
    a. Glucagon b. Cortisol
    c. Epinephrine d. GH
23. **Biotin is a coenzyme for**
    a. Oxidases b. Decarboxylases
    c. Oxygenases d. Carboxylases
24. **Breakdown of 1 gram of hemoglobin produces**
    a. 20 mg of bilirubin b. 35 mg of bilirubin
    c. 50 mg of bilirubin d. 70 mg of bilirubin
25. **The immunoglobulin can fix complement is**
    a. IgM b. IgM
    c. IgA d. IgD
26. **Characteristic intestinal pathogen in AIDS is**
    a. Salmonella b. Isospora
    c. Cryptosporidium d. Strongylosis
27. **The first IOL implantation was carried out by**
    a. Binkhorst b. Ridley
    c. Cholyce d. Strampelli
28. **Strawberry vaginitis is seen in infection with**
    a. *Gonococcus* b. *Trichomonas vaginalis*
    c. *Haemophilus vaginalis* d. *Candida albicans*
29. **Vitiligo involving distal digits, periorificial areas is named as**
    a. Vitiligo vulgaris b. Focal vitiligo
    c. Acrofacial vitiligo d. Universal vitiligo
30. **The sign of increased ICP in a child, 18-month old is**
    a. Increased irritability b. Narrowing pulse pressure
    c. Pinpoint pupils d. Tachycardia
31. **Pseudounipolar neurons are seen in**
    a. Retina b. Olfactory mucosa
    c. Spinal cord d. Spinal ganglion
32. **The following is atavistic epiphysis**
    a. Coracoid process
    b. Trochanter of femur
    c. Lower end fibula
    d. Greater tubercle of humerus
33. **Example of multipinnate muscle**
    a. Dorsal interossei b. Flexor pollicis longus
    c. Rectus femoris d. Subscapularis
34. **The following denotes the toxicity of medications may cause a client to see a green halo around the light**
    a. Digoxin b. Furosemide
    c. Metoprolol d. Enlapril
35. **The morbidity indicator, which is equivalent to number of years of full health, a newborn can expect to live based on current rate of its health?**
    a. HALE b. DALY
    c. Sullivan's index d. IMR
36. **Giving instructions for breast self-examination, is particularly important for client with the following medical problem**
    a. Cervical dysplasia b. Dermoid cyst
    c. Endometrial polyp d. Ovarian cancer
37. **The following vitamins is used to enhance absorption of calcium from GI tract**
    a. Vitamin A b. Vitamin C
    c. Vitamin D d. Vitamin E
38. **A client with following condition is likely to develop rectal cancer**
    a. Adenomatous polyps b. Diverticulitis
    c. Hemorrhoids d. PUD
39. **Osteomyelitis most commonly results from which of the following mechanisms?**
    a. Immune suppression b. IV drug use
    c. Surgery d. Trauma
40. **For a client having an episode of acute narrow angle glaucoma, a nurse expects to give the following medication**
    a. Acetazolamide b. Atropine
    c. Furosemide d. Urokinase

41. A client with cancer develops pleural effusion. During chest auscultation, the following breath sounds should be expected to hear

a. Cackles
b. Rhonchi
c. Diminished breath sounds
d. Wheeze

42. According to the psychological theorist such as Freud and Jung, treatment of symptoms should involve the following action

a. Modifying the behavior by manipulating the environment
b. Using desensitization
c. Uncovering past events
d. Using family therapy

43. Norepinephrine has been linked to pTSD, because it plays a role in which of the following activities?

a. ANS activity
b. Glutamate metabolism
c. Excitatory neurotransmitter inhibition
d. Pain regulation

44. The term applied to tiny, blanched, slightly raised end arterioles found on the face, neck, arms and chest

a. Epulis b. Linea nigra
c. Striae gravidarum d. Telangiectasis

45. In a complete hydatidiform mole, which of the following karyotypes is typically found?

a. 46 XX b. 69 XXY
c. 69 XXX d. 69 XYY

46. The method of pain control incorporates effleurage as a technique to displace pain

a. Bradley method b. Hydrotherapy
c. Lamaze method d. Nubain method

47. The following Leopold's maneuvers assess the descent of the presenting part into pelvis

a. First b. Second
c. Third d. Fourth

48. When attempting to interact with a neonate experiencing drug withdrawal, which behavior would indicate that the neonate's willing to interact?

a. Gaze aversions b. Hiccups
c. Quiet alert state d. Yawning

49. The GI disorder most suggestive of cystic fibrosis

a. Duodenal obstruction b. Jejunal atresia
c. Malrotation d. Meconium ileus

50. Name the operation recommended to correct tricuspid atresia

a. Blalock-Taussig operation
b. Fontan procedure
c. Jutune procedure
d. Patch closure

51. The following is the most frequent site of internal bleeding associated with hemophilia

a. Brain tissue b. GI tract
c. Joint cavities d. Spinal cord

52. The following percentages represent a case of congenital hip dysplasia involving both hips

a. 10% b. 25%
c. 50% d. 75%

53. Quality assurance refers to

a. Standard practice b. Measurement scale
c. Evaluation scale d. Rating scale

54. When it comes to sodium, for a healthy diet, sodium should be limited to

a. 4000 mg/day b. 3000 mg/day
c. 2400 mg/day d. 2300 mg/day

55. Pinel is known for

a. Psychoanalysis
b. Moral treatment of patient
c. Cognitive therapy
d. Group psychotherapy

56. A 34-year-old female has recently been diagnosed with autoimmune disease. She has also recently discovered that she is pregnant, the immunoglobulin that will provide protection to the fetus in the womb is

a. IgA b. IgG
c. IgM d. IgE

57. A 35-year-old male has been an insulin dependent diabetic for last 5 years and is now unable to urinate. The following is most likely to suspect

a. Atherosclerosis b. Diabetic nephropathy
c. Autonomic neuropathy d. Somatic neuropathy

58. A 24-year-old female is admitted to casualty with confusion. The patient has a history of myeloma. Now she has the complaints of constipation, severe abdominal pain, and polyurea. The condition is

a. Diverticulitis
b. Hypercalcemia
c. Hypocalcemia
d. Irritable bowel syndrome

59. **"Totem and Toboo" is the work of**
a. Freud b. Jung
c. Mead d. Erikson

60. **'Widemark formula' is used to determine the quantity of**
a. Alcohol b. Barbiturates
c. Cannabis d. Diazepam

61. **'Amotivational syndrome' has been associated with long-term use of**
a. Alcohol b. Benzodiazepines
c. Cannabis d. Barbiturates

62. **Angel dust is**
a. Amphetamine b. Phencyclidine
c. Heroin d. LSD

63. **The rate is produced by dividing the number of deaths during one year by estimated midyear population**
a. Crude death rate
b. Morbidity incidence
c. Mortality prevalence
d. Proportional population rate

64. **Within epidemiological framework, interrelationships among a multitude of factors, constitute**
a. Confounding variables
b. Natural history of disease causation
c. Systems effect
d. Web of causation

65. **Mittelschmerz is pain associated with**
a. Vomiting b. Ovulation
c. Defecation d. Sexual intercourse

66. **A statistical source for population age distributions, dependency ratios and SES characteristics is**
a. Census data b. Morbidity data
c. Service utilization data d. Vital statistics

67. **During the first trimester of pregnancy, the source of elevated estrogen and progesterone is**
a. Fetal adrenal glands b. Fetal liver
c. Corpus luteum d. Maternal ovaries

68. **Regarding fetal development, lungs are capable of breathing air at**
a. 22nd weeks of pregnancy
b. 25th weeks of pregnancy
c. 30th weeks of pregnancy
d. 18th weeks of pregnancy

69. **SHBG is decreased in**
a. Cirrhosis b. Hirsutism
c. Pregnancy d. Estrogen therapy

70. **The nursing intervention, most appropriate for promoting the environment safety of client with cognitive disorder is**
a. Applying an identification bracelet on the client
b. Maintaining daily routine care to the client
c. Placing a clock and daily shedule in the client's room
d. Using short sentences when speaking with client

71. **When disposing plastic bags, tubings, syringes and gloves used to administer antineoplastic drugs, the nurse should implement which nursing intervention?**
a. Avoiding contact with the equipment by allowing housekeeping to remove it
b. Discarding all used equipment in a container marked "Isolation"
c. Dispose all equipments in a container marked "Biohealth Hazard"
d. Disposing all used equipments in the regular trash receptacles

72. **Triphasic K-complex is seen in which phase of sleep?**
a. Stage-I b. Stage-II
c. Stage-III d. REM Sleep

73. **The following problem does not typically result from uncontrolled gestational diabetes mellitus**
a. Maternal hypoglycemia
b. Fetal demise
c. Insufficient amniotic fluid
d. Maternal hypertension

74. **'Knock-out drops' or 'Mickey Finn' stands for**
a. Methyl alcohol b. Ethylene glycol
c. Chloroform d. Chloral hydrate

75. The client with a rectovaginal fistula is at risk of infection. The intervention, most important in preventive aspect of nursing care is

a. Administering antibiotics
b. Ensuring adequate rest to enhance healing
c. Monitoring temperature and WBC count
d. Performing perineal care

76. A patient with bipolar disorder becomes verbally aggressive in a group therapy session, which of the following response by the nurse would be the best?

a. "You are behaving in an unacceptable manner, and you need to control yourself"
b. "If you continue like that, no one will want to be around you"
c. "You are fighting everyone in the group, leave room immediately"
d. "Other people are disturbed by your profanity. I will walk with you down the hall to help release some of that energy"

77. The natural hormone produced by the pineal gland that induces sleep

a. Amphetamine b. Melatonin
c. Methylphenidate d. Pemoline

78. "Let likes be cured by likes". This law similar in the concept of

a. Ayurveda b. Biofield therapeutics
c. Chiropractic medicine d. Homeopathy

79. The nurse suspects that laboring client may have been physically abused by her male partner. The most appropriate interventions is

a. Confront the male partner
b. Question the women in front of her partner
c. Contact hospital security
d. Collaborate with the physician to make a referral to social services

80. One of the action, best explains the main role of surfactant in the neonate is

a. Assists the ciliary body maturation in the upper airways
b. Helps to maintain rhythmic breathing pattern
c. Promotes clearing mucus from the respiratory tract
d. Helps the lung remain expanded after the initiation of breathing

81. Free base is a form of

a. LSD b. Brown sugar
c. Cocaine d. Heroin

82. Aminopterin is antivitamin of

a. Pyridoxine b. Niacin
c. Folic acid d. Riboflavin

83. The following medication has been connected with development of Reye's syndrome

a. Amphetamine b. Melatonin
c. Aspirin d. Ibuprofen

84. Pelkan's spur is seen in

a. Rickets b. Scurvy
c. Hypothyroidism d. Hypopituitarism

85. Bruxism refers to

a. Nightmares b. Nocturnal enuresis
c. Sleep walking d. Tooth grinding

86. Father of epidemiology

a. Hippocrates b. Robert Wilson
c. Hohn Snow d. John Alex

87. The goal of oxygen therapy for a client with pulmonary embolism is to obtain

a. $PaCO_2$ above 40 mm Hg
b. $PaCO_2$ above 60 mm Hg
c. $PaCO_2$ below 40 mm Hg
d. $PaCO_2$ below 60 mm Hg

88. A client with a pulmonary embolism may have an umbrella filter, placed in the venacava to

a. Prevents further clot formation
b. Collects clots, so they do not go to the lungs
c. Break up clots into insignificantly small pieces
d. Contains anticoagulants that are slowly released, releasing the clots

89. Frankel's line in the X-ray is seen in

a. Scurvy b. Rickets
c. Congenital syphilis d. None of the above

90. Theophylline is prescribed for a client with chronic bronchitis, the substance increases the elimination of theophylline leading to sub-therapeutic levels of the drug is

a. Caffeine containing beverages
b. Oral contraceptives
c. Corticosteroids
d. Marijuana

91. A client is presented with an embolic stroke. Which of the following condition places the client at the risk of thrombo embolic stroke?

a. Atrial fibrillation b. Bradycardia
c. Deep vein thrombosis d. History of myocardial infarction

92. "Education is the natural harmonious and progressive development of man's innate powers", said by

a. John Dewy b. Pestalozi
c. Heward Joyce d. Rousseau

93. At which stage, should initial screening for idiopathic juvenile scoliosis take place?

a. 7 years b. 10 years
c. 13 years d. 17 years

94. The following committee was given recommendations to start college of nursing in India

a. Bhore committee
b. Kartar Singh Committee
c. S Radhakrishnan Committee
d. Mudhaliar Committee

95. The statistical synthesis of the datas from a set of comparable studies of a problem, and it yields a quantitative summary of the period of the pooled results is

a. Meta synthesis b. Meta analysis
c. Concept mapping d. Concept synthesis

96. FIGLU test is used to detect

a. Vitamin A intoxication b. Niacin acid deficiency
c. Folic acid deficiency d. Vitamin B_{12} deficiency

97. Accrediting body "responsible for the specialized accreditation of nursing educational programs, both postsecondary and higher degree (Master's degree, Baccalurate Degree, Associate Degree, Diploma, and Practical Nursing Program)"

a. NLNAC b. TNAI
c. NABH d. NAE

98. "It may seem a strange principle to enunciate as the very first requirement in a hospital that it should do the sick no harm". This famous quote is of

a. Florence Nightingale b. Cass Canfield
c. Carrie Latet d. Virginia Henderson

99. The aspiration of theory "the fully functional person, the best approach for the facilitator to assist the learners to perform their full potential, is to know them well"

a. Levin's theory
b. Roger's theory
c. King goal attainment theory
d. Peplau's theory

100. A client attorney can file a law suit within which time frame

a. Discovery role
b. Statute of limitations
c. Grace period
d. Alternative dispute resolution.

ANSWER KEY

1. b	2. b	3. a	4. d	5. b	6. b.	7. a	8. c	9. a	10. a	11. c	12. c
13. b	14. b	15. a	16. b	17. a	18. d	19. d	20. b	21. b	22. a	23. d	24. b
25. b	26. c	27. b	28. b	29. c	30. a	31. c	32. a	33. c	34. a	35. a	36. d
37. c	38. a	39. d	40. a	41. c	42. c	43. a	44. d	45. a	46. b	47. c	48. d
49. d	50. b	51. c	52. a	53. a	54. c	55. b	56. b	57. c	58. b	59. a	60. a
61. c	62. b	63. a	64. d	65. b	66. a	67. c	68. a	69. b	70. c	71. c	72. b
73. d	74. d	75. d	76. d	77. b	78. d	79. d	80. a	81. c	82. c	83. c	84. b
85. d	86. a	87. b	88. b	89. b	90. a	91. c	92. b	93. b	94. b	95. b	96. d
97. a	98. a	99. b	100. b								

Rank Making Points

1. The erectile structure in the female which is analogous to penis in male
2. Most important muscle group supporting pelvic organs
3. Bacilli present in vaginal secretion
4. Major side effect of haloperidol
5. The causative organism of dengue fever
6. A viral disease that begins with respiratory symptoms and skin rash and may result in grave complication
7. Immunity by antibody formation during the course of a disease
8. One of the most important symptoms of salicylate toxicity
9. Pulse pressure
10. Reason for chest pain associated with myocardial infarction
11. The virus causing chickenpox can also produce
12. Transparent mucoprotein covering of ovum
13. The part of uterine tube where fertilization occurs
14. The measure of health status of children in a community
15. Drug given to reduce extrapyramidal reactions
16. A patient receiving warfarin should report to the doctor
17. A viral disease caused by one of the smallest human viruses that infect the motor cells of the anterior horn of a spinal cord
18. Kartar Singh Committee is otherwise known as
19. Gingival hyperplasia is a complication of
20. The desired quantity of 'free residual chlorine' in drinking water
21. False ideas or beliefs that the patient accepts as real
22. Imaginary perceptions
23. A child with a Wilms' tumor should not be subjected to
24. Recommended maximum noise level for human beings
25. A side effect of amitriptyline
26. Muscular layer of the uterus
27. The compression-ventilation ratio for two rescuer CPR
28. The serious side effect of vincristine
29. Pouch of Douglas
30. Fertilization span of oocyte
31. Average weight of placenta
32. Average weight of uterus
33. ECT may be used to treat
34. Fear of situations or places that may be difficult or embarrassing to leave
35. Drug of choice to treat leukemia
36. The best method of refuse disposal in a hospital
37. World Heart Day is observed on
38. Most important complication of mumps in adolescent boys
39. The personality disorder that is characterized primarily by mistrust
40. The chest pain resulting from inadequate blood supply to myocardium
41. Triple antigen denotes
42. Causative organism of malaria
43. To qualify for the diagnosis of anorexia nervosa, the patient's weight must drop below
44. Pent up blood inside the vagina behind the hymen
45. Color of amniotic fluid in Rh-incompatibility
46. Digoxin toxicity occurs when serum level of digoxin exceeds
47. Time required to measure the Mantoux test
48. The drug given to relieve pain in myocardial infarction
49. The birth weight of the baby doubles at the age of
50. Antisterility vitamin
51. Koplik's spot is seen in
52. The assessment finding that strongly suggests IV drug abuse
53. Collected blood in the fallopian tubes
54. Average heart rate of newborn
55. The amount of blood ejected per minute by rhythmic ventricular contraction
56. Lifespan of fetal RBC
57. The drug used for morphine induced respiratory depression

58. The ability of the body to recognize, destroy and eliminate antigenic material
59. A child with tracheoesophageal fistula will have
60. A fibrinolytic agent
61. Trisomy 21
62. Separation of an infected person from non-infected persons
63. Simian crease is a characteristic feature of
64. The apical pulse is located at
65. Lecithin-Sphingomyelin ratio in amniotic fluid that indicates lung maturity
66. Hypertrophied sebaceous glands around nipples during pregnancy
67. Menopausal women are at risk for
68. Oxytocin is produced from
69. Drug used to treat bradycardia
70. The most important parameter of APGAR score
71. Immunoglobulin present in human milk
72. Currently married couple, where woman is in the reproductive age
73. Sudden uncontrollable attack of deep sleep even during eating and lasting up to 20 minutes
74. The test used to find out syphilis
75. The first stool of newborn
76. The position used to treat shock and decreased blood pressure
77. Color of urine in glomerulonephritis
78. Characteristics of stool in Hirschsprung's disease
79. The parameter that should be monitored in patients after heart valve replacement
80. Pigmentation around neck, forehead and around eyes found during pregnancy
81. Boot shaped heart in X-ray is seen in
82. Life threatening complication of hyperbilirubinemia in newborn
83. A non-living object may replace a human partner in a patient with
84. Hemolytic disease in new born is due to
85. The science of health and its preservation
86. Distorted or invented words that have meaning only for the patient
87. Folic acid deficiency in pregnancy predisposes to
88. Pernicious anemia is due to
89. Pulse rate less than 60 beats per minute
90. Normal respiratory rate in the newborn
91. Right ventricular enlargement due to pulmonary problem
92. World breastfeeding week is celebrated on
93. An outbreak of disease in a community in excess of normal expectation
94. The type of cell division occurring in the germ cell
95. Average total weight gain during pregnancy
96. The strongest joint in the human body
97. Children with prolonged diarrhea are prone for
98. Ruptured graphian follicle after ovulation
99. Displacement of negative feelings onto another person
100. Telescoping of one part of bowel to another part
101. World blood donation day is celebrated on
102. World hypertension day is celebrated on

ANSWER KEY

1. Clitoris
2. Levator ani
3. Doderlein bacilli
4. Extrapyramidal reactions
5. Arbovirus
6. Rubeola
7. Active natural immunity
8. Ringing in ears
9. Difference between diastolic and systolic pressure
10. Decreased oxygen in heart muscle
11. Herpes zoster
12. Zona pellucida
13. Ampulla
14. Infant mortality rate (IMR)
15. Benztropine
16. Bleeding from any sites
17. Polio myelitis
18. Multipurpose workers committee
19. Phenytoin
20. 0.5 mg/L
21. Delusion
22. Hallucinations
23. Renal biopsy
24. 85 dB
25. Agranulocytosis
26. Myometrium
27. 5:1

28. Neurotoxicity
29. Rectouterine pouch
30. 12–24 hours
31. 500 grams
32. 50 grams
33. Major depressive disorder
34. Agoraphobia
35. Vincristine
36. Incineration
37. 28th September
38. Sterility
39. Paranoid personality disorder
40. Angina pectoris
41. DPT
42. Plasmodium
43. 85% of ideal body weight
44. Cryptomenorrhea
45. Golden yellow color
46. 2 mg/dL
47. 24–48 hours
48. Morphine sulfate
49. 6 months
50. Vitamin E
51. Measles
52. Skin lesions
53. Hematosalpinx
54. 120–140 beats/min
55. Cardiac output
56. 80 days
57. Naloxone
58. Immunity
59. Excessive drooling of saliva
60. Streptokinase
61. Down's syndrome
62. Isolation
63. Down's syndrome
64. 5th left intercostals space
65. 2:1
66. Montgomery's tubercle
67. Osteoporosis
68. Posterior pituitary
69. Atropine
70. Heart rate
71. Ig A
72. Eligible couple
73. Narcolepsy
74. VDRL
75. Meconium
76. Trendelenburg position
77. Cola colored
78. Ribbon shaped stools
79. Prothrombin time
80. Chloasma
81. Tetralogy of Fallot
82. Kernicterus
83. Fetishism
84. Rh-incompatibility
85. Hygiene
86. Neologism
87. Neural tube defects
88. Vitamin B_{12} deficiency
89. Bradycardia
90. 30–60 breaths per minute
91. Corpulmonale
92. August 1st week
93. Epidemic
94. Meiosis
95. 10-12 kg
96. Sacroiliac joint
97. Metabolic acidosis
98. Corpus luteum
99. Projection
100. Intussusception
101. 14th June
102. May 17

MODEL QUESTION PAPERS

MODEL QUESTION PAPER I

1. **Hypocalcemia causes**
   a. Tetanus b. Tetany
   c. Tinnitus d. Tenesmus
2. **The common complaint of a woman with IUCD is**
   a. Vaginal bleeding b. Pelvic infection
   c. Uterine perforation d. Abdominal pain
3. **The umbilical cord contains**
   a. One artery and one vein
   b. Two arteries and one vein
   c. One artery and two veins
   d. Two arteries and two veins
4. **Hypotension in postoperative period leads to**
   a. Hypoxia b. Hypovolemia
   c. Cardiac arrhythmias d. TAO
5. **Subarachnoid hemorrhage is bleeding between**
   a. Skull and dura mater b. Dura and pia mater
   c. Arachnoid and pia mater
   d. Skull and arachnoid mater
6. **An important mineralocorticoid by adrenal cortex**
   a. Androgen b. Aldosterone
   c. Cortisone d. Corticosterone
7. **Koplik's spots are characteristic of**
   a. Mumps b. Oral thrush
   c. Oral cancer d. Measles
8. **Cholelithiasis is stone formation in the**
   a. Kidneys b. Gallbladder
   c. Urinary bladder d. Spleen
9. **Normal level of $PaCO_2$ is**
   a. 35–45 mm of Hg b. 45–55 mm of Hg
   c. 40–60 mm of Hg d. 80–100 mm of Hg
10. **A positive sign of pregnancy is**
    a. Morning sickness b. Hegar's sign
    c. Fetal heart sounds d. Chadwick's sign
11. **Acromegaly is due to the over production of**
    a. Testosterone b. ACTH
    c. FSH d. Growth hormone
12. **Painless, irregular contractions occurring in uterus in pregnancy**
    a. Osiander's sign
    b. Chadwick's sign
    c. False pains
    d. Braxton Hick's contractions
13. **Imaginary perception is**
    a. Illusion b. Hallucination
    c. Imagination d. Echolalia
14. **Clay colored stools are seen in**
    a. Obstructive jaundice b. Food poisoning
    c. Lactic intolerance d. Cirrhosis
15. **The inflammation of the tongue is called**
    a. Stomatitis b. Glossitis
    c. Glossodynia d. Halitosis
16. **The non-pregnant uterus weighs**
    a. 40 g b. 60 g
    c. 80 g d. 100 g
17. **Lecithin: Sphingomyelin ratio in amniotic fluid that indicates lung maturity**
    a. 1:1 b. 1:2
    c. 2:1 d. 2:2
18. **A permanent colostomy is usually made in**
    a. Sigmoid colon b. Transverse colon
    c. Ascending colon d. Descending colon
19. **Average heart rate of newborn**
    a. 100–120 bpm b. 120–140 bpm
    c. 140–160 bpm d. >160 bpm
20. **Pigeon chest is seen in**
    a. Osteoporosis b. Ricketts
    c. Osteosarcoma d. Costochondritis

21. Simon-Binet test is used for measuring
a. Aptitude b. Intelligence
c. Attitude d. Memory

22. CSF is secreted by
a. Cerebral aqueduct b. Arachnoid granulations
c. Choroid plexus d. Falx cerebri

23. Accepted ways of behaving in the society are called
a. Customs b. Norms
c. Folkways d. Culture

24. Adverse effect of Streptomycin
a. Ototoxicity b. Nephrotoxicity
c. Hepatitis d. Diarrhea

25. Area where the optic nerve leaves the eye is called
a. Macula lutea b. Choroid
c. Ciliary body d. Optic disk

26. The process of destroying microorganisms including spores is called
a. Disinfection b. Sterilization
c. Infection control d. Isolation

27. Dumping syndrome is a postoperative complication of
a. Appendicectomy b. Cholecystectomy
c. Gastrostomy d. Gastrectomy

28. Bell's palsy is due to the compression of
a. Olfactory nerve b. Optic nerve
c. Facial nerve d. Oculomotor nerve

29. The amount of salt needed to make one liter of 0.9 % normal saline
a. 19 g b. 18 g
c. 9 g d. 90 g

30. The position immediately after tonsillectomy
a. Trendelenburg b. Sim's
c. Prone d. Dorsal recumbent

31. World AIDS day is on
a. 1st October b. 1st December
c. 10th October d. 10th December

32. Deficient salivation is called
a. Xerophthalmia b. Xerostomia
c. Ptyalism d. Halitosis

33. Hormone stimulating gastric acid production
a. Renin b. Gastrin
c. Erythropoietin d. Thiamine

34. Largest gland in the body
a. Pituitary b. Hypothalamus
c. Liver d. Skin

35. Cancer of pigmented skin cells
a. Myeloma b. Melanoma
c. Osteosarcoma d. Retinoblastoma

36. Antisterility vitamin is
a. Vitamin A b. Vitamin B
c. Vitamin C d. Vitamin E

37. Indian Red Cross society was established on
a. 1920 b. 1924
c. 1928 d. 1930

38. IDRV is a vaccine for
a. Rubella b. Chickenpox
c. Rabies d. Meningitis

39. Wound dehiscence is
a. Wound infection
b. Delayed wound healing
c. Protrusion of the contents through the wound
d. Separation of wound edges

40. SLE is a disease of
a. Bone b. Erythrocytes
c. Connective tissue d. Joints

41. Lack of oxygen in the blood stream is
a. Anoxemia b. Anoxia
c. Asphyxia d. Hypoxia

42. Specialized type of cartilage in which collagen is being impregnated with calcium
a. Bone b. Fibrocartilage
c. Hyaline cartilage d. Elastic cartilage

43. Shape of human placenta
a. Oval b. Dome shaped
c. Circular d. Discoid

44. Substances used to counteract the effect of poison
a. Antidotes b. Antiseptics
c. Antibiotics d. Antifungal

45. Voiding during normal sleeping hours is termed as
a. Dysuria b. Nocturia
c. Anuria d. Oliguria

46. The temperature for the sponge bath
a. 110°–115°F b. 100°–110°F
c. 90°–100°F d. 120°–125°F

47. **Lifespan of fetal RBC**
a. 70 days b. 80 days
c. 100 days d. 120 days

48. **Inborn all round mental efficiency of an individual is called**
a. Emotion b. Intelligence
c. Behavior d. Drives

49. **The part of uterine tube where fertilization occurs**
a. Ampulla b. Infundibulum
c. Cornua d. Fimbriae

50. **Sudden severe attack of shivering in which the body temperature rises rapidly**
a. Stadium b. Fastigium
c. Crisis d. Rigor

51. **The most common symptoms of hypoglycemia are**
a. Nervousness and diaphoresis
b. Anorexia and incoherent speech
c. Kussmaul's respiration and confusion
d. Bradycardia and blurred vision

52. **Progesterone is secreted by**
a. Corpus luteum b. Corpus albicans
c. Pituitary gland d. Graafian cells

53. **Hormones are produced by**
a. Exocrine glands b. Endocrine glands
c. Holocrine glands d. Apocrine glands

54. **The male sex hormone is called**
a. Vasopressin b. Gonadotropic hormone
c. FSH d. Testosterone

55. **The blood vessel in which the oxygen content is highest in the fetus is**
a. Aorta b. Umbilical vein
c. Pulmonary artery d. Inferior vena cava

56. **The measure of health status of children in a community is**
a. Infant mortality rate b. Maternal mortality rate
c. Crude birth rate d. Crude death rate

57. **Which of the following signs and symptoms indicate salicylate toxicity?**
a. Chest pain b. Pink colored urine
c. Slow pulse rate d. Ringing in ears

58. **Urinary bladder is lined with**
a. Simple epithelium
b. Stratified epithelium
c. Transitional epithelium
d. Pseudostratified epithelium

59. **Which of the following is a potassium sparing diuretic?**
a. Furosemide b. Aldactone
c. Mannitol d. Dimox

60. **The position, most suited for an unconscious patient is**
a. Fowler's position b. Prone position
c. Supine position d. Semiprone position

61. **39°C is equal to**
a. 100.2°F b. 102.2°F
c. 101.2°F d. 103.2°F

62. **The vitamin which is involved in fat, protein and carbohydrate metabolism**
a. Riboflavin b. Folic acid
c. Niacin d. Thiamine

63. **The hormonal contraceptives are**
a. Oral b. Injectable
c. Implant d. All of them

64. **Poliomyelitis is transmitted through**
a. Water b. Air
c. Blood d. Vectors

65. **MCH service includes**
a. Prenatal and postnatal care
b. Under fives care
c. Family planning service
d. All of the above

66. **The recommended maximum noise level for human beings**
a. 85 dB b. 50 dB
c. 110 dB d. 160 dB

67. **The master gland of the body is**
a. Liver b. Pituitary
c. Thyroid d. Adrenal

68. **Causative organism of malaria is**
a. Cryptococcosis b. Leishmania
c. Plasmodium d. Klebsiella

69. **Sepsis means**
   a. Absence of infection
   b. Presence of pathogenic organisms
   c. Destruction of pathogenic organisms
   d. Infection in the blood

70. **Father of antiseptic surgery**
   a. Joseph Lister b. Louis Pasteur
   c. William Harvey d. Ronald Ross

71. **Vaccines and toxoids produce**
   a. Natural immunity b. Active immunity
   c. Passive immunity d. Acquired immunity

72. **A disease caused by bacteria**
   a. Cold b. Typhoid
   c. Typhus fever c. Chickenpox

73. **The cells that are responsible for the production of antibodies are**
   a. Red blood cells b. Platelets
   c. Plasma d. White blood cells

74. **A healthy person can donate blood ....or .... times a year.**
   a. Six or seven b. Five or six
   c. Three or four d. Two or three

75. **Radioactive cobalt and radium are used for the treatment of**
   a. Cholera b. Hemophilia
   c. Cancer d. Sickle cell anemia

76. **World Health Day is on ....**
   a. 12th May b. 7th April
   c. 30th April d. 18th December

77. **To relieve from dyspnea the appropriate position to be used is**
   a. Prone position b. Supine position
   c. Side-lying position d. Fowler's position

78. **Peurparium is the period begins**
   a. As soon as the placenta is expelled and last for 6 to 8 weeks
   b. As soon as the baby is expelled and last for 6 to 8 weeks
   c. As soon as the membrane ruptures and last for 6 to 8 weeks
   d. As soon as the placenta is expelled and last for 10 to 12 weeks

79. **When the umbilical cord lies in front of the presenting part and the membranes are intact, it is known as**
   a. Cord prolapse b. Cord presentation
   c. Cord pulsation d. Cord delivery

80. **Starting of menstrual cycle is called**
   a. Ovulation b. Menstruation
   c. Menarche d. Menopause

81. **Normal blood urea level is**
   a. 40–60 mg% b. 20–40 mg%
   c. 10–20 mg% d. 80–120 mg%

82. **One gram of carbohydrate yields**
   a. 4 calories b. 8 calories
   c. 9 calories d. 1 calorie

83. **A method of making the victim to breath passively**
   a. Artificial respiration b. Spontaneous respiration
   c. Deep breathing d. Kussmaul's breathing

84. **Minute, thin walled blood vessels between the ends of the arteries and beginning of veins is called**
   a. Arteries b. Veins
   c. Capillaries d. Alveoli

85. **A waste gas produced by the body and exhaled through the lungs is**
   a. Carbon dioxide b. Carbon monoxide
   c. Nitrogen peroxide d. Oxygen

86. **A condition characterized by moving of bones, out of joint**
   a. Fracture b. Sprain
   c. Strain d. Dislocation

87. **A tube of muscular tissue carrying ingested food from the mouth to stomach**
   a. Esophagus b. Duodenum
   c. Trachea d. Pharynx

88. **A red pigment in the blood cells which combines with oxygen and carbon dioxide for carrying them**
   a. Red blood cells b. Hemoglobin
   c. Platelet d. Plasma

89. **Information given by the sufferer about his illness**
   a. Sign b. Symptom
   c. Observation d. Diagnosis

90. **Normal respiratory rate in adults is**
   a. 20–40/min b. 40–60/min
   c. 16–20/min d. 10–15/min

91. Characteristic of the blood flow due to arterial bleeding is the following except

a. Bright red in color
b. Spurts at each contraction of the heart
c. Flow is pulsatile
d. Dark red in color

92. An agent that has the power to kill microorganism

a. Bacteriostatic b. Bactericide
c. Antiseptic d. Bacteriostasis

93. Following are predisposing cause for bedsore except

a. Impaired circulation b. Lowered vitality
c. Emaciation d. Anorexia

94. Inability to sleep is termed as

a. Dyspepsia b. Dyspnea
c. Anorexia d. Insomnia

95. Tobacco contains a poisonous substance called

a. Nicotine b. Narcotics
c. Alcohol d. Caffeine

96. A disease caused by allergic disease is

a. Asthma b. Tuberculosis
c. Cancer d. Gastroenteritis

97. Deficiency of thyroxin in adults leads to a condition called

a. Tetani b. Cretinism
c. Myxedema d. Graves diseases

98. The hormone that is injected to pregnant women at the time of delivery is

a. Vasopressin b. Oxytocin
c. Androgen d. Estrogen

99. The outer layer of the eye ball is

a. Sclera b. Choroids
c. Retina d. Conjunctiva

100. The smallest bone in the human body is

a. Malleus b. Incus
c. Stapes d. Sternum

ANSWER KEY

1. b	2. a	3. b	4. c	5. c	6. b	7. d	8. b	9. a	10. c	11. d	12. d
13. b	14. a	15. b	16. b	17. c	18. a	19. b	20. b	21. b	22. c	23. b	24. a
25. d	26. b	27. d	28. d	29. c	30. b	31. b	32. b	33. b	34. c	35. b	36. d
37. a	38. c	39. d	40. c	41. a	42. a	43. d	44. a	45. b	46. a	47. b	48. b
49. a	50. d	51. a	52. a	53. b	54. d	55. b	56. a	57. d	58. c	59. b	60. d
61. b	62. c	63. d	64. a	65. d	66. a	67. b	68. c	69. b	70. a	71. d	72. b
73. d	74. c	75. c	76. b	77. d	78. a	79. b	80. c	81. b	82. a	83. a	84. c
85. a	86. d	87. a	88. b	89. b	90. c	91. d	92. b	93. d	94. d	95. a	96. a
97. c	98. b	99. a	100. c								

MODEL QUESTION PAPER II

1. **Difficulty in getting off to sleep or in maintaining sleep**
   a. Amnesia b. Insomnia
   c. Narcolepsy d. Hypersomnia
2. **Goiter, exophthalmos and hyperthyroidism are characteristic symptoms of**
   a. Grave's disease b. Thyroiditis
   c. MNG d. Thyroid adenoma
3. **A complication of prolonged bed rest**
   a. Jaundice b. Diarrhea
   c. Kidney stone d. Fever
4. **Repair of tympanic membrane is**
   a. Tympanoplasty b. Myringoplasty
   c. Myringotomy d. Septoplasty
5. **A hereditary form of arthritis where there is excess uric acid in the blood**
   a. Syringomyelia b. Still's disease
   c. Gout d. Spondylitis
6. **Expected weight of a 1-year-old child whose birth weight was 3 kg is**
   a. 7 kg b. 9 kg
   c. 10.5 kg d. 12 kg
7. **Dysphagia is difficulty in**
   a. Swallowing b. Speech
   c. Walk d. Breathing
8. **A basic document for organizing family planning work is**
   a. Eligible couple register b. MCH record
   c. Family record d. Birth and death register
9. **Children assumes squatting posture when they have**
   a. PDA b. Tetralogy of Fallot
   c. Constipation d. Abdominal cramps
10. **A patient can become hypoxic if a tracheostomy suction is done for more than**
    a. 30 seconds b. 60 seconds
    c. 10–15 seconds d. 20–30 seconds
11. **A high malignant sarcoma that arises in the bone marrow**
    a. Osteosarcoma b. Multiple myeloma
    c. Ewing's tumor d. Osteochondritis
12. **Drug of choice in leukemia**
    a. Melphalan b. Vincristine
    c. Vancomycin d. Methotrexate
13. **A common type of fracture in children**
    a. Simple fracture b. Compound fracture
    c. Greenstick fracture d. Collis fracture
14. **Tarry stool indicates**
    a. Hemorroids b. Anal fissure
    c. Gastric bleeding d. Intestinal obstruction
15. **Normal CVP is**
    a. 4–10 cm of water b. 60–120 cm of water
    c. 20–40 cm of water d. 40–60 cm of water
16. **Rice water stool is found in**
    a. Amebic dysentery b. Bacillary dysentery
    c. Food poisoning d. Cholera
17. **Bluish discoloration of vagina during pregnancy**
    a. Jacquemier's sign b. Chadwick's sign
    c. Osiander's sign d. Goodell's sign
18. **Placental abruption is a complication of**
    a. Gestational diabetes b. PPH
    c. PIH d. GTD
19. **Commonly used drug for angina pectoris is**
    a. Lasix b. Nitroglycerine
    c. Analgesics d. Anticoagulants
20. **Anasarca is**
    a. General malaise b. Periorbital edema
    c. Pitting edema d. Generalized edema
21. **Persistent irrational fear of an object is**
    a. Obsession b. Illusion
    c. Phobia d. Hallucination
22. **Infection of the body by pus forming bacteria**
    a. Asepsis b. Sepsis
    c. Inflammation d. Immunosuppression
23. **Duration of a cardiac cycle is**
    a. 0.8 seconds b. 10 seconds
    c. 8 seconds d. 1.2 seconds
24. **Acetone in urine is tested by**
    a. Smith's test b. Hey's test
    c. Rothera's test d. Benedict's test

25. **Color of amniotic fluid in Rh-incompatibility**
    a. Pale straw colored
    b. Golden yellow colored
    c. Greenish yellow colored
    d. Dark brown colored

26. **Offensive odor of breath due to poor oral hygiene**
    a. Dental caries b. Plaque
    c. Calculus d. Halitosis

27. **Hospital acquired infection is known as**
    a. Droplet infection b. Opportunistic infection
    c. Nosocomial infection d. Contamination

28. **Florence Nightingale was born on**
    a. 12th May b. 10th May
    c. 15th June d. 12th June

29. **Transparent mucoprotein covering of ovum**
    a. Hyaluronidase b. Zona pellucida
    c. Corona radiata d. Chorionic leave

30. **The vector of malaria**
    a. Culex mosquito b. Tiger mosquito
    c. Tsetse fly d. Anopheles mosquito

31. **Branch of medicine dealing with the problems of ageing and diseases of the elderly**
    a. Geriatrics b. Pediatrics
    c. Gerontologic nursing d. Gerentology

32. **Abnormal condition of the vertebral column characterized by increased convexity in the thoracic spine**
    a. Kyphosis b. Scoliosis
    c. Lordosis d. Sertorius

33. **Excessive menstrual flow during menstruation with regular cycles is known as**
    a. Dysmenorrhea b. Menorrhagia
    c. Metrorrhagia d. Premenstrual syndrome

34. **Inner force which moves an individual to a certain action**
    a. Motive b. Attitude
    c. Behavior d. Mind

35. **The valve that lies between right atrium and right ventricle**
    a. Aortic valve b. Bicuspid valve
    c. Mitral valve d. Tricuspid valve

36. **The tendency of an organism to behave in the same way as it has behaved before**
    a. Motive b. Drive
    c. Behavior d. Habit

37. **Beriberi is caused by the deficiency of**
    a. Vitamin A b. Vitamin B
    c. Vitamin C d. Vitamin D

38. **The most reliable investigation in CAD is**
    a. Cardiac catheterization
    b. Echocardiography
    c. Coronary angiography
    d. Computerized tomography

39. **The best method for hospital refused disposal is**
    a. Dumping b. Incineration
    c. Controlled pitting d. Landfill

40. **Incubation period of cholera**
    a. Few hours to 5 days b. One week
    c. 10 days d. 15 days

41. **Longest and strongest bone in human body is**
    a. Femur b. Humerus
    c. Radius d. Tibia

42. **Universally recognized type of marriage is**
    a. Exogamy b. Monogamy
    c. Endogamy d. Polygamy

43. **Chikungunya is transmitted by**
    a. Aedes aegypti b. Tsetse fly
    c. Culex d. Anopheles

44. **The opening in the occipital bone through which the cranial cavity communicates with the vertebral canal**
    a. Fontanelles b. Foramen magnum
    c. Mastoid antrum d. Cribriform plate

45. **An abnormal curvature of the spine where the spine is found twisted**
    a. Kyphosis b. IVDP
    c. Lordosis d. Scoliosis

46. **Muscle present at the back of the thigh which helps in the flexion of the knees**
    a. Quadriceps femoris b. Sartorius
    c. Gastrocnemius d. Hamstring

47. **Epidemic affecting large population is called**
    a. Pandemic b. Endemic
    c. Disaster d. Hazard

48. Presence of ketone in urine is

a. Ketosis b. Azotemia
c. Ketonuria d. Proteinuria

49. Collection of pus in pleural cavity

a. Emphysema b. Bronchitis
c. Bronchiectasis d. Empyema

50. Loss of hair is called

a. Alopecia b. Urticaria
c. Acrochordon d. Paronychia

51. A common symptom of active tuberculosis

a. Marked weight loss b. Dyspnea on exertion
c. Mental status changes d. Constipation

52. Cessation of menstrual cycle is called

a. Ovulation b. Puberty
c. Menopause d. Implantation

53. Islets of Langerhans are present in

a. Brain b. Stomach
c. Ovary d. Pancreas

54. Number of spinal nerves in man are

a. 11 pairs b. 12 pairs
c. 31 pairs d. 33 pairs

55. The cerebellum is concerned with

a. Coordination of muscular movements
b. Perception
c. Memory
d. Vision

56. Removal of gallbladder in man could lead to

a. Impairment of fat digestion
b. Impairment of digestion of protein
c. Jaundice
d. Increased acidity in intestine

57. India's National Health Policy was approved in the parliament in

a. 1961 b. 1980
c. 1983 d. 1991

58 Which of the following food constituents are more required by pregnant woman?

a. Iron b. Calcium
c. Potassium d. Vitamin C

59. An antenatal mother is ordered to have a diet that contains 90 grams of protein each day. How many calories will the protein contribute to her daily weight?

a. 180 calories b. 360 calories
c. 540 calories d. 810 calories

60. The antidote of magnesium sulfate is

a. Calcium gluconate b. Diazepam
c. Calcium chloride d. Nalorphine hydrochloride

61. Sprain is due to pulling of

a. Muscles b. Tendons
c. Ligaments d. Nerves

62. Rickets is due to deficiency of

a. Vitamin D b. Vitamin A
c. Vitamin B d. Vitamin C

63. Which of the following is a mechanical method of contraception?

a. Vasectomy b. Mala-D
c. Condom d. MTP

64. Kartar Singh Committee is otherwise known as

a. Multipurpose Workers Committee
b. Health Survey and Development Committee
c. Health Survey and Planning Committee
d. Committee on Medical Education

65. Sand bags are used to prevent

a. Foot drop
b. Wrist drop
c. Internal rotation of thigh
d. All of the above

66. Hemoptysis is

a. Blood in urine b. Blood in vomitus
c. Blood in sputum d. Blood in feces

67. For continuous oxygen administration for longer period, the nasal catheter should be changed

a. Every 6 hours b. Every 12 hours
c. Every 24 hours d. Every 48 hours

68. The causative organism of dengue fever is

a. Enteric virus b. Arbovirus
c. Variola virus d. Influenza virus

69. The desired quantity of 'free residual chlorine' in drinking water is

a. 1 mg./L b. 0.5 mg/L
c. 2 mg/L d. 0.25 mg/L

70. Which of the following combination of blood types is most likely to produce hemolytic disease of the new born

a. Negative mother and Positive father
b. Positive mother and Negative father
c. Negative mother and Negative father
d. Positive mother and Positive father

71. **The vein which will most likely be used to give exchange transfusion in the**
   a. Jugular vein b. Femoral vein
   c. Temporal vein d. Umbilical vein

72. **Which of the following is not an occupational disease?**
   a. Asbestosis b. Pneumoconiosis
   c. Japanese encephalitis d. Silicosis

73. **Carbohydrate is stores in the liver as**
   a. Glucose b. Sucrose
   c. Glycogen d. Galactose

74. **Which of the following signs and symptoms indicate salicylate toxicity?**
   a. Chest pain b. Pink colored urine
   c. Slow pulse rate d. Ringing in ears

75. **Which of the following symptoms might indicate that a client is developing tetany following subtotal thyroidectomy?**
   a. Backache b. Hoarseness
   c. Dyspnea d. Tingling in the fingers

76. **Which of the following vitamin deficiency results in scurvy?**
   a. Vitamin C b. Vitamin B
   c. Vitamin D d. Vitamin A

77. **An example of a congenital cyanotic heart disease is**
   a. Rheumatic heart disease
   b. Ventricular septal defect
   c. Aortic stenosis
   d. Tetrology of Fallot

78. **Approximate time for introduction of solid food in the diet of a child is**
   a. 1–3 months b. 5–6 months
   c. 6–8 months d. 10–12 months

79. **Expected time of closure of anterior fontanel is**
   a. 4–6 weeks b. 6–8 months
   c. 9–12 months d. 16–18 months

80. **Wilm's tumor is a condition affecting**
   a. Kidney b. Bone
   c. Blood d. Brain stem

81. **Most common side effect of blood transfusion**
   a. Urine output b. Skin turgor
   c. Anaphylactic reaction d. Level of consciousness

82. **Which of the following symptoms must be reported to the doctor by a patient receiving warfarin?**
   a. Hematuria b. Constipation
   c. Dyspnea d. Pruritus

83. **In a patient receiving peritoneal dialysis, which of the following signs indicate peritonitis?**
   a. Swelling in the legs
   b. Redness at the catheter insertion site
   c. Poor drainage of the dialysate fluid
   d. Cloudy dialysate fluid

84. **Non-invasive method of oxygen saturation monitoring can be done by**
   a. Arterial blood gas studies
   b. Capillary blood gas studies
   c. Venoclysis
   d. Pulse oxymetry

85. **Drug of choice for respiratory depression in a newborn whose mother received morphine during labor**
   a. Naloxone b. Digoxin
   c. Lidocaine d. Adrenaline

86. **Site for Mantoux test**
   a. Outer and upper quadrant of gluteus maximus
   b. Deltoid region
   c. Posterior right forearm
   d. Anterior left forearm

87. **Media of transmission of bovine type of tubercle bacilli**
   a. Milk b. Water
   c. Air d. Food

88. **Painful micturition**
   a. Enuresis b. Dysuria
   c. Rentetion of urine d. Diarrhea

89. **Drugs used to relieve pain**
   a. Anti-inflammatory b. Antipyretics
   c. Analgesics d. Thrombolytics

90. **Number of chromosome in a cell**
   a. 23 b. 44
   c. 46 d. 40

91. **A water soluble vitamin**
   a. Vitamin A b. Vitamin K
   c. Vitamin B d. Vitamin D

92. Quickening means

a. The movement of the fetus in the uterus felt by the mother
b. Sudden cessation of menstruation
c. Hearing of the fetal heart sound
d. Nausea and vomiting in the morning

93. Cholera is caused by a bacterium called

a. *Tubercle bacillus* b. *Vibrio cholerae*
c. *Protozoa* d. *Entamoeba histolytica*

94. Drinking of alcohol will severely effects the

a. Kidney b. Brain
c. Stomach d. Liver

95. A raised solid lesion of more than 1 cm

a. Vesicle b. Nodule
c. Papule d. Pustule

96. The method of applying medication to the skin

a. Inhalation b. Ingestion
c. Injection d. Inunction

97. The normal rate of oxygen inhalation

a. 1–2 liters per minute b. 4–6 liters per minute
c. 6–8 liters per minute d. 8–10 liters per minute

98. Average length of umbilical cord

a. 20 cm b. 30 cm
c. 50 cm d. 75 cm

99. The following minerals are needed for the synthesis of Hb except

a. Zinc b. Iron
c. Cobalt d. Copper

100. Spalding sign is characteristic of

a. Fetal distress b. IUGR
c. IUD d. Breech presentation

ANSWER KEY

1. b	2. a	3. c	4. b	5. c	6. b	7. a	8. a	9. b	10. c	11. b	12. b
13. c	14. c	15. a	16. d	17. a	18. c	19. b	20. d	21. c	22. b	23. a	24. c
25. b	26. d	27. c	28. a	29. b	30. d	31. a	32. a	33. b	34. a	35. d	36. d
37. b	38. c	39. b	40. a	41. a	42. b	43. a	44. b	45. d	46. d	47. a	48. c
49. d	50. a	51. a	52. c	53. d	54. c	55. a	56. a	57. c	58. b	59. b	60. a
61. c	62. a	63. c	64. a	65. a	66. c	67. c	68. b	69. b	70. a	71. d	72. c
73. c	74. d	75. d	76. a	77. d	78. c	79. d	80. b	81. c	82. a	83. d	84. d
85. a	86. d	87. a	88. b	89. c	90. c	91. c	92. a	93. b	94. d	95. b	96. d
97. b	98. c	99. a	100. c								

MODEL QUESTION PAPER III

1. **Time required for maturation of spermatozoa**
   a. 16 days b. 31 days
   c. 45 days d. 61 days
2. **Vestibule contains openings except**
   a. Urethra b. Vagina
   c. Bartholin's glands d. Perineum
3. **The Mental Status Examination (MSE) investigates all of the following except the patient's**
   a. LOC
   b. Mood, affect and perceptions
   c. Medication effects
   d. ADL
4. **Food constituents, more required by pregnant woman**
   a. Iron b. Calcium
   c. Potassium d. Vitamin C
5. **The virus causing chickenpox can also produce**
   a. Athlete's foot b. Infectious hepatitis
   c. Herpes zoster d. German measles
6. **Edema is due to**
   a. Increased permeability of capillary walls
   b. Reduced return of lymph
   c. Increased capillary pressure
   d. All of the above
7. **Fertilization span of oocyte**
   a. 12–24 hours b. 24–48 hours
   c. 48–72 hours d. > 72 hours
8. **Skine's glands are homologous to**
   a. Testis b. Epididymis
   c. Prostate d. Penis
9. **The test for assessing patient's orientation and recall**
   a. Beck depression inventory
   b. Thematic apperception test
   c. Mini-mental status examination
   d. Millon clinical multiaxial inventory III
10. **Drug which is not used in the treatment of leprosy**
    a. Streptomycin b. Rifampicin
    c. Clofaximin d. INH
11. **MTP Act was passed in the year**
    a. 1983 b. 1977
    c. 2000 d. 1972
12. **A viral disease caused by one of the smallest human viruses that infect the motor cells of the anterior horn of a spinal cord**
    a. Rubeola b. Rubella
    c. Chickenpox d. Poliomyelitis
13. **Reason for chest pain associated with myocardial infarction**
    a. Decreased oxygen in heart muscle
    b. Left ventricular overload
    c. Circulatory collapse
    d. Electrolyte imbalance
14. **Color of amniotic fluid in postmaturity**
    a. Pale straw colored
    b. Golden yellow colored
    c. Greenish yellow colored
    d. Dark brown colored
15. **Pouch of Douglas is**
    a. Uterovesical pouch b. Rectouterine pouch
    c. Urethrovesical pouch d. Rectovesical pouch
16. **Signs and symptoms of ADHD include the following except**
    a. Inattention b. Impulsiveness
    c. Hyperactivity d. Good concentration
17. **Which of the following is not an occupational disease?**
    a. Asbestosis b. Pneumoconiosis
    c. Japanese encephalitis d. Silicosis
18. **Gingival hyperplasia is a complication of**
    a. Phenobarbitone b. Phenytoin
    c. Diazepam d. Amoxicillin
19. **A patient receiving warfarin should report to the doctor**
    a. Hematuria b. Constipation
    c. Dyspnea d. Pruritus

20. A child is getting 5% dextrose 1000 mL IV in 24 hours, The minidropper delivers 60 drops/mL. The rate of flow will be

a. 30 drops per minute b. 32 drops per minute
c. 38 drops per minute d. 42 drops per minute

21. Carbohydrate is stores in the liver as

a. Glucose b. Sucrose
c. Glycogen d. Galactose

22. Priority area while caring for a child with depression

a. Developing strength and improving self-esteem
b. Addressing ways to learn to complete tasks
c. Determining strategies to help handle fear
d. Developing communication skills

23. Surfactant is secreted by

a. Alveolar epithelium b. Cuboidal epithelium
c. Squamous epithelium d. Keratinized epithelium

24. Hypertrophied sebaceous glands around nipples during pregnancy

a. Montgomery's tubercle b. Sebaceous cyst
c. Chloasma d. Linea nigra

25. Cryptomenorrhea is

a. Early menarche
b. Late menarche
c. Pent up blood inside the vagina behind the hymen
d. Narrow introitus

26. The child is getting injection morphine 20 mg and the vial contains 50 mg/mL. The amount to be given to get the ordered dose

a. 0.6 mL b. 0.4 mL
c. 0.8 mL d. 1.0 mL

27. Postnatally, striae gravidarum becomes

a. Linea nigra b. Linea albicans
c. Striae gravidarum d. Striae albicans

28. Permanent cessation of menstruation

a. Menarche b. Menopause
c. Menorrhagia d. Metrorhagia

29. Major side effect of haloperidol

a. Drowsiness b. Extrapyramidal reactions
c. Dry mouth d. Anorexia

30. One gram of fat yields

a. 9 calories b. 6 calories
c. 8 calories d. 4 calories

31. Antisterility vitamin is

a. Vitamin A b. Vitamin E
c. Vitamin D d. Vitamin K

32. The best indication that fluid replacement for the client in hypovolemic shock is adequate

a. Skin feels warm
b. Systolic BP above 100 mm Hg
c. Diastolic BP above 90 mm Hg
d. Urine output greater than 30 mL/h

33. A medication given to a patient with angina

a. Digoxin b. Sorbitrate
c. Metoprolol d. Lidocaine

34. The serious side effect of vincristine

a. Neurotoxicity b. Irreversible alopecia
c. Fever and anemia d. GIT symptoms

35. Immunization against DPT should be administered via

a. Oral route b. Intramuscular route
c. Subcutaneous route d. Intradermal route

36. World No Tobacco Day is observed on

a. 5th June b. 31st May
c. 10th August d. 7th April

37. A drug for treating depression

a. Methylphenidate b. Fluoxetine
c. Benztropine d. Pemoline

38. Menopausal symptoms include the following except

a. Dry vagina b. Hot flushes
c. Dysuria d. S. estradiol > 100 pg/mL

39. Total iron requirement during pregnancy

a. 500 g b. 750 g
c. 1000 g d. 1500 g

40. The obstetrical conjugate measures

a. 10 cm b. 11 cm
c. 12 cm d. 13 cm

41. Normal hemoglobin level

a. 4–8 g% b. 1–5 g%
b. 15–25 g% d. 10–14 g%

42. Digoxin toxicity occurs when serum level of digoxin exceeds

a. 1.5 mg/dL b. 1.8 mg/dL
c. 2.0 mg/dL d. 2.5 mg/dL

43. **Chickenpox can be fatal if the child is receiving**
a. Antibiotics b. Steroids
c. Anticonvulsants d. Insulin

44. **Most important complication of mumps in adolescent boys**
a. Hypothyroidism b. Hypopituitarism
c. Sterility d. Cachexia

45. **The ability of the body to recognize, destroy and eliminate antigenic material**
a. Energy b. Immunity
c. Adaptation d. Resistance

46. **Water soluble vitamin.**
a. Vitamin A b. Vitamin B complex
c. Vitamin D d. Vitamin K

47. **Epidemiological triad comprises of**
a. Agent, host and disease
b. Agent, host and organism
c. Agent, host and environment
d. Agent, host and infection

48. **Name of the oral polio vaccine**
a. BCG b. TAB
c. Salk d. Sabin

49. **Age related cognitive decline may grow more significant by about age**
a. 60 b. 65
c. 70 d. 75

50. **Flattening of emotions refers to**
a. Anhedonia b. Associality
c. Blunted affect d. Regression

51. **Which of the following is a complication of prolonged bed rest?**
a. Jaundice b. Diarrhea
c. Kidney stone d. Fever

52. **Acetone in urine is tested by**
a. Hey's test b. Smith's test
c. Rothera's test d. Benedict's test

53. **Inner force that moves the individual to a certain action**
a. Motive b. Attitude
c. Behavior d. Mind

54. **The temperature for sponge bath**
a. 110°–115°F b. 100°–110°F
c. 90°–100°F d. 120°–125°F

55. **Dumping syndrome is a postoperative complication of**
a. Cholecystectomy b. Gastrostomy
c. Appendicectomy d. Gastrectomy

56. **A group of drug to treat extrapyramidal side effect is**
a. Antipsychotic drugs b. Antiparkinsonism drugs
c. Antidepressant drugs d. Anticonvulsants

57. **The best time for administration of diuretics is**
a. 9 am b. 1 pm
c. 4 pm d. 6 pm

58. **Inborn all round mental efficiency of an individual is called**
a. Emotion b. Intelligence
c. Behavior d. Drives

59. **The strongest joint in the human body**
a. Sacroiliac joint b. Symphysis pubis
c. Sacrococcygeal joint d. Sacrospinous joint

60. **The common complaint of a woman with IUD is**
a. Vaginal bleeding b. Pelvic infection
c. Uterine perforation d. Abdominal pain

61. **Condition in which the endometrial cells seeded outside the uterine cavity is**
a. Endometritis b. Fibroid
c. Procidentia d. Endometriosis

62. **For a patient with pulmonary edema, the oxygen flow rate should be at**
a. 2 L b. 6 L
c. 8 L d. 10 L

63. **Difficulty in getting off to sleep or in maintaining sleep is called**
a. Amnesia b. Insomnia
c. Narcolepsy d. Hypersomnia

64. **An elevated ASO titer is seen in which of the following conditions**
a. Nephrotic syndrome b. Rheumatic fever
c. Gastric ulcer d. Ulcerative colitis

65. **Genital anomalies in which the urethral opening is below its normal location on the glans of the penis is termed**
a. Epispadias b. Hypospadias
c. Chordee d. Phimosis

66. **Children with Tetralogy of Fallot assumes**
a. Squatting b. Fowler's
c. Sitting d. Legs down

67. **CSF is secreted by**
a. Cerebral aqueduct b. Arachnoid granulations
c. Choroid plexus d. Falx cerebri

68. **Do not suction the patient more than 10–15 seconds at a time after tracheostomy because there is the danger of**
a. Anoxia b. Hypoxia
c. Anorexia d. Ataxia

69. **A basic document for organizing family planning work is**
a. Family record b. Eligible couple register
c. MCH record d. Birth and death register

70. **Hypocalcemia causes**
a. Tetanus b. Tetany
c. Tinnitus d. Tenesmus

71. **A hereditary form of arthritis with an excess of uric acid in the blood occurs in**
a. Syringomyelia b. Still's disease
c. Gout d. Spondylitis

72. **Expected weight of a child at one year whose birth weight was 3 kg is**
a. 7 kg b. 9 kg
c. 10.5 kg d. 12 kg

73. **Accidental removal of a parathyroid gland during thyroidectomy would cause**
a. Myxedema
b. Tetany
c. Hypovolemic shock
d. Adrenocortical stimulation

74. **The client with gastric lavage or prolonged vomiting must be assessed for**
a. Acidosis
b. Alkalosis
c. Loss of oxygen from the blood
d. Loss of osmotic pressure of the blood

75. **Dysphasia is a defect that cause difficulty in**
a. Walk b. Speech
c. Swallowing d. Vision

76. **Goiter, hyperthyroidism and exophthalmos are characteristic symptoms of**
a. Grave's disease b. Thyroiditis
c. MNG d. Thyroid adenoma

77. **Repair of tympanic membrane is**
a. Tympanoplasty b. Myringoplasty
c. Myringotomy d. Septoplasty

78. **Primary effect of cold application**
a. Vasodilation b. Violation
c. Ventilation d. Vasoconstriction

79. **The best method of sterilizing gloves**
a. Boiling b. Drying
c. Soaking d. Steam under pressure

80. **The patient with liver cirrhosis and hepatic coma should be assessed for**
a. Icterus b. Urticaria
c. Uremic frost d. Hemangioma

81. **Pathological imitation of movements of one person by another person is**
a. Echopraxia b. Echolalia
c. Catalepsy d. Stupor

82. **Which of the following developmental milestone is expected from a 2-year-old child**
a. Uses a spoon to eat
b. Uses a cup to drink
c. Uses a knife for cutting food
d. Pour milk into a cup

83. **Worm that is transmitted through meat is**
a. Hookworm b. Tapeworm
c. Round worm d. Pinworm

84. **The nurse should position a client recovering from general anesthesia in a**
a. Supine position b. Side-lying position
c. High Fowler's position d. Trendelenburg position

85. **IUCDs are introduced postpartum at**
a. 4 weeks b. 6–8 weeks
c. 3 months d. 6 months

86. **A group of drug to treat extrapyramidal side effect is**
a. Antipsychotic drugs b. Antiparkinsonism drugs
c. Antidepressant drugs d. Anticonvulsants

87. **The strongest joint in the human body**
a. Sacroiliac joint b. Symphysis pubis
c. Sacrococcygeal joint d. Sacrospinous joint

88. **What is the compression-ventilation ratio for one rescuer CPR?**
a. 4:2 b. 5:1
c. 5:2 d. 15:2

89. **Genital anomalies in which the urethral opening is below its normal location on the glans of the penis is termed**
   a. Epispadias b. Hypospadias
   c. Chordee d. Phimosis

90. **Normal hemoglobin level**
   a. 4–8 g% b. 1–5 g%
   b. 15–25 g% d. 10–14 g%

91. **An elevated ASO titer is seen in which of the following conditions**
   a. Nephrotic syndrome b. Rheumatic fever
   c. Gastric ulcer d. Ulcerative colitis

92. **The amount of blood ejected per minute by rhythmic ventricular contraction**
   a. Cardiac output b. Tidal volume
   c. Vital capacity d. Stroke volume

93. **Pigeon chest is seen in**
   a. Osteoporosis b. Ricketts
   c. Osteosarcoma d. Costochondritis

94. **The common complaint of a woman with IUD is**
   a. Vaginal bleeding b. Pelvic infection
   c. Uterine perforation d. Abdominal pain

95. **Physical examination using a stethoscope**
   a. Auscultation b. Percussion
   c. Palpation d. Vibration

96. **Do not suction the patient more than 10–15 seconds at a time after tracheostomy because there is the danger of**
   a. Anoxia b. Hypoxia
   c. Anorexia d. Ataxia

97. **The client with gastric lavage or prolonged vomiting must be assessed for**
   a. Acidosis b. Alkalosis
   c. Loss of oxygen from the blood
   d. Loss of osmotic pressure of the blood

98. **Dysphasia is a defect that cause difficulty in**
   a. Walk b. Speech
   c. Swallowing d. Vision

99. **The drug of choice in controlling convulsions in eclamptic seizures**
   a. Diazepam b. Phenobarbitone
   c. Eptoin sodium d. Sodium valproate

100. **Trendelenburg's test is simple non-invasive diagnostic tool to assess**
   a. Varicose veins b. TAO
   c. Raynaud's disease d. Thrombophlebitis

ANSWER KEY

1. d	2. d	3. c	4. a	5. c	6. a	7. a	8. c	9. c	10. c	11. d	12. d
13. a	14. c	15. b	16. d	17. c	18. b	19. a	20. d	21. c	22. a	23. a	24. a
25. c	26. b	27. d	28. b	29. b	30. a	31. b	32. b	33. b	34. a	35. b	36. b
37. b	38. d	39. c	40. a	41. d	42. c	43. b	44. c	45. b	46. b	47. c	48. d
49. d	50. c	51. c	52. c	53. a	54. a	55. d	56. b	57. a	58. b	59. a	60. a
61. d	62. a	63. b	64. b	65. b	66. a	67. c	68. b	69. b	70. b	71. c	72. b
73. b	74. b	75. b	76. a	77. a	78. d	79. d	80. a	81. a	82. b	83. b	84. b
85. b	86. b	87. a	88. d	89. b	90. d	91. b	92. a	93. b	94. a	95. a	96. b
97. b	98. b	99. a	100. a								

MODEL QUESTION PAPER IV

1. **Paul-Bunnell test is used to diagnose**
   a. Cytomegalo virus infection
   b. Infectious mononucleosis
   c. Herpes simplex infection
   d. Ca cervix

2. **A sesamoid bone**
   a. Femur b. Radius
   c. Fibula d. Carpal bone

3. **The waste product of ammonia metabolism**
   a. Urea b. Protein
   c. Amino acid d. Fatty acid

4. **Epinephrine is secreted by the**
   a. Adrenal medulla b. Adrenal cortex
   c. Posterior pituitary d. Anterior pituitary

5. **Hormone responsible for ovulation**
   a. FSH b. LH
   c. Estrogen d. Progesterone

6. **Inflammation of a joint**
   a. Adenitis b. Bursitis
   c. Arthritis d. Osteoporosis

7. **1 g of fat provides**
   a. 4 calories b. 6 calories
   c. 7 calories d. 9 calories

8. **Branch of medicine dealing with the problems of the aged and the disease of the elderly**
   a. Gerontology b. Geriatrics
   c. Pediatrics d. Psychology

9. **Semisolid preparation of a drug**
   a. Ointment b. Liniment
   c. Lotion d. Powder

10. **Drugs that contract pupil of the eye is called**
    a. Miotic b. Mydriatics
    c. Lozenges d. Demulcents

11. **Lifespan of RBC is**
    a. 80 days b. 90 days
    c. 120 days d. 130 days

12. **Position used for dyspneic patients**
    a. Dorsal recumbent position
    b. Left lateral position
    c. Orthopneic position
    d. Sim's position

13. **Normal serum sodium level**
    a. 120–126 mEq/L b. 135–145 mEq/L
    c. 145–150 mEq/L d. 150–160 mEq/L

14. **Vomiting center is located in**
    a. Cerebrum b. Cerebellum
    c. Thalamus d. Medulla

15. **Instrument used to measure joint ROM**
    a. Stadiometer b. Goniometer
    c. Pelvimeter d. Hemoglobinometer

16. **Amount of blood ejected by ventricle per minute**
    a. Stroke volume b. Cardiac output
    c. Vital capacity d. FEV1

17. **Drugs that reduce blood glucose level is called**
    a. Hyperglycemics b. Hypoglycemics
    c. Antihypertensives d. Cardiac glycosides

18. **Minimum score in GCS scale**
    a. 1 b. 2
    c. 3 d. 4

19. **The length of thermometer that should be inserted to rectum to take rectal temperature**
    a. 1 inch b. 1.5 inches
    c. 2 inches d. 2.5 inches

20. **Inflammation of the tongue**
    a. Mastitis b. Mastoiditis
    c. Stomatitis d. Glossitis

21. **The radiological study of bile duct**
    a. Cholecystogram b. Cholangiogram
    c. Pancreaticodeodenoscopyd. Endoscopy

22. **BMI is assessed by**
    a. Wt in kg / Ht in m_2 b. Wt in Kg/ Ht in cm_2
    c. Wt in Lb/Ht in m_2 d. Wt in Lb/ Ht in feet

23. **Telescoping of the bowel**
    a. Megacolon b. Intussusception
    c. Diverticulum d. Borborygmi

24. **Irrigation of the stomach**
    a. Gastric lavage b. Gastric gavage
    c. Jejunostomy d. Gastrostomy

25. **Clay colored stools are characteristic of**
    a. Food poisoning b. Enteritis
    c. Obstructive jaundice d. Gastric bleeding

26. **Apoptosis means**
    a. Neoadjuvant chemotherapy
    b. Programmed cell death
    c. Teletherapy
    d. Excision biopsy

27. **Cancer of pigmented skin cells**
    a. Myeloma b. Lymphoma
    c. Melanoma d. Seminoma

28. **Indian Red Cross Society was established in**
    a. 1910 b. 1920
    c. 1925 d. 1936

29. **Cyanocobalamine is**
    a. Vitamin B_1 b. Vitamin B_2
    c. Vitamin B_6 d. Vitamin B_{12}

30. **Fear of animals**
    a. Pedophobia b. Nectophobia
    c. Agoraphobia d. Zoophobia

31. **Increased sweating is termed as**
    a. Diuresis b. Diarrhea
    c. Diaphoresis d. Ptyalism

32. **1 ounce is equal to**
    a. 20 mL b. 30 mL
    c. 50 mL d. 60 mL

33. **Occupational disease due to inhalation of sugar cane dust**
    a. Byssinosis b. Bagassosis
    c. Anthracosis d. Silicosis

34. **Difficulty in performing voluntary movements**
    a. Dyslalia b. Dysthymia
    c. Dyskinesia d. Dyspepsia

35. **Lower motor neuron facial paralysis**
    a. Bell's palsy b. Erb's palsy
    c. Trigeminal neuralgia d. Opisthotonus

36. **The most common cause of amenorrhea**
    a. Fibroid uterus b. OCP use
    c. DUB d. Pregnancy

37. **Amount of calcium in one liter of milk**
    a. 500 mg b. 1 g
    c. 1500 mg d. 2 g

38. **Oral thrush is caused by**
    a. Treponema pallidum b. Candida albicans
    c. Staph aureus d. Chlamydia trachomatis

39. **The term dementia praecox was coined by**
    a. Sigmund Freud b. Eugin Bleuler
    c. Kraepelin d. Leon Festinger

40. **Professional negligence also known as**
    a. Maloccurrence b. Malpractice
    c. Torticollis d. Euthanasia

41. **The "four A's" of schizophrenia diagnosis includes all, except**
    a. Associational loosening
    b. Ambivalence
    c. Autism
    d. Affect appropriateness

42. **Bone age is less than chronological age in all, except**
    a. Malnutrition b. Chondrodystrophies
    c. Hypopituitarism d. Hypoaldosteronism

43. **Omega sign is noticed in patients with**
    a. OCD b. Depression
    c. Schizophrenia d. Dementia

44. **The most frequent complication arising from hyperviscosity of polycythemia is**
    a. Leukemia b. Pulmonary fibrosis
    c. Thrombosis d. Cardiomyopathy

45. **Wernicke's encephalopathy is attributed to**
    a. Severe riboflavin deficiency
    b. Excessive blood alcohol content
    c. Severe thiamine deficiency
    d. Excessive GGT levels

46. **Name the operation recommended to correct tricuspid atresia**
    a. Fontan procedure
    b. Blalock-Taussig operation
    c. Ramsted's surgery
    d. Patch closure

47. The following is the most frequent site of internal bleeding associated with hemophilia

a. GI tract b. Brain tissue
c. Spinal cord d. Joint cavities

48. Mittelschmerz is pain associated with

a. Sexual intercourse b. Defecation
c. Vomiting d. Ovulation

49. During the first trimester of pregnancy, the source of elevated estrogen and progesterone is

a. Maternal ovaries b. Corpus luteum
c. Fetal adrenal glands d. Fetal liver

50. The following problem does not typically result from uncontrolled gestational diabetes mellitus

a. Insufficient amniotic fluid
b. Maternal hypoglycemia
c. Maternal hypertension
d. Fetal demise

51. The natural hormone produced by the pineal gland that induces sleep

a. Melanin b. Amphetamine
c. Melatonin d. Adrenaline

52. X-ray study of bile duct

a. Cholecystography b. Cholangiography
c. Cholecystectomy d. Barium enema

53. Night blindness occurs due to the deficiency of

a. Vitamin B_2 b. Vitamin B_6
c. Vitamin A d. Vitamin C

54. Drinking water should have hardness at the range of

a. 100–150 mg/L b. 200–250 mg/L
c. 300–350 mg/L d. 325–400 mg/L

55. Incubation period of cholera

a. up to 5 days b. 5–15 days
c. 15–20 days d. more than 20 days

56. Tobacco juice color of meconium is seen in

a. IUGR b. IUD
c. Fetal distress d. Rh-incompatibility

57. Mark left on the skin after healing is called

a. Keloid b. Scar
c. Wound d. Abrasion

58. Cervical secretions are

a. Acidic b. Neutral
c. Alkaline d. None of the above

59. Medicines introduced into the subcutaneous tissue is called

a. Intramuscular b. Intravenous
c. Intradermal d. Hypodermal

60. Normal platelet count

a. 1.5–4 lakhs per mm^3 b. 5–7 lakhs per mm^3
c. 10–12 lakhs per mm^3 d. 12–15 lakhs per mm^3

61. Time required to read Mantoux test

a. 12–24 hours b. 24–48 hours
c. 48–72 hours d. More than 72 hours

62. Humoral immunity is transmitted through

a. T cells b. B cells
c. Alpha cells d. Beta cells

63. Weil's disease is transmitted through

a. Algae b. Fungi
c. Spirochetes d. Yersinia pestis

64. Inflammation of urinary bladder

a. Cystitis b. Cystoscopy
c. Urethritis d. Ureteritis

65. Which of the following medication may be suspected as a possible cause of bronchial asthma?

a. Acetylsalicylic acid (aspirin)
b. Milk of magnesia
c. Famotidine
d. Diphenhydramine

66. Penicillinase-resistant penicillins include

a. Benzylpenicillin b. Phenoxymethylpenicillin
c. Cloxacillin d. Ampicillin

67. Quickening means

a. Hearing of the fetal heart sound
b. Sudden cessation of menstruation
c. The movement of the fetus in the uterus felt by the mother
d. Nausea and vomiting in the morning

68. The diseases notifiable to the WHO under the International Regulation Act are all except

a. Cholera b. Plague
c. Yellow fever d. Diphtheria

69. Fear of strangers

a. Arachnophobia b. Acrophobia
c. Xenophobia d. Claustrophobia

70. **The longest vein in the body**
a. SVC b. Long saphenous vein
c. Short saphenous vein d. IVC

71. **RNTCP is started on**
a. 1990 b. 1991
c. 1992 d. 1993

72. **Modifiable risk factors in case of hypertension include all, except**
a. Age b. Obesity
c. Salt intake d. Alcohol intake

73. **Measles vaccine is given under the National Immunization Program**
a. 6 weeks b. 6 months
c. 9 months d. 18 months

74. **FIGLU test is used to detect**
a. Vitamin B_{12} deficiency b. Vitamin A intoxication
c. Niacin acid deficiency d. Folic acid deficiency

75. **Frankel's line in the X-ray is seen in**
a. Congenital syphilis b. Scurvy
c. Rickets d. None of the above

76. **Coracoid process is on**
a. Pelvic girdle b. Humerus
c. Scapula d. Femur

77. **The bones that participate in the formation of the anterior cranial fossa are all the following, except**
a. Temporal bone
b. Sphenoid bone
c. Ethmoid bone
d. Orbital part of the frontal bone

78. **Ziehl-Neelsen staining is used to diagnose**
a. Methicillin-resistant Staphylococcus aureus (MRSA) infection
b. Clostridium perfringens infection
c. Acid-fast tubercle bacilli infection
d. Neisseria meningitidis infection

79. **Asthmatic attacks can be precipitated by**
a. Sympathomimetics
b. Digitalis glycosides
c. Aminoglycoside antibiotics
d. Beta-adrenoceptor blockers

80. **Glucose-6-phosphate dehydrogenase (G6PD) activity is important to the integrity of the**
a. Platelets b. White blood cells
c. Red blood cells d. Mast cells

81. **Physical signs indicative of poor nutrition are all, except**
a. Spongy, bleed easily, marginal redness, recession gums
b. Dental caries, mottled appearance (fluorosis), malpositioned
c. Brittle, depigmented, easily plucked; thin and sparse hair
d. Tongue—deep red in appearance; surface papillae present

82. **The term used for normal respiratory rhythm and depth**
a. Eupnea b. Apnea
c. Bradypnea d. Tachypnea

83. **The term used for a high-pitched musical sound in clients during a respiratory assessment?**
a. Sigh b. Stridor
c. Crowing d. Wheezing

84. **When recording blood pressure, the sounds which can be heard with a stethoscope placed over the artery is termed as**
a. Wheeze b. Murmurs
c. Crackle sounds d. Korotkoff sounds

85. **Number of births divided by total population including men, women and children (1000s) is**
a. Crude birth rate
b. General fertility rate
c. Age-specific fertility rates
d. Total period fertility rate

86. **A hypothesis which a researcher tries to disprove is**
a. Positive hypothesis b. Research hypothesis
c. Null hypothesis d. Alternate hypothesis

87. **Electroencephalogram (EEG) rhythm** was first recorded by
a. Gaillard L b. William Einthovan
c. Egas Moniz d. Hans Berger

88. **Gingival hyperplasia is associated with use of**
a. Phenylephidrine b. Phenytoin
c. Carbamazepine d. Phenhydramine

89. The characteristic EEG findings in seizure disorders is

a. Slow waves
b. Spikes, sharp waves
c. Alpha rhythm
d. Asynchronous EEG rhythm

90. Amount of solution used for evacuant enema

a. 250–500 mL b. 100–200 mL
c. 500–1000 mL d. 50–100 mL

91. Which is a specific investigation of diagnosing seizure disorder?

a. EMG b. EEG
c. EOG d. ECT

92. Classification of glaucoma includes all, except

a. Wide angle b. Closed angle
c. Open angle d. Congenital

93. Digoxin causes

a. Scotoma b. Optic neuritis
c. Retinal pigmentation d. Blue vision

94. Which of the following NSAIDs is a propionic acid derivative

a. Indomethacin b. Ibuprofen
c. Mephanamic acid d. Diclofenac

95. Therapeutic serum drug level of theophylline is

a. 0.8 to 2 ng/mL b. 0.8 to 1.2 mEq/dL
c. 5 to 20 µg/mL d. 50 to 100 µg/mL

96. Which microorganism is associated with cervical cancer?

a. Pneumocystis carinii b. Human papiloma virus
c. Mycobacterium avium d. Cytomegalovirus

97. HIV is a

a. Retrovirus b. Rotavirus
c. Arbovirus d. Papilomavirus

98. Giardiasis, an opportunistic infection in AIDS patients, is a

a. Bacterial infection b. Parasitic infection
c. Fungal infection d. Viral infection

99. Glisson's capsule is associated with

a. Kidney b. Lung
c. Liver d. Pancreas

100. Number of milk teeth in a toddler

a. 10 b. 20
c. 30 d. 32

ANSWER KEY

1. b	2. d	3. a	4. a	5. b	6. c	7. d	8. b	9. a	10. a	11. c	12. c
13. b	14. d	15. b	16. b	17. b	18. c	19. b	20. d	21. b	22. a	23. b	24. a
25. c	26. b	27. c	28. b	29. d	30. d	31. c	32. b	33. b	34. c	35. a	36. d
37. b	38. b	39. c	40. b	41. d	42. b	43. b	44. c	45. c	46. a	47. d	48. d
49. b	50. c	51. c	52. b	53. c	54. b	55. a	56. b	57. b	58. c	59. d	60. a
61. c	62. b	63. c	64. a	65. a	66. c	67. c	68. a	69. c	70. b	71. c	72. a
73. c	74. a	75. c	76. c	77. a	78. c	79. d	80. c	81. d	82. a	83. d	84. d
85. a	86. c	87. d	88. b	89. b	90. c	91. b	92. a	93. d	94. b	95. c	96. b
97. a	98. b	99. c	100. b								

Index

Page numbers followed by *f* refer to figure

A

Abdominal
- bloating 220
- pain 229
- scar following hysterectomy 228
- wall 69

Abdominoperineal resection 57
Abduction 69
Abnormal
- menstrual bleeding 221
- volume of pulse 84

Abnormalities of placenta and cord 203
Abortion 200, 216
Abruptio placenta 201
Acetazolamide 21
Acetic acid 81
Acid
- base imbalances 8
- fast bacilli 81

Acquired immunodeficiency syndrome 175, 219
- related complex 219

Acute
- closed angle glaucoma 20
- glomerulonephritis 144
- gonorrhea 217
- hepatitis 175
- pain 4
- renal failure 64
- respiratory infection 161
- spasmodic laryngitis 143

Acyanotic heart defects 139
Adduction 69
Adenohypophysis 147
Adrenal
- arteries 27
- cortex 73
- genital syndrome 232
- medulla 73

Adrenocorticotropic hormone 147
Adrenogenital syndrome 233
Aggregation of platelets 27
Agoraphobia 106
Air pollution 164
Akinetic seizures 136
Alanine 263
Alcohol
- abuse 102
- addictions 102

Alcoholics anonymous 103
Alpha adrenergic receptor blocker 32
Alprazolam 96
Alzheimer's disease 102
Amenorrhea 195, 196, 217
Aminoglycosides 4
Amitriptyline hydrochloride 97
Ammonia 261
Ammonium sulphate 81
Anaerobic exercise 86
Androblastoma 227
Androgen insensitivity syndrome 233
Anemia 132, 141, 161, 230
- during pregnancy 204

Angina pectoris 30
Angioplasty 30
Angiotensin converting enzyme inhibitor 32
Anopheles mosquito 164
Anorexia 86, 135, 217
- nervosa 99

Antepartum hemorrhage 201
Antianginal drugs 33
Antiarrhythmic drugs 35
Anticholinesterase drugs 18
Antidepressants 97
Antidiuresis 73
Antidiuretic hormone 5, 97
Antifungal drugs 4
Antihypertensive therapy 32
Antimicrobial drugs 3
Anti-retroviral therapy 175, 219
Antisocial personality disorder 108
Antitubercular drugs 4
Anuria 217
Anxiety disorder 106
Aortic stenosis 140
Arteries 27
Ascariasis 174
Ascites 58
Ascorbic acid 250, 261
Asepsis 1, 78
Aspartate 263
Aspermia 224
Asphyxia
- livida 131
- neonatorum 131
- pallida 131

Assisted reproductive technology 224
Asthenospermia 224
Ataxia 137
Atelectasis 45
Athetosis 137
Atrial
- fibrillation 31
- septal defect 139

Atrophy of muscles 85
Atropine sulfate 34
Attention defect hyperactivity disorder 98
Augmentation of labor 204
Autistic disorder 98
Autoclaving 2
Autonomic nervous system 13-15
Autosomal recessive disorder 232
Azoospermia 224

B

Bacterial infectious disease 44
Barbiturate sedatives 97
Barlow's
- sign 145
- test 145

Barriers of communication 77
Bartholin's ducts 216
Basal
- ganglia 14
- metabolism 132

Bell's palsy 19
Benedict's
 solution 81
 test 81
Benign
 lesions of ovary 226
 prostatic hypertrophy 65
Benzalkalonium chloride 2
Beta adrenergic blocker 32
Bhore committee 179
Biceps
 brachii 69
 femoris 69
Bigeminal pulse 84
Bilateral
 tubal ligation 205
 vasectomy 205
Biliary system 53
Bilirubin 261
Bishop's score 204
Bitot's spots 248
Bleeding gums 82
Blindness 137
Blood
 cells 25
 circulation 27
 clotting process 27
 coagulation 27
 components 25
 groups 26
 isolation 3
 parameters 200
 pressure 9, 85
 test reference range chart 261
 urea nitrogen 263
 vessels 27
 volume 261
Bluish discoloration of
 cervix 195
 vagina 195
Body dysmorphic disorder 107
Boggy uterus 202
Bones 68, 145
 of body 68
Bony pelvis 197
Borderline personality disorder 109
Bordetella pertussis 171
Bottle mouth syndrome 82
Bounding pulse 84
Bowel surgery 57
Brachialis 69
Brachioradialis 69
Brain 13
 abscess 19
Brainstem 14
Branches of
 carotid artery 28*f*
 common iliac arteries 28*f*
Breast 235
 changes 196
 tenderness 220
Broad ligament 212
Bronchial asthma 44, 143
Bronchiectasis 44
Bronchitis 44
Bronchopulmonary dysplasia 131
Brudzinski's sign 18
Brush field's spots 133
Buerger's disease 33
Bulimia nervosa 99

C

Cachexia 230
Cancer of
 colon/rectum 56
 esophagus 54
 larynx 46
 pancreas 60
 stomach 56
Cancrum oris 82
Candida albicans 218
Captopril 32
Carbohydrates 8, 247
Carbon dioxide pressure 261
Carcinoma cervix 221, 229
Cardiac
 catheterization 25
 enzymes 24
 glycosides 33
 stimulants 34
 tamponade 32
Cardiovascular system 86
Carditis 141
Cataract 20
Causes of
 acyclic bleeding 221
 hardness 163
 infertility 223
 intermenstrual bleeding 221
 pain 220
Cavity of uterus 211
Cecostomy 57
Celomic metaplasia 229
Central
 nervous system 13, 94
 venous pressure 25
Cephalosporins 3
Cerebellum 14
Cerebral palsy 137
Cerebrospinal fluid 14
Cerebrovascular accident 17
Cervical
 cysts 225
 defense 215
 endometriosis 221
 erosion 224
 eversion 225
 intraepithelial neoplasia 229
 tear 225
Cervix 211
Chadha committee 179
Chadwick's sign 195, 196
Chancroid 175, 218
Cheilosis 82
Chemotherapy 54
Chest
 drainage systems 45
 pain 172
 trauma 44
 wall 69
Cheyne-Stokes' respiration 85
Chickenpox 169
Child
 health nursing 130
 survival and safe motherhood 161, 162
Chlamydia trachomatis 216, 218
Chlordiazepoxide hydrochloride 96
Chlorpromezine hydrochloride 96
Chlorprothixene 96
Cholecystitis 59
Cholelithiasis 59
Cholera 173
Cholesterol synthesis 36
Chorionic somatomammotrophin 195
Chronic
 closed angle glaucoma 20
 hepatitis 175
 liver disease 173
 obstructive pulmonary disease 44
 open angle glaucoma 20
 pain 4
 pelvic pain 217
 renal failure 64
Circle of Willis 28
Circulatory system 198
Cirrhosis of liver 58
Clamping chest tube 46
Classification of
 disinfectants 169
 enema 86
 fats 246
 foods 245
 immunity 166
 ovarian tumor 227

shock 8
vitamins 248
Cleavage 194
Cleft
lip 133
palate 133
Clitoris 210
Clomiphene induced cycles 224
Clorazepate dipotassium 96
Clostridium botulinum 174
Clubfoot 146
Coarctation of aorta 140
Coitus interruptus 205
Cold
application 87
chain 168
Collapsing pulse 84
Colonization 1
Combined vaccines 167
Common
electrolytes 6
pulse sites 84
sites of pressure sores 82
tests of urine 81
Communicable disease 161, 166
Community health nursing 160
Complete
abortion 200
blood cell count 261
perineal tear 232
stroke 17
Complication of benign ovarian tumors 228
Composition of human body 245
Concurrent disinfection 2, 169
Conduct disorders 99
Conduction system of heart 24
Condyloma acuminata 175, 218
Confirmation of pregnancy 196
Congenital
adrenal hyperplasia 232
aganglionic megacolon 134
dislocation of hip 145
heart defects 139
hypothyroidism 147
Congestive cardiac failure 31, 139, 203
Conjunctivitis 137
Consequences of population growths 176
Constituents of
food 245
urine 80
Contents of broad ligament 213
Continent ileostomy 57
Continuous
ambulatory peritoneal dialysis 65
fever 172
Contraceptive methods 176, 205
Control of infectious diseases 168
Conversion disorder 107
Coronary
angiography 25
artery 24
bypass graft 30
disease 29
Corpus
callosum 14
luteum cyst 226
Correlation of dysplasia and CIN 229
Corrigan's pulse 84
Corynebacterium diphtheriae 170
Covering of blood vessels 27
Crab louse 218
Cranial nerves 15
Crippling disease 161
Crohn's disease 232
Cross infection 1
Culex mosquito 164
Cutaneous ureterostomy 64
Cyanotic heart defects 139, 140
Cystecomy removal of urinary bladder 64
Cystitis 63

D

Deafness 138
Decubitus ulcer 82, 221
Deep
tendon reflexes 20
vein thrombosis 86
Defense of
genital tract 215
vagina 215
Deficiency of
niacin 250
riboflavin 250
Degrees of retroversion 222
Delayed puberty 214
Delirium 101
Dementia of Alzheimers 102
Dengue fever 164
Dental
caries 82
plaque 82
Deodorant 168
Depression 220
Depressive episode 105
Depth of respiration 84
Dermoid cyst 228
Development of embryo 194
Diabetes mellitus 147
Diaphoresis 30
Diaphragm 69, 205
Diarrhea 132
Diarrheal diseases 161
Diazepam 96
Diencephalon 14
Dietary sources of vitamin 248, 249
Digestive system 198
Digitalis 9, 35
Digoxin 33
Diphtheria 170, 171
Dipyridamole 34
Direct
acting vasodilators 32, 34
observed treatment, short course 172
Diseases and disorders of
cardiovascular system 24
central nervous system 13
endocrine system 73
gastrointestinal system 53
genitourinary system 63
musculoskeletal system 68
respiratory system 43
Diseases
cycle 165
transmission 166
Disinfection 2, 3, 78, 168
of wells 163
Disorders of gonadal development 233
Displacement of uterus 222
Disruptive behavior disorders 98
Disseminated intravascular coagulation 200
Distribution of total body water 5
Dobutamine 9
Doderlein's bacillus 215
Donovania granulomatis 218
Dopamine 9
Double-barrelled colostomy 57
Down's syndrome 102, 133
Doxepin hydrochloride 97
Droplet infection 2
Drug 20
in emotional disorders 96
in shock 9
used in induction of ovulation 224
Dry heat 2
sterilization 78
Ductus
arteriosus 139
venosum 138
Duhamel's surgery 135
Dumping syndrome 56
Duodenal ulcer 55
Dust diseases 177
Dysfunctional uterine bleeding 221
Dysgerminoma 228

Dysmenorrhea 219, 229
Dyspareunia 220, 229
Dyspnea 30, 31
Dysrhythmias 30

E

Eating disorders 99
Echocardiogram 25
Eclampsia 200
Ectopic pregnancy 201
Electrocardiogram 25
Electrolytes 6
Elimination disorders 100
Elongation of cervix 225
Embryonic period 194
Emphysema 44
Enalapril 32
Encephalitis 18
Endemic goitre 161
Endometrial
- carcinoma 221
- cyst 227
- sinus tumor 228

Endometrioid tumors 227
Endometriosis 228
Endometriotic cysts 225
Endotoxic shock 217
Enema 86
Enlarged placenta 132
Enlargement of uterus 196
Enteric
- fever 161, 174
- isolation 3

Environmental
- health 162
- sanitation 161, 162

Epidemiology of disease 164
Epididymitis 65
Epimenorrhea 221
Epinephrine 21
Episiotomy 205
Episode excessive drinking 102
Epithelial tumor 227
Erythema marginatum 141
Erythroblastosis foetalis 131
Erythrocyte sedimentation rate 261
Erythropoiesis 132
Esophageal varices 54
Esophagojejunostomy 56
Esophagus 53
Essential fatty acids 247
Ethambutol 4
Ethyl alcohol 2
Ethylene oxide 2
Excoriation 86
Excretory system 199
Exomphalus 134
Expiratory reserve volume 43
External
- ear 16*f*
- genitalia 210
- rotation of head 197

Extracellular fluid 5, 7

F

Fallopian tubes 211
Family
- planning 176
- welfare 176

Fascia 212
Fat soluble vitamins 248
Fatigue 196
Febrile seizures 136
Fecal vomiting 135
Feelings of worthlessness 105
Fertility rate 178
Fertilization 194
Fetal circulation 194
Fever 83, 134
Fibrin 27
Fibroid 225
Fibroma 227
FIGO staging of carcinoma cervix 230, 231
Filaria 161
First generation cephalosporins 3
Fish liver oils 248
Flail chest 45
Flexion 69
Fluid and electrolyte balance 5
Fluorosis 161
Fluoxetine hydrochloride 97
Folic acid 250
Follicle stimulating hormone 193, 213
Follicular cyst 226
Food
- and Agricultural Organization 181
- poisoning 174

Foot drop 85
Foramen ovale 138
Forced expiratory volume 43
Formation of
- gametes 194
- RBCs and granulocytes 26*f*

Fractures 70
Fredet-Ramstedt surgery 134
Frequency of micturition 229
Frequent periods of apnea 132
Fresh blood transfusion 54
Fumigation 78
Functional cysts 226
Functions of
- fats 247
- food 245
- pelvic floor 212
- proteins 246

G

Gastrectomy 56
Gastric
- surgery 55
- ulcers 55

Gastritis 55
Gastrocnemius 69
Gastroduodenostomy 56
Gastrointestinal system 195
Gastrojejunostomy 56
Gate control theory 4
Genital
- fistula 231
- herpes 175, 218
- prolapse 222
- tuberculosis 217

Genitourinary system 86
Germ cell tumor 228
German measles 170
Gestational diabetes 203
Gigantism 73
Glaucoma 20
Glomerular filtration rate 132
Glomerulonephritis 63
Glossitis 82
Gonadal dysgenesis 133, 233
Gonadoblastoma 228
Gonadotropic
- hormones 194
- releasing hormone 213

Gonorrhea 175
Goodell's sign 195, 196
Gout 70
Granuloma inguinale 175, 218
Granulosa cell tumors 227
Growth hormone 73, 1943
- releasing hormone 213

Guillain Barre syndrome 20
Gynandroblastoma 227

H

Habitual excessive drinking 102
Haemophilus
- *ducreyi* 175, 218
- *vaginalis* 218

Halitosis 82
Hamstring group 69
Hardness of water 163
Hay's test 81
Hazards of diabetes during pregnancy 203
Headache 220
Health
- education 178
- hazards 235

problems of India 161
promotion of workers 176
statistics 177
Heart 24
disease in pregnancy 203
rate 132
Heat
sterilization 2
test 81
Hegar's sign 195, 196
HELLP syndrome 200
Helmenthiasis 161
Hemodialysis 65
Hemoglobin 262
Hemolytic disease of newborn 131
Hemophilia
A 142
B 142
C 142
Hemoptysis 172
Hemorrhage 230
Hemorrhagic fever 164
Hemorrhoidectomy 57
Hemostasis 27
Hemothorax 45
Heparin sodium 34
Hepatic
artery 27
encephalopathy 59
Hepatitis 58
A 58, 173
B 58, 173
virus 173, 175, 218
C 58, 173
virus 173
E 163, 173
virus 173
Hepatolenticular disease 101
Herpes
genitalis 218
simplex virus 175, 218, 229
Hiatus hernia 55
High density lipids 25
Hirschsprung's disease 134
Histrionic personality disorder 109
Hormone 73
regulation 73
replacement therapy 235
Hospital acquired infection 2, 175
Hot
air oven 2
and cold applications 87
Human
chorionic gonadotropin 194
gammaglobulin 167, 218, 219
immunodeficiency virus 219
papillomavirus 175, 218
infection 229
placental lactogen 194
Hydatidiform mole 201
Hydralazine 32
Hydrogen peroxide 2
Hydronephrosis 145, 230
Hydrophobia 174
Hydroxyzine hydrochloride 96
Hyoid bone 68
Hyperbilirubinemia 131
Hypercalcemia 7, 73
Hyperkalemia 7, 73
Hypernatremia 7, 73
Hypersecretion of growth hormone 148
Hypersomnia 105
Hypertension 32
Hypertonicity 2
Hypocalcemia 7, 73
Hypochondriasis 107
Hypoglycemia 132
Hypokalemia 7, 73
Hypomenorrhea 221
Hypomotility and constipation 86
Hyponatremia 7, 73
Hypoplastic left heart syndrome 140
Hypostatic pneumonia 86
Hypothalamic pituitary ovarian axis 214
Hypothalamus 14, 213

I

Idiopathic thrompocytopenic purpura 142
Ileostomy 57
Iliopsoas 69
Imipramine hydrochloride 97
Imperforate anus 135
Implantation 88, 194
Importance of
perineum 212
water 162
Incompetent cervix 201
Incomplete abortion 200
Incubation period 1, 165, 166
Inevitable abortion 200
Infant mortality rate 177
Infection
chain 1, 1*f*
control 1
Infection of neighboring structures 82
Infertility 217, 223, 229
Infundibulopelvic ligament 212
Insipidus 73
Insomnia 105, 220
Inspiratory capacity 43
Instillation 88
Integumentary system 85, 199
Interaction of circulatory system 6
Internal genital organs 210
International Council of Nursing 77
Intestinal obstruction 134
Intracellular fluid 5
Intracranial pressure 16
Intracystic hemorrhage 228
Intrauterine devices 205
Intussusception 134
Invasive carcinoma 230
Iodine solution 81
Iris 15
Iron
deficiency anemia 141
sorbitol-citric acid complex 204
Islets of Langerhans 73
Isokinetic exercise 86
Isolation 2, 166
Isometric exercise 86
Isoniazid 4
Isopropyl alcohol 2
Isoproterenol 9, 34
Isotonic exercise 86
Isthmus 211

J

Jacquemier's sign 195, 196
Jaundice 132
Joints 68
Jones' criteria 141

K

Kaposi's sarcoma 219
Kartar Singh committee 179
Keratomalacia 248
Kernig's sign 18
Klinefelter's syndrome 133, 234
Kock's pouch 57
Kupffer cells 53
Kyphosis 85

L

Lactate 262
Lactic
acid 262
dehydrogenase 262
Lamivudine 219
Large intestine 53
Latissimus dorsi 69
Layers of
fallopian tube 211
ovary 212
uterus 211
Leprosy 161
Leukorrhea 195

Level of consciousness 9
Lidocaine 35
Life threatening complication of fibroids 226
Liquor ammonia 81
Liver function tests 262
Loop colostomy 57
Lordosis 85
Loss of muscle tone 235
Low
- density lipids 25
- grade fever 132

Lower
- arm flexion 69
- respiratory tract 43

Lung volumes 43
Lutein cyst 227
Luteinizing hormone-releasing hormone 213
Lymph
- nodes 29
- vessels 29

Lymphatic
- system 29
- theory 229

Lymphogranuloma venereum 218

M

Malaria 161, 164
- action program 161

Male reproductive system 63
Malignant ovarian tumor 230
Management of intersex 234
Manipulation 80
Maternal mortality rate 178
Mean corpuscular
- hemoglobin 262
- volume 262

Measles 169, 170
Medical
- asepsis 78
- supervision during pregnancy 196
- surgical nursing 1
- termination of pregnancy 206

Meig's syndrome 228
Melanocyte stimulating hormone 213
Meniere's disease 21
Meninges 14
Meningitis 18, 161
Meningocele 136
Meningococcal meningitis 172
Meningomyelocele 136
Menometrorrhagia 221
Menopause 206, 234
Menorrhagia 217, 220, 221, 229
Menstrual
- cycle 193
- extraction 206
- regulation 206

Menstruation 193, 235
Mental
- health nursing 94
- retardation 98

Mesometrium 213
Mesonephroid Brenner tumor 227
Mesosalpinx 213
Metabolic
- acidosis 8
- alkalosis 8

Method of
- collecting sputum specimen 81
- group teaching 179

Metrorrhagia 221
Milky white appearance of pupil 20*f*
Missed abortion 200
Mittelschmerz's syndrome 220
Mixed
- epithelial tumors 227
- gonadal dysgenesis 233

Mode of
- infection 216
- spread 230, 231
- transmission 1, 166

Moist heat 2
Molluscum contagiosum 218
Monilial vaginitis 218
Monoamine oxidase inhibitors 97
Mood disorders 104
Mosquito borne diseases 164
Mucinous cyst adenoma 227, 228
Mucous polyp of cervix 221
Mudaliar committee 179
Mukherji committee 179
Multiple pregnancy 202
Mumps 170
Muscles 68, 212
Musculoskeletal system 85
Myasthenia gravis 17, 18
Mycobacterium tuberculosis 44, 171
Mycoplasma hominis 216, 218
Myelodysplasia 136
Myocardial infarction 29, 30
Myoclonic seizures 136
Myometrium 211

N

Naegele's rule 196
Narcissistic personality disorder 109
Narcotic analgesics 4
National
- AIDS Control Program 161, 175
- Anti-Malaria Program 161
- Family Welfare Program 162
- Filaria Control Program 161
- Health Policy 180
- Immunization Schedule 167, 168
- Leprosy Eradication Program 161
- Malaria Control Program 161
- Program for Prevention of Blindness 162
- TB Control Program 161

Nausea 135, 196
Nebothian cyst 225
Necrophilia 108
Necrospermia 224
Necrotizing enterocolitis 131
Necrozoospermia 224
Neisseria
- *gonorrhea* 175, 216, 217
- *meningitidis* 172

Neonatal
- mortality rate 177
- respiratory distress 131
- sepsis 132

Nephrectomy 64
Nephrolithiasis 63
Nephrostomy 64
Nephrotic syndrome 144
Nerve block 19
Nervous system 13, 13*f*
Niacin 250
Nifedipine 35
Night blindness 248
Non-communicable disease 166
Non-gonococcus urethritis 218
Non-Hodgkin's lymphoma 219
Non-hormonal treatment 235
Non-menstrual bleeding 222
Non-narcotic analgesics 5
Norepinephrine 9
- blockers 97

Nortriptyline hydrochloride 97
Nose and throat secretions 168
Nosocomial infection 2

O

Obsessive
- compulsive disorder 106
- compulsive personality disorder 109

Obstructive disease 44
Occupational
- cancer 177
- dermatitis 177
- diseases 177
- health 176

Odor 81
Oligohydramnios 202
Oligomenorrhea 217, 221
Oligospermia 224
Oligozoospermia 224
Oliguria 217

Omphalocele 134
Open pneumothorax 45
Opisthotonus 18
Oral
  cancer 47, 54
  contraceptives 205
  hygiene 82
Organic mental syndromes and disorders 101
Orthostatic hypotension 86
Ortolani's sign 145
Osiander's sign 195
Osmoreceptor system 5
Osteoarthritis 70
Osteogenesis imperfecta 146
  congenita 146
  tarda 146
Otitis media 138
Otosclerosis 21
Ovarian tumors 227
Ovaries 73, 211, 213, 228
Ovular bleeding 221
Ovulatory pain 220
Oxazepam 96
Oxygen
  pressure 262
  saturation 262

P

Pain in dysmenorrhea 219
Palpitations 30
Pancreas 53, 73
Pancreatitis 59
Paradoxical pulse 84
Paraldehyde 97
Parametritis 217
Paranoid personality disorder 108
Parathyroid
  hormone 73
  regulation of calcium 6
Parkinson's disease 17, 101
Paroxysmal nocturnal dyspnea 31
Partial thromboplastin time 36
Parts of
  broad ligament 212
  ear 16*f*
  fallopian tube 211
Passive aggressive personality disorder 109
Patent ductus arteriosus 139
Pediculosis pubis 218
Pelvic
  floor 212
  infections 215
  inflammatory disease 215
  pain 229
  peritoneum 212
Penicillins 3
Perimetrium 211
Perinatal mortality rate 178
Periodontal diseases 82
Peripheral
  acting adrenergic neuron blockers 32
  nervous system 13, 14
  vasodilators 33
Peritoneal dialysis 65
Peritonitis 57, 217
Permanent
  colostomy 57
  hardness 163
  methods of family planning 205
Personality disorders 108
Pertussis 171
Pervasive developmental disorders 98
Phenothiazine derivates 97
Phobic disorders 105
Phrenic arteries 27
Phthirus pubis 218
Pilocarpine 21
Pituitary dwarfism 147
Placenta 194
  previa 201
Plan of care 78
Plantar flexion 69
Plasmapheresis 18
Plasmodium falciparum 161
Platelet count 262
Pneumoconiosis 177
Pneumonia 46
Pneumothorax 45
Polio vaccine 173
Poliomyelitis 163, 172
Polyarthritis 141
Polycystic ovarian syndrome 227
Polyembryoma 228
Polyhydramnios 202
Polymenorrhea 221
Portal circulation 27, 29
Positive bar body 233
Posterior pituitary 73, 213
Postpartum hemorrhage 202
Post-traumatic stress disorder 106
Pouch of Douglas 212, 228
Pox virus 218
Precocious
  pseudopuberty 214
  puberty 214
Pregnancy induced hypertension 200
Preinvasive carcinoma 230
Premature
  rupture of membranes 204
  ventricular contraction 31
Premenstrual syndrome 220
Pressure
  sore 82, 83
  ulcer 85
Prevention of occupational diseases 177
Primary
  dysmenorrhea 219
  health care 160
Principles of
  community health nursing 160
  health education 178
Procainamide 35
Prochlorperazine 96
Prodromal period 165
Progressive disease 59
Prophylactic disinfection 169
Prostaglandins 206
Prostate specific antigen 262
Prostatic surgery 65
Prostatitis 65
Protein 8, 246
  calorie malnutrition 161
  deficiency 246
  requirements 246
Prothrombin time 36
Pseudomyxoma peritonei 228
Psychomotor retardation 105
Puberty 193
  menorrhagia 215
Pulmonary
  artery 27
  circulation 27, 29
  edema 31
  embolism 86, 217
  stenosis 140
  tuberculosis 44, 81
  veins 27
Pulse polio immunization 162, 173
Pulses alterans 84
Purification of water on
  large scale 163
  small scale 163
Purified protein derivative 172
Pyelonephritis 230
Pyloric stenosis 134
Pyloromyotomy 134
Pyloroplasty 56
Pyometra 230
Pyorrhea 82
Pyrazinamide 4
Pyrexia 217
Pyridoxine 250
Pyruvic acid 263

Q

Quadratus lumborum 69
Quadriceps femoris group 69

Quarantine 2, 166
Quinidine 35

R

Rabies 174, 175
Radiation therapy 54
Ranges of fever 83
Recommended protein allowances 247
Rectovaginal
 fistula 230, 232
 septum 228
Rectus
 abdominis 69
 femoris 69
Red blood cell 25
 count 263
Regulatory function of kidney 63
Removal of hardness 163
Renal
 arteries 27
 calculi 86
Reproductive
 and child health program 161
 system 198
Reserpine 32
Respiration 9, 84
Respiratory
 acidosis 8
 alkalosis 8
 distress 143
 isolation 2
 rate 132
 system 86, 196
Retina 15
Retinal detachment 21
Retrograde menstruation 229
Retrolental fibroplasias 131
Retroversion 222
Revised National Tuberculosis Control Program 161, 172
Reyes syndrome 136
Rheumatic fever 141
Rheumatoid arthritis 70
Rhizotomy 19
Rhythm method 205
Riboflavin 250
Rifampicin 4
Root abscess 82

S

Safe period method 205
Saline injection 206
Salmonella
 enteritidis 174
 food poisoning 174
 typhi 174
Sarcoptes scabiei 218
Scabies 218
Schick test 171
Schizoid personality disorder 108
Schizophrenic disorders 104
Schizotypal personality disorder 108
Sclerotherapy 54
Scoliosis 85, 146
Secondary dysmenorrhea 219
Seizure disorders 136
Sengstaken-Blakemore tube insertion 54
Sepsis 2, 230
Serological test 218
Serous
 cyst adenoma 228
 tumor 227
Serum
 electrolytes 24
 lipids 24, 25
Severe
 abdominal pain 134
 acute respiratory syndrome 171
Sex cord stromal tumors 227
Sexual disorders 108
Sexually transmitted diseases 175, 217, 218
Shock 8, 230
Short course chemotherapy 172
Shrivastav Committee 180
Sickle cell anemia 141
Signs of
 DIC 202
 hypotension 202
 pregnancy 196
Silver nitrate 2
Simple phobia 106
Simpson's theory 229
Sinus
 bradycardia 30
 tachycardia 30
Small intestine 53
Smallpox 169
Smith's test 81
Social phobia 106
Sodium
 bicarbonate 173
 chloride 173
 nitroprusside 9, 32, 81
Soft sore 175
Softening of
 cervix 195
 lower uterine segment 195
Sources of
 air pollution 164
 carbohydrates 247
 infection 166
 proteins 246
 water 162
Specific death rate 177
Speech disorders 100
Spina bifida 136
 occulta 136
Spinal cord 14
 injury 18
Splenic artery 27
Spontaneous
 cycles 224
 pneumothorax 45
Spread of communicable diseases 164
Stages of development of CVA 17
Staphylococcal food poisoning 174
Staphylococcus
 aureus 174
 pyogenes 216
Status epilepticus 136
Sterilization 2, 3, 168
Sternocleidomastoid 69
Stomach 53
Stomatitis 54, 82
Streptomycin 4
Stress test 25
Stressors 101
Stridor 85
Structural scoliosis 146
Structure of eye 15*f*
Subcutaneous nodules 141
Submucous fibroid 221
Superficial veins 28
Superior mesenteric arteries 27
Supports of uterus 222
Surgery of urinary system 64
Surgical
 asepsis 78
 sterilization 205
Sydenhams' chorea 141
Syphilis 175, 218
Systemic
 circulation 27
 lupus erythematosus 70

T

Telephone scatologia 108
Temporary colostomy 57
Tension pneumothorax 45
Tensor fasciae latae 69
Teratoma 228
Teratospermia 224
Teratozoospermia 224
Terminal disinfection 2, 169
Testicular feminization 233
Testing of reflexes 80
Testosterone 73
Tetracyclines 4
Tetralogy of Fallot 140
Thalamus 14

Thecoma 227
Therapeutic uses of
- cold application 87
- hot application 87

Thioridazine 96
Thiothixene 96
Third generation cephalosporins 3
Threadworm hydatid disease 163
Threatened abortion 200
Thromboangiitis obliterans 33
Thrombophlebitis 33, 217
Thymectomy 18
Thyroid 73
- cartilage of larynx 43
- stimulating hormone 147, 263

Thyrotrophin releasing hormone 213
Tibialis anterior 69
Timing of IUI 224
Tonsillitis 143
Torsion of pedicle 228
Transient ischemic attack 17
Transposition of great vessels 140
Transurethral resection of prostate 65
Tranyl cypromine sulfate 97
Trapezius 69
Treadmill test 25
Treatment of
- acute closed angle glaucoma 21
- chronic closed angle glaucoma 21
- depressive episode 105
- female infertility 224
- male infertility 224
- manic episode 105
- pre-eclampsia 200
- VVF 232

Treponema pallidum 175, 218
Triceps brachii 69
Trichloroacetic acid 97
Trichomonas vaginitis 218
Trifluoperazine 96
Trigeminal neuralgia 19
Triglycerides 25, 262
Truncus arteriosus 140
Tubal defense 215
Tuberculosis 161, 171
Tubo-ovarian mass 217
Turner's syndrome 133, 233
Types of
- disinfection 169
- drainage systems 45
- fever 83
- food poisoning 174
- muscles 68
- placenta previa 201

Typhoid
- and paratyphoid fever 163
- fever 174

U

Ulcerative colitis 56
Umbilical cord 194
Unclassified epithelial tumors 227
Under five mortality rate 178
United Nations Development Program 181
United International Children's Emergency Fund 180
United States Agency for International Development 181
Universal Immunization Program 162
Upper respiratory tract 43
Uremia 230
Ureters 63
Urethra 63
Urethral caruncle 221
Uric acid 263
Urinary
- diversions 64
- frequency 196
- LH detection 224
- system 63
- tract infection 86, 143

Urolithiasis 63
Uterine
- defense 215
- polyps 221
- prolapse 222
- tubes 211

Uterosacral ligament 228
Uterus 210, 235

V

Vaccines 167
Vacuum aspiration 206
Vagina 210, 235
Vaginal
- defense 215
- discharge 81
- prolapse 222
- sponge 205

Vagotomy 55
Vancomycin 4
Varicella 169
Vascular theory 229
Veins 27, 28
Venereal diseases 175
Ventricles of brain 14*f*
Ventricular
- septal defect 139
- tachycardia 31

Verapamil 35
Vertebral column 68
Vesicoureteral reflux 143
Vesicovaginal fistula 230, 231
Vesicular mole 201
Vibrio cholerae 173
Viral hepatitis 218
Vision 15
Visual pathway 15, 16*f*
Vital
- capacity 43
- signs 83, 199

Vitamin 247
- A 248, 263
  - deficiency 248
- B_1 or thiamine 249
- B_{12} 250
- B_1 250
- B6 250
- C 250
- D 249
  - deficiency 249
- E 249
- K 249
  - therapy 54

Vomiting 132, 134, 196
- in pregnancy 202

Vulva 235
Vulval
- defense 215
- inspection 231

W

Warfarin sodium 35
Water
- hammer pulse 84
- pollution 163
- related diseases 163
- soluble vitamins 248

Waterborne disease 163, 173
Weil's disease 163
Wheeze 85
White blood cell 26
- count 263

Whooping cough 171
Wrist drop 85

X

Xerophthalmia 248

Y

Yellow fever 164

Z

Zidovudine 219
Zoonosis 166